Instructional Course Lectures
Pediatrics

Instructional Course Lectures Pediatrics

Edited by
John Birch, MD, FRCSC
Assistant Chief of Staff
Texas Scottish Rite Hospital for Children
Clinical Professor
Department of Orthopaedic Surgery
University of Texas Southwestern Medical School
Dallas, Texas

Developed with support from
Pediatric Orthopaedic Society of North America

Published by the
American Academy
of Orthopaedic Surgeons
6300 North River Road
Rosemont, IL 60018

American Academy of Orthopaedic Surgeons

The material presented in the *Instructional Course Lectures Pediatrics* has been made available by the American Academy of Orthopaedic Surgeons for educational purposes only. This material is not intended to present the only, or necessarily best, methods or procedures for the medical situations discussed, but rather is intended to represent an approach, view, statement, or opinion of the author(s) or producer(s), which may be helpful to others who face similar situations.

Some drugs or medical devices demonstrated in Academy courses or described in Academy print or electronic publications have not been cleared by the Food and Drug Administration (FDA) or have been cleared for specific uses only. The FDA has stated that it is the responsibility of the physician to determine the FDA clearance status of each drug or device he or she wishes to use in clinical practice.

Furthermore, any statements about commercial products are solely the opinion(s) of the author(s) and do not represent an Academy endorsement or evaluation of these products. These statements may not be used in advertising or for any commercial purpose.

Some of the authors or the departments with which they are affiliated have received something of value from a commercial or other party related directly or indirectly to the subject of their chapter.

First Edition
Copyright 2006 by the American Academy of Orthopaedic Surgeons
ISBN 10: 0-89203-418-1
ISBN 13: 978-0-89203-418-5

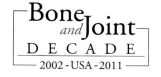

Editorial Board

Contributors

David B. Aronsson, MD
Professor
Department of Orthopaedics and Rehabilitation
University of Vermont College of Medicine
Burlington, Vermont

Peter F. Armstrong, MD, FRCSC, FAAP
Director of Medical Affairs
Shriners Hospitals for Children
Shriners International Headquarters
Tampa, Florida

Donald S. Bae, MD
Resident in Orthopaedic Surgery
Harvard Combined Orthopaedic Residency Program
Massachusetts General Hospital
Boston, Massachusetts

John Birch, MD, FRCSC
Assistant Chief of Staff
Texas Scottish Rite Hospital for Children
Clinical Professor
Department of Orthopaedic Surgery
University of Texas Southwestern Medical School
Dallas, Texas

Keith H. Bridwell, MD
Asa C. and Dorothy W. Jones Professor
Chief, Orthopaedic Spine Surgery
Department of Orthopaedic Surgery
Washington University
St. Louis, Missouri

R. Jay Cummings, MD
Chairman
Department of Orthopaedics
Nemours Children's Clinic
Jacksonville, Florida

Jon R. Davids, MD
Assistant Chief of Staff
Director
Motion Analysis Laboratory
Shriners Hospitals for Children
Greenville, South Carolina

Richard S. Davidson, MD
Associate Clinical Professor
The Children's Hospital of Philadelphia
University of Pennsylvania
Philadelphia, Pennsylvania

Roy B. Davis III, PhD, PE
Director
Motion Analysis Laboratory
Shriners Hospitals for Children
Greenville, South Carolina

Peter A. DeLuca, MD
Medical Director
Center for Motion Analysis
Connecticut Children's Medical Center
Hartford, Connecticut

Frederick R. Dietz, MD
Professor of Orthopaedic Surgery
Department of Orthopaedic Surgery
University of Iowa Hospital and Clinics
Iowa City, Iowa

Matthew B. Dobbs, MD
Resident Physician
Department of Orthopaedic Surgery
University of Iowa Hospital and Clinics
Iowa City, Iowa

John P. Dormans, MD
Chief of Orthopaedic Surgery
The Children's Hospital of Philadelphia
Professor of Orthopaedic Surgery
Division of Orthopaedic Surgery
University of Pennsylvania
Philadelphia, Pennsylvania

Howard R. Epps, MD
Fondren Orthopaedic Group, LLP
Texas Orthopaedic Hospital
Houston, Texas

John M. Flynn, MD
Attending Surgeon
The Children's Hospital of Philadelphia
Assistant Professor of Orthopaedic Surgery
University of Pennsylvania
Philadelphia, Pennsylvania

Laura L. Forese, MD, MPH
Associate Clinical Professor
Department of Orthopaedic Surgery
Columbia University
New York, New York

Freddie H. Fu, MD
David Silver Professor and Chairman
Department of Orthopaedic Surgery
University of Pittsburgh School of Medicine
Pittsburgh, Pennsylvania

Theodore J. Ganley, MD
Attending Surgeon
The Children's Hospital of Philadelphia
Assistant Professor of Orthopaedic Surgery
University of Pennsylvania
Philadelphia, Pennsylvania

Mark C. Gebhardt, MD
Frederick W. and Jane M. Ilfeld Professor of
  Orthopaedic Surgery
Harvard Medical School
Department of Orthopaedic Surgery, Children's
  Hospital
Orthopaedic Surgeon-in-Chief
Beth Israel Daemen Medical Center
Boston, Massachusetts

Robert N. Hensinger, MD
Professor
Department of Orthopaedic Surgery
University of Michigan Health System
Ann Arbor, Michigan

Martin J. Herman, MD
Assistant Professor of Orthopaedic Surgery
Drexel University College of Medicine
St. Christopher's Hospital for Children
Philadelphia, Pennsylvania

John A. Herring, MD
Chief of Staff
Texas Scottish Rite Hospital for Children
Professor of Orthopaedic Surgery
Department of Orthopaedic Surgery
University of Texas Southwestern Medical School
Dallas, Texas

John E. Herzenberg, MD, FRCSC
Head of Pediatric Orthopaedics
Sinai Hospital of Baltimore
Co-Director, International Center for Limb Lengthening
Rubin Institute for Advanced Orthopedics
Baltimore, Maryland

Johnny Huard, PhD
Henry J. Mankin Associate Professor
Department of Orthopaedic Surgery
University of Pittsburgh
Pittsburgh, Pennsylvania

Mary Lloyd Ireland, MD
President and Orthopaedic Surgeon
Kentucky Sports Medicine
Lexington, Kentucky

Robert M. Kay, MD
Assistant Professor of Orthopaedic Surgery
University of Southern California
Keck School of Medicine
Los Angeles, California

Scott H. Kozin, MD
Associate Professor
Temple University
Shriners Hospital for Children
Department of Orthopaedic Surgery
Philadelphia, Pennsylvania

Wallace B. Lehman, MD
Chief Emeritus, Pediatric Orthopaedic Surgery
Professor, Clinical Orthopaedic Surgery
New York University School of Medicine
Pediatric Orthopaedic Surgery
Hospital for Joint Diseases
New York University Hospitals Center
New York, New York

K. Kellie Leitch, MD, FRCSC
Department of Orthopedics
Children's Hospital Los Angeles
Los Angeles, California

Laura Powers Lemke, MD
Clinical Fellow-Pediatric Orthopaedic Surgery
Children's Memorial Hospital
Northwestern University
Chicago, Illinois

Lawrence G. Lenke, MD
The Jerome J. Gelden Professor of Orthopaedic Surgery
Department of Orthopaedic Surgery
Columbia Presbyterian Medical Center
New York, New York

Tzu-Shang Thomas Liu, MD, PhD
Resident
Orthopaedic Surgery
Department of Orthopaedic Surgery
University of Pittsburgh
Pittsburgh, Pennsylvania

Randall T. Loder, MD
Chief of Staff
Shriners Hospitals for Children
Minneapolis, Minnesota

Thomas G. Lowe, MD
Clinical Professor
University of Colorado Health Sciences Center
Orthopaedic Spine Surgery
Woodridge Orthopaedic and Spine Center PC
Wheat Ridge, Colorado

James J. McCarthy, MD
Assistant Chief of Staff
Shriners Hospital for Children
Assistant Professor
Temple University
Department of Orthopaedics
Philadelphia, Pennsylvania

Peter L. Meehan, MD
Clinical Associate Professor
Department of Orthopaedic Surgery
Emory University School of Medicine
Atlanta, Georgia

Lyle J. Micheli, MD
Director
Division of Sports Medicine
Children's Hospital
Boston, Massachusetts

Arya W. Moti, DO
Resident
Department of Orthopaedic Surgery
Botsford General Hospital
Farmington Hills, Michigan

Scott J. Mubarak, MD
Clinical Professor of Orthopaedics
University of California San Diego Children's Hospital
San Diego, California

Peter O. Newton
Chief of Scoliosis Service and Orthopedic Research
Children's Hospital at San Diego
Associate Clinical Professor
University of California, San Diego
San Diego, California

Sylvia Ounpuu, MSc
Director/Kinesiologist
Center for Motion Analysis
Connecticut Children's Medical Center
Hartford, Connecticut

Stefan Parent, MD, PhD
Pediatric Orthopedic Spine Fellow
Department of Pediatric Orthopedics
Children's Hospital at San Diego
San Diego, California

Stephan G. Pill, MS, PT
Medical Student
University of Pennsylvania
Philadelphia, Pennsylvania

Peter D. Pizzutillo, MD
Director
Orthopaedic Surgery
St. Christopher's Hospital for Children
Philadelphia, Pennsylvania

Charles T. Price, MD
Surgeon-In-Chief
Orthopaedic Division
Nemours Children's Clinic
Orlando, Florida

B. Stephens Richards, MD
Assistant Chief of Staff
Professor, Orthopaedic Surgery
Texas Scottish Rite Hospital for Children
Dallas, Texas

Bruce T. Rougraff, MD
Orthopedic Surgeon
Orthopedics Indianapolis
St. Vincent Hospital
Indianapolis, Indiana

Dennis Roy, MD
Professor of Orthopaedic Surgery
Associate Director, Pediatric Orthopaedics
Department of Orthopaedics
Children's Hospital Medical Center
Cincinnati, Ohio

John F. Sarwark, MD
Professor
Orthopedic Surgery
Department of Orthopedic Surgery
Northwestern University
Chicago, Illinois

David L. Skaggs, MD
Assistant Professor of Orthopedic Surgery
University of Southern California Children's Hospital
Los Angeles, California

Paul D. Sponseller, MD
Professor and Head, Pediatric Orthopaedics
Johns Hopkins Medical Institution
Baltimore, Maryland

Daniel J. Sucato, MD MS
Texas Scottish Rite Hospital for Children
Dallas, Texas

Kenneth B. Tepper, MD
Sports Medicine Fellow
Kentucky Sports Medicine
Lexington, Kentucky

George H. Thompson, MD
Professor
Orthopaedic Surgery and Pediatrics
Director
Pediatric Orthopaedics
Rainbow Babies and Children's Hospital
Case Western Reserve University
Cleveland, Ohio

John R. Tongue, MD
Clinical Assistant Professor
Department of Orthopaedics and Rehabilitation
Oregon Health Sciences University
Portland, Oregon

Peter M. Waters, MD
Director, Hand and Upper Extremity Surgery
Associate Professor
Harvard Medical School
Department of Orthopaedic Surgery
Children's Hospital
Boston, Massachusetts

Stuart L. Weinstein, MD
Ponseti Professor of Orthopaedic Surgery
Department of Orthopaedic Surgery
University of Iowa Hospital and Clinics
Iowa City, Iowa

Kurt R. Weiss, MD
Resident Surgeon
Department of Orthopaedic Surgery
University of Pittsburgh
Pittsburgh, Pennsylvania

Dennis R. Wenger, MD
Director, Pediatric Orthopedics
Children's Hospital at San Diego
Clinical Professor of Orthopedic Surgery
University of California
San Diego, California

Kaye E. Wilkins, DVM, MD
Professor of Orthopedics and Pediatrics
University of Texas Health Science Center
 at San Antonio
San Antonio, Texas

Preface

To identify prospective articles for this volume, I reviewed the *Instructional Course Lectures* published between 2000 and 2006. From many excellent lectures, I selected 27 that I believed most pertinent to the practice of pediatric orthopaedics. I organized these into seven sections and selected a section editor for each. I knew that each would provide a wise, insightful, and contemporary commentary on the lectures in their respective sections.

Dr. Tony Herring has guided a prospective clinical study of Legg-Pérthes disease for nearly 25 years and has made significant contributions to our understanding of developmental dysplasia of the hip and slipped capital femoral epiphysis. He reviews the five articles covering these three subjects.

Dr. John Herzenberg has made significant contributions to our understanding of the three-dimensional nature of clubfoot deformity, among the many other contributions he has made to orthopaedic knowledge. He is a skilled proponent and educator of the Ponseti method of clubfoot deformity correction and has contributed to our further understanding and application of this resurgent method. He has ably and insightfully provided commentary on the two articles in this volume that address clubfoot management.

Dr. Kaye Wilkins is the acknowledged "grandfather" of the management of orthopaedic injuries in children and has served as coeditor of the first three editions of *Fractures in Children*. He comments on five articles that review management of upper and lower extremity injuries, advances in knee injury management, and recent advances in treatment of musculoskeletal infections in children.

Dr. Dan Sucato is expert in and has made significant contributions to recent advances in the surgical management of spinal deformity. He has ably reviewed the largest section of this work, seven articles covering almost all aspects of spinal deformity management, including adolescent idiopathic scoliosis, Scheuermann's kyphosis, and spondylolisthesis.

Dr. Robert Hensinger requires no introduction to any professional orthopaedic circle. He developed the *Journal of Pediatric Orthopedics*

25 years ago and remains a senior editor. His contributions to orthopaedic knowledge, particularly in the area of the cervical spine, are legendary. He was an obvious choice to provide commentary on the three articles pertaining to cervical spinal injury and torticollis.

Dr. Mark Gebhardt is a leader in the field of malignant and benign tumors. His insightful comments with respect to the management of benign bone tumors incorporates his thoughts regarding the two excellent articles that review benign tumors and simple cyst fracture management.

Without specific personal credentials to do so, it was my pleasure to provide commentary on the final three articles, which did not neatly fit into one of the previous six sections, and therefore fall into the somewhat ignobly termed "miscellaneous" section. From my own view, these lectures particularly merited inclusion in this compendium. The three that I selected include a superb review on gene therapy and tissue engineering in orthopaedics, the optimization of walking ability in children with cerebral palsy, and the always valuable art of communications skills, an area in which we all can use improvement.

I would like to personally thank Perry Schoenecker, MD, President of the Pediatric Orthopaedic Society of North America and Richard Kyle, MD, President of the American Academy of Orthopedic Surgeons, for providing me the opportunity to supervise the collation of this volume. I also want to particularly thank Lynne Shindoll, Managing Editor in the Academy's Publications Department, for her able and enthusiastic support and coordination of this project and for making me look better at my task than I deserve. Any shortcomings you find in this volume are my own. I sincerely hope you enjoy reading this collection as much as I did, and I hope this collection of outstanding articles leaves you with satisfying sense of knowing "what's up" in the areas of pediatric orthopaedics they address.

John Birch, MD
Editor

Contents

Section 7 Miscellaneous Issues in Pediatric Orthopaedics

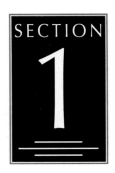

SECTION 1

Congenital Disorders About the Hip

Congenital Disorders About the Hip

The articles in this section provide an overview of our understanding of the three common hip disorders in the pediatric population: slipped capital femoral epiphysis (SCFE), Legg-Calvé-Perthes disease, and developmental dysplasia of the hip (DDH). These articles are useful for the generalist in that they summarize important information about the diagnosis and management of these disorders and implications that each condition has for early and late degenerative hip pathology. The reader will appreciate that much remains to be learned about the natural course of these hip abnormalities in the decades after childhood. For the pediatric orthopaedist, this collection of articles presents the existing knowledge base concerning these hip disorders. Young surgeons should appreciate the opportunities for future clinical research presented in areas in which our understanding is incomplete. Clearly, we still do not know precisely which imperfect hips will require early arthroplasty and which will last most of a lifetime. Despite this fact, these articles outline the best known methods to produce relatively normal hip architecture, which remains our best approach to prevention of adult hip disability.

The first of the two articles on SCFE by Dobbs and Weinstein and Loder and associates provides an excellent review of the natural history and long-term outcomes of the affected hip. The reader should appreciate that even though the article is authored by the true world experts in the field, the natural history of the condition remains either controversial or unknown. One study reports that 5% of patients who require total hip arthroplasty have had prior slipped epiphyses, whereas another reports 40% had prior slips. The heart of the disagreement lies in the interpretation of the "pistol grip" deformity of the femoral neck and head. At this time, it is unclear whether this deformity represents a previously asymptomatic slipped epiphysis or is an anatomic consequence of "idiopathic" degenerative arthritis.

This dilemma has become even more relevant in the years since publication of this work. Ganz popularized the concept that an offset deformity of the femoral neck may regularly predispose the hip to impingement between the neck and the acetabulum. This impingement causes a labral injury and may progress to delamination of the acetabular cartilage, resulting in early degenerative hip disease. With this concept in mind, Carney and Weinstein's work requires careful review; in their study, only 4 of 31 untreated patients had significant late hip symptoms. In their 41-year follow-up study, all of the patients with mild slips had an Iowa Hip Score higher than 80, and 64% of the patients with moderate and severe slips had higher scores. Yet by the Ganz philosophy, a large percentage of such hips should be presenting with symptoms in their third decade. This area is ripe for further investigation; young investigators should take notice.

The authors point out another contradiction that remains unresolved. The realignment procedures for SCFE, initially designed by Southwick and others, were devised to realign the anatomy in an effort to prevent future degenerative disease. Current corrective procedures are based on the same premise. Yet, well-done studies show an opposite effect. The realigned hips had the greater incidence of arthritic decline, whereas the hips treated with in situ pinning did the best. The realignment procedures studied were from an earlier era, which may account for some of the discrepancy. Still, the findings are disconcerting and await future study.

The second article on SCFE by Loder and associates reviews demographic characteristics and treatment concepts, and its authors have done most of the scholarly work in this area. The etiologic roles of obesity, race, and skeletal maturity are described. The authors note that when a younger patient presents with a slip, a second or contralateral slip is likely. Later work clearly relates this to pelvic bone age, and currently prophylactic pinning of the other hip is recommended for less skeletally mature patients. The most useful classification system divides the disorder into stable and unstable types based on weightbearing ability following onset of symptoms; this system should replace the other classification of acute, subacute, and chronic.

Management is well presented in this article. Stable slips are best treated with in situ screw fixation, and the authors provide an excellent review of the surgical technique. Attention to the details presented provides the patient with a safe and predictable procedure, and only the more severely displaced hips require secondary realignment. Realignment procedures are discussed in some detail.

Unstable slips typically are treated with fixation after "positioning" on the fracture table, which usually results in partial reduction of the displacement. Unfortunately, the incidence of osteonecrosis ranges between 30% and 40% with this technique. Open reduction with strict attention to the femoral head blood supply and vascular tension recently has become popular in some centers, and early results are promising. Future investigation should clarify the management that provides the

best results and fewest complications for the unstable slipped epiphysis.

Legg-Calvé-Perthes disease is the focus of the next article by Thompson and associates. Current concepts about etiology are discussed, with emphasis on disorders of clotting mechanisms, the role of passive smoking, and the likelihood that these children have a systemic disorder. The discussion of pathogenesis and anatomy provides a basic understanding of the nature of the disease. The way in which the classification of severity has evolved is reviewed, beginning with Catterall's groups and risk factors, Salter and Thompson's analysis of subchondral fracture, Herring's lateral pillar classification, and the scintigraphic classification of Dias and Conway.

The authors thoroughly review the various treatment alternatives used over the years. Bracing, which for many years was the mainstay of treatment, largely has been shown to lack effectiveness. Proximal femoral varus osteotomy is discussed in detail, with considerable information about technique. Other procedures, including pelvic osteotomies, shelf procedures, and combined osteotomies, are reviewed with relevant analyses of outcome studies.

Weinstein and associates address DDH in the final two articles of the section. In their first article, the authors review the relevant

anatomy and pathophysiology of DDH and describe the important embryology of the hip, noting the role of the femoral head in producing a concave acetabulum. The role of the acetabular labrum in developing acetabular depth and femoral head coverage also is emphasized in an effort to eliminate the practice of labral excision. Such excision, which was popular in early times, results in irreversible growth disturbance of the acetabulum. The early abnormalities of DDH are described and noted to be reversible with simple treatment. The natural history also is considered relative to the dislocated hip, the hip with subluxation, and the hip with acetabular dysplasia.

The methods of early and late diagnosis are discussed, as is relevant radiographic evaluation. I found the description of the ultrasound findings in DDH especially useful. The authors described role of selective and universal ultrasound screening, noting that at present in North America, the standard is to recommend ultrasound evaluation for patients with risk factors for DDH and for those with abnormal physical findings.

The final article presents a thorough review of treatment, beginning with the Pavlik harness. Even the experienced practitioner will benefit from the careful review of techniques, results, and pitfalls of

Pavlik harness management. For the recalcitrant or later presenting hip dislocation, the use of traction and closed reduction is outlined. Next, the authors fully describe the methods of surgical treatment, including an excellent review of medial approaches and anterior open reduction with capsulorrhaphy. The authors' extensive experience makes these descriptions classic in the field. Acetabular redirection by the Salter procedure and others also are covered, and acetabular correction at the time of reduction is recommended for children older than 18 months. Femoral shortening and acetabular redirection combined with open reduction is the treatment of choice for children older than age 2 years at presentation.

These articles reiterate the fact that these conditions affecting the hips of children, adolescents, and subsequently adults, remain challenging to treat. In a perfect world, our treatment would result in completely normal hip anatomy and function. In the real world, however, the usual treatment sometimes fails; there are patients who are diagnosed late, and there are disorders that simply fail to respond to our efforts. In addition, we still lack full knowledge of the natural history of the conditions, with and without our intervention. One of my former fellows is fond of saying that she will return to repeat the fellowship when we finally completely understand DDH. We can hope that these deficiencies will be resolved in the not-too-distant future, and they continue to offer wide avenues for future investigation.

John A. Herring, MD
Chief of Staff
Texas Scottish Rite Hospital
 for Children
Dallas, Texas

Natural History and Long-Term Outcomes of Slipped Capital Femoral Epiphysis

Matthew B. Dobbs, MD
Stuart L. Weinstein, MD

Introduction

Slipped capital femoral epiphysis (SCFE) is a disorder in which there is a displacement of the capital femoral epiphysis from the metaphysis through the physeal plate. The term slipped capital femoral epiphysis is actually a misnomer, because the head of the femur is held in the acetabulum by the ligamentum teres, and thus it is actually the neck that comes upward and outward while the head remains in the acetabulum. In the majority of cases, there is a varus relationship between the head and neck, but occasionally the slip is into a valgus position, with displacement superiorly and posteriorly in relation to the neck.[1,2]

Classification

Traditionally, on the basis of the patient's history, physical examination, and radiographs, SCFE can be classified into four clinical categories: preslip, acute, acute on chronic, and chronic.

In the preslip stage, patients usually have a limp, complain of weakness in the leg, or have exertional pain in the groin or knee with prolonged standing or walking. On physical examination, the most consistent positive finding is lack of medial rotation. Radiographs reveal generalized bone atrophy of the hemipelvis and upper femur only in those patients who limped or limited their activity. There may be some widening and irregularity of the physeal plate region.[3]

An acute slip is an abrupt displacement through the proximal physeal cartilaginous plate in which there was a preexisting epiphyseolysis.[4] Acute slips account for only 10% to 15% of the slips in most large reported series.[5,6] The clinical criteria for having an acute slip include the onset of symptoms for less than 2 weeks. Physical examination demonstrates an external rotation deformity, shortening, and marked limitation of motion secondary to pain. In general, the greater the amount of slip, the greater the motion restriction. However, 67% of patients with acute slips give a history of mild prodromal symptoms for 1 to 3 months before their acute episode, indicating that they probably had a preslip or mild slip preceding their acute episode.[1,4,5,7,8] The traumatic episode may be as trivial as turning over in bed. The pain is usually severe enough to prevent weight bearing. Slips in those patients with a history of mild prodromal symptoms may be better classified as acute-on-chronic slips.

An acute-on-chronic SCFE is one associated with chronic symptoms initially and with subsequent development of acute symptoms as well as a sudden increase in the degree of slip.

Chronic slips are by far the most common type, accounting for 85.5% of all slips.[6] Patients with chronic SCFE generally have a history of groin or medial thigh pain for months to years. They may have a history of exacerbations and remissions of the pain and limp. Importantly, 46% will have knee or lower thigh pain as their initial symptom, emphasizing the importance of a hip examination in any child complaining of knee pain.[9,10] All of these patients demonstrate limited motion, particularly medial rotation.

A newer and more clinically useful classification of slips is stable versus unstable.[6,11,12] Unstable slips are those in which weight bearing is not possible, with or without crutches, and stable slips are those in which weight bearing is possible, with or without crutches. The reason this classification is important is that in a large series of patients with acute symptomatology classified as stable versus unstable (all treated with pinning in situ), the incidence of aseptic necrosis in the unstable slip was significantly greater than in those patients with stable slips. The traditional classification of acute versus chronic is considered to be misleading because it does not consider hip stability. The high complication rates in the unstable slip are most likely secondary to vascular injury caused at the time of the initial displacement.[6,11]

Slips can also be classified radiographically by the amount of displacement anteriorly, posteriorly, or laterally.[13] The minimal slip is classified as one with maximal displacement of less than one third of the diameter of the neck. Moderate slip is greater than 1 cm of displacement but less

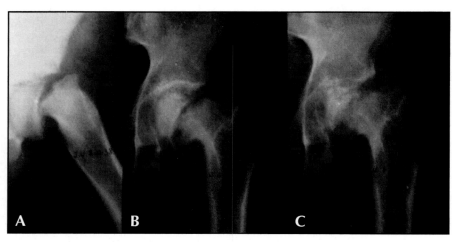

Fig. 1 A, Radiograph of the left hip in a 14-year-old boy with immediate severe hip pain following acute trauma, without prior hip symptoms. **B** and **C,** Follow-up radiographs over a 1-year period showing the rapid development of severe degenerative changes.

than one half the diameter of the neck, and a severe slip is displacement greater than half the diameter of the neck. This classification is probably most important when considering long-term prognosis, because mild and moderate slips have an excellent long-term prognosis when treated by pinning in situ, whereas severe slips tend to deteriorate with time.[9,14]

Natural History

Howarth[15] stated that SCFE is probably the most frequent cause of degenerative joint disease of the hip in middle-aged patients and is a common source of pain and disability, but there are few long-term studies of patients with slipped capital femoral epiphysis, and included in these are few untreated patients.[3,5,9,14,16-18] However, there are some data on the natural history of true acute slips. The acute episode is followed by a 2- to 3-week period of intolerance to weight bearing. As the pain and spasm subside, some motion returns, though the hip remains moderately painful in external rotation. Degenerative changes develop within only a few months and the patient is left with residual flexion, adduction, and external rotation contractures[3] (Fig. 1).

In reviewing a large series of patients with degenerative joint disease, the number of patients with known SCFE is small, averaging around 5%.[19-21] Murray,[20] however, reported an association with SCFE in 40% of 200 patients thought to have primary degenerative joint disease. He described a tilt deformity caused by bone resorption laterally with new bone formation medially and thought this to be compatible with old SCFE. Stulberg and associates[22] also described a similar deformity, the pistol grip deformity, in 40% of patients without known prior hip disease undergoing total hip arthroplasty. This deformity was also thought to be compatible with old SCFE. Resnick,[23] however, refuted this theory in a pathologic study of 48 femoral heads of patients with a tilt deformity on radiographs. The specimens suggested that the deformity was solely related to the remodeling changes of osteoarthritis. In summary, whether subclinical forms of SCFE lead to early osteoarthritis remains uncertain because of the controversy over its incidence.

The severity of deformity does correlate with the overall long-term prognosis with regard to the development of degenerative joint disease and function.[9,14,17,18,24,25] Oram[17] reported results of 22 untreated slips, 11 of which were observed for more than 15 years. Patients with moderate slips retained good function for years, whereas those with severe slips developed early degenerative joint disease with resultant poor function. Poor results are occasionally seen even with minimal slips.[5,9,14,18]

Carney and Weinstein[14] reported results in 31 hips in 28 patients with SCFE observed without surgical intervention. The mean duration of patient follow-up from the onset of symptoms was 41 years. The mean patient age was 54 years at review. Complications occurred in four slips: displacement to a severe degree occurred in two hips; chondrolysis and aseptic necrosis in one hip each. In this natural history group, chondrolysis, defined as early loss of width of the joint space, was seen in one mild slip, and osteonecrosis, defined as collapse of some portion of the femoral head, was seen in one severe slip. The mean Iowa Hip Rating (100-point scale) for the entire group was 89 points. The mild slips had a mean rating of 87 points and the severe slips had a mean Iowa Hip Rating of 75. At the 41-year follow-up, all mild slips had an Iowa Hip Rating of more than 80 points, whereas only 64% of moderate and severe slips had similar ratings. Mild slips had good long-term results regarding Iowa Hip Rating and degenerative disease rating. There were no degenerative changes in 36% of the mild slips; however, all moderate and severe slips had evidence of degenerative joint disease.

In an earlier study, Carney and associates[9] reported on 35 slips that were observed initially. After the time of initial diagnosis, additional displacement occurred in six (17%), five of which became severe. Two of these six were untreated. The other four slips were stabilized surgically and excluded from the natural history study. Eleven of the original 35 patients had an acute episode superimposed on the chronic slip. These 11 slips all progressed to severe displacement and were stabilized surgically and also were excluded from the natural history study.[9]

Ordeberg and associates[26] studied a series of patients with slipped capital femoral epiphyses without primary treatment, from 20 to 40 years after diagnosis. Few patients had restrictions in working capacity or social life.

In summary, the natural history of chronic SCFE is favorable provided that displacement is mild and remains so. Jerre[24,25] and Ross and associates[18] reported a decline in favorable results with older age at follow-up. Both groups reported many patients doing well early on but having increasing symptoms and decreasing function with increasing age.

Long-Term Results

Carney and associates[9] reported long-term results for 155 hips in 124 patients who were reviewed at a mean follow-up of 41 years after the onset of symptoms.[5] The slips were classified by duration of symptoms as acute, chronic, or acute on chronic. As determined by the head shaft angle,[27] 42% of slips were mild, 32% were moderate, and 26% were severe. Reduction was performed on 39 hips and realignment in 65 hips. Treatment of chronic slips included symptomatic treatment only in 25% of the hips, spica cast in 30%, pinning in situ in 24%, and osteotomy in 20%. The Iowa Hip Rating and radiographic classification of degenerative joint disease were determined at follow-up and both worsened with increasing severity of the slip and where reduction or realignment had been done (Fig. 2). Osteonecrosis (12%) and chondrolysis (16%) were also more common with increasing severity of the slip. Poor results were common when either reduction or realignment had been performed. Deterioration over time was most marked with increasing severity of the slip. The authors reported that the long-term natural history of malunited slips is mild

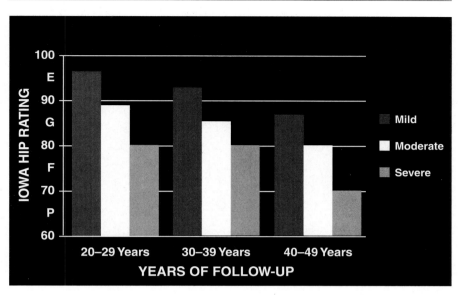

Fig. 2 Bar graph depicting worsening scores on the Iowa Hip Rating when following a group of patients long term with SCFE. Deterioration over time was most marked with increasing severity of the slip. (Adapted with permission from Carney BT, Weinstein SL, Noble J: Long-term follow-up of slipped capital femoral epiphysis. *J Bone Joint Surg* 1991;73: 667-674.)

deterioration related to the severity of the slip and complications.

Realignment techniques are associated with risk of appreciable complications and adversely affect the natural history of the disease. Regardless of the severity of the slip, pinning in situ provided the best long-term function and delay of degenerative arthritis with a low risk of complications. Although limb-length discrepancy and motion in abduction and internal rotation were affected by the severity of the slip, function was not significantly impaired.

Wilson and associates[28] reviewed the results of 300 hips in 240 patients who had been seen for SCFE at the Hospital for Special Surgery between 1936 and 1960. Of these hips, 187 had been treated by pinning in situ, with good clinical results in 81% and good radiographic results in 77%. The results were worse (60% good clinical results and 55% good radiographic results) for the 76 hips in which correction of the deformity had been attempted. Hall[16] reported on 100 patients from a study of the British

Orthopaedic Association as well as an additional 38 patients in regard to the results of various types of treatment. The best results were obtained with the use of multiple pins: 16 of 20 patients (80%) had excellent results. The worst results were seen after realignment had been attempted with manipulation or osteotomy. Osteotomy of the femoral neck was followed by a poor result in 36% of the hips and osteonecrosis in 38%.

Patients with SCFE in southern Sweden were observed for more than 30 years.[9,26,29] Symptomatic treatment or pinning in situ resulted in high clinical ratings and few radiographic changes, with only 2% of the hips requiring a secondary reconstructive procedure. When closed reduction and spica cast were used, the combined rate of osteonecrosis and chondrolysis was 13% and reconstructive procedures were needed in 35% of the hips. Osteotomy through the femoral neck was followed by a combined rate of osteonecrosis and chondrolysis of 30%, and reconstructive procedures were necessary in 15% of the hips.

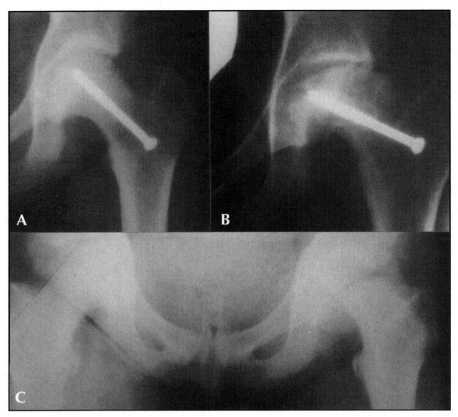

Fig. 3 A and **B,** Radiographs of the the left hip of a 13-year-old girl with immediate severe hip pain after running sprints, without prior hip symptoms. Patient was thought to have an acute slip and was therefore placed on the fracture table and in situ pinning was performed in the operating room. **C,** Follow-up radiograph demonstrates aseptic necrosis with collapse of the femoral head.

to the severity of the slip and the complications of treatment. Realignment is associated with the risk of substantial complications and adversely affects the natural course of disease. Regardless of the severity of the slip, pinning in situ provides the best long-term function with a low risk of complications and most effectively delays the development of degenerative arthritis. Remodeling of the metaphyseal prominence is seen in many radiographs during the course of time.

The development of aseptic necrosis is the most devastating complication of SCFE (Fig. 3). The factors noted to be responsible for the development of aseptic necrosis are acute slips, unstable slips, overreduction of acute slips, attempts at reduction of the chronic component of an acute-on-chronic slip, placement of pins in the superolateral quadrant of the femoral head, or osteotomies of the femoral neck.[9,12,31-34]

The etiology of chondrolysis in the treatment of SCFE is unknown. Clinically, chondrolysis presents with loss of range of motion, pain, limp, and joint contracture. The question of whether it is an autoimmune phenomenon or has some factors interfering with cartilage nutrition is yet to be defined. Risk factors leading to chondrolysis include cast immobilization, unrecognized pin penetration (only if the pin is left in the joint), severe slips, and long duration of symptoms before treatment. The treatment of chondrolysis is difficult, with most patients requiring anti-inflammatory agents and bed rest with skeletal traction to relieve their contractures. Rarely, patients may require surgical capsulectomy and continuous passive motion.[9,11,35-37]

The treatment of SCFE is somewhat controversial, but most authors now agree that pinning in situ offers the best long-term results, with secondary corrective osteotomies as necessary to relieve mechanical symptoms or pain once the physis is closed. In general, patients with

In several series, the use of multiple pins in situ resulted in good or excellent results in more than 90% of the hips. The high percentage of good results has been attributed to remodeling of the femoral neck. However, difficulty with pin removal and a relatively high incidence of unrecognized penetration of the joint space by pins have also been reported. Because of the significant prevalence of early osteoarthritis, reduction by closed or open means currently is not advocated.[4,9,30]

Carney and associates[9] reported on a series of 39 slips that had been reduced. Their mean Iowa Hip Rating was 72 points, and the mean radiographic degenerative score was 2.4 of 3 (0 = no degenerative disease, 3 = severe degenerative disease). Osteonecrosis developed in 12 of the hips (31%) and chondrolysis in 11 (28%). For the 116 hips that had not been reduced, the mean Iowa Hip Rating was 85 points and the mean radiographic grade was 1.7 of 3. Osteonecrosis developed in 7 hips (6%) and chondrolysis in 14 (12%). Results of this long-term study support the use of pinning in situ as the treatment of choice for SCFE. Twenty-seven hips in which the slip was chronic were so treated, and at the most recent follow-up the mean Iowa Hip Rating was 90 points and the mean radiographic degenerative score was 1.5 of 3. Osteonecrosis developed in one of these hips and chondrolysis did not develop in any.

The natural history of a malunited slip is one of mild deterioration that is related

the condition do well over the long term if the slip is of mild or moderate degree and good congruity between the femoral head and the acetabulum remains. It is only in the severe slips that the deterioration occurs with degenerative changes over time.

SCFE differs from other pediatric hip disorders such as Legg-Calvé-Perthes disease and developmental dysplasia of the hip in that slips occur at an age when the majority of acetabular development is completed. Because of the maturity of the acetabulum, no adaptation to head deformity can occur. Mild and most moderate slips may cause some incongruity and eventually lead to degenerative disease. Aseptic necrosis and chondrolysis, which may also compromise outcome, are associated with a high incidence of degenerative disease.

References

1. Schein AJ: Acute severe slipped capital femoral epiphysis. *Clin Orthop* 1967;51:151-166.

2. Segal LS, Weitzel PP, Davidson RS: Valgus slipped capital femoral epiphysis: Fact or fiction? *Clin Orthop* 1996;322:91-98.

3. Ponseti I, Barta CK: Evaluation of treatment of slipping of the capital femoral epiphysis. *Surg Gynecol Obstet* 1948;86:87-97.

4. Fahey JJ, O'Brien ET: Acute slipped capital femoral epiphysis: Review of the literature and report of ten cases. *J Bone Joint Surg Am* 1965;47:1105-1127.

5. Boyer DW, Mickelson MR, Ponseti IV: Slipped capital femoral epiphysis: Long-term follow-up and study of one hundred and twenty-one patients. *J Bone Joint Surg Am* 1981;63:85-95.

6. Loder RT, Aronson DD, Greenfield ML: The epidemiology of bilateral slipped capital femoral epiphysis: A study of children in Michigan. *J Bone Joint Surg Am* 1993;75:1141-1147.

7. Aadalen RJ, Weiner DS, Hoyt W, Herndon CH: Acute slipped capital femoral epiphysis. *J Bone Joint Surg Am* 1974;56:1473-1487.

8. Casey BH, Hamilton HW, Bobechko WP: Reduction of acutely slipped upper femoral epiphysis. *J Bone Joint Surg* Br 1972;54:607-614.

9. Carney BT, Weinstein SL, Noble J: Long-term follow-up of slipped capital femoral epiphysis. *J Bone Joint Surg Am* 1991;73:667-674.

10. Jacobs B: Diagnosis and natural history of slipped femoral capital epiphysis. *Instr Course Lect* 1972;21:167-173.

11. Aronsson DD, Loder RT: Treatment of the unstable (acute) slipped capital femoral epiphysis. *Clin Orthop* 1996;322:99-110.

12. Loder RT, Richards BS, Shapiro PS, Reznick LR, Aronson DD: Acute slipped capital femoral epiphysis: The importance of physeal stability. *J Bone Joint Surg Am* 1993;75:1134-1140.

13. Wedge JH, Wasylenko MJ: The natural history of congenital dislocation of the hip: A critical review. *Clin Orthop* 1978;137:154-162.

14. Carney BT, Weinstein SL: Natural history of untreated chronic slipped capital femoral epiphysis. *Clin Orthop* 1996;322:43-47.

15. Howorth B: Slipping of the capital femoral epiphysis: History. *Clin Orthop* 1966;48:11-32.

16. Hall JE: The results of treatment of slipped femoral epiphysis. *J Bone Joint Surg Br* 1957;39:659-673.

17. Oram V: Epiphysiolysis of the head of the femur: A follow-up examination with special reference to end results and the social prognosis. *Acta Orthop Scand* 1953;23:100-120.

18. Ross PM, Lyne ED, Morawa LG: Slipped capital femoral epiphysis: Long-term results after 10-38 years. *Clin Orthop* 1979;141:176-180.

19. Johnston RC, Larson CB: Results of treatment of hip disorders with cup arthroplasty. *J Bone Joint Surg Am* 1969;51:1461-1479.

20. Murray RO: The aetiology of primary osteoarthritis of the hip. *Br J Radiol* 1965;38: 810-824.

21. Solomon L: Patterns of osteoarthritis of the hip. *J Bone Joint Surg Br* 1976;58:176-183.

22. Stulberg SD, Cordell LD, Harris WH: Unrecognized Childhood Hip Disease: A Major Cause of Idiopathic Osteoarthritis of the Hip, in *The Hip: Proceedings of the Third Open Scientific Meeting of the Hip Society*. St. Louis, MO, CV Mosby 1975, pp 212-230.

23. Resnick D: The 'tilt deformity' of the femoral head in osteoarthritis of the hip: A poor indicator of previous epiphysiolysis. *Clin Radiol* 1976;27:355-363.

24. Jerre T: A study in slipped upper femoral epiphysis: With special reference to the late functional and roentgenological results and the value of closed reduction. *Acta Orthop Scand* 1950;6(suppl):5-157.

25. Jerre T: Early complications after osteosynthesis with a three flanged nail in situ for slipped epiphysis. *Acta Orthop Scand* 1958;27:126-134.

26. Ordeberg G, Hansson LI, Sandstrom S: Slipped capital femoral epiphysis in southern Sweden: Long-term result with no treatment or symptomatic primary treatment. *Clin Orthop* 1984;191:95-104.

27. Southwick WO: Osteotomy through the lesser trochanter for slipped capital femoral epiphysis. *J Bone Joint Surg Am* 1967;49:807-835.

28. Wilson PD, Jacobs B, Schecter L: Slipped capital femoral epiphysis: An end-result study. *J Bone Joint Surg Am* 1965;47:1128-1145.

29. Mickelson MR, Ponseti IV, Cooper RR, Maynard JA: The ultrastructure of the growth plate in slipped capital femoral epiphysis. *J Bone Joint Surg Am* 1977;59:1076-1081.

30. Billing L, Severin E: Slipping epiphysis of the hip: A roentgenological and clinical study based on a new roentgen technique. *Acta Radiol* 1959;174(suppl):5-76.

31. Brodetti A: The blood supply of the femoral neck and head in relation to the damaging effects of nails and screws. *J Bone Joint Surg Br* 1960;42:794-801.

32. Claffey TJ: Avascular necrosis of the femoral head: An anatomical study. *J Bone Joint Surg Br* 1960;42:802-809.

33. Dietz FR: Traction reduction of acute and acute-on-chronic slipped capital femoral epiphysis. *Clin Orthop* 1994;302:101-110.

34. Krahn TH, Canale ST, Beaty JH, Warner WC, Lourenco P: Long-term follow-up of patients with avascular necrosis after treatment of slipped capital femoral epiphysis. *J Pediatr Orthop* 1993;13:154-158.

35. Frymoyer JW: Chondrolysis of the hip following Southwick osteotomy for severe slipped capital femoral epiphysis. *Clin Orthop* 1974;99:120-124.

36. Ingram AJ, Clarke MS, Clarke CS Jr, Marshall WR: Chondrolysis complicating slipped capital femoral epiphysis. *Clin Orthop* 1982;165: 99-109.

37. O'Brien ET, Fahey JJ: Remodeling of the femoral neck after in situ pinning for slipped capital femoral epiphysis. *J Bone Joint Surg Am* 1977;59:62-68.

Reference to Video

Moseley C, Canale ST, Morrissy R: Pediatric: At issue in orthopaedics. *Slipped Capital Femoral Epiphysis (SCFE): Diagnosis, Treatment, and Postoperative Care.* Rosemont, IL, American Academy of Orthopaedic Surgeons, 1994.

Slipped Capital Femoral Epiphysis

Randall T. Loder, MD
David D. Aronsson, MD
Matthew B. Dobbs, MD
Stuart L. Weinstein, MD

Slipped capital femoral epiphysis (SCFE) is a well-known disorder of the hip in adolescents that is characterized by displacement of the capital femoral epiphysis from the metaphysis through the physis. The term SCFE is a misnomer because the epiphysis is held in the acetabulum by the ligamentum teres, and thus it is actually the metaphysis that moves upward and outward while the epiphysis remains in the acetabulum. In most patients, there is an apparent varus relationship between the head and the neck, but occasionally the slip is into a valgus position, with the epiphysis displaced superiorly in relation to the neck.[1,2] In the vast majority of cases, the etiology is unknown. Although the condition may be associated with a known endocrine disorder,[3-5] with renal failure osteodystrophy,[6] or with previous radiation therapy,[4,7] this chapter deals only with idiopathic SCFE.

Etiology

Multiple theories have been proposed for the etiology of idiopathic SCFE, and it is likely a result of both biomechanical and biochemical factors.[8] The combination of these factors results in a weakened physis with subsequent failure.

Mechanical factors[9] associated with the disorder are obesity,[10,11] increased femoral retroversion,[9,12,13] and increased physeal obliquity.[14] The vast majority of children with an SCFE are obese, which increases the shear stress across the physis. Obesity is also associated with femoral retroversion, with anteversion averaging 10.6° in adolescents with normal weight but only 0.40° in obese adolescents.[12] This femoral retroversion increases the stress across the physis.[9] Children with an SCFE also have a more vertical proximal femoral physis (an increase of 8° to 11° compared with that in children without the disorder) even in the contralateral, normal hip. The combination of mechanical forces resulting from femoral retroversion and increased physeal slope is enough to cause an SCFE.[9] The mean shear load to failure of the proximal femoral physis in adolescents of normal weight is 4.0 times body weight; the mean shear load to failure in adolescents who are running, who are obese, or who have neutral version (or 10° of relative retroversion) is 5.1 times body weight. Finally, recent data[15] have shown that children with the disorder have deeper acetabula (a mean center-edge angle of Wiberg[16] of 37° compared with a mean of 33° in control subjects). Greater coverage of the femoral head yields more shear stress across the physis.

Biochemical factors are also likely involved. SCFE is a disease of puberty,[17] when many hormonal changes occur;[18] this raises the possibility of an association between the disorder and endocrine function. The increased prevalence of SCFE in children who have hypothyroidism, who are receiving growth hormone supplementation, or who have hypogonadism also suggests an association between the disorder and endocrine dysfunction. Rapid longitudinal growth occurs during puberty in response to growth hormone. This is due to the increased physiologic activity of the physis and is associated with widening of the physis. Decreased physeal strength occurs at puberty;[18] the cause is not clear, but it may be because of the increased cartilage width of the hypertrophic zones and to provisional calcification.[19]

The effects of the gonadotropins on the physis may explain the male predominance of SCFE; estrogen reduces physeal width and increases physeal strength,[20] whereas testosterone reduces physeal strength.[18] This probably also accounts for the fact that the disorder is extremely rare in girls after menarche.[21] Although most children with an SCFE do not have a demonstrable endocrine disorder,[22-26] a subtle but as yet undiagnosable endocrinopathy may be present. In some children, there is a delay in bone age compared with chronological age,[18-21] which further supports this concept.

SCFE does not appear to be a heritable disorder. Rennie[27] discovered that the risk of an SCFE in a second family member was 7.1% and that 14.5% of patients with an SCFE had a close relative who also had the disorder. A few families with the disorder may have an autosomal dominant inheritance with incomplete penetrance.[27] The findings of HLA-typing in children with an SCFE have varied.[28,29]

Routine histologic evaluation and electron microscopy studies of SCFE demonstrate a deficiency and abnormality in the supporting collagenous and proteoglycan framework of the physis. Both the hypertrophic and the proliferative zones are abnormal. Whether these abnormalities represent the cause or the effect of the SCFE is not known. Chondrocyte clustering and disarray occur in a thickened hypertrophic zone,[30,31] and ultrastructural studies have demonstrated defective collagen fibrils and defects in collagen banding in this zone.[32] The proliferative zone demonstrates changes in proteoglycan and glycoprotein concentrations, with increased glycoprotein staining in the territorial matrix and increased proteoglycan staining in the extraterritorial matrix.

Epidemiology and Demographics

The prevalence of SCFE is not completely known. The prevalence has been reported as 0.2 per 100,000 in eastern Japan,[33] as 2.13 per 100,000 in the southwestern United States, and as high as 10.08 per 100,000 in the northeastern United States.[34] Most series have demonstrated a male predominance. Early in the 20th century, 90% of the children with the disorder were boys, but more recently male predominance has decreased to 60%.[35] The mean duration of symptoms before the diagnosis of chronic SCFE is 5 months, with no difference noted with respect to gender. The mean age at diagnosis is 13.5 years for boys and 12.0 years for girls, with a typical age range of 9 to 16 years.[11] The majority of the children are obese; at least 50% of the children with the disorder are over the 95th percentile for weight according to age.[10,11]

The age at onset decreases with increasing obesity.[11] The mean age at onset for children over the 95th percentile for weight according to age is 12.4 years; the mean age for children under the 10th percentile for weight according to age is 14.3 years. Although the chronologic age at the onset of SCFE varies, the physiologic age range appears to be smaller, with a "narrow window" of time during which it can occur.[36] In latitudes north of 40°, the onset of SCFE occurs more frequently in the summer and autumn months.[18,37-40]

The reported prevalence of bilaterality varies and depends on the study, the method of radiographic measurement, race, and possibly the type of treatment. In most series, a prevalence of 18% to 50% has been reported;[11] however, recent studies with follow-up into adulthood have demonstrated a prevalence of bilaterality as high as 63%.[39,41,42] The percentage of bilaterality has been found to be higher in black children (34%) than in Hispanic children (17%), white children (17%), and Asian children (18%), according to a study of 1,630 children.[11] Treatment may affect the prevalence of bilaterality. In one study,[43] the prevalence was 36% in 169 patients treated with in situ pinning and 7% in 30 treated with a spica cast. Therefore, it is mandatory that close attention be paid to the contralateral, normal hip in children who have a unilateral SCFE treated with in situ pinning.

Between 50% and 60% of patients with bilateral involvement have it when they are first seen.[11] Eighty-two percent of second cases of SCFE that develop in patients who initially presented with unilateral involvement are seen within 18 months after the first presentation.[11,21,39,44-46] In addition, children who are seen first with unilateral involvement and in whom bilateral SCFE later develops have a younger age at presentation than do children in whom the disorder does not develop bilaterally.[11,44,45,47,48] This difference is seen in both the chronologic age (12 compared with 13 years) and the pelvic bone age. Of those

with unilateral involvement, 60% have an SCFE in the left hip.[11]

The predilection for SCFE varies by race. The relative racial frequency of SCFE is 1.0 for whites, 4.5 for Pacific Islanders, 2.2 for blacks, 1.05 for Amerindian peoples (Native Americans and Hispanics), 0.5 for Indonesian-Malay peoples (Chinese, Japanese, Thai, Vietnamese, and so on), and 0.1 for Indo-Mediterranean peoples (those of Near East, North African, or Indian subcontinent ancestry).[11] There are at least two possible explanations for these racial differences. One is that they reflect the mean body weight for each racial group, which further supports the theory that obesity is a major factor in the cause of the disorder.[11] The second explanation is that there is a racial variability in acetabular depth and femoral head coverage; the acetabula in adolescent black children are deeper than those in white children.[15]

Classification

SCFE is classified according to both the clinical nature and the magnitude of the disorder. The traditional clinical categories are preslip, acute, chronic, and acute-on-chronic.[49-53] Classification into these four categories depends on the patient's history, physical examination, and radiographs.

In the preslip stage, patients usually complain of weakness in the leg, limping, or pain in the groin or the knee on exertion. Prolonged standing or walking may produce these symptoms. On physical examination, the most consistent positive finding is lack of internal rotation. On radiographs, there may be generalized osteopenia of the hemipelvis and the proximal part of the femur in patients who limp or who have limited their activity. There may be widening and irregularity of the physis.[54]

An acute SCFE is an abrupt displacement through the proximal physis in which there was a preexisting epiphysiolysis.[52] Ten percent to 15% of

SCFEs have been acute in most large series.[45,51] The clinical criteria for an acute SCFE include a duration of symptoms of less than 3 weeks and demonstration of an external rotation deformity, shortening, and marked limitation of motion secondary to pain on physical examination. In general, the greater the amount of slip, the more the motion is restricted. However, 67% of patients with an acute SCFE have a 1- to 3-month history of mild prodromal symptoms before the acute episode, indicating that there was a preslip or a mild SCFE prior to the acute episode.[1,49,51,52,55] The traumatic episode may be as trivial as turning over in bed. The pain is usually severe enough to prevent weight bearing.

Chronic SCFEs are by far the most common and account for 85% of all slips.[45] Patients with a chronic SCFE have pain in the groin, thigh, and knee that varies in duration, often ranging from months to years. They may have a history of exacerbations and remissions of the pain and limp. Physical examination demonstrates an antalgic gait, with loss of internal rotation, abduction, and flexion of the hip.[56] In more severe cases, patients have a limb-length discrepancy and a natural positioning of the lower extremity in external rotation. As the hip is flexed, the lower extremity spontaneously moves into a position of increased external rotation. Importantly, 46% of the patients have pain in the knee or the distal part of the thigh as the initial symptom, emphasizing the importance of a hip examination in a child who complains of knee pain.[57,58]

An acute-on-chronic SCFE is one associated with chronic symptoms initially and with subsequent development of acute symptoms as well as a sudden increase in the degree of slip.

The traditional classification depends on the memory of the child or parent, or both, and may be inaccurate; it also does not give a prognosis with regard to the potential for osteonecrosis.

Two newer and more clinically useful classifications, one clinical and one radiographic, depend on physeal stability. The clinical classification depends on the ability of the child to walk.[59] The SCFE is considered stable when the child is able to walk with or without crutches, and it is considered unstable when the child cannot walk with or without crutches. The radiographic classification depends on the presence or absence of a hip effusion on ultrasonography.[60,61] If the ultrasound demonstrates the absence of metaphyseal remodeling and the presence of an effusion, an acute event is likely to have occurred and the SCFE is considered unstable. If the ultrasound demonstrates metaphyseal remodeling and the absence of an effusion, an acute event has not occurred and the SCFE is considered stable.

This classification is important because it is predictive of the prognosis. The traditional classification of slips as acute or chronic is misleading because it does not consider the stability of the hip, which is highly predictive of the development of osteonecrosis. Unstable SCFEs have a much higher prevalence of osteonecrosis (up to 50% in some series) compared with stable SCFEs (nearly 0%).[59] The high rates of complications with unstable slips are most likely secondary to vascular injury caused at the time of the initial displacement.[59,62] The development of osteonecrosis is associated with the findings on bone scans made before treatment. A cold bone scan (demonstrating an absence of vascularity) essentially is seen only in unstable cases. When a patient has such a bone scan, the risk of subsequent development of osteonecrosis is 80% to 100%.[63] The symptoms of a child with an unstable SCFE mimic those of a child with a hip fracture, and indeed the SCFE may be considered a type of Salter-Harris type I fracture.[64] The child has severe pain and resists any passive or active attempt to move the lower extremity. The extrem-

ity is held in a flexed and externally rotated position.

Radiographs demonstrate an inferior and posterior slip of the proximal femoral epiphysis relative to the metaphysis. In a gradual slip, there are radiographic signs of superior and anterior remodeling on the femoral metaphysis and of periosteal new bone formation at the epiphyseal-metaphyseal junction posteriorly and inferiorly. In an early slip, the changes can be subtle, and both AP and lateral radiographs must be made. The epiphysis typically slips posteriorly[56] and as such is often seen only on a lateral radiograph in the earlier stages. Other helpful radiographic signs are the metaphyseal blanch sign of Steel[65] and Klein's line[66] (Fig. 1). The metaphyseal blanch sign of Steel is a double density seen at the level of the metaphysis on an AP radiograph; the double density reflects the posterior cortical lip of the epiphysis as it is beginning to slip posteriorly and is radiographically superimposed on the metaphyseal density. Klein's line is drawn on a radiograph along the anterior or superior aspect of the femoral neck; the epiphysis should normally intersect this line. In an early SCFE, the epiphysis is flush with or even below this line.

Other imaging methods may be needed in the evaluation of a child with an SCFE. A bone scan[63] and an MRI scan allow earlier diagnosis of osteonecrosis and chondrolysis. Advances in ultrasonography have allowed visualization of an effusion in the hip (a sign of an unstable SCFE) and remodeling of the femoral neck (a sign of a stable SCFE). CT scanning provides three-dimensional imaging of an SCFE, creating an awareness that the epiphysis remains in the acetabulum while the femoral neck displaces anteriorly. This process results in a retroversion deformity of the proximal part of the femur.

The severity of an SCFE is commonly assessed by two different methods. The first is evaluation of the amount of displacement of the epiphysis on the

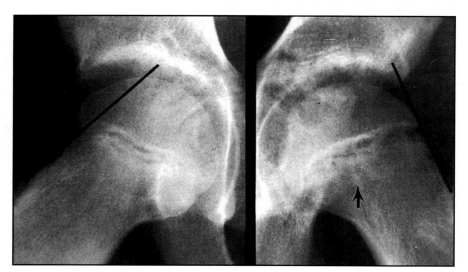

Fig. 1 AP radiographs showing the metaphyseal blanch sign and Klein's line. The metaphyseal blanch sign is a radiographic double density seen at the level of the metaphysis (*arrow*); this double density reflects the posterior cortical lip of the epiphysis as it is beginning to slip posteriorly and is radiographically superimposed on the metaphyseal density. Klein's line is drawn along the anterior or superior aspect of the femoral neck; the epiphysis should normally intersect this line (*left*). In an early SCFE, the epiphysis is flush with or even below this line (*right*).

metaphysis. The disorder is considered mild when the epiphyseal-metaphyseal displacement is less than one third of the width of the femoral neck, moderate when the displacement is one third to one half of the width of the femoral neck, and severe when the displacement is greater than one half of the width of the femoral neck.[58] However, because of the remodeling associated with a gradual slip,[67] this method is less accurate than the angular measurement method, which typically involves measurement of the epiphyseal shaft angle on the frog-leg lateral radiograph as described by Southwick.[68] The angle of slip can also be categorized into groups. Slip angles of less than 30° are considered mild; those of 30° to 50°, moderate; and those of more than 50°, severe.[51] This classification is probably most important with regard to long-term prognosis. Mild and moderate slips have an excellent long-term prognosis with regard to the Iowa hip score when treated with in situ pinning, whereas severe slips are associated

with a more rapid decline in Iowa hip scores over time.[57,69]

Treatment

The most important priority in the management of a patient with an SCFE is primum non nocere (first, do no harm).[70] Most investigators agree that once an SCFE has been diagnosed, treatment is indicated to prevent progression of the slip. The goal of treatment is to prevent additional slippage while avoiding the complications of osteonecrosis and chondrolysis. Chondrolysis is defined as narrowing of the joint space to at least one half of that in the contralateral hip in unilateral cases and as narrowing of the joint space to less than 3 mm in bilateral cases.[58,71,72] There are several treatment methods, and each has its own advantages and disadvantages.

The treatment of a patient with an SCFE has changed because of improved imaging techniques. Twenty-five years ago, radiographs were the only imaging technique used to evaluate a patient with

the disorder. Patients were often treated with in situ fixation with multiple pins, and intraoperative spot radiographs were used to control pin placement. Pin placement was not always ideal with this technique, and malpositioned pins were associated with complications, including additional slippage, chondrolysis, and osteonecrosis in 20% to 40% of patients.[70,73] The high rate of complications associated with in situ fixation with multiple pins led others to try treatment with a hip spica cast, open epiphysiodesis, or femoral osteotomy. The development of intraoperative fluoroscopy to assist in the placement of internal fixation devices has markedly lowered the complication rate associated with internal fixation.

Stable Slipped Capital Femoral Epiphysis

The current treatment methods for a patient with a stable (chronic) SCFE include (1) immobilization in a hip spica cast,[74] (2) in situ stabilization with single or multiple pins or screws,[50,53,70,75] (3) open epiphysiodesis with iliac crest[76,77] or allogeneic[78] bone graft, (4) open reduction with a corrective osteotomy through the physis and internal fixation with use of multiple pins,[79,80] (5) compensating base-of-neck osteotomy with in situ stabilization of the SCFE with use of multiple-pin fixation,[81,82] and (6) intertrochanteric osteotomy with internal fixation.[68] The advantages and disadvantages of each method are discussed below.

Hip Spica Cast Immobilization in a bilateral hip spica cast avoids the complications associated with a surgical procedure. The prevalence of bilateral SCFE is approximately 20% to 40%,[11,39,41,42] and a hip spica cast also provides prophylactic treatment of the contralateral hip. Hurley and associates[43] compared the results of in situ pinning in 169 patients with those of immobilization in a hip spica cast in 30 patients. After a mean follow-up of 2.8 years, SCFE had developed in

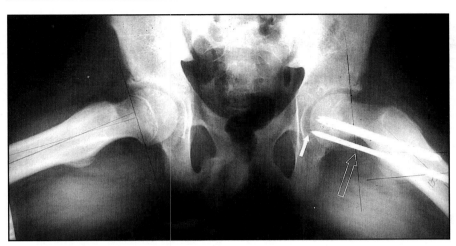

Fig. 2 Radiograph showing a pin (*open arrow*) exiting the posterior part of the femoral neck and entering the posterior aspect of the epiphysis. The pin also penetrates the femoral head and protrudes into the hip joint (*solid arrow*).

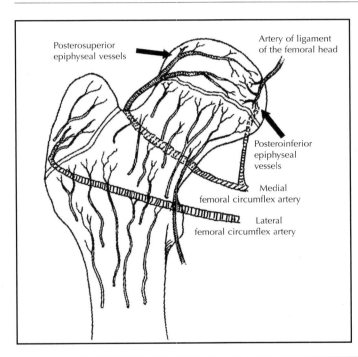

Posterosuperior epiphyseal vessels

Artery of ligament of the femoral head

Posteroinferior epiphyseal vessels

Medial femoral circumflex artery

Lateral femoral circumflex artery

Fig. 3 Drawing showing the blood supply to the femoral head. The most important contribution to this blood supply is from the posterosuperior epiphyseal vessels that originate from the medial femoral circumflex artery.

the contralateral hip of 61 patients (36%) treated with in situ pinning. After a mean follow-up of 3.6 years, SCFE had developed in the contralateral hip of two patients (7%) treated with a hip spica cast. Betz and associates[74] evaluated 32 patients (37 hips) treated with a hip spica cast. A reduction was not attempted, and the cast was worn until the metaphyseal lucency adjacent to the physis was no longer visible on radiographs. The duration of immobilization in the cast averaged 12 weeks. Osteonecrosis did not develop in any hip, but the slip progressed in two hips (5%) and chondrolysis developed in seven (19%). Meier and associates[83] evaluated 13 patients (17 hips) who were treated with a hip spica cast for a mean of 12 weeks. The slip progressed in three hips, chondrolysis developed in nine, and full-thickness cast pressure sores developed in two. In total, complications occurred in 14 of the 17 hips, which led those authors to abandon the hip spica cast as a treatment for SCFE. In addition to the high rate of complications, the hip spica cast is awkward and cumbersome for the family, particularly if the patient is obese. The hip spica cast does not stabilize the SCFE, and most investigators have reported progression of the slip in 5% to 10% of patients, despite immobilization in the cast.[74,83] For all of these reasons, a hip spica cast for treatment of SCFE is not recommended.

In Situ Stabilization With Use of Single or Multiple Pins or Screws Since O'Brien and Fahey[84] reported on the remodeling potential of the proximal part of the femur in patients with an SCFE, in situ fixation with multiple pins has been the most popular treatment method. Long-term follow-up studies of in situ fixation have shown that postoperative remodeling occurs and that the loss of internal rotation of the hip in most patients is not clinically relevant.[85,86] In the past, the three-dimensional anatomy of SCFE was not well understood and reliable intraoperative imaging techniques were not available. As a result, insertion of the pins often was started on the lateral aspect of the femoral shaft, a technique similar to that used in treating a hip fracture in an adult. Because the proximal part of the femur is retroverted in a patient with an SCFE, the pins were often placed in the anterosuperior aspect of the epiphysis, achieving suboptimal fixation. To improve fixation, clinicians angled the pins more posteriorly. The pins often exited the posterior aspect of the femoral neck and entered the epiphysis in the posterosuperior quadrant, which jeopardized the blood supply to the femoral head (Fig. 2).

The most important contribution to the blood supply to the femoral head is from the lateral epiphyseal vessels.[87]

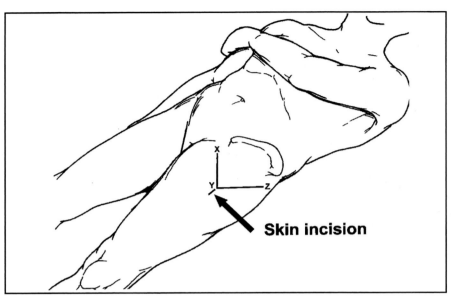

Fig. 4 Drawing showing the technique used for positioning the skin incision. The line X-Y represents a line overlying the center of the femoral head and perpendicular to the physis on the AP fluoroscopic image. The line Y-Z represents a line overlying the center of the femoral head and perpendicular to the physis on the lateral fluoroscopic image. The skin incision is made at the intersection of these lines.

Brodetti[88] demonstrated that the lateral epiphyseal vessels enter the femoral head in the posterosuperior quadrant and anastomose with the vessels from the round ligament at the junction of the medial and central thirds of the femoral head (Fig. 3). The ideal position for a screw, therefore, is in the central area or neutral zone of the femoral head. If a pin is placed in the posterosuperior quadrant, the risk of damage to the epiphyseal blood supply is increased. This risk is minimized by placement of a single screw in the center of the epiphysis, perpendicular to the physis.[50] A comparison of single-screw fixation and double-screw fixation in a calf model demonstrated only a slight increase in stiffness with two screws, which does not justify the increased risk of complications associated with the use of two screws.[89]

Another reason to use as few pins or screws as possible is that, even with the use of AP and true lateral radiographs, there is an area (the "blind spot") that cannot be seen.[73] This blind spot is often the site of unrecognized pin protrusion. Pin protrusion can be associated with the development of chondrolysis and subchondral bone changes. With multiple pins, the possibility that one or more will protrude into the joint is increased; this risk is lowered when a single screw is used.[53,90,91] The advantages of single-screw fixation in a patient with a stable SCFE include a high rate of success and a low prevalence of additional slippage and of complications.[50,92,93] It is presently the most common treatment for SCFE in North America.

Surgical Technique The technique for percutaneous insertion of a single screw has been described.[50,91] The patient is positioned on a fracture table or radiolucent table in the supine position to allow simultaneous biplane AP and lateral fluoroscopic imaging. It is important to emphasize that the technique is image-dependent, so excellent observation of the femoral head and neck is required before the procedure is begun. Because the procedure is performed percutaneously through a small skin incision with use of a cannulated screw, it is important to locate the proper starting position for the guide pin. To determine the starting point, a guide pin is placed on the skin overlying the proximal part of the femur and, under AP fluoroscopic guidance, the pin is positioned such that it projects over the center of the femoral neck and head, crossing the physis in a perpendicular fashion. Once this pin position has been obtained, a marking pen is used to draw a line on the skin reflecting the pin position on the AP image. The same procedure is used for the lateral fluoroscopic image, and a 1-cm skin incision is made at the intersection of the two lines (Fig. 4). The guide pin is advanced freehand through the soft tissues to engage the anterolateral femoral cortex. The position and angulation of the guide pin are adjusted, with fluoroscopic guidance, to obtain the proper alignment before the guide pin is drilled into the bone. It is ideal to advance the guide pin into the center of the femoral head, perpendicular to the physis, as seen on both the AP and the lateral fluoroscopic images on the first attempt, since multiple drill-holes can weaken the bone, causing a fracture through an unused hole.[94] After the appropriate screw length has been determined, a 7.3-mm stainless-steel cannulated screw is placed over the guide pin and is advanced until five threads engage the epiphysis (Fig. 5). The screw should not be left protruding beyond the lateral aspect of the femoral shaft, where it can be toggled by the soft tissues, leading to screw loosening.[95] After surgery, the patient begins partial weight bearing with use of crutches and gradually advances to full weight bearing as tolerated. Most patients can walk without crutches within 2 to 4 days.

The results of single-screw fixation in patients with SCFE have been gratifying. Aronson and Carlson[50] reported excellent or good results in 36 (95%) of

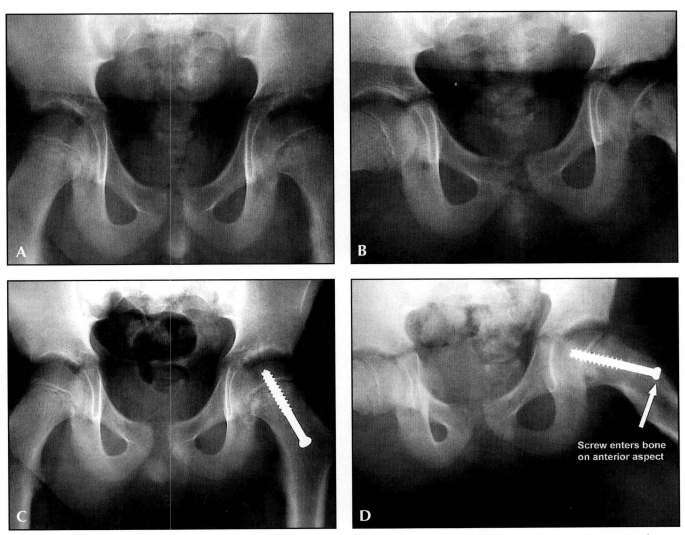

Fig. 5 A 10-year-old boy with a stable (chronic) mild SCFE involving the left hip. **A,** Preoperative AP pelvic radiograph. **B,** Preoperative frog-leg lateral pelvic radiograph. **C,** Postoperative AP radiograph. **D,** Pelvic radiograph showing placement of the screw perpendicular to the physis.

38 mild slips, 10 of 11 moderate slips, and 8 of 9 severe slips. Osteonecrosis developed in only one patient (2%), with an unstable SCFE, and chondrolysis developed in none. Ward and associates[53] reported on 42 patients (53 hips) with an SCFE treated with single-screw fixation. After a mean follow-up of 32 months, 92% of the patients demonstrated physeal fusion and were able to participate in full activities. Neither chondrolysis nor osteonecrosis developed in any patient. Samuelson and Olney,[96] using a similar percutaneous technique, reported excellent results in seven patients treated with two Knowles pins and in 17 patients treated with a single Knowles pin.

Open Epiphysiodesis With Iliac Crest or Allogeneic Bone Graft Open epiphysiodesis with iliac crest bone graft to stabilize the SCFE was first reported by Ferguson and Howorth[38] in 1931. This procedure avoids the complications associated with internal fixation, including unrecognized pin protrusion, damage to the lateral epiphyseal vessels, and hardware failure. The surgical technique involves an anterior iliofemoral exposure of the hip joint. A rectangular window of bone is removed from the anterior aspect of the femoral neck. A hollow mill is used to create a cylindrical tunnel across the physis, and multiple corticocancellous strips of iliac crest bone graft are driven into the tunnel as bone pegs across the proximal femoral physis (Fig. 6). Weiner and associates[77] reported on their 30-year experience with this technique, which they used to treat 159

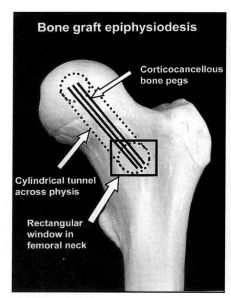

Bone graft epiphysiodesis

Corticocancellous bone pegs

Cylindrical tunnel across physis

Rectangular window in femoral neck

Fig. 6 Illustration showing the technique for performing an open epiphysiodesis. A rectangular window of bone is removed from the anterior aspect of the femoral neck, and a cylindrical tunnel is created across the physis. Multiple strips of corticocancellous bone from the iliac crest are then driven into the tunnel as bone pegs across the physis.

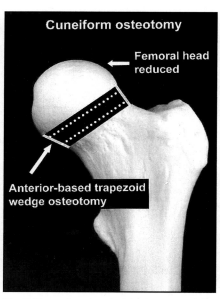

Cuneiform osteotomy

Femoral head reduced

Anterior-based trapezoid wedge osteotomy

Fig. 7 Illustration showing the location of the anterior-based trapezoid wedge of bone that is removed from the metaphysis of the femoral neck during the cuneiform osteotomy. The epiphysis is then gently reduced and internally fixed with three pins.

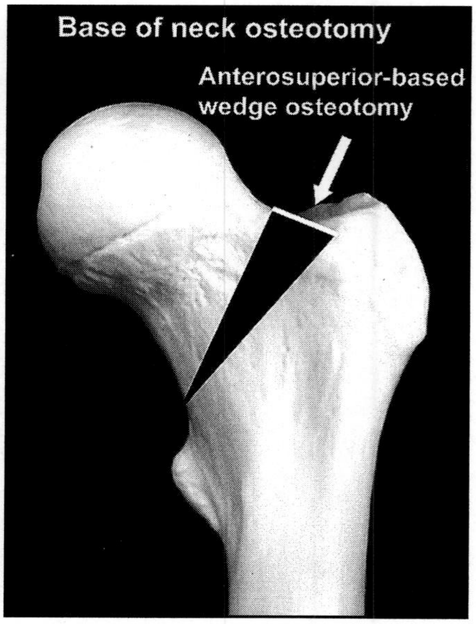

Base of neck osteotomy

Anterosuperior-based wedge osteotomy

Fig. 8 Illustration showing the location of the anterosuperior-based wedge of bone that is removed during the compensating base-of-neck osteotomy. The osteotomy site is internally fixed with multiple pins.

patients (185 hips) who had an SCFE. Additional slipping developed in four hips (2%); osteonecrosis, in one (1%); and chondrolysis, in none.

An advantage of open epiphysiodesis with iliac crest bone graft is that the graft is inserted at the correct angle in the center of the femoral head, minimizing the risk of damage to the blood supply of the femoral head. The graft is not inserted as deeply as is recommended for internal fixation, so there is less risk of graft protrusion into the hip joint. However, the fixation provided by the iliac crest bone graft is not as secure as that achieved by internal fixation. Rao and associates[76] evaluated 43 patients (64 hips) treated by open bone-peg epiphysiodesis. At the time of healing, 27 hips (42%) had had additional slipping. Osteonecrosis developed in four hips (6%); chondrolysis, in three (5%); and additional complications, in 14 (22%). Other disadvantages of open

bone-peg epiphysiodesis include increased blood loss, a longer duration of anesthesia, and a larger scar. As a result of these complications, Rao and associates[76] stated that they no longer recommend open bone-peg epiphysiodesis as the initial treatment for SCFE.

Schmidt and associates[78] developed a technique to percutaneously place a freeze-dried, irradiated cortical strut allograft across the physis. The technique is similar to that used for the percutaneous insertion of a single screw but, instead of a screw, a 10-mm cannulated reamer is placed over the guide pin to ream a channel to within 2 mm of the subchondral bone. A cortical strut allograft then is passed into the channel and is advanced until at least 1 cm is across the physis. Schmidt and associates[78] evaluated 31 patients (38 hips) who had a mean follow-up of 3 years and 6 months and reported that the Harris hip rating was excellent for 35 hips, good for one, and fair for two. Six patients (19%) had a major complication,

including osteonecrosis, chondrolysis, femoral neck fracture, subtrochanteric hip fracture, bilateral coxa vara deformity, and unilateral coxa vara deformity in one patient each. Despite these complications, those authors still recommended this technique, particularly for a patient with a severe SCFE.

Open Reduction With Corrective Osteotomy Through the Physis and Internal Fixation With Use of Multiple Pins
A cuneiform osteotomy through the physis is the ideal method with which to correct the retroversion deformity of the femoral neck, but is it safe? The surgical technique involves an anterior Smith-Petersen[79] or anterolateral[80] exposure of the hip. A wedge of bone is removed from the metaphysis of the femoral neck. This allows the epiphysis to be anatomically repositioned on the metaphysis without creating tension on the epiphyseal vasculature (Fig. 7). The osteotomy is created with use of osteotomes, rongeurs, curets, and a Kerrison punch (Codman, Raynham, MA). After the femoral neck is suf-

ficiently shortened, the epiphysis is reduced and internally fixed with the use of three pins. Fish[97] performed the cuneiform osteotomy in 61 patients (66 hips) and reported that 55 hips (83%) had an excellent result; six (9%), a good result; two (3%), a fair result; and three (5%), a poor result. DeRosa and associates[79] evaluated 23 patients (27 hips) with a severe SCFE treated by cuneiform osteotomy. After a mean follow-up of 8 years and 5 months, no hip had an excellent result; 19 hips (70%) had a good result; four (15%), a fair result; and four, a poor result. Osteonecrosis developed in four hips (15%) and chondrolysis, in eight (30%). In addition, two patients (7%) lost fixation and required additional surgery, a skin erosion developed over one of the pins and required pin removal, and a buttock pressure sore developed in another patient. Despite the 15% rate of osteonecrosis in their study, DeRosa and associates[79] stated that they would still recommend the cuneiform osteotomy for patients with a severe SCFE.

Velasco and associates[80] evaluated 65 patients (66 hips) treated with open reduction of an SCFE. In 60 hips, the open reduction of the slip was combined with a cuneiform subcapital wedge resection of the femoral neck according to the technique described by Dunn and Angel.[98] At a mean of 16 years, chondrolysis had developed in eight hips (12%) and osteonecrosis, in seven (11%). Of the 48 hips that had been followed for a minimum of 10 years (mean, 20.6 years), 22 (46%) had a good result; 16 (33%), a moderate result; and 10 (21%), a poor result. Degenerative arthritis was seen in 19 (40%) of the 48 hips. Because of the high risk of osteonecrosis and subsequent poor results in most series, a physeal cuneiform osteotomy as the initial treatment of SCFE is not recommended.

Compensating Base-of-Neck Osteotomy With In Situ Stabilization of the SCFE With Use of Multiple-Pin Fixation Kramer and associates[82] described an

anterosuperior-based wedge osteotomy of the femoral neck. They stabilized both the osteotomy site and the SCFE with multiple pins (Fig. 8). They reported on 55 patients (56 hips) who all had had a positive preoperative Trendelenburg test and had walked with a lurching gait. After the osteotomy, 48 patients (87%) had a negative Trendelenburg test. Nine hips (16%) had a poor result because of pain, a limp, or a decreased range of motion. Osteonecrosis developed in two patients (4%) and chondrolysis, in one (2%). Barmada and associates[81] described an extracapsular basilar neck osteotomy that was performed in an attempt to repair an SCFE while avoiding the risk of osteonecrosis. The prevalence of osteonecrosis associated with basilar neck osteotomy is less than that associated with cuneiform osteotomy. However, only 35° to 55° of correction is possible with this technique.[99] One benefit of the basilar neck osteotomy is improvement in hip motion. A disadvantage is that it shortens the femoral neck, which may result in impingement of the greater trochanter against the lateral aspect of the acetabulum during hip abduction. If there is premature closure of the proximal femoral physis, as is often seen in patients with an SCFE, shortening of the femoral neck may aggravate a limb-length discrepancy.

Intertrochanteric Osteotomy With Internal Fixation Southwick[68] described an intertrochanteric osteotomy through the lesser trochanter. This osteotomy improves hip motion and is not associated with osteonecrosis. The technique advocated by Crawford[100] involves an intertrochanteric osteotomy with flexion, abduction, and internal rotation of the distal fragment (Fig. 9). The osteotomy site is fixed with a compression hip screw, and the SCFE, if it is unstable, is fixed with a percutaneous cannulated screw. The intertrochanteric osteotomy is also a compensating osteotomy with correction limited to 45° on the AP radiograph and

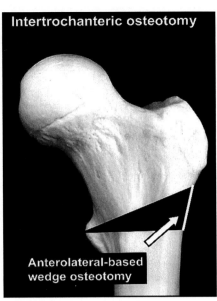

Fig. 9 Illustration showing the location of the anterolateral-based wedge of bone that is removed during the intertrochanteric osteotomy. This osteotomy includes flexion, abduction, and internal rotation of the distal fragment. The osteotomy site is internally fixed with a compression hip screw.

to 60° on the lateral radiograph as measured by the Southwick method.[101] An anterolateral wedge of bone is removed, so this osteotomy is also a shortening procedure. There is a risk that a limb-length discrepancy will be created if considerable correction is achieved. Schai and associates[102] evaluated 51 patients who had an SCFE of 30° to 60° that was treated with an intertrochanteric osteotomy and followed for a mean of 24 years. Moderate osteoarthritis developed in 14 patients (27%) and severe osteoarthritis, in nine (18%). Thirty-five patients (69%) had a shorter limb on the affected side, and two patients (4%) had a limb-length equalization procedure. Osteonecrosis developed in only one patient (2%). A summation of the results of these series indicates that intertrochanteric osteotomy with use of the Southwick technique is not the ideal initial treatment for an SCFE because the outcome of the procedure is relatively

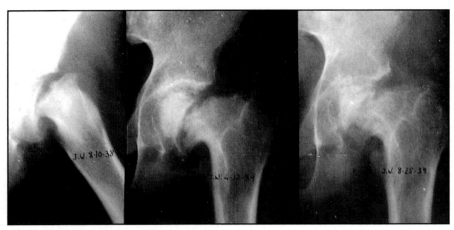

Fig. 10 Radiographs of the left hip of a 14-year-old boy who had immediate severe hip pain following acute trauma, without prior hip symptoms. The radiograph on the left was made at presentation. Those in the middle and on the right were made during a 1-year follow-up period and show the rapid development of osteonecrosis and severe degenerative changes.

poor compared with that of current techniques of in situ single-screw fixation.

Jerre and associates[103] evaluated the results of different realignment procedures in 36 patients (37 hips) after a mean follow-up of 33.8 years (range, 26 to 42 years). Serious short-term complications developed in seven (32%) of the 22 hips treated with subcapital osteotomy, 3 of the 11 hips treated with intertrochanteric osteotomy, and 3 of the 4 hips treated with manipulative reduction. Jerre and associates[103] reported that 41% of the hips treated with subcapital osteotomy, four of those treated with intertrochanteric osteotomy, and none of those treated with manipulative reduction had an excellent or good result.

Unstable Slipped Capital Femoral Epiphysis

The treatment of an unstable SCFE (acute or acute-on-chronic) is similar to that of a stable SCFE but is considerably more controversial. The role of immediate reduction compared with delayed reduction is controversial, as is the role of preoperative traction. Loder and associates[59] compared the results of treatment in 25 hips (24 patients) that had a stable SCFE with those in 30 hips (30 patients) that had an unsta-

ble SCFE. The result was satisfactory in 96% of the 25 hips that had a stable SCFE and in 47% of the 30 hips that had an unstable SCFE. Osteonecrosis developed in none of the hips in the former group and in 14 hips (47%) in the latter group. de Sanctis and associates[104] evaluated 70 patients (81 hips) who had an unstable SCFE (acute or acute-on-chronic) that was treated with a gentle closed reduction and fixation with use of one or two screws or pins. A complication developed in eight hips: three (4%) had chondrolysis, three had a wound infection, and two (2%) had osteonecrosis. de Sanctis and associates[104] concluded that a gentle reduction with percutaneous single-screw fixation is a stable, safe, and reliable method for treating patients who have an unstable SCFE.

Herman and associates[105] evaluated the cases of 21 patients (21 hips) with a severe SCFE (a displacement of more than 50%) after a mean follow-up of 2.8 years. Fifteen patients had an unstable SCFE; nine of them were treated with a gentle closed reduction and internal fixation with use of either one or two screws. Five of the nine hips had a complete reduction of the SCFE, and osteonecrosis developed in three of them. Four hips had an incomplete reduction, and none had osteonecro-

sis. The authors hypothesized that injury to the epiphyseal vasculature occurs at the time of the acute SCFE.

Peterson and associates[106] evaluated 91 patients (91 hips) with an unstable SCFE after a mean of 44 months. Forty-two hips had a closed reduction performed less than 24 hours after presentation, and osteonecrosis developed in three (7%). Forty-nine hips had a closed reduction performed more than 24 hours after presentation, and osteonecrosis developed in 10 (20%). The authors hypothesized that the acute displacement of the femoral head may kink the posterior blood vessels, compromising the blood flow to the epiphysis. In this situation, a timely reduction of the SCFE may restore blood flow to the epiphysis. In contrast, Loder and associates[59] assigned patients who had an acute slip into two groups on the basis of the time interval between the onset of symptoms and the surgical stabilization. Osteonecrosis developed in seven of eight hips that had surgical stabilization less than 48 hours after the onset of symptoms and in seven (32%) of 22 hips that had surgical stabilization more than 48 hours after the onset of symptoms. However, the present data cannot be used to develop guidelines with regard to the exact timing of surgical stabilization because the cause-and-effect relationship between the timing of surgical stabilization and the development of osteonecrosis cannot be determined. It is not known whether a hip with a more severe unstable SCFE, which would likely be associated with a higher risk of osteonecrosis, was stabilized sooner in an effort to reduce the child's discomfort as quickly as possible, or whether a hip with a less severe unstable SCFE, which theoretically might be associated with a lower risk of osteonecrosis, was stabilized later because the child may have been more comfortable.

Complications
Osteonecrosis

Osteonecrosis is the most devastating complication of SCFE (Fig. 10). The factors responsible for the development of osteonecrosis are an acute unstable SCFE, overreduction of an acute SCFE, attempts at reduction of the chronic component of an acute-on-chronic SCFE, placement of pins in the superolateral quadrant of the femoral head, and femoral neck osteotomy.[57,59,87,88,107,108] The frequency of osteonecrosis is increased if a cuneiform or basilar neck osteotomy is performed prior to physeal closure. The complication of osteonecrosis is rare in patients with a stable SCFE, but it occurs frequently in patients with an unstable SCFE.[59] A patient with osteonecrosis typically complains of pain in the groin or knee. On physical examination, there is a loss of motion of the hip, particularly internal rotation, and the hip is irritable on passive internal and external rotation. Plain radiographs are unremarkable early in the course of the disorder, but changes diagnostic of osteonecrosis (collapse of the femoral head with cyst formation and sclerosis) develop after a few months. All cases of osteonecrosis after SCFE are radiographically apparent within 1 year. An early bone scan[109] or MRI often shows asymmetry between the femoral heads, predicting the eventual development of osteonecrosis.

The treatment of osteonecrosis is not particularly rewarding for the patient or the clinician. Non–weight-bearing walking with crutches, range-of-motion exercises, and anti-inflammatory medication may help to minimize symptoms and epiphyseal collapse. An internal fixation device that protrudes into the hip joint should be backed out of the joint or removed, if the physis is closed, to reduce additional damage to the hip. In severe cases, a hip arthrodesis or joint arthroplasty may be needed.

Chondrolysis
The etiology of chondrolysis in SCFE is unknown. The possible role of an autoimmune phenomenon or some factor interfering with cartilage nutrition is yet to be defined. Risk factors leading to chondrolysis include immobilization in a cast, unrecognized permanent pin penetration, severe SCFE, and prolonged symptoms before treatment.

The prevalence of chondrolysis in patients with an SCFE is 5% to 7%.[110,111] A patient typically complains of pain in the groin or knee, and physical examination demonstrates a loss of hip motion, particularly internal rotation. The diagnosis is confirmed by radiographs that demonstrate a decrease in the width of the joint space of greater than 50% compared with the uninvolved side or, in patients who have bilateral involvement, a joint space of less than 3 mm. Hips that demonstrate increased uptake with premature closure of the greater trochanter on an early bone scan have been associated with an increased risk for the development of chondrolysis.[111] The prevalance of chondrolysis increases with the increasing severity of the SCFE, but it is not increased in the black population,[112-115] as previously reported.[110,116,117] The frequency of chondrolysis can be reduced with use of single-screw fixation rather than fixation with multiple screws or pins. With multiple pins or screws, the possibility that one or more may protrude into the joint is increased, and pin protrusion has been associated with an increased risk of chondrolysis.[118] The frequency of chondrolysis can also be reduced by not using a hip spica cast[83] and by waiting until physeal closure prior to performing a subtrochanteric osteotomy.[119]

As is the case with osteonecrosis, the treatment of chondrolysis is not particularly rewarding for the patient or the clinician. Non–weight-bearing walking with crutches, range-of-motion exercises, and anti-inflammatory medication may help to alleviate the symptoms. If there is pin protrusion, backing the pin out of the joint or removing it, if the physis is closed, helps to minimize damage to the hip. Some have recommended lengthening of the contracted muscle or muscles if a hip contracture develops. Arthrodesis may also be necessary in severe cases.

Internal Fixation Devices
The frequency of problems related to internal fixation devices (slip progression, pin breakage, and joint penetration by the pins) is decreasing with the use of fluoroscopic guidance and cannulated single-screw fixation. The risk of fracture through an unused pinhole can be avoided with use of fluoroscopy to position the guide pin correctly on the first attempt and by entering the bone proximal to the lesser trochanter.

Natural History Without Treatment
Two major issues arise when SCFE is untreated: the risk of additional progression and the risk of degenerative joint disease in adult life. Unfortunately, there are few long-term studies of patients with an SCFE and even fewer that have included untreated patients.[51,54,57,69,120-122]

Risk of Progression
The natural history of SCFE is unpredictable, and the risk of additional progression is difficult to ascertain. Ordeberg and associates[123] studied a series of patients 20 to 60 years after diagnosis of SCFE without primary treatment. Few patients had restrictions in working capacity or social life. However, there was a risk of slip progression as long as the physis remained open.[124] Carney and associates[57] reported on 36 cases of SCFE that were initially observed. Additional displacement occurred in six hips (17%) after the initial diagnosis; the SCFE became severe in five of them. Of these six hips, two were untreated and the other four were stabilized surgically. Eleven of the original 36 patients had an acute episode superimposed on the chronic SCFE. All 11 slips progressed to severe displacement and required surgical stabilization.

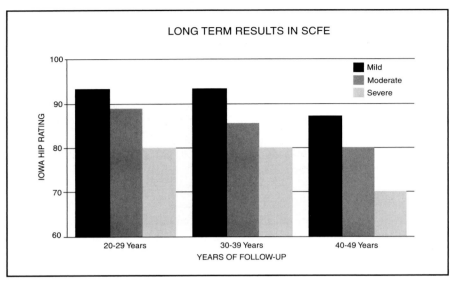

Fig. 11 Graph showing the worsening mean scores on the Iowa hip-rating scale for a group of 124 patients (155 hips) with an SCFE.[19]

Risk of Degenerative Joint Disease

Little is known about the risk of degenerative joint disease. Howorth[125] stated that SCFE is likely the most frequent cause of degenerative joint disease of the hip in middle-aged patients, and it is a common source of pain and disability. However, this theory is not necessarily supported by other studies. In reviews of a large series of patients with degenerative joint disease, the numbers of patients who were known to have an SCFE have been small, averaging approximately 5%.[126-128] Murray,[127] however, reported an association with SCFE in 40% of his 200 patients who were thought to have primary degenerative joint disease. He described a tilt deformity caused by bone resorption laterally with new bone formation medially, which he thought was compatible with an old SCFE. Stulberg and associates[129] described a similar deformity, the pistol-grip deformity, in 40% of patients without known prior hip disease who had total hip arthroplasty. This deformity was also thought to be compatible with an old SCFE. Resnick,[130] however, refuted this theory in a pathologic study of 48 femoral heads from patients with evidence of a tilt

deformity on radiographs. The specimens suggested that the deformity was solely related to the remodeling changes of osteoarthritis. In summary, whether subclinical forms of SCFE lead to early osteoarthritis remains uncertain because of the controversy over the prevalence of the disorder.

What is known is that the severity of the untreated SCFE correlates with the long-term prognosis with regard to degenerative joint disease.[57,69,102,121,131,132] Oram[121] reported on 22 hips with an untreated SCFE, 11 of which were observed for more than 15 years. The hips with a moderate SCFE retained good function for years, whereas degenerative joint disease with resultant poor function developed within 15 years in the hips with a severe SCFE. Jerre[131,132] and Ross and associates[122] reported increasingly poor results with longer follow-up. In those studies, many patients did well early on, but symptoms increased and function decreased with increasing age. Carney and Weinstein[69] also studied the natural history of untreated, chronic SCFE. They evaluated 31 hips in 28 patients who had a mean age of 54 years and had been fol-

lowed for a mean of 41 years. The mean Iowa hip rating score was 89 points for the entire group, 92 points for the 17 hips in which the SCFE was mild, 87 points for the 11 hips in which it was moderate, and 75 points for the three hips in which it was severe. There were four complications: displacement to a severe degree in two hips, and chondrolysis and osteonecrosis in one hip each. The chondrolysis developed in a hip in which the SCFE was mild and the osteonecrosis, in a hip in which it was severe. Although patients with a mild SCFE appear to have a favorable prognosis, patients in whom the disorder is moderate or severe have a high prevalence of degenerative joint disease. At a mean of 41 years after the diagnosis, all hips with a mild SCFE had an Iowa hip rating score of more than 80 points, whereas only 64% of the hips with a moderate or severe disorder had similar ratings. Thirty-six percent of the hips in which the disorder was mild had no degenerative changes; however, all of the hips in which the SCFE was moderate or severe had evidence of degenerative joint disease. Poor results, however, can occasionally be seen even with a minimal SCFE.[51,57,69,122] In summary, the natural history of chronic (stable) SCFE is favorable provided that displacement is mild and remains so.

Few data are available on the natural history of untreated acute SCFE. The acute episode is followed by a 2- to 3-week period of intolerance to weight bearing. As the pain and spasm subside, some motion returns, although the hip remains moderately painful in a position of external rotation. Degenerative changes (joint-space narrowing, subchondral bone cysts, and epiphyseal collapse) develop within a few months, and the patient is left with residual flexion, adduction, and external rotation contractures[54] (Fig. 10).

Long-Term Results of Treatment

Wilson and associates[46] reviewed the results in 300 hips in 240 patients treated between 1936 and 1960; 187 were treated with in situ pinning, with good clinical results in 81% and good radiographic results in 77%. Seventy-six hips in which correction of the deformity had been attempted had poorer results (60% had good clinical results, and 55% had good radiographic results). Hall,[120] in a study of 138 patients, reported that the best results were obtained with the use of multiple pins; 16 (80%) of 20 patients had an excellent result. The worst results were seen after realignment had been attempted with manipulation or osteotomy. Osteotomy of the femoral neck led to a poor result in 36% of the hips and to osteonecrosis in 38%.

Patients with an SCFE in southern Sweden were followed for more than 30 years.[35] Symptomatic treatment or in situ pinning resulted in high clinical ratings and few radiographic changes, with a secondary reconstructive procedure needed in only 2% of the hips. When closed reduction and a spica cast were used, the combined rate of osteonecrosis and chondrolysis was 16%, and a reconstructive procedure was needed in 35% of the hips. When femoral neck osteotomy was performed, the combined rate of osteonecrosis and chondrolysis was 30%, and a reconstructive procedure was necessary in 15% of 33 hips.

Carney and associates[57] reported on 155 hips in 124 patients who were followed for a mean of 41 years and were assessed with use of the Iowa hip rating system and a radiographic classification of degenerative joint disease, with grade 0 indicating no degenerative disease and grade 3 indicating severe degenerative disease. The SCFE was classified as acute, chronic, or acute-on-chronic. According to the head-shaft angle,[68] the degree of the slip was mild in 42%, moderate in 32%, and severe in 26%. Twenty-five percent of the hips that had a chronic SCFE received symptomatic treatment only; 30% were managed with a spica cast; 24%, with in situ pin-

ning; and 20%, with osteotomy. The results worsened as the severity of the slip increased and when realignment had been performed (Fig. 11). Osteonecrosis, which developed in 12% of the hips, and chondrolysis, which developed in 16%, were more common with increasing severity of the slip. Reduction was performed in 39 hips and realignment, in 65 hips. For the 116 hips that had not been reduced, the mean Iowa hip rating was 85 points and the mean radiographic grade was 1.7. Osteonecrosis developed in seven (6%) of those hips, and chondrolysis, in 14 (12%). For the 39 hips with an SCFE that had been reduced, the mean Iowa hip rating score was 72 points and the mean radiographic grade was 2.4. Osteonecrosis developed in 12 of those hips (31%) and chondrolysis, in 11 (28%). Twenty-seven hips with a chronic SCFE that had in situ pinning demonstrated a mean Iowa hip rating score of 90 points and a mean radiographic grade of 1.5. Osteonecrosis developed in one of those hips and chondrolysis, in none. The long-term results of that study support the use of in situ pinning as the treatment of choice for SCFE. Realignment was associated with appreciable complications and had an adverse effect on the outcome. Regardless of the severity of the slip, in situ pinning provided the best long-term function and the longest delay of degenerative arthritis with the lowest risk of complications. Although limb-length discrepancy and motion in abduction and internal rotation were affected by the severity of the slip, function was not significantly impaired.

In conclusion, these series demonstrate that, regardless of the severity of the slip, in situ pinning provides the best long-term function, the lowest risk of complications, and the most effective delay of degenerative arthritis. Many patients with an SCFE respond well to this treatment, as seen at the time of

long-term follow-up, if the SCFE is mild or moderate in severity, good congruity is maintained between the femoral head and the acetabulum, and osteonecrosis and chondrolysis do not develop. Hips with a severe SCFE and those with osteonecrosis or chondrolysis undergo more rapid deterioration with degenerative changes. SCFE differs from other pediatric disorders of the hip, such as Legg-Calvé-Perthes disease and developmental hip dysplasia, in that SCFE occurs at an age when the majority of acetabular development is completed and acetabular adaptation to a deformity of the femoral head cannot occur.

References

1. Schein AJ: Acute severe slipped capital femoral epiphysis. *Clin Orthop* 1967;51:151-166.

2. Segal LS, Weitzel PP, Davidson RS: Valgus slipped capital femoral epiphysis: Fact or fiction? *Clin Orthop* 1996;322:91-98.

3. Loder RT, Wittenberg B, DeSilva G: Slipped capital femoral epiphysis associated with endocrine disorders. *J Pediatr Orthop Am* 1995;15:349-356.

4. McAfee PC, Cady RB: Endocrinologic and metabolic factors in atypical presentations of slipped capital femoral epiphysis: Report of four cases and review of the literature. *Clin Orthop* 1983;180:188-197.

5. Wells D, King JD, Roe TF, Kaufman FR: Review of slipped capital femoral epiphysis associated with endocrine disease. *J Pediatr Orthop Am* 1993;13:610-614.

6. Loder RT, Hensinger RN: Slipped capital femoral epiphysis associated with renal failure osteodystrophy. *J Pediatr Orthop Am* 1997;17:205-211.

7. Loder RT, Hensinger RN, Alburger PD, et al: Slipped capital femoral epiphysis associated with radiation therapy. *J Pediatr Orthop Am* 1998;18:630-636.

8. Weiner D: Pathogenesis of slipped capital femoral epiphysis: Current concepts. *J Pediatr Orthop Br* 1996;5:67-73.

9. Pritchett JW, Perdue KD: Mechanical factors in slipped capital femoral epiphysis. *J Pediatr Orthop Am* 1988;8:385-388.

10. Kelsey JL, Acheson RM, Keggi KJ: The body build of patients with slipped capital femoral epiphysis. *Am J Dis Child* 1972;124:276-281.

11. Loder RT: The demographics of slipped capital femoral epiphysis: An international multicenter study. *Clin Orthop* 1996;322:8-27.

12. Galbraith RT, Gelberman RH, Hajek PC, et al: Obesity and decreased femoral anteversion in adolescence. *J Orthop Res* 1987;5:523-528.

13. Gelberman RH, Cohen MS, Shaw BA, Kasser JR, Griffin PP, Wilkinson RH: The association of femoral retroversion with slipped capital femoral epiphysis. *J Bone Joint Surg Am* 1986;68:1000-1007.

14. Mirkopulos N, Weiner DS, Askew M: The evolving slope of the proximal femoral growth plate relationship to slipped capital femoral epiphysis. *J Pediatr Orthop Am* 1988;8:268-273.

15. Kitadai HK, Milani C, Nery CA, Filho JL: Wiberg's center-edge angle in patients with slipped capital femoral epiphysis. *J Pediatr Orthop Am* 1999;19:97-105.

16. Wiberg G: Studies on dysplastic acetabula and congenital subluxation of the hip joint: With special reference to the complication of osteoarthrosis. *Acta Chir Scand* 1939; 58(suppl):7.

17. Exner GU: Growth and pubertal development in slipped capital femoral epiphysis: A longitudinal study. *J Pediatr Orthop Am* 1986;6:403-409.

18. Morscher E: Strength and morphology of growth cartilage under hormonal influence of puberty: Animal experiments and clinical study on the etiology of local growth disorders during puberty. *Reconstr Surg Traumatol* 1968;10: 3-104.

19. Speer DP: Experimental epiphysiolysis: Etiologic models of slipped capital femoral epiphysis, in Nelson JP (ed): *The Hip: Proceedings of the Tenth Open Scientific Meeting of the Hip Society*. St. Louis, MO, CV Mosby, 1982, pp 68-88.

20. Harris WR: The endocrine basis for slipping of the upper femoral epiphysis: An experimental study. *J Bone Joint Surg Br* 1950;32:5-11.

21. Sørensen KH: Slipped upper femoral epiphysis: Clinical study on aetiology. *Acta Orthop Scand* 1968;39:499-517.

22. Brenkel IJ, Dias JJ, Iqbal SJ, Gregg PJ: Thyroid hormone levels in patients with slipped capital femoral epiphysis. *J Pediatr Orthop Am* 1988;8:22-25.

23. Eisenstein A, Rothschild S: Biochemical abnormalities in patients with slipped capital femoral epiphysis and chondrolysis. *J Bone Joint Surg Am* 1976;58:459-467.

24. Mann DC, Weddington J, Richton S: Hormonal studies in patients with slipped capital femoral epiphysis without evidence of endocrinopathy. *J Pediatr Orthop Am* 1988;8:543-545.

25. Razzano CD, Nelson C, Eversman J: Growth hormone levels in slipped capital femoral epiphysis. *J Bone Joint Surg Am* 1972;54:1224-1226.

26. Wilcox PG, Weiner DS, Leighley B: Maturation factors in slipped capital femoral epiphysis. *J Pediatr Orthop Am* 1988;8:196-200.

27. Rennie AM: The inheritance of slipped upper femoral epiphysis. *J Bone Joint Surg Br* 1982;64:180-184.

28. Bednarz PA, Stanitski CL: Slipped capital femoral epiphysis in identical twins: HLA predisposition. *Orthopedics* 1998;21:1291-1293.

29. Günal I, Ates E: The HLA phenotype in slipped capital femoral epiphysis. *J Pediatr Orthop Am* 1997;17:655-656.

30. Agamanolis DP, Weiner DS, Lloyd JK: Slipped capital femoral epiphysis: A pathological study. I: A light microscopic and histochemical study of 21 cases. *J Pediatr Orthop Am* 1985;5:40-46.

31. Ponseti IV, McClintock R: The pathology of slipping of the upper femoral epiphysis. *J Bone Joint Surg Am* 1956;38:71-83.

32. Agamanolis DP, Weiner DS, Lloyd JK: Slipped capital femoral epiphysis: A pathological study. II: An ultrastructural study of 23 cases. *J Pediatr Orthop Am* 1985;5:47-58.

33. Ninomiya S, Nagasaka Y, Tagawa H: Slipped capital femoral epiphysis. A study of 68 cases in the eastern half area of Japan. *Clin Orthop* 1976;119:172-176.

34. Kelsey JL, Keggi KJ, Southwick WO: The incidence and distribution of slipped capital femoral epiphysis in Connecticut and southwestern United States. *J Bone Joint Surg Am* 1970;52:1203-1216.

35. Hansson LI, Hägglund G, Ordeberg G: Slipped capital femoral epiphysis in southern Sweden 1910-1982. *Acta Orthop Scand* 1987; 226(suppl):1-67.

36. Loder RT, Farley FA, Herzenberg JE, Hensinger RN, Kuhn JL: Narrow window of bone age in children with slipped capital femoral epiphyses. *J Pediatr Orthop Am* 1993;13:290-293.

37. Andrén L, Borgström K-E: Seasonal variation of epiphysiolysis of the hip and possibility of causal factor. *Acta Orthop Scand* 1958;28:22-26.

38. Ferguson AB, Howorth MB: Slipping of the upper femoral epiphysis: A study of 70 cases. *JAMA* 1931;97:1867-1872.

39. Hägglund G, Hansson LI, Ordeberg G: Epidemiology of slipped capital femoral epiphysis in southern Sweden. *Clin Orthop* 1984;191:82-94.

40. Loder RT: A worldwide study on the seasonal variation of slipped capital femoral epiphysis. *Clin Orthop* 1996;322:28-36.

41. Jerre R, Billing L, Hansson G, Wallin J: The contralateral hip in patients primarily treated for unilateral slipped upper femoral epiphysis: Long-term follow-up of 61 hips. *J Bone Joint Surg Br* 1994;76:563-567.

42. Jerre R, Billing L, Hansson G, Karlsson J, Wallin J: Bilaterality in slipped capital femoral epiphysis: Importance of a reliable radiographic method. *J Pediatr Orthop Br* 1996;5:80-84.

43. Hurley JM, Betz RR, Loder RT, Davidson RS, Alburger PD, Steel HH: Slipped capital femoral epiphysis: The prevalence of late contralateral slip. *J Bone Joint Surg Am* 1996;78: 226-230.

44. Dreghorn CR, Knight D, Mainds CC, Blockey NJ: Slipped upper femoral epiphysis: A review of 12 years of experience in Glasgow (1972-1983). *J Pediatr Orthop Am* 1987;7:283-287.

45. Loder RT, Aronson DD, Greenfield ML: The epidemiology of bilateral slipped capital femoral epiphysis: A study of children in Michigan. *J Bone Joint Surg Am* 1993;75:1141-1147.

46. Wilson PD, Jacobs B, Schecter L: Slipped capital femoral epiphysis: An end-result study. *J Bone Joint Surg Am* 1965;47:1128-1145.

47. Segal LS, Davidson RS, Robertson WW Jr, Drummond DS: Growth disturbances of the proximal femur after pinning of juvenile slipped capital femoral epiphysis. *J Pediatr Orthop Am* 1991;11:631-637.

48. Stasikelis PJ, Sullivan CM, Phillips WA, Polard JA: Slipped capital femoral epiphysis: Prediction of contralateral involvement. *J Bone Joint Surg Am* 1996;78:1149-1155.

49. Aadalen RJ, Weiner DS, Hoyt W, Herndon CH: Acute slipped capital femoral epiphysis. *J Bone Joint Surg Am* 1974;56:1473-1487.

50. Aronson DD, Carlson WE: Slipped capital femoral epiphysis: A prospective study of fixation with a single screw. *J Bone Joint Surg Am* 1992;74:810-819.

51. Boyer DW, Mickelson MR, Ponseti IV: Slipped capital femoral epiphysis: Long-term follow-up of one hundred and twenty-one patients. *J Bone Joint Surg Am* 1981;63:85-95.

52. Fahey JJ, O'Brien ET: Acute slipped capital femoral epiphysis: Review of the literature and report of ten cases. *J Bone Joint Surg Am* 1965;47:1105-1127.

53. Ward WT, Stefko J, Wood KB, Stanitski CL: Fixation with a single screw for slipped capital femoral epiphysis. *J Bone Joint Surg Am* 1992;74:799-809.

54. Ponseti I, Barta CK: Evaluation of treatment of slipping of the capital femoral epiphysis. *Surg Gynecol Obstet* 1948;86:87-97.

55. Casey BH, Hamilton HW, Bobechko WP: Reduction of acutely slipped upper femoral epiphysis. *J Bone Joint Surg Br* 1972;54:607-614.

56. Rab GT: The geometry of slipped capital femoral epiphysis: Implications for movement, impingement, and corrective osteotomy. *J Pediatr Orthop Am* 1999;19:419-424.

57. Carney BT, Weinstein SL, Noble J: Long-term follow-up of slipped capital femoral epiphysis. *J Bone Joint Surg Am* 1991;73:667-674.

58. Jacobs B: Diagnosis and natural history of slipped femoral capital epiphysis. *Instr Course Lect* 1972;21:167-173.

59. Loder RT, Richards BS, Shapiro PS, Reznick LR, Aronson DD: Acute slipped capital femoral epiphysis: The importance of physeal stability. *J Bone Joint Surg Am* 1993;75: 1134-1140.

60. Kallio PE, Paterson DC, Foster BK, Lequesne GW: Classification in slipped capital femoral epiphysis: Sonographic assessment of stability and remodeling. *Clin Orthop* 1993;294:196-203.

61. Kallio PE, Mah ET, Foster BK, Paterson DC, LeQuesne GW: Slipped capital femoral epiphysis: Incidence and clinical assessment of physeal instability. *J Bone Joint Surg Br* 1995;77:752-755.

62. Aronsson DD, Loder RT: Treatment of the unstable (acute) slipped capital femoral epiphysis. *Clin Orthop* 1996;322:99-110.

63. Rhoad RC, Davidson RS, Heyman S, Dormans JP, Drummond DS: Pretreatment bone scan in SCFE: A predictor of ischemia and avascular necrosis. *J Pediatr Orthop Am* 1999;19:164-168.

64. Salter RB, Harris WR: Injuries involving the epiphyseal plate. *J Bone Joint Surg Am* 1963;45:587-622.

65. Steel HH: The metaphyseal blanch sign of slipped capital femoral epiphysis. *J Bone Joint Surg Am* 1986;68:920-922.

66. Klein A, Joplin RJ, Reidy JA, Hanelin J: Slipped capital femoral epiphysis: Early diagnosis and treatment facilitated by "normal" roentgenograms. *J Bone Joint Surg Am* 1952;34:233-239.

67. Loder RT, Blakemore LC, Farley FA, Laidlaw AT: Measurement variability of slipped capital femoral epiphysis. *J Orthop Surg* 2000;7:33-42.

68. Southwick WO: Osteotomy through the lesser trochanter for slipped capital femoral epiphysis. *J Bone Joint Surg Am* 1967;49:807-835.

69. Carney BT, Weinstein SL: Natural history of untreated chronic slipped capital femoral epiphysis. *Clin Orthop* 1996;322:43-47.

70. Aronson DD, Peterson DA, Miller DV: Slipped capital femoral epiphysis: The case for internal fixation in situ. *Clin Orthop* 1992;281:115-122.

71. Maurer RC, Larsen IJ: Acute necrosis of cartilage in slipped capital femoral epiphysis. *J Bone Joint Surg Am* 1970;52:39-50.

72. Vrettos BC, Hoffman EB: Chondrolysis in slipped upper femoral epiphysis: Long-term study of the aetiology and natural history. *J Bone Joint Surg Br* 1993;75:956-961.

73. Walters R, Simon SR: Joint destruction: A sequel of unrecognized pin penetration in patients with slipped capital femoral epiphyses, in Riley LH Jr (ed): *The Hip: Proceedings of the Eighth Open Scientific Meeting of the Hip Society.* St. Louis, MO, CV Mosby, 1980, pp 145-164.

74. Betz RR, Steel HH, Emper WD, Huss GK, Clancy M: Treatment of slipped capital femoral epiphysis: Spica-cast immobilization. *J Bone Joint Surg Am* 1990;72:587-600.

75. Strong M, Lejman T, Michno P, Sulko J: Fixation of slipped capital femoral epiphyses with unthreaded 2-mm wires. *J Pediatr Orthop Am* 1996;16:53-55.

76. Rao SB, Crawford AH, Burger RR, Roy DR: Open bone peg epiphysiodesis for slipped capital femoral epiphysis. *J Pediatr Orthop Am* 1996;16:37-48.

77. Weiner DS, Weiner S, Melby A, Hoyt WA Jr: A 30-year experience with bone graft epiphysiodesis in the treatment of slipped capital femoral epiphysis. *J Pediatr Orthop Am* 1984;4:145-152.

78. Schmidt TL, Cimino WG, Seidel FG: Allograft epiphysiodesis for slipped capital femoral epiphysis. *Clin Orthop* 1996;322:61-76.

79. DeRosa GP, Mullins RC, Kling TF Jr: Cuneiform osteotomy of the femoral neck in severe slipped capital femoral epiphysis. *Clin Orthop* 1996;322:48-60.

80. Velasco R, Schai PA, Exner GU: Slipped capital femoral epiphysis: A long-term follow-up study after open reduction of the femoral head combined with subcapital wedge resection. *J Pediatr Orthop Br* 1998; 7:43-52.

81. Barmada R, Bruch RF, Gimbel JS, Ray RD: Base of the neck extracapsular osteotomy for correction of deformity in slipped capital femoral epiphysis. *Clin Orthop* 1978;132:98-101.

82. Kramer WG, Craig WA, Noel S: Compensating osteotomy at the base of the femoral neck for slipped capital femoral epiphysis. *J Bone Joint Surg Am* 1976;58:796-800.

83. Meier MC, Meyer LC, Ferguson RL: Treatment of slipped capital femoral epiphysis with a spica cast. *J Bone Joint Surg Am* 1992;74:1522-1529.

84. O'Brien ET, Fahey JJ: Remodeling of the femoral neck after in-situ pinning for slipped capital femoral epiphysis. *J Bone Joint Surg Am* 1977;59:62-68.

85. Bellemans J, Fabry G, Molenaers G, Lammens J, Moens P: Slipped capital femoral epiphysis: A long-term follow-up, with special emphasis on the capacities for remodeling. *J Pediatr Orthop Br* 1996;5:151-157.

86. Jerre R, Billing L, Karlsson J: Loss of hip motion in slipped capital femoral epiphysis: A calculation from the slipping angle and the slope. *J Pediatr Orthop Br* 1996;5:144-150.

87. Claffey TJ: Avascular necrosis of the femoral head: An anatomical study. *J Bone Joint Surg Br* 1960;42:802-809.

88. Brodetti A: The blood supply of the femoral neck and head in relation to the damaging effects of nails and screws. *J Bone Joint Surg Br* 1960;42:794-801.

89. Karol LA, Doane RM, Cornicelli SF, Zak PA, Haut RC, Manoli A II: Single versus double screw fixation for treatment of slipped capital femoral epiphysis: A biomechanical analysis. *J Pediatr Orthop Am* 1992;12:741-745.

90. Blanco JS, Taylor B, Johnston CE II: Comparison of single pin versus multiple pin fixation in treatment of slipped capital femoral epiphysis. *J Pediatr Orthop Am* 1992;12:384-389.

91. Morrissy RT: Slipped capital femoral epiphysis: Technique of percutaneous in situ fixation. *J Pediatr Orthop Am* 1990;10:347-350.

92. Goodman WW, Johnson JT, Robertson WW Jr: Single screw fixation for acute and acute-on-chronic slipped capital femoral epiphysis. *Clin Orthop* 1996;322:86-90.

93. Stevens DB, Short BA, Burch JM: In situ fixation of the slipped capital femoral epiphysis with a single screw. *J Pediatr Orthop Br* 1996;5:85-89.

94. Canale ST, Azar F, Young J, Beaty JH, Warner WC, Whitmer G: Subtrochanteric fracture after fixation of slipped capital femoral epiphysis: A complication of unused drill holes. *J Pediatr Orthop Am* 1994;14:623-626.

95. Maletis GB, Bassett GS: Windshield-wiper loosening: A complication of in situ screw fixation of slipped capital femoral epiphysis. *J Pediatr Orthop Am* 1993;13:607-609.

96. Samuelson T, Olney B: Percutaneous pin fixation of chronic slipped capital femoral epiphysis. *Clin Orthop* 1996;326:225-228.

97. Fish JB: Cuneiform osteotomy of the femoral neck in the treatment of slipped capital femoral epiphysis: A follow-up note. *J Bone Joint Surg Am* 1994;76:46-59.

98. Dunn DM, Angel JC: Replacement of the femoral head by open operation in severe adolescent slipping of the upper femoral epiphysis. *J Bone Joint Surg Br* 1978;60:394-403.

99. Crawford AH: Role of osteotomy in the treatment of slipped capital femoral epiphysis. *J Pediatr Orthop Br* 1996;5:102-109.

100. Crawford AH: Osteotomies in the treatment of slipped capital femoral epiphysis. *Instr Course Lect* 1984;33:327-349.

101. Southwick WO: Compression fixation after biplane intertrochanteric osteotomy for slipped capital femoral epiphysis: A technical improvement. *J Bone Joint Surg Am* 1973;55:1218-1224.

102. Schai PA, Exner GU, Hansch O: Prevention of secondary coxarthrosis in slipped capital femoral epiphysis: A long-term follow-up study after corrective intertrochanteric osteotomy. *J Pediatr Orthop Br* 1996;5:135-143.

103. Jerre R, Hansson G, Wallin J, Karlsson J: Long-term results after realignment operations for slipped upper femoral epiphysis. *J Bone Joint Surg Br* 1996;78:745-750.

104. de Sanctis N, Di Gennaro G, Pempinello C, Corte SD, Carannante G: Is gentle manipulative reduction and percutaneous fixation with a single screw the best management of acute and acute-on-chronic slipped capital femoral epiphysis? A report of 70 patients. *J Pediatr Orthop Br* 1996;5:90-95.

105. Herman MJ, Dormans JP, Davidson RS, Drummond DS, Gregg JR: Screw fixation of Grade III slipped capital femoral epiphysis. *Clin Orthop* 1996;322:77-85.

106. Peterson MD, Weiner DS, Green NE, Terry CL: Acute slipped capital femoral epiphysis: The value and safety of urgent manipulative reduction. *J Pediatr Orthop Am* 1997;17:648-654.

107. Dietz FR: Traction reduction of acute and acute-on-chronic slipped capital femoral epiphysis. *Clin Orthop* 1994;302:101-110.

108. Krahn TH, Canale ST, Beaty JH, Warner WC, Lourenco P: Long-term follow-up of patients with avascular necrosis after treatment of slipped capital femoral epiphysis. *J Pediatr Orthop Am* 1993;13:154-158.

109. Strange-Vognsen H, Wagner A, Dirksen K, et al: The value of scintigraphy in hips with slipped capital femoral epiphysis and the value of radiography and MRI after 10 years. *Acta Orthop Belg* 1999;65:33-38.

110. Ingram AJ, Clarke MS, Clark CS Jr, Marshall WR: Chondrolysis complicating slipped capital femoral epiphysis. *Clin Orthop* 1982;165:99-109.

111. Mandell GA, Keret D, Harcke HT, Bowen JR: Chondrolysis: Detection by bone scintigraphy. *J Pediatr Orthop Am* 1992;12:80-85.

112. Aronson DD, Loder RT: Slipped capital femoral epiphysis in black children. *J Pediatr Orthop Am* 1992;12:74-79.

113. Bishop JO, Oley TJ, Stephenson CT, Tullos HS: Slipped capital femoral epiphysis: A study of 50 cases in black children. *Clin Orthop* 1978;135:93-96.

114. Kennedy JP, Weiner DS: Results of slipped capital femoral epiphysis in the black population. *J Pediatr Orthop Am* 1990;10:224-227.

115. Spero CR, Masciale JP, Tornetta P III; Star MJ, Tucci JJ: Slipped capital femoral epiphysis in black children: Incidence of chondrolysis. *J Pediatr Orthop Am* 1992;12:444-448.

116. Orofino C, Innis JJ, Lowrey CW: Slipped capital femoral epiphysis in Negroes: A study of ninety-five cases. *J Bone Joint Surg Am* 1960;42:1079-1083.

117. Tillema DA, Golding JSR: Chondrolysis following slipped capital femoral epiphysis in Jamaica. *J Bone Joint Surg Am* 1971;53:1528-1540.

118. Gonzalez-Moran G, Carsi B, Abril JC, Albinana J: Results after preoperative traction and pinning in slipped capital femoral epiphysis: K wires versus cannulated screws. *J Pediatr Orthop Br* 1998;7:53-58.

119. Frymoyer JW: Chondrolysis of the hip following Southwick osteotomy for severe slipped capital femoral epiphysis. *Clin Orthop* 1974;99:120-124.

120. Hall JE: The results of treatment of slipped femoral epiphysis. *J Bone Joint Surg Br* 1957;39:659-673.

121. Oram V: Epiphysiolysis of the head of the femur: A follow-up examination with special reference to end results and the social prognosis. *Acta Orthop Scand* 1953;23:100-120.

122. Ross PM, Lyne ED, Morawa LG: Slipped capital femoral epiphysis: Long-term results after 10-38 years. *Clin Orthop* 1979;141:176-180.

123. Ordeberg G, Hansson LI, Sandström S: Slipped capital femoral epiphysis in southern Sweden: Long-term result with no treatment or symptomatic primary treatment. *Clin Orthop* 1984;191:95-104.

124. Jerre R, Karlsson J, Romanus B, Wallin J: Does a single device prevent further slipping of the epiphysis in children with slipped capital femoral epiphysis? *Arch Orthop Trauma Surg* 1997;116:348-351.

125. Howorth B: Slipping of the capital femoral epiphysis: History. *Clin Orthop* 1966;48:11-32.

126. Johnston RC, Larson CB: Results of treatment of hip disorders with cup arthroplasty. *J Bone Joint Surg Am* 1969;51:1461-1479.

127. Murray RO: The aetiology of primary osteoarthritis of the hip. *Br J Radiol* 1965;38:810-824.

128. Solomon L: Patterns of osteoarthritis of the hip. *J Bone Joint Surg Br* 1976;58:176-183.

129. Stulberg SD, Cordell LD, Harris WH: Unrecognized childhood hip disease: A major cause of idiopathic osteonecrosis of the hip, in *The Hip: Proceedings of the Third Open Scientific Meeting of the Hip Society*. St Louis, MO, CV Mosby, 1975, pp 212-230.

130. Resnick D: The "tilt deformity" of the femoral head in osteoarthritis of the hip: A poor indicator of previous epiphysiolysis. *Clin Radiol* 1976;27:355-363.

131. Jerre T: A study in slipped upper femoral epiphysis: With special reference to the late functional and roentgenological results and to the value of closed reduction. *Acta Orthop Scand* 1950;6(suppl):5-157.

132. Jerre T: Early complications after osteosynthesis with a three flanged nail in situ for slipped epiphysis. *Acta Orthop Scand* 1958;27:126-134.

Legg-Calvé-Perthes Disease: Current Concepts

George H. Thompson, MD
Charles T. Price, MD
Dennis Roy, MD
Peter L. Meehan, MD
B. Stephens Richards, MD

Introduction

Legg-Calvé-Perthes disease (LCPD) is a relatively common but controversial pediatric hip disorder. Despite almost 100 years of research and a general appreciation of the pathophysiology, clinical characteristics, radiographic features, and natural history of LCPD, the etiology of the disease still is not understood, and efficacy of treatment remains a subject of controversy.

Etiology

The etiology of LCPD remains unknown: infection, trauma, and transient synovitis have been proposed but unsubstantiated. There is, however, disruption of the blood supply to the capital femoral epiphysis (CFE). The blood supply of the proximal femur is provided by an extracapsular arterial ring supplied by the medial and lateral circumflex femoral arteries. The lateral circumflex femoral artery contributes to the anterior anastomotic network while the posterior, medial, and lateral networks are supplied by the medial femoral circumflex artery. The extracapsular arterial ring gives off retinacular or ascending cervical arteries, which then provide branches to the metaphysis and epiphysis. The most important vessel is the lateral ascending cervical artery, which is the termination of the medial circumflex femoral artery.[1-3] This artery crosses the posterior trochanteric fossa through an area that tends to be constricted in children younger than 8 years, and it may be prone to injury. The anterior anastomotic network is less extensive than the posterior network and is more often incomplete in boys.[2]

Disruption of the blood supply has been suggested to occur by either extravascular or intravascular means: obliterative vascular thickening has been reported on pathologic specimens, and obstruction of the retinacular arteries has been seen angiographically.[4] Based on animal models and pathologic specimens, two (and perhaps more) infarctions are necessary to cause this disorder.[5] Reports of recurrent LCPD are supportive evidence for this theory. An increase in blood viscosity has been reported,[6] as has intraosseous venous hypertension.[7] Disturbances in the clotting mechanism also have been proposed.[8] Factors leading to thrombophilia, an increased tendency to develop thrombosis and hypofibrinolysis, and a reduced tendency to lyse thrombi have been identified: factor V Leiden mutation, protein C and S deficiency, lupus anticoagulant, anticardiolipin antibodies, antitrypsin, and plasminogen activator may play a role in the abnormal clotting mechanism,[9-13] although studies have failed to corroborate the initial findings.[14-22] LCPD in multiple family members has, however, been reported with the factor V Leiden mutation.[23] Exposure to secondhand smoke has been reported as an association in children with LCPD.[24,25] In adults, smoke exposure is a known factor in producing hypofibrinolysis.

A contrasting theory to disruption of the blood supply to the proximal femur is that the disorder may be a reflection of an underlying systemic disorder. Children with LCPD have delayed skeletal maturation and are shorter than normal. Abnormalities of thyroid hormone and insulin-like growth factors have been reported.[26] Radiographically, changes in the contralateral femoral head[27] and sites of other ossification abnormalities, such as the tarsal navicular, provide further evidence. Histologic changes also have been reported in other epiphyses (greater trochanter).[28] The role of apparent hyperactivity in this disorder remains to be clarified.[29]

Histologic findings in the CFE reveal various stages of bone necrosis and repair. Perthes in 1913 described the pathology as "a self limiting, noninflammatory condition, affecting the capital femoral epiphysis with stages of degeneration and regeneration leading to a restoration of the bone nucleus."[30] Histopathologic descriptions by Catterall and associates[28,31] and Ponseti and associates[32] suggest two possible pathways for the bone necrosis: that the vascular event or events are primary, or that there may be a primary disorder of epiphyseal cartilage, with collapse and necrosis as a result.

Pathogenesis of Deformity

The deformity can occur by four mechanisms.[26] The first is a growth disturbance in the CFE and physis. A central arrest of the physis leads to a short neck (coxa breva) and trochanteric overgrowth. A lateral physeal arrest tilts the head externally and into valgus, and there is trochanteric overgrowth. The second mechanism for deformity involves the repair process itself. The deformity can occur related to the asymmetric repair process and the applied stresses on the femoral head. There may be a molding action of the acetabulum on the femoral head, and a deformed femoral head may deform the acetabulum. The third mechanism for deformity is related to the disease process. The superficial layers of articular cartilage continue to "overgrow" as they are nourished by the synovial fluid. The deeper layers are, however, devitalized by the disease process, leading to epiphyseal trabecular collapse and deformity. The repair process proceeds from the periphery inward, contributing to asymmetric growth. The fourth mechanism is iatrogenic and is caused by trying to contain, either nonsurgically or surgically, a noncontainable femoral head.

Once the repair process is completed, residual deformity includes coxa magna, a premature physeal arrest pattern, deformed or out-of-round femoral head, and osteochondritis dissecans in the central area of the femoral head. Osteo-chondritis dissecans occurs infrequently and is reported in approximately 3% of cases. Coxa breva and trochanteric overgrowth are other sequelae of growth disturbance.

Clinical Characteristics

Children usually present between the ages of 4 and 8 years; however, LCPD has been reported in patients from ages 2 to 12 years.

It occurs more commonly in boys in a ratio of 4:1 to 5:1. LCPD is more common in whites, Asians, and Central Europeans and is unusual in blacks and Native Americans.

The most common presenting symptom is a painless limp of a varying period of time. Pain, if present, usually is activity related and may be localized in the groin, anterior thigh, or knee. Less commonly, the onset may be much more acute and may be associated with a failure to ambulate. Parents often report that symptoms were initiated by a traumatic event.

On physical examination, an antalgic or Trendelenburg gait may be observed. Generally, motion, primarily internal rotation and abduction, is limited. A mild hip flexion contracture of 10° to 20° also may be present. Atrophy of the muscles of the thigh, calf, or buttock may be evident. There might be an apparent lower extremity length inequality because of an adduction contracture or from true shortening on the involved side because of CFE collapse. Clinical at-risk factors include an older child, obesity, female sex, and marked restriction of motion. Female sex recently has been shown not to be as much a factor as initially presumed.[33]

The differential diagnosis during the initial evaluation includes inflammatory or infectious etiologies, such as toxic synovitis, septic arthritis, or juvenile arthritis. Other known causes of osteonecrosis include sickle cell anemia, thalassemia, hemophilia, idiopathic thrombocytopenia purpura, leukemia, and Gaucher's disease. In bilateral symmetrical cases, a skeletal dysplasia should be considered, such as multiple or spondyloepiphyseal dysplasia. Endocrinopathies, such as hypothyroidism, also may produce bilateral symmetrical involvement.[34] Some genetic syndromes, such as trichorhinophalangeal syndrome, may have LCPD-like changes.

Radiographic Evaluation

Routine radiographs are the primary imaging tool for LCPD. AP and Lauenstein (frog-lateral) views are used

to diagnose, stage, provide prognosis, follow the course of the disease, and assess results. Ultrasound has been proposed to observe changes in the shape of the femoral head and to diagnose synovitis,[35] but it is not widely used. In the absence of changes on plain radiographs, a technetium Tc 99m bone scan may reveal the avascularity of the CFE. Transient photopenia, however, may give a false diagnosis. Periodic technetium Tc 99m bone scans have been used for prognosis and to follow the course of the disease.[36] MRI also is useful for diagnosis; its use as a prognostic tool is not proven.

The radiographic stages of LCPD are based on the initial scheme of Waldenström: the disease process is divided into initial, fragmentation, reossification or repair, and healed stages. During the initial stage, the radiographic changes include a decreased size of the ossification center, widening of the medial joint space, a subchondral fracture, and physeal irregularity. In the fragmentation stage, the epiphysis appears fragmented, and there are areas of increased radiolucency and radiodensity. The bone density returns to normal during the reossification or repair stage. Once reossification is complete, the shape of the femoral head is representative of the healed phase.

Classification Systems

Attempts to classify the severity of LCPD and evaluate prognosis by plain radiography have been developed from three classifications. In 1971, Catterall[37] proposed a four-group classification, based on the amount of CFE involvement and a set of radiographic "head at risk" signs. Group I hips have anterior CFE involvement of approximately 25%, no sequestrum, and no metaphyseal abnormalities. Group II hips have up to 50% involvement, with a clear demarcation between involved and uninvolved segments. Metaphyseal cysts may be present. Group III hips display up to 75% involvement with a large sequestrum. In group IV, the entire femoral head is involved. There appears to be a high degree of interobserver variability in using this classification scheme.[38]

In 1984, Salter and Thompson[39] reported a two-group classification based on the extent of the subchondral fracture, which corresponded to the amount of subsequent resorption. In group A, less than 50% of the femoral head is involved; in group B, more than 50% of the femoral head is involved. A distinguishing feature between group A and group B is the presence or absence of an intact viable lateral margin of the epiphysis. A disadvantage of the Salter-Thompson classification is that not all patients are diagnosed early during the phase of the subchondral fracture. However, this classification scheme has good interobserver reliability.

The newest classification was proposed in 1992 by Herring and associates.[40] In this classification, the height of the lateral 15% to 33% of the involved epiphysis is compared with the height of the contralateral normal epiphysis on an AP radiograph. This classification is applied in the early fragmentation phase of the disease. In group A, there is no involvement of the lateral pillar; in group B, the lateral pillar maintains at least 50% of its height; and in group C, there is a loss of more than 50% of the original height of the lateral pillar. The lateral pillar classification has been found to be prognostic, and it has good interobserver reliability.[41-43]

Prognostic Factors

As mentioned, radiographic head-at-risk signs were introduced by Catterall.[37] He described four radiographic findings to use in conjunction with the amount of femoral head involvement: Gages sign, a radiolucent V in the lateral portion of the epiphysis; calcification lateral to the epiphysis; lateral CFE subluxation; and a horizontal physis. Waldenström, much earlier, reported lateralization of the femoral head and metaphyseal lucency as risk signs. Dickens and Menelaus[44] reported that the extent of uncovering of the femoral head, Catterall classification, lateral calcification, and lateral CFE displacement were prognostic. The value or accuracy of these head-at-risk signs remains controversial.

Controversy also continues about the exact location and significance of metaphyseal cysts;[45,46] however, the prognosis appears to be worse when they are present. They most likely represent more severe disease, and their juxtaphyseal location probably portends the significance of the disease and a future growth disturbance.

Physeal changes are common. Bowen and associates[47] reported two patterns of growth arrest and suggested growth arrest as a prognostic factor. An early radiographic sign is a narrowed physeal plate with an overlying avascular epiphysis and a marked metaphyseal reaction below. Bony metaphyseal projections into either the central or lateral portions of the epiphysis denote a bony bridge. Acetabular changes usually parallel the shape and position of the femoral head.

A standing AP radiograph of the pelvis will give better information about extrusion and subluxation. The extrusion index has been used as a method of quantifying the amount of uncovering. The extrusion index is the width of the involved epiphysis lateral to the lateral margin of the acetabulum divided by the width of the uninvolved epiphysis. As the femoral head extrudes or subluxates, hinge abduction becomes more of a possibility. An AP radiograph of the pelvis, with the involved hips in maximal abduction, may allow for early diagnosis of hinge abduction. This likewise can be evaluated by arthrography or dynamic MRI.[48]

Classification of Radiographic Results

Once the patient is skeletally mature, the shape of the femoral head can be measured by two radiographic techniques.

Mose[49] used a radiolucent template with concentric circles that was placed over the femoral head on the AP and lateral radiographs. The sphericity was then measured. A good result was one in which the femoral head sphericity did not deviate more than 1 mm; a fair result was within 2 mm; and a poor result was 3 mm or more of deviation.

Stulberg and associates[50,51] developed a radiographic classification based on residual femoral head shape and the development of subsequent degenerative joint disease. They described five classes (Stulberg classes).[51] In class I, the femoral head is round and equal in size to the opposite, uninvolved hip. Class II is a spherical femoral head with coxa magna, coxa breva, and/or a steep acetabulum. In class III, the femoral head is nonspherical but not flat (mushroom shaped) and is associated with the abnormalities of the femoral head, neck, and acetabulum seen in class II results; the hip joint, however, is congruous. Class IV is a flat femoral head associated with the same abnormalities of the femoral head, neck, and acetabulum; the hip joint, again, is congruous. Class V is a flat femoral head with a normal femoral neck and acetabulum. Classes I and II are described as being spherically congruent and having a good long-term prognosis. These are typically Mose's good and fair results. Classes III and IV are described as being aspherically congruent and having an intermediate prognosis. These hips represent Mose's poor results. Class V hips are aspherically incongruent and are destined to early degenerative joint disease. Whether class III is a satisfactory or unsatisfactory result is controversial; the ovoid femoral head has a lower incidence of osteoarthritis than do the flat class IV and V heads.

A computed method of following the shape of the femoral head and acetabulum has been proposed as a method of evaluation.[52] It has not gained popularity.

Natural History

No long-term natural history studies of LCPD have been published. In the classic article by Catterall in 1971,[37] the follow-up ranged from 4 to 16 years and included treated patients. A subsequent study of 95 untreated patients had a short-term mean follow-up of 6 years.[53] In this study, 92% of group I and II hips had a good result, whereas 91% of group III and IV hips had a poor result. In their natural history study in 1981, Stulberg and associates[51] reported on two groups of patients (divided into three different nonsurgical treatment groups) with mean follow-ups of 30 and 40 years. Thus, this was not truly a natural history study.

McAndrew and Weinstein[54] presented the results of 32 untreated patients with a mean long-term follow-up of 48 years. Forty percent of these patients had an Iowa hip rating of greater than 80 points, in contrast with a previous review of the same patients at an average of 36 years' follow-up, in which 92% had Iowa hip ratings above 80 points.[55] Forty percent had had an arthroplasty, and 10% were awaiting an arthroplasty. McAndrew and Weinstein found the prognostic factors to include the age at onset, the number of Catterall head-at-risk signs, the ratio of unaffected-to-affected femoral head size in regard to width, and a decrease in joint space over time.

Prognosis

From a prognostic standpoint, long-term follow-up studies of patients with LCPD show that most hips do well until the fifth decade of life.[37,54] Because of remodeling potential, the shape of the femoral head can improve until maturity.[56] At maturity, deformity and congruency are the key factors, as Stulberg and associates[51] reported. Age at onset is also prognostic. Children younger than 6 years generally do well, although not all do.[57-59] The remodeling potential is higher in younger children; however, the extent of CFE involvement and duration of the disease

process must play a role in the poor outcomes of these younger children.

During the disease process, prognosis is related to the extent of involvement of the femoral head. Hips at risk for a poor prognosis are those classified as Catterall groups III and IV, Salter-Thompson group B, and lateral pillar group C. Lateral pillar group B hips in older children are likewise at increased risk. Head-at-risk factors include lateralization (subluxation) of the femoral head, metaphyseal lesions (especially in the juxtaphyseal region), and involvement of the physis.

Treatment

The efficacy of treatment is the most controversial aspect of LCPD.[60] Salter[61] in 1984 outlined the methods of treatment that are still used as guidelines today. These include (1) observation or no treatment, (2) intermittent symptomatic treatment, (3) containment, (4) late surgery for deformity, and (5) late surgery for osteoarthritis.

Containment, which can be either nonsurgical or surgical, is the most controversial. The purpose of containment is to contain the femoral head within the acetabulum to prevent deformity, permit physiologic motion, and promote remodeling. The current indications for containment methods of treatment include (1) age at clinical onset of 6 to 10 years (perhaps 5 years in girls), (2) greater than one-half CFE involvement (Catterall groups III and IV, Salter-Thompson group B, and lateral pillar groups B and C), and (3) loss of femoral head containment (subluxation) on the AP radiograph.[60,61] The prerequisites include (1) a good to full range of hip motion, especially abduction in extension, (2) minimal or no residual hip irritability, and (3) a minimally deformed femoral head.

Nonsurgical Treatment

Most abduction orthoses are based on the Petrie abduction cast principle. A number of orthoses have been developed to affect

containment including the Newington,[62] Toronto,[63] Tachdjian,[64] Scottish Rite,[65] and others.[66-69] The Scottish Rite orthosis was developed in 1971, with modifications made to the hinge system in 1974. It or modifications of it are widely used for the nonsurgical management of LCPD.

Scottish Rite Abduction Orthosis This orthosis was developed to contain the femoral head in the acetabulum while permitting a child to engage relatively normally in activities. The knees are not included in the Scottish Rite orthosis. Knee stiffness, which potentially accompanied the Petrie cast method of treatment, is obviated.

Management Protocol Before an orthosis can be applied, hip range of motion must be regained. For the Scottish Rite orthosis to function satisfactorily, the affected hip must be able to be abducted in extension to 40° to 45°. If the orthosis is applied to a hip with 20° of abduction, the nonaffected hip will be abducted 60° to 70°, assuming that the orthosis has a total arc of abduction of 90°.

Restoration of full range of motion can be difficult. Previously, patients were admitted to the hospital for supervised bed rest and skin traction, but prolonged hospitalization is no longer possible for most patients. Bed rest in traction in the home setting, in the best of circumstances, is difficult. The use of a wheelchair as a means of restricting activity, with the use of oral anti-inflammatory medication, is an alternative. For recalcitrant hips, abduction casts offer an alternative. The use of physical therapy may be of benefit for a child who has an adduction contracture; however, the routine use of physical therapy may be counterproductive because the basis for the restricted range of motion is synovitis. In this circumstance, it is impossible for physical therapy to decrease the underlying inflammation.

Following the restoration of motion, the patient can be fitted with the orthosis. After the orthosis is applied, an AP radiograph of the pelvis is obtained to ensure that the hips are abducted symmetrically and that the affected femoral head is contained within the acetabulum. To be effective, the orthosis must be worn full-time. Follow-up clinical and radiographic examinations every 3 to 4 months are advised. Radiographs are made with the patient in the orthosis to be certain that the hip remains contained within the acetabulum. Clinical examination determines whether the hip range of motion is being maintained. Loss of range of motion must be treated to restore full abduction of the hip.

The use of the orthosis is continued until subchondral reossification is demonstrated on the AP radiograph.[70,71] Serial radiographs facilitate making this determination. Generally, the active phase of the disease that requires an orthosis is 9 to 18 months.

Results A large number of patients with LCPD do well without treatment. Those younger than 5 or 6 years with any extent of CFE involvement generally have a good prognosis; children older than 6 years at onset with a substantial portion of the CFE involved are at risk for a poor result and may benefit from treatment.

Two published series[65,72] question the effectiveness of the Scottish Rite abduction orthosis in altering the natural history of the disease process. Meehan and associates[65] reported on 34 children from the Atlanta Scottish Rite Medical Center who were 6 years old at the time of disease onset and had Catterall group III (27 hips) or IV (7 hips) involvement. In 7 of 34 children (21%), the Catterall grouping was changed during the first 6 months of management. All patients were followed for 2 years after treatment was discontinued. The mean follow-up was 6 years, 9 months (range, 2 years to 15 years, 8 months). The orthosis was discontinued when subchondral new bone formation in the CFE was demonstrated on AP or lateral radiographs. There were 3

Stulberg class II (9%), 24 class III (71%), 6 class IV results (18%), and 1 class V result (3%). No patient had a class I, or spherical, femoral head. Statistical correlation between calcification lateral to the epiphysis, the epiphyseal extrusion index on the initial radiograph, and end result was not found. A break in Shenton's line on the initial films was suggestive but not statistically associated with a poor outcome.

In the other series, Martinez and associates[72] at the University of Iowa reported on 31 patients with 34 involved hips. All patients had either Catterall group III (5 hips) or IV (29 hips) involvement. The mean age of onset was 6 years (range, 3 to 12 years). The orthosis was discontinued when the patient reached the reossification phase of the disease. The mean follow-up was 7 years (range, 2 to 13 years). There were no Stulberg class I, 14 class II (41%), 9 class III (27%), 9 class IV (27%), and 2 class V results (6%). The authors of both studies concluded that the Scottish Rite orthosis did not alter the natural history of LCPD and therefore they did not recommend its use.

Current Application Whenever possible, it is important to compare the effect of treatment with the known natural history of a condition. We therefore analyzed the illustrations and descriptions in Catterall's series of 95 untreated patients[37,53] and correlated the resulting categories (good, fair, and poor) with the radiographic femoral head classification scheme of Stulberg and associates,[51] which had not been published when

Catterall published the results of his series. Thirty-six of the 95 patients in Catterall's series had group III or IV involvement. In Table 1, these 36 hips are compared with the results of orthotic treatment from the Scottish Rite Medical Center study by Meehan and associates[65] and the University of Iowa study by Martinez and associates.[72] Class III hips are considered to be unsatisfactory results, emphasizing the controversy regarding class III hips.

For several reasons, this type of abduction orthosis may not be effective in providing containment of the femoral head. The orthosis causes flexion and external rotation of the hip; this results in increased posterior coverage of the femoral head at the expense of anterior coverage. The anterior and lateral portion of the CFE is predominately affected in LCPD, and the design of the Scottish Rite orthosis does not permit containment or coverage of the part of the femoral head at risk. Using gait analysis and computer modeling, Rab and associates[73] analyzed the amount and location of femoral head containment in both normal children and children with LCPD. Their containment index, representing the percentage of the area of the femoral head contained at some time during the gait cycle, was not significantly altered when children wearing the Scottish Rite orthosis were compared with children walking without the orthosis. The mean containment index for normal children was 64%; this increased to 75% with use of the orthosis. Another important finding was that coverage did

Table 1
Results in Untreated Versus Orthotically Treated LCPD Patients

| | No. (%) Hips | | | |
| | Catterall[37] groups III and IV | Stulberg et al[51] classification | | |
Study		I	II	III–V
Untreated Catterall[37,53]	36(100)	4(11)	11(31)	21(43)
Treated Meehan et al[65]	34(100)	0(0)	3(9)	31(91)
Martinez et al[72]	34(100)	0(0)	14(41)	20(59)

not increase over the normal gait cycle in children who had 20° loss of motion. Loss of motion is a frequent problem in nonsurgical management of this disorder.

Age of the patient at the onset of disease is one of the most important variables in LCPD. The difference in results between the series of Meehan and associates and Martinez and associates may be related to the older age of the patients in the Meehan and associates series. However, based on these data, the role of this type of abduction orthosis is questioned for the treatment of LCPD in children 6 years old and older at time of disease onset and with severe involvement. Such devices, however, may have a use in patients with lesser degrees of CFE involvement and in younger patients.

Proximal Femoral Osteotomy

Proximal femoral osteotomy has been widely used in the surgical treatment of LCPD.[74-83] A varus osteotomy of the proximal femur is the most common procedure. It also can be used in combination with pelvic osteotomy when containment cannot be obtained by proximal femoral varus osteotomy alone.[84,85] In contrast, valgus osteotomy of the proximal femur has been recommended in the later stages of LCPD when the deformed, extruded femoral head causes pain and an adduction deformity.[86,87]

Proximal Femoral Osteotomy in the Early and Fragmentation Stages Proximal femoral varus osteotomy is an effective method of containment in the early and fragmentation stages of the disease process.[75-81,88-90] Axer[74] introduced this method of management in 1965, and many authors have demonstrated that it can prevent femoral head deformity and restore spherical congruity, provided that the femoral head can be contained in the acetabulum and that growth remains to allow femoral head remodeling.[74,76-81,88-90] Eckerwall and associates[91] made MRI studies before and after proximal femoral varus osteotomies in 21 children who

demonstrated poor containment, anterolateral CFE flattening, and deformation of the femoral head before osteotomy. Over a period of 3 years, the authors noted continuous improvement of femoral head sphericity in all children and no deterioration of sphericity in any patient. Hoikka and associates,[79] in a study of 112 intertrochanteric osteotomies for LCPD, concluded that satisfactory results were obtained in all children younger than 9 years when the surgery was done during the first 8 months after the onset of symptoms. This is consistent with the results reported by other authors.[76,89,92]

The limitations of femoral varus osteotomy are similar to the limitations inherent in all methods of containment. Several authors have observed that the outcome of femoral varus osteotomy is worse in patients operated on during the healing phase of disease, in patients operated on at 9 years of age or older, and when the femoral head could not be contained by the osteotomy.[76,79,92,93] Noonan and associates[94] and Hoikka and associates[79] in separate studies noted that femoral varus osteotomy did not produce a good result in patients who had surgery at 10 years of age or more. Mazda and associates[95] noted that satisfactory results in older children (older than 12 years) may be achieved by containment as long as the triradiate cartilage is open at the time of surgery.

Advantages As mentioned earlier, proximal femoral varus osteotomy can be done even when there is flattening or incongruity of the femoral head as long as the disease is in the early or fragmentation stages and the femoral head can be contained in the acetabulum. In contrast, pelvic osteotomies or shelf procedures are indicated only when the femoral head is still round and without deformity.[61,90,96-98] Also, pelvic osteotomies require full range of motion before surgical intervention,[61,96,97] whereas a proximal femoral varus osteotomy can be done

when mild to moderate limitation of motion is present preoperatively.[81,82,99] Thus, the prerequisites for proximal femoral varus osteotomy are not as strict as the prerequisites for pelvic osteotomy.

Another theoretic advantage is that proximal femoral varus osteotomy is done on the affected side of the hip joint. Varization increases the functional length of the femoral neck, shortens the length of the femur, and reduces the joint reaction forces acting on the femoral head.[74,89,100] In contrast, pelvic osteotomies increase the resting length of several muscles and lateralize the acetabular segment[75,101] and thus may increase the joint reaction forces and the pressure on the femoral head.

Proximal femoral osteotomy also decreases the venous congestion of the femoral neck, which has been demonstrated in LCPD and other conditions;[102,103] it resolves after intertrochanteric osteotomy.[102-104] The significance of this finding is unclear. Even though the venous circulation is normalized after femoral osteotomy, this does not shorten the time for healing.[105,106]

Disadvantages The potential disadvantage of proximal femoral varus osteotomy for LCPD is that failure of remodeling may result in persistent varus angulation, trochanteric prominence, and lower extremity length inequality.[83,99,107] Parents should be advised that the principle objective of containment surgery is to achieve a spherical, concentric femoral head but that residual deformities after femoral varus osteotomy may require additional surgery if remodeling is incomplete. Attention to certain technical pitfalls may reduce the need for further corrective surgery. Parents also should be instructed that limping will be noticeable in the first year or two after femoral varus osteotomy because the joint forces and mechanics of the hip will be altered until remodeling occurs and the disease process heals.

Most patients have mild residual varus with neck-shaft angles of 127° to

129° after remodeling is complete.[83,88,107] The mean improvement in the femoral neck-shaft angle ranges from 11° to 21°.[83,88,107] Persistent varus angulation is most likely to occur in patients who are older than 9 years at the time of surgery or when the neck-shaft angle is reduced below 105°. Additional risk factors for persistent varus include severe disease, osteotomy performed in the later stages of disease, and premature closure of the femoral neck physis.[47,83,88,93,99] Contributing factors for early physeal closure include excessive varus angulation, lack of containment, or physeal damage from internal fixation. It is difficult to assess these contributing factors because early physeal arrest has often been observed in patients without surgical intervention.[47,77,108] Residual femoral varus does not increase the risk of pain or later osteoarthritis,[77,79,93] but it does contribute to trochanteric prominence and potential abductor muscle weakness.

Trochanteric prominence with a positive or delayed-positive Trendelenburg sign has been noted in 20% to 25% of patients more than a year after femoral varus osteotomy.[77,83,99] Some patients may require trochanteric advancement or valgus osteotomy after the LCPD has resolved, but the amount of trochanteric overgrowth does not always correlate with the Trendelenburg sign.[77,93] Persistent trochanteric prominence occurs more often in older patients and in patients with greater degrees of varus angulation.[93,99,107] Trochanteric apophyseodesis at the time of surgery has been recommended to improve functional and radiographic outcomes.[82,83] Children younger than 8 years with coxa vara benefit from trochanteric apophyseodesis.[109,110] Older children may not benefit from the procedure, but delayed skeletal maturation is common in LCPD, and there is little additional risk from trochanteric apophyseodesis at the time of femoral varus osteotomy.

Lower extremity length inequality of more than than 2 cm has been reported in 4% to 6% of patients treated by varus femoral osteotomy.[77,83,99,111] Several authors have reported a similar incidence of lower extremity length discrepancy in patients who were treated nonsurgically.[47,76,99,111] Kitakoji and associates[107] stated that "femoral varus osteotomy itself does not have a disadvantage for leg length discrepancy in the treatment of Legg-Calvé-Perthes disease." Several authors share this opinion.[47,80,112-114] Varus osteotomy creates an immediate shortening, but progressive remodeling of the neck-shaft angle and growth stimulation from the osteotomy lead to recovery of length when the CFE remains open and there is sufficient growth remaining for remodeling to occur. Therefore, residual shortening after osteotomy is more likely to occur in older patients when varus is excessive and when a closing wedge osteotomy has been done.[76,99,111] All children with LCPD should be followed with serial scanograms to assess lower extremity length inequality so that an epiphysiodesis can be done at an appropriate age, if necessary.

Kitakoji and associates[107] noted that some children develop a valgus femoral-tibial angle after femoral varus osteotomy. When osteotomy is done without medial displacement of the distal fragment, the mechanical axis shifts to the medial side of the knee. The growing child remodels the femoral-tibial axis into valgus to shift the mechanical axis to the center of the knee. This phenomenon can be reduced by medial displacement of the distal fragment at time of osteotomy.[107]

Technical Considerations As previously mentioned, treatment of any type is unnecessary for most children with LCPD who are younger than 6 years of age unless subluxation develops. Likewise, treatment rarely is required for patients 6 to 9 years of age who have minimal involvement because they are unlikely to develop subluxation or femoral head deformity. Children 9 years of age or older require treatment regardless of the amount of necrosis because the prognosis is poor for all untreated patients in this age group.[40,51,54,115]

The three prerequisites for successful containment by proximal femoral varus osteotomy are the following: (1) The child must be in the early or fragmentation stage of disease. Osteotomy in the ossification, or healing, stage of disease is too late to be effective and may cause further damage. (2) A fair to good presurgical range of hip motion is required. A stiff, irritable hip is a contraindication to surgery; a minimum of 30° abduction and no more than 10° of hip flexion contracture are preferred. When range of motion is completely normal presurgically, a hip spica cast is unnecessary. However, a hip spica cast usually is preferred postoperatively to maintain the leg in a neutral position, with the femoral head contained for 4 to 6 weeks until synovitis and muscle spasm subside. (3) Containment must be possible without hinge abduction. This can be verified by preoperative radiographs or by arthrography at the time of surgery.[116]

The optimal amount of varus reduction is approximately 20° in most patients (Fig 1). The neck-shaft angle must be reduced enough to contain the femoral head without creating excessive varus. Therefore, the neck-shaft angle should not be reduced below 105°.[83,107] In children younger than 5 years, the risk of growth arrest of the CFE after proximal femoral varus osteotomy is greater than in older children.[77,93] Barnes[93] suggested that excessive abduction in a plaster spica after osteotomy might obstruct blood flow to the CFE. Care therefore should be taken in these younger, smaller children to avoid excessive abduction and to avoid injury to the physis with the instrumentation. In children older than 8 years, Barnes recommends that the femoral neck-shaft angle be maintained at more than 115°. If greater varus is required for containment, the surgeon should consid-

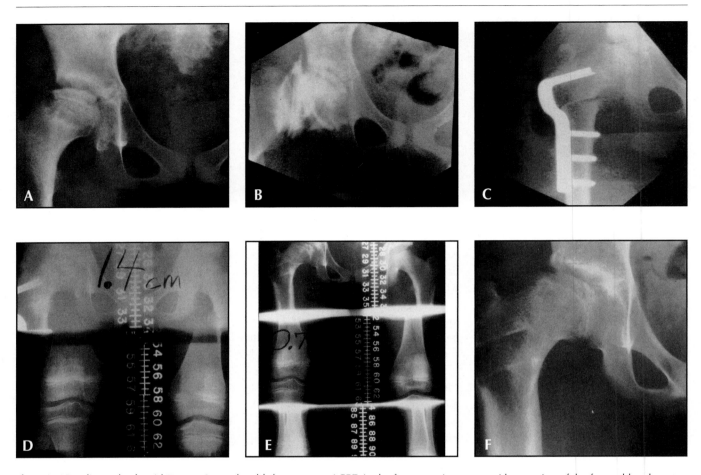

Fig. 1 A, AP radiograph of a girl 7 years 8 months old shows severe LCPD in the fragmentation stage, with extrusion of the femoral head, metaphyseal cysts, and lateral subluxation of the hip. **B,** Arthrogram shows that the femoral head can be contained in the acetabulum. **C,** Varus osteotomy with medial displacement. **D,** Scanogram 3 months after surgery shows 1.4 cm of discrepancy. **E,** Scanogram 20 months after surgery shows 0.7 cm of discrepancy. **F,** AP radiograph 20 months after femoral varus osteotomy. The femoral head demonstrates improved sphericity, continued healing, and a contained femoral head.

er substituting a shelf procedure or adding a pelvic osteotomy.

Several types of internal fixation have been successful for maintaining alignment.[31,117,118] The 90° fixed-angle blade plate allows medial displacement of the distal fragment more easily than do other devices (Fig. 2).[118,119] Kitakoji and associates[107] advise medial displacement to prevent the development of femoral-tibial valgus during remodeling. Also, the 90° fixed-angle blade plate can be inserted to obtain 10° to 15° of extension of the distal fragment to facilitate containment of the anterior femoral head (Fig. 3). However, the choice of device in most

cases depends on the experience and preference of the surgeon.

Opening wedge osteotomy was recommended by Mirovsky and associates[111] to reduce the early limb shortening that is produced by proximal varus femoral osteotomy (Fig. 4). They reported that the mean residual shortening was 1.1 cm after closing wedge resection compared with 0.4 cm after an opening wedge technique.

Derotation at the time of surgery is not recommended. Derotation of the proximal femur does not change the mechanics or position of the proximal fragment unless the derotation is com-

bined with capsulorrhaphy or muscle-redirecting procedures, such as might be done in surgery for developmental dysplasia of the hip. With an isolated femoral osteotomy, derotation will affect only the position of the distal fragment in a manner similar to a fracture that is reduced with the distal fragment externally rotated. This can lead to an external rotation gait without achieving additional containment of the femoral head.[120]

When these principles and techniques are followed, a high percentage of satisfactory results can be expected from proximal femoral varus osteotomy for LCPD in the early and fragmentation stages of disease.

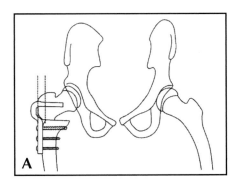

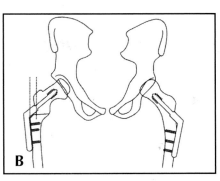

Fig. 2 Difference in medial displacement of the distal fragment with two types of internal fixation devices. **A,** A 90° fixed-angle blade plate facilitates medial displacement of the distal fragment. **B,** Lateralization may occur with screw-plate devices. (Reproduced with permission from Hau R, Dickens DR, Nattrass GR, O'Sullivan M, Torode IP, Graham HK: Which implant for proximal femoral osteotomy in children? A comparison of the AO (ASIF) 90 fixed-angle blade plate and the Richards intermediate hip screw. *J Pediatr Orthop* 2000;20:336-343.)

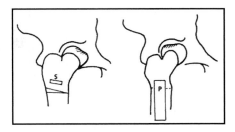

Fig. 3 Left, Fixation technique to produce extension of the distal fragment for improved coverage of the anterior portion of the femoral head. The insertion slot (s) is oblique to facilitate extension of the distal fragment. **Right,** Following osteotomy, application of the plate (p) to the diaphysis reduces the anterior portion of the femoral head under the lip of the acetabulum. (Reproduced with permission from Olney BW, Asher MA: Combined innominate and femoral osteotomy for the treatment of severe Legg-Calvé-Perthes disease. *J Pediatr Orthop* 1985;5:645-651.)

Valgus Extension Osteotomy of the Proximal Femur for Hinge Abduction
Hinge abduction in LCPD was first described by Moseley in 1980.[100] This occurs in later stages when the extruded, deformed femoral head impinges on the lateral margin of the acetabulum during abduction of the hip, preventing containment and causing the medial surface of the femoral head to pull away from the medial wall of the acetabulum during attempted abduction (Fig. 5). Lateral hinging may occur during the early stages of subluxation, before the deformed femoral head is fully ossified.[100,116]

Clinical symptoms of hinge abduction are increasing pain, limp, and restriction of movement during the fragmentation or resorption stages. Arthrography under general anesthesia can confirm the presence of hinge abduction. Using plain radiographs in the clinic setting, Reinker[116] and Kruse and associates[121] suggested that the hinge abduction may be determined by obtaining an AP radiograph of the pelvis with the patellae facing anteriorly. This is then compared with an AP radiograph of the pelvis with the hips in extension and maximal abduction with the patellae directly anterior. Failure of the femoral head to be contained under the lateral aspect of the

acetabulum, or widening of the medial joint space by more than 2 mm on the abduction radiograph, suggests that hinge abduction is present.[100,116]

The presence of hinge abduction indicates a very poor prognosis unless treatment is initiated.[86,116] In the early stages of hinge abduction, it may be possible to restore motion and contain the femoral head as long as the disease process is still in the fragmentation stage and there is potential for remodeling. In this situation, a child may benefit from preliminary traction, adductor tenotomy, iliopsoas recession, and medial capsulotomy to reduce the femoral head into the acetabulum.[15,116,122] The femoral head is then maintained in the acetabulum by Petrie casts for 2 to 4 months. This allows improved sphericity of the femoral head. The hip can then be contained by a surgical procedure, such as proximal varus femoral osteotomy, Salter osteotomy, or both.

When the hinge abduction is fixed, the options are a shelf acetabuloplasty, Chiari osteotomy, or valgus extension proximal femoral osteotomy.[86,87,121,122] The shelf procedure and Chiari osteotomy are not designed to reduce lateral impingement during abduction. However, these two procedures result in improved coverage

and pain relief in some patients.[121,123] In contrast, valgus extension osteotomy of the proximal femur unloads the lateral aspect of the femoral head and reestablishes the abductor mechanism while relieving impingement. Relief of pain and restoration of motion occur in 80% to 90% of patients.[86,87] Bankes and associates[86] defined failure as total hip arthroplasty, arthrodesis, or repeat osteotomy after valgus extension osteotomy. They reported a cumulative survival rate of 75% at 18 years after proximal femoral valgus extension osteotomy. These authors also noted femoral head remodeling with improved sphericity in 23% of hips. Remodeling was associated with open triradiate cartilage at the time of surgery. They postulated that the favorable remodeling was the result of the unloading of the lateral part of the femoral head.[86] Our preference is a valgus extension proximal femoral osteotomy when hinge abduction is diagnosed by arthrography (Fig. 6).

Pelvic Osteotomies
Pelvic osteotomies in LCPD are divided into three categories: (1) acetabular rota-

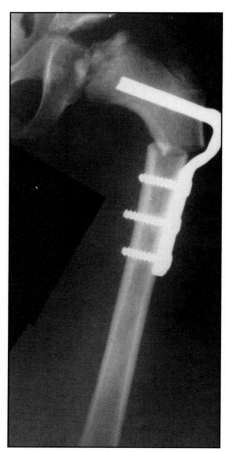

Fig. 4 Femoral varus osteotomy with a 90° fixed-angle blade plate. An opening wedge osteotomy is recommended to reduce the amount of extremity shortening.

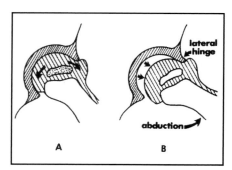

Fig. 5 A, Hinge abduction. Lateral extrusion and deformity of the femoral head impinges on the acetabular margin. **B,** Abduction of the hip produces lateral hinging with separation of the medial joint surface. (Reproduced with permission from Moseley CF: The biomechanics of the pediatric hip. *Orthop Clin North Am* 1980;11:3-16.)

tional osteotomies, (2) shelf procedures, and (3) medial displacement or Chiari osteotomies. The osteotomy most commonly done is the Salter acetabular rotational osteotomy.[61,96,97,124-132] Other rotational osteotomies include those described by Sutherland and Green-field[133] (double) and Steel[134] (triple). Shelf procedures recently have been used in LCPD as a method to gain additional lateral coverage of the femoral head.[98,121,135,136] The medial displacement osteotomy of Chiari usually is done for salvage of deformed femoral heads.[112,114,123,137-141] Any of these pelvic osteotomies can be combined with a proximal femoral varus osteotomy when severe deformity of the femoral head cannot be contained by a pelvic or proximal femoral varus osteotomy alone.[84,85,142] The shelf procedure also can be combined with an acetabular rotational osteotomy or Chiari osteotomy to gain further lateral coverage of the femoral head.[135]

Salter Osteotomy This procedure is done as described for developmental dislocation of the hip.[143,144] The Salter innominate osteotomy and the other rotational osteotomies are designed to gain anterior and lateral coverage of the femoral head by acetabular rotation;[101,145] the anterior and anterolateral region of the hip is the area of greatest stress concentration. Containment is never absolute because the femoral head is larger than the acetabulum. The improved anterior coverage is gained at the expense of posterior coverage of the femoral head. This osteotomy also displaces the acetabulum 1 to 1.5 cm medially (although it is difficult to visualize radiographically), thereby decreasing the biomechanical compression forces across the hip joint.[101,144] Ideal rotation and alignment occur when the acetabulum is displaced anteriorly 1 to 1.5 cm and a triangular-shaped iliac crest bone graft with a 30° to 35° apical angle is used.[101]

The Salter osteotomy depends on rotation occurring at the pubic symphysis, whereas in the double osteotomy described by Sutherland and Green-field,[133] rotation occurs at the osteotomy of the superior and inferior pubic rami. The triple osteotomy described by Steel[134] divides the ilium, the superior pubic ramus, and ischial ramus separately; it allows for maximal rotation of the acetabulum but is more difficult to stabilize. Postoperatively, it is desirable to maintain hip motion to minimize stiffness and enhance remodeling. The use of crutches and partial weight bearing in reliable children is recommended after a Salter osteotomy. A hip spica cast may be necessary to maintain alignment until sufficient healing has occurred in unreliable children. Once complete healing has occurred, the internal fixation devices, usually threaded Steinmann pins, can be removed. The child is then allowed to return to normal activities, including sports, as tolerated.

In 1980, Salter[130] compared the results of innominate osteotomy in 110 hips treated over a 15-year period with 38 hips treated years earlier by a weight-relieving sling (noncontainment treatment). All children in both groups were older than 6 years at clinical onset, had extensive CFE involvement (Catterall group III or IV), and mild subluxation, but the head had not become significantly deformed. The radiographic results were assessed by the Mose circle criteria.[49] The radiographic results in the 110 osteotomized hips were 77% good and 17% fair—that is, 94% were satisfactory results and only 6% were poor or unsatisfactory results. In the 38 hips treated by noncontainment, the results were 37% good and 29% fair—that is, 66% were satisfactory results and 34% were poor or unsatisfactory. Salter and Brown[131] expanded this series to 159 patients in 1988. Using the same criteria,[130] 79% of results were rated good and 16% fair (96% satisfactory); only 4% were rated poor. Clinically, 93% of the patients were asymptomatic.

In 1982, Ingman and associates[126]

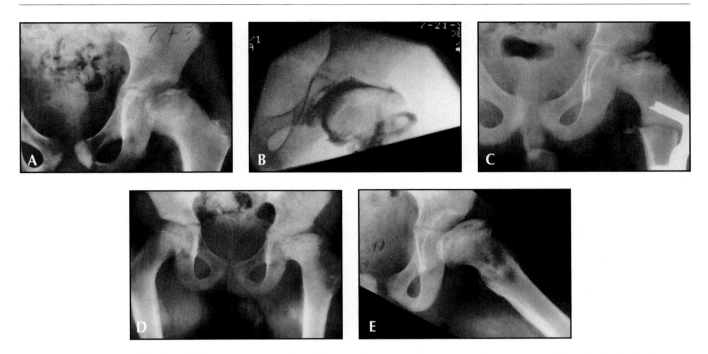

Fig. 6 A, AP radiograph of the hip of a boy 7 years, 3 months old 1 year after onset of symptoms, demonstrating subluxation in the late fragmentation stage of LCPD. The patient complained of pain and difficult gait caused by fixed flexion-adduction deformity of the hip. **B,** Arthrogram under general anesthesia with the hip in maximal abduction demonstrates widening of the medial joint and compression of the labrum without containment of the femoral head in the acetabulum. **C,** A valgus extension femoral osteotomy was done. AP **(D)** and lateral **(E)** radiographs 2 years and 4 months after osteotomy demonstrate an oval femoral head without impingement. The patient was asymptomatic.

compared the results of 38 Salter osteotomies with 33 patients treated by recumbency in hip spica casts. The authors used their own clinical criteria and the Mose circle criteria radiographically to assess their results. They reported satisfactory results (good and fair) in 75% of the patients treated by innominate osteotomy, compared with satisfactory results in 82% of patients treated by conservative treatment. However, when some of these patients, plus additional patients, were reevaluated in 1991 by Paterson and associates,[96] the incidence of satisfactory results in the patients treated by Salter osteotomy increased to 96%. The authors suggested that this improvement was the result of femoral head remodeling with subsequent growth.

In an unpublished study of 40 hips in 40 patients older than 6 years with LCPD treated by a Salter osteotomy, all patients were Catterall group III (35 patients) or IV (5 patients), Salter-Thompson group B, or lateral pillar group C. At a mean follow-up of 7.2 years (range, 3 to 17 years), results were satisfactory in 97% of patients (either Stulberg class II [28 hips] or III [11 hips]) (Fig. 7). There was only one Stulberg class IV, or unsatisfactory, result (3%) (GH Thompson, MD, and S. Scherl, MD, unpublished data, 2001).

Other studies regarding the Salter osteotomy have shown similar rates of satisfactory clinical and radiographic results.[97,125,127,128,132,146-148] Canale and associates[149] and Cotler and Donahue[150] used a trapezoidal rather than a triangular shape and reported results similar to those of the Salter osteotomy. There are few reports on the efficacy of the Sutherland and Greenfield[133] (double) or Steel[134] (triple) innominate osteotomy in LCPD.[151]

Shelf Procedures A shelf procedure provides a congruous extension of the acetabulum by bone grafting the anterolateral, lateral, and posterolateral aspects of the acetabulum. It is a common method of treatment of LCPD.[16,98,113,121,151-153] Plastic construction of the acetabulum, or the shelf procedure, was originally described by Gill in 1935[154] for developmental hip dislocation with instability persisting after closed reduction. The slotted acetabular augmentation developed by Staheli and Chew[135] is the most common technique currently used. A 1-cm deep trough is created at the capsular attachments to the acetabulum and grafted in an overlapping fashion with cancellous bone strips obtained from the lateral aspect of the ipsilateral iliac crest. The grafts are held in position by repairing the reflected head of the rectus femoris tendon. A thick augmentation is then developed superiorly with additional graft material. No metallic internal fixation is necessary. As healing occurs the interposed capsule undergoes

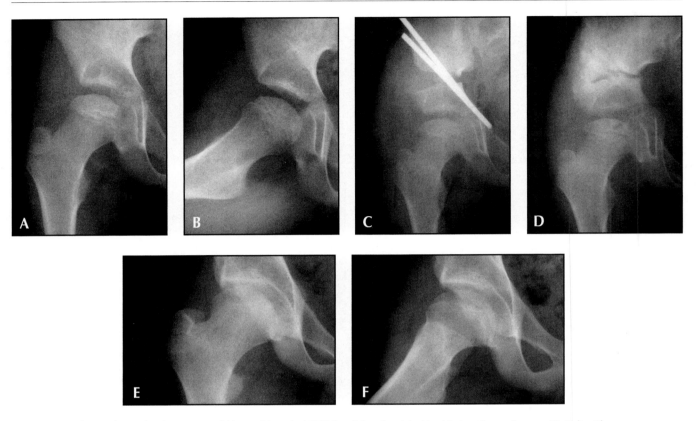

Fig. 7 A, AP pelvic radiograph of an 8-year-old boy with early LCPD involving the right hip. He has Catterall group III, Salter-Thompson group B, or lateral pillar (Herring and associates[40]) group C involvement. There is no subluxation of the uninvolved medial pillar because Shenton's line is intact. B, The Lauenstein (frog-lateral) radiograph. C, Postoperative radiograph after a Salter osteotomy. The threaded Steinmann pins are directed posterior and medial to the acetabulum. The increased coverage of the femoral head is the result of acetabular rotation. D, Three months postoperatively, the osteotomy is healed, and the Steinmann pins have been removed. The extent of CFE involvement is now more clearly evident. E, AP radiograph of the right hip 7 years postoperatively. The patient is now skeletally mature and has a Stulberg class II result. The femoral head is round, but coxa magna and coxa breva are apparent. The femoral head is well covered, and Shenton's line is intact. The patient is asymptomatic, with essentially a full range of hip motion. F, Lauenstein (frog-lateral) radiograph.

fibrocartilage metaplasia. How much weight bearing occurs across the grafted area is debatable; because the position of the acetabulum is unchanged, no decrease in the hip joint biomechanical compression forces occurs. A major disadvantage of the shelf procedure is that children require spica cast immobilization until healing is complete, usually 6 to 8 weeks. Protected weight bearing is allowed until a satisfactory range of hip motion has been restored.

Willett and associates[98] reported improved results with shelf procedures done early in LCPD in 20 children 8 years of age or older at clinical onset with extensive CFE involvement, compared with 14 similar children with no treatment. The authors used their own clinical and radiographic rating systems, so their results are not comparable with other studies. The mean follow-up for both groups was short, with a mean of 22 and 28 months in the treated and untreated groups, respectively. Willett and associates thought that the shelf procedure produced better early results than the results in the untreated group. Similar improved results were reported by van der Heyden and van Tongerloo.[136] Staheli and Chew[135] thought the slotted acetabulum augmentation to be beneficial in the late stages of LCPD, when rotational osteotomies may be contraindicated because of possible incongruity between the femoral head and acetabulum.

Kruse and associates[121] reported a long-term study of 20 hips in 19 patients with LCPD treated with shelf procedures to increase the volume of the acetabulum and improve coverage of subluxated femoral heads. They used the technique described by Gill[154] and later by Kamhi and MacEwen.[155] Fourteen hips had had hinge abduction preoperatively. Thus, in this group, the criteria were similar to those for the Chiari medial displacement osteotomy, and the procedure was undertaken predominantly for salvage. Nineteen hips underwent surgery during the reossification phase and one during the remodeling phase. The results at a mean follow-up of 19 years (range, 7 to 45 years) were compared with a matched control group of 18 hips in 17 patients treated conservatively and followed for a mean of 20 years (range, 7 to 45 years). The clinical and radiographic results were distinctly better in the patients who underwent shelf procedures. Hinge abduction was corrected in 11 of 14 patients; Mose circle sphericity and the center-edge angle measurements were improved; and by the Iowa hip rating system, the treated patients had a mean of 91 points compared with 81 points in the control group. The Stulberg rating was applicable in 15 hips and showed two class II, seven class III, and five class IV hips, and one class V hip. The shelf resorbed in 2 hips and was adequate in 18. In the control group, Stulberg ratings could be applied to only 12 hips and showed four class II, five class III, and three class IV hips. The better results in the shelf-procedure group were statistically significant with respect to Mose circle sphericity, center-edge angle, and Iowa hip rating scores ($P \leq 0.001$, $P \leq 0.05$, and $P \leq 0.05$, respectively) but not by the Stulberg rating.

Daly and associates[152] in 1999 reported 27 hips in 26 children whose onset of the disease process was after 8 years of age and who were treated with shelf procedures. The authors reported that 22 hips (81%) achieved Stulberg class I, II, or III at skeletal maturity. Poor results tended to occur in older children (older than 11 years), in girls, and with extensive femoral head involvement (Catterall group IV, Salter-Thompson group B, and lateral pillar group C). Van Der Geest and associates[153] reported similar results in 30 hips followed for a mean of 12 years. Eighteen hips had reached skeletal maturity: 6 with Stulberg class I or II results, 10 with class III results, and only 2 with class IV or V results.

Medial Displacement Osteotomy The osteotomy described by Chiari[138,139] is an extra-articular domed osteotomy at the capsular attachment of the acetabulum along the anterolateral, lateral, and posterolateral margins. It is done primarily for salvage of a deformed femoral head. The osteotomy is angulated cephalad or superiorly 10° to 15° from lateral to medial. The acetabulum is displaced medially and slightly superiorly, which allows the ilium to come into contact with the superior aspect of the hip capsule. The medial displacement of the acetabulum also decreases the biomechanical compression forces across the hip joint. The femoral head should be completely contained radiographically and situated medial to Perkin's line, using the osteotomized margin of the ilium as the new lateral margin of the acetabulum. If there is an exposed area of capsule between the ilium and acetabular segments, this can be grafted with bone obtained from the lateral aspect of the ilium.[112,137] Also, if there is not good contact between the hip capsule and the ilium anteriorly, additional graft material, usually cancellous, can be inserted. The interposed capsule, which is now under compression during weight bearing, undergoes metaplasia to fibrocartilage. Although this is not as durable as normal hyaline articular cartilage, medial displacement osteotomy is useful as a salvage procedure for deformed femoral heads. Internal fixation with two or three threaded Steinmann pins is necessary to eliminate the need for postoperative immobilization.[112,123,137] It is important that motion be preserved to enhance remodeling and the capsular fibrocartilage metaplasia. When healing is complete, the internal fixation devices are removed. However, Chiari[139] reported that, without internal fixation, immobilization in a hip spica cast was necessary for only 3 weeks before sufficient healing occurred to allow initiation of the rehabilitation program.

Bennett and associates[123] reported the results of 18 Chiari osteotomies in 17 patients with painful subluxation of the femoral head as sequelae of LCPD. Their clinical results in 13 patients personally examined by the authors demonstrated no pain during normal physical activities and an adequate range of motion at a mean follow-up of 4.3 years (range, 2 to 8 years). The mean range of motion was moderately restricted, with 105° of flexion, 33° of abduction, 5° of internal rotation, and 10° of external rotation. There were no good radiographic results according to the Mose circle criteria, but there was significant improvement in the center-edge angle and the percentage of coverage of the femoral head. Similar results have been published by others after Chiari osteotomy for the treatment of painful subluxated hips with incongruency in older children or adolescents.[114,137,140,141,156] The advantage of this procedure is that it increases the volume of the acetabulum to contain an enlarged, deformed femoral head. Significant remodeling of the femoral head can be anticipated with growth. Unfortunately, no long-term results of the Chiari osteotomy in LCPD have been published.

Combined Proximal Femoral and Pelvic Osteotomies

The combined procedures usually are a Salter osteotomy and a proximal femoral varus (110° to 115°) derotation osteotomy.[84,85] Most patients are immobilized in a hip spica cast for 3 to 6 weeks postoperatively. Vukasinovic and associates[157] recommended a combination of a Salter osteotomy and femoral shortening.

The results of combined Salter and proximal femoral varus derotation osteotomies for severe LCPD have been reported by Olney and Asher[85] and by Crutcher and Staheli.[84] The results of these studies were more standardized than most and allow appropriate comparative analysis. Olney and Asher studied nine patients at a mean follow-up of 4.2 years (range, 1.7 to 7.7 years). They used the clinical criteria of Ratliff[158] and the radiographic criteria of Mose[49] and Lloyd-Roberts and associates[81] in evaluating their results. The Ratliff criteria include pain, limited range of motion, and a limp. A patient is rated good when none of these findings is present, fair when one is present, and poor when two or three are present. Postoperatively, Olney and Asher reported seven (78%) good and two (22%) fair clinical results. The two patients with fair results had a persistent limp because of abductor muscle weakness from greater trochanteric overgrowth. No patient had significant pain or a functional loss of hip motion. By the Mose circle criteria, there were five satisfactory (three good and two fair) and four poor or unsatisfactory results. The criteria adapted from Lloyd-Roberts and associates[81] improved the radiographic results to eight (89%) satisfactory results (four good and four fair) and only one poor or unsatisfactory result. A good result implied that the femoral head was round and congruous and had minimal loss of epiphyseal height. A fair result indicated that the femoral head was not completely spherical but was congruous, had no more than one fifth of the femoral head uncovered, and had a mild loss of epiphyseal height. A poor result had obvious flattening of the femoral head with loss of congruity, greater than one fifth lateral extrusion, and secondary acetabular changes.

Similar results were found by Crutcher and Staheli[84] in 14 patients using the same preoperative and postoperative clinical and radiographic criteria, with the exception that they also included the Stulberg rating in their postoperative radiographic evaluation. They reported seven Stulberg class II hips and six class III hips (for 93% satisfactory results) and only one class IV hip at a mean follow-up of 8 years (range, 5 to 10.5 years). This indicated a significant salvage rate of hips with a potentially poor prognosis. They observed that 11 of

14 hips had documentable improvement in femoral head sphericity with growth because of remodeling.

Currently, the short-term results of pelvic osteotomies appear to alter the natural history of untreated LCPD. The published studies indicate improved sphericity of the femoral head, which may be related to the continuous containment of the femoral head compared with short-term containment for individuals treated with an abduction orthosis. With the improved sphericity of the femoral head should come a decreased risk for degenerative osteoarthritis in adulthood. The advantages of the acetabular rotational osteotomies, specifically the Salter osteotomy, over proximal femoral varus osteotomy include better anterior and lateral coverage of the femoral head that (1) does not result in further shortening of the femoral neck (coxa breva), (2) increases the length of the involved extremity by approximately 1 cm rather than causing further shortening, and (3) improves the Trendelenburg gait. Other advantages include (4) easier metal removal and (5) no risk for pathologic fracture through seven holes in the proximal femur.[61,159] However, pelvic osteotomies require significant experience. These are technically demanding procedures, especially the rotational osteotomies described by Salter, Sutherland, and Steel. The shelf procedures are more easily accomplished and may be a more appropriate alternative for individuals with less experience.

A comparison of the results of proximal femoral varus osteotomies and Salter osteotomies indicates similar results with respect to femoral head sphericity. Moberg and associates[146] in 1997 found similar radiographic results between 16 hips treated with proximal femoral varus osteotomies and 18 treated with Salter osteotomies at 6 and 8 years of follow-up, respectively. They did not use the Stulberg criteria; however, the center-edge angle was better in the hips treated with Salter osteotomies.

Similar results were published by Sponseller and associates[132] in 1988 in an analysis of 42 femoral osteotomies and 49 Salter osteotomies. All hips were Catterall group III or IV, and patients had a mean age of 7 years at clinical onset. At a mean follow-up of 9 years (range, 3 to 17 years), there was no difference by Stulberg classification between the two groups. In the femoral osteotomy group there were 8 Stulberg class I, 20 class II, and 5 class III results (79% satisfactory) and 2 class IV and 7 class V results (21% unsatisfactory). Six of the seven patients with class V hips were more than 10 years of age at diagnosis. In the Salter osteotomy group, there were 7 Stulberg class I, 27 class II, and 13 class III results (96% satisfactory) and 1 each class IV and class V result (4% unsatisfactory). Only one patient in the Salter group was more than 10 years of age at diagnosis (class III). However, the authors also found that the center-edge angle, neck-shaft angle, lower extremity lengths, range of abduction, and total range of motion were closer to normal after a Salter osteotomy.

Multicenter Prospective Legg-Calvé-Perthes Disease Study

A prospective multicenter study was undertaken in 1981 to compare, in the short term and through skeletal maturity, the results in patients with LCPD who had surgical treatment, nonsurgical treatment, or no treatment at all. The goal of the study was to establish firm criteria to be used by clinicians in determining the most appropriate care for patients with LCPD. The results of the study will be finalized and published when nearly all of the patients in the study have reached skeletal maturity.

Thirty-six pediatric orthopaedic surgeons from 28 institutions participated in the study. Because preferred treatment options existed at numerous institutions, it became evident early in the study that randomization of patients was not possible. Therefore, the criteria for inclusion into the study included (1) a uniform treatment method at each center; (2) the use of one of five standard treatment methods (no treatment, range of motion, Scottish Rite abduction orthosis, proximal femoral varus osteotomy, and Salter osteotomy); and (3) patients enrolled only when they were chronologically 6 years of age and older, with (4) no prior treatment, (5) disease in the increased radiodensity or fragmentation stage, and (6) no other disorders present that were associated with osteonecrosis of the CFEs. The period of enrollment extended from 1984 through 1992.

The data were submitted to and evaluated at one site (Texas Scottish Rite Hospital, Dallas, TX). Numerous variables were examined, separately and in combination: Catterall classification, lateral pillar classification, chronologic age at the onset of disease, skeletal age at the onset of disease, patient sex, and method of treatment. The skeletal age was determined from a wrist radiograph or by the Oxford method from a pelvic radiograph when no wrist radiograph was available.[160]

A total of 389 patients are enrolled in the study. All of their femoral heads are sufficiently healed to determine a probable Stulberg result, but only three fourths of the group at last analysis were fully skeletally mature. When all available data are accumulated, the study will be completed. Definitive recommendations for management can then be made based on significant ($P < 0.05$) differences found between the five treatment methods. Our current approach, based on the information available at this time, is to do the following.

For patients with Catterall groups I and II or lateral pillar group A involvement and those with Catterall group II or lateral pillar group B hips whose onset of disease was at a skeletal age of 6 years or less, symptomatic care is all that is required. Children with Catterall groups I and II or lateral pillar group A involvement usually can be recognized because they rarely experience persistent loss of joint motion or major symptoms. Initial management should focus on pain relief, with reduction of activities and the use of anti-inflammatory medications, with short periods of bed rest during major episodes of pain or loss of joint motion.

Patients with Catterall group III or lateral pillar group B involvement whose onset occurred after skeletal age 6 years, and all children with Catterall group IV or lateral pillar group C hips, currently are treated with surgical containment once joint range of motion has been achieved by symptomatic means. Salter osteotomy and femoral varus osteotomy produce similar results in terms of femoral head shape. Salter osteotomies occasionally result in stiffness of the hip, especially in patients older than 10 years at the onset of the disease process. However, femoral osteotomy results in elevation of the greater trochanter with a tendency toward abductor dysfunction. Patients older than 9 years with Catterall groups III and IV or lateral pillar group B and C hips may benefit from combined femoral and pelvic osteotomies, but the success rate is unpredictable in this population regardless of the treatment methods applied.

References

1. Atsumi T, Yamano K, Muraki M, Yoshihara S, Kajihara T: The blood supply of the lateral epiphyseal arteries in Perthes' disease. *J Bone Joint Surg Br* 2000;82:392-398.

2. Chung SM: The arterial supply of the developing proximal end of the human femur. *J Bone Joint Surg Am* 1976;58:961-970.

3. Gautier E, Ganz K, Krügel N, Gill T, Ganz R: Anatomy of the medial femoral circumflex artery and its surgical implications. *J Bone Joint Surg Br* 2000;82:679-683.

4. Theron J: Angiography in Legg-Calvé-Perthes disease. *Radiology* 1980;135:81-92.

5. Inoue A, Freeman MA, Vernon-Roberts B, Mizuno S: The pathogenesis of Perthes' disease. *J Bone Joint Surg Br* 1976;58:453-461.

6. Kleinman RG, Bleck EE: Increased blood viscosity in patients with Legg-Perthes disease: A preliminary report. *J Pediatr Orthop* 1981;1:131-136.

7. Green NE, Griffin PP: Intra-osseous venous pressure in Legg-Perthes disease. *J Bone Joint Surg Am* 1982;64:666-671.

8. Roy DR, Glueck CJ: The etiology of osteonecrosis: The role of coagulopathies. *APLAR Journal of Rheumatology* 1999;2:260-261.

9. Glueck CJ, Crawford A, Roy D, Freiberg R, Glueck H, Stroop D: Association of antithrombotic factor deficiencies and hypofibrinolysis with Legg-Perthes disease. *J Bone Joint Surg Am* 1996;78:3-13.

10. Glueck CJ, Brandt G, Gruppo R, et al: Resistance to activated protein C and Legg-Perthes disease. *Clin Orthop* 1997;338:139-152.

11. Gregosiewicz A, Okonski M, Stolecka D, Kandzierski G, Szponar M: Ischemia of the femoral head in Perthes' disease: Is the cause intra- or extravascular? *J Pediatr Orthop* 1989;9:160-162.

12. Arruda VR, Belangero WD, Ozelo MC, et al: Inherited risk factors for thrombophilia among children with Legg-Calvé-Perthes disease. *J Pediatr Orthop* 1999;19:84-87.

13. Eldridge J, Dilley A, Austin H, et al: The role of protein C, protein S, and resistance to activated protein C in Legg-Perthes disease. *Pediatrics* 2001;107:1329-1334.

14. Gallistl S, Reitinger T, Linhart W, Muntean W: The role of inherited thrombotic disorders in the etiology of Legg-Calvé-Perthes disease. *J Pediatr Orthop* 1999;19:82-83.

15. Hayek S, Kenet G, Lubetsky A, Rosenberg N, Gitel S, Wientroub S: Does thrombophilia play an aetiological role in Legg-Calvé-Perthes disease? *J Bone Joint Surg Br* 1999;81:686-690.

16. Herndon WA: Association of antithrombotic factor deficiencies and hypofibrinolysis with Legg-Perthes disease. *J Bone Joint Surg Am* 1997;79:1114-1115.

17. Hunt DM, Holmes Z, Pickering W, Cohen H: Association of antithrombotic factor deficiencies and hypofibrinolysis with Legg-Perthes disease. *J Bone Joint Surg Am* 1998;80:604-606.

18. Kahle WK: Letter. Association of antithrombotic factor deficiencies and hypofibrinolysis with Legg-Perthes disease. *J Bone Joint Surg Am* 1997;79:1114-1115.

19. Kealey WD, Mayne EE, McDonald W, Murray P, Cosgrove AP: The role of coagulation abnormalities in the development of Perthes' disease. *J Bone Joint Surg Br* 2000;82:744-746.

20. Liesner RJ: Does thrombophilia cause Perthes' disease in children? *J Bone Joint Surg Br* 1999;81:565-566.

21. Sirvent N, Fisher F, el Hayek T, Appert A, Giudicelli H, Griffet J: Absence of congenital prethrombotic disorders in children with Legg-Perthes disease. *J Pediatr Orthop* 2000;9:24-27.

22. Thomas DP, Morgan G, Tayton K: Perthes' disease and the relevance of thrombophilia. *J Bone Joint Surg Br* 1999;81:691-695.

23. Gruppo R, Glueck CJ, Wall E, Roy D, Wang P: Legg-Perthes disease in three siblings, two heterozygous and one homozygous for the Factor V Leiden mutation. *J Pediatr* 1998;132:885-888.

24. Glueck CJ, Freiberg RA, Crawford A, et al: Secondhand smoke, hypofibrinolysis, and Legg-Perthes disease. *Clin Orthop* 1998;352:159-167.

25. Mata SG, Aicua EA, Ovejero AH, Grande MM: Legg-Calvé-Perthes disease and passive smoking. *J Pediatr Orthop* 2000;20:326-330.

26. Weinstein SL: Legg-Calvé-Perthes syndrome, in Morrissy RT, Weinstein SL (eds): *Pediatric Orthopaedics*, ed 4. Philadelphia, PA, Lippincott-Raven, 1996, vol 2, pp 951-991.

27. Harrison MH, Blakemore ME: A study of the "normal" hip in children with unilateral Perthes' disease. *J Bone Joint Surg Br* 1980;62:31-36.

28. Catterall A, Pringle J, Byers PD, et al: A review of the morphology of Perthes' disease. *J Bone Joint Surg Br* 1982;64:269-275.

29. Loder RT, Schwartz EM, Hensinger RN: Behavioral characteristics of children with Legg-Calvé-Perthes disease. *J Pediatr Orthop* 1993;13:598-601.

30. Herring JA (ed): *Legg-Calvé-Perthes Disease*. Rosemont, IL, American Academy of Orthopaedic Surgeons, 1996.

31. Catterall A, Pringle J, Byers PD, Fulford GE, Kemp HB: Perthes' disease: Is the epiphysial infarction complete? *J Bone Joint Surg Br* 1982;64:276-281.

32. Ponseti IV, Maynard JA, Weinstein SL, Ippolito EG, Pous JG: Legg-Calvé-Perthes disease: Histochemical and ultrastructural observations of the epiphyseal cartilage and physis. *J Bone Joint Surg Am* 1983;65:797-807.

33. Guille JT, Lipton GE, Szoke G, Bowen JR, Harcke HT, Glutting JJ: Legg-Calvé-Perthes disease in girls: A comparison of the results with those seen in boys. *J Bone Joint Surg Am* 1998;80:1256-1263.

34. Roy DR: Perthes'-like changes caused by acquired hypothyroidism. *Orthopedics* 1991;14:901-904.

35. Suzuki S, Awaya G, Okada Y, Ikeda T, Tada H: Examination by ultrasound of Legg-Calvé-Perthes disease. *Clin Orthop* 1987;220:130-136.

36. Tsao AK, Dias LS, Conway JJ, Straka P: The prognostic value and significance of serial bone scintigraphy in Legg-Calvé-Perthes disease. *J Pediatr Orthop* 1997;17:230-239.

37. Catterall A: The natural history of Perthes' disease. *J Bone Joint Surg Br* 1971;53:37-53.

38. Van Dam BE, Crider RJ, Noyes JD, Larsen LJ: Determination of the Catterall classification in Legg-Calvé-Perthes disease. *J Bone Joint Surg Am* 1981;63:906-914.

39. Salter RB, Thompson GH: Legg-Calvé-Perthes disease: The prognostic significance of the subchondral fracture and a two-group classification of the femoral head involvement. *J Bone Joint Surg Am* 1984;66:479-489.

40. Herring JA, Neustadt JB, Williams JJ, Early JS, Browne RH: The lateral pillar classification of Legg-Calvé-Perthes disease. *J Pediatr Orthop* 1992;12:143-150.

41. Farsetti P, Tudisco C, Caterini R, Potenza V, Ippolito E: The Herring lateral pillar classification for prognosis in Perthes disease: Late results in 49 patients treated conservatively. *J Bone Joint Surg Br* 1995;77:739-742.

42. Podeszwa DA, Stanitski CL, Stanitski DF, Woo R, Mendelow MJ: The effect of pediatric orthopaedic experience on interobserver and intraobserver reliability of the Herring lateral pillar classification of Perthes disease. *J Pediatr Orthop* 2000;20:562-565.

43. Ritterbusch JF, Shantharam SS, Gelinas C: Comparison of the lateral pillar classification and Catterall classification of Legg-Calvé-Perthes disease. *J Pediatr Orthop* 1993; 13:200-202.

44. Dickens DR, Menelaus MB: The assessment of prognosis in Perthes' disease. *J Bone Joint Surg Br* 1978;60:189-194.

45. Hoffinger SA, Henderson RC, Renner JB, Dales MC, Rab GT: Magnetic resonance evaluation of "metaphyseal" changes in Legg-Calvé-Perthes disease. *J Pediatr Orthop* 1993;13:602-606.

46. Song HR, Dhar S, Na JB, et al: Classification of metaphyseal change with magnetic resonance imaging in Legg-Calvé-Perthes disease. *J Pediatr Orthop* 2000;20:557-561.

47. Bowen JR, Schreiber FC, Foster BK, Wein BK: Premature femoral neck physeal closure in Perthes' disease. *Clin Orthop* 1982;171:24-29.

48. Weishaupt D, Exner GU, Hilfiker PR, Hodler J: Dynamic MR imaging of the hip in Legg-Calvé-Perthes disease: Comparison with arthrography. *AJR Am J Roentgenol* 2000;174:1635-1637.

49. Mose K: Methods of measuring in Legg-Calvé-Perthes disease with special regard to the prognosis. *Clin Orthop* 1980;150:103-109.

50. Stulberg SD, Salter RB: The natural course of Legg-Perthes' disease and its relationship to degenerative arthritis of the hip: A long-term follow-up study. *Orthop Trans* 1977;1:105-106.

51. Stulberg SD, Cooperman DR, Wallensten R: The natural history of Legg-Calvé-Perthes disease. *J Bone Joint Surg Am* 1981;63:1095-1108.

52. Harry JD, Gross RH: A quantitative method for evaluating results of treating Legg-Perthes syndrome. *J Pediatr Orthop* 1987;7:671-676.

53. Catterall A: Radiological features, in Catterall A (ed): *Legg-Calvé-Perthes Disease*. Edinburgh, Scotland, Churchill Livingstone, 1982, pp 39-64.

54. McAndrew MP, Weinstein SL: A long-term follow-up of Legg-Calvé-Perthes disease. *J Bone Joint Surg Am* 1984;66:860-869.

55. Gower WE, Johnston RC: Legg-Perthes disease: Long-term follow-up of thirty-six patients. *J Bone Joint Surg Am* 1971;53:759-768.

56. Herring JA, Williams JJ, Neustadt JN, Early JS: Evolution of femoral head deformity during the healing phase of Legg-Calvé-Perthes disease. *J Pediatr Orthop* 1993;13:41-45.

57. Clarke NM, Harrison MH: Painful sequelae of coxa plana. *J Bone Joint Surg Am* 1983;65:13-18.

58. Keret D, Harrison MH, Clarke NM, Hall DJ: Coxa plana: The fate of the physis. *J Bone Joint Surg Am* 1984;66:870-877.

59. Snyder CR: Legg-Perthes disease in the young hip: Does it necessarily do well? *J Bone Joint Surg Am* 1975;57:751-759.

60. Herring JA: The treatment of Legg-Calvé-Perthes disease: A critical review of the literature. *J Bone Joint Surg Am* 1994;76:448-458.

61. Salter RB: The present status of surgical treatment for Legg-Perthes disease. *J Bone Joint Surg Am* 1984;66:961-966.

62. Curtis BH, Gunther SF, Gossling HR, Paul SW: Treatment for Legg-Calvé-Perthes disease with the Newington ambulation-abduction brace. *J Bone Joint Surg Am* 1974;56:1135-1146.

63. Bobechko WP, McLaurin CA, Motloch WM: Toronto orthosis for Legg-Perthes disease. *Artif Limb* 1968;12:36-41.

64. Tachdjian MO, Jouett LD: Abstract: Trilateral socket hip abduction orthosis for the treatment of Legg-Perthes disease. *J Bone Joint Surg Am* 1968;50:1272-1273.

65. Meehan PL, Angel D, Nelson JM: The Scottish Rite abduction orthosis for the treatment of Legg-Perthes disease: A radiographic analysis. *J Bone Joint Surg Am* 1992;74:2-12.

66. Donovan MM, Urquhart BA: Legg-Calvé-Perthes syndrome: Treatment with ambulatory abduction brace. *Orthop Rev* 1979;8:147-151.

67. Harrison MH, Turner MH, Nicholson FJ: Coxa plana: Results of a new form of splinting. *J Bone Joint Surg Am* 1969;51:1057-1069.

68. Harrison MH, Turner MH: Abstract: Containment splintage for Perthes' disease of the hip. *J Bone Joint Surg Br* 1974;56:199.

69. Katz JF: Letter. Nonoperative therapy in Legg-Calvé-Perthes disease. *Orthop Rev* 1979;8:69-74.

70. Ferguson AB, Howorth MB: Coxa plana and related conditions at the hip. *J Bone Joint Surg* 1934;16:781-803.

71. Thompson GH, Westin GW: Legg-Calvé-Perthes disease: Results of discontinuing treatment in the early reossification phase. *Clin Orthop* 1979;139:70-80.

72. Martinez AG, Weinstein SL, Dietz FR: The weight-bearing abduction brace for the treatment of Legg-Perthes disease. *J Bone Joint Surg Am* 1992;74:12-21.

73. Rab GT, Wyatt M, Sutherland DH, Simon SR: A technique for determining femoral head containment during gait. *J Pediatr Orthop* 1985 ;5:8-12.

74. Axer A: Subtrochanteric osteotomy in the treatment of Perthes' disease: A preliminary report. *J Bone Joint Surg Br* 1965;47:489-499.

75. Axer A, Gershuni DH, Hendel D, Mirovski Y: Indications for femoral osteotomy in Legg-Calvé-Perthes disease. *Clin Orthop* 1980;150:78-87.

76. Canario AT, Williams L, Wientroub S, Catterall A, Lloyd-Roberts GC: A controlled study of the results of femoral osteotomy in severe Perthes' disease. *J Bone Joint Surg Br* 1980;62:438-440.

77. Coates CJ, Paterson JM, Woods KR, Catterall A, Fixsen JA: Femoral osteotomy in Perthes' disease: Results at maturity. *J Bone Joint Surg Br* 1990;72:581-585.

78. Friedlander JK, Weiner DS: Radiographic results of proximal femoral varus osteotomy in Legg-Calvé-Perthes disease. *J Pediatr Orthop* 2000;20:566-571.

79. Hoikka V, Lindholm TS, Poussa M: Intertrochanteric varus osteotomy in Legg-Calvé-Perthes disease: A report of 112 hips. *J Pediatr Orthop* 1986;6:600-604.

80. Joseph B, Srinivas G, Thomas R: Management of Perthes' disease of late onset in southern India: The evaluation of a surgical method. *J Bone Joint Surg Br* 1996;78:625-630.

81. Lloyd-Roberts GC, Catterall A, Salamon PB: A controlled study of the indications for and the results of femoral osteotomy in Perthes' disease. *J Bone Joint Surg Br* 1976;58:31-36.

82. Matan AJ, Stevens PM, Smith JT, Santora SD: Combination trochanteric arrest and intertrochanteric osteotomy for Perthes' disease. *J Pediatr Orthop* 1996;16:10-14.

83. Weiner SD, Weiner DS, Riley PM: Pitfalls in treatment of Legg-Calvé-Perthes disease using proximal femoral varus osteotomy. *J Pediatr Orthop* 1991;11:20-24.

84. Crutcher JP, Staheli LT: Combined osteotomy as a salvage procedure for severe Legg-Calvé-Perthes disease. *J Pediatr Orthop* 1992;12:151-156.

85. Olney BW, Asher MA: Combined innominate and femoral osteotomy for the treatment of severe Legg-Calvé-Perthes disease. *J Pediatr Orthop* 1985;5:645-651.

86. Bankes MJ, Catterall A, Hashemi-Nejad A: Valgus extension osteotomy for 'hinge abduction' in Perthes' disease: Results at maturity and factors influencing the radiological outcome. *J Bone Joint Surg Br* 2000;82 :548-554.

87. Urlus M, Stoffelen D, Fabry G: Hinge abduction in avascular necrosis of the hip: Diagnosis and treatment. *J Pediatr Orthop Part B* 1992;1:67-71.

88. Evans IK, Deluca PA, Gage JR: A comparative study of ambulation-abduction bracing and varus derotation osteotomy in the treatment of severe Legg-Calvé-Perthes disease in children over 6 years of age. *J Pediatr Orthop* 1988;8 :676-682.

89. Heikkinen E, Puranen J: Evaluation of femoral osteotomy in the treatment of Legg- Calvé-Perthes disease. *Clin Orthop* 1980;150:60-68.

90. Wang L, Bowen JR, Puniak MA, Guille JT, Glutting J: An evaluation of various methods of treatment for Legg-Calvé-Perthes disease. *Clin Orthop* 1995;314:225-233.

91. Eckerwall G, Hochbergs P, Wingstrand H, Egun N: Magnetic resonance imaging and early remodeling of the femoral head after femoral varus osteotomy in Legg-Calvé-Perthes disease. *J Pediatr Orthop Br* 1997;6:239-244.

92. Bayliss N, Margetts M, Taylor JF: Intertrochanteric femoral osteotomy for Legg-Calvé-Perthes disease. *J Pediatr Orthop Part B* 1994;3:15-17.

93. Barnes JM: Premature epiphysial closure in Perthes' disease. *J Bone Joint Surg Br* 1980;62:432-437.

94. Noonan KJ, Price CT, Kupiszewski SJ, Pyevich M: Results of femoral varus osteotomy in children older than 9 years of age with Perthes' disease. *J Pediatr Orthop* 2001;21:198-204.

95. Mazda K, Pennecot GF, Zeller R, Taussig G: Perthes' disease after the age of twelve years: Role of the remaining growth. *J Bone Joint Surg Br* 1999;81:696-698.

96. Paterson DC, Leitch JM, Foster BK: Results of innominate osteotomy in the treatment of Legg-Calvé-Perthes disease. *Clin Orthop* 1991;266:96-103.

97. Stevens PM, Williams P, Menelaus M: Innominate osteotomy for Perthes' disease. *J Pediatr Orthop* 1981;1:47-54.

98. Willett K, Hudson I, Catterall A: Lateral shelf acetabuloplasty: An operation for older children with Perthes' disease. *J Pediatr Orthop* 1992;12:563-568.

99. Leitch JM, Paterson DC, Foster BK: Growth disturbance in Legg-Calvé-Perthes disease and the consequences of surgical treatment. *Clin Orthop* 1991;262:178-184.

100. Moseley CF: The biomechanics of the pediatric hip. *Orthop Clin North Am* 1980;11:3-16.

101. Rab GT: Biomechanical aspects of Salter osteotomy. *Clin Orthop* 1978;132:82-87.

102. Heikkinen E, Lanning P, Suramo I, Puranen J: The venous drainage of the femoral neck as a prognostic sign in Perthes' disease. *Acta Orthop Scand* 1980;51:501-503.

103. Iwasaki K: The change of the venous circulation of the proximal part of the femur after varus osteotomy in Perthes' disease. *Nippon Seikeigeka Gakkai Zasshi* 1986;60:237-249.

104. Arnoldi CC, Lemperg R, Linderholm H: Immediate effect of osteotomy on the intramedullary pressure in the femoral head and neck in patients with degenerative osteoarthritis. *Acta Orthop Scand* 1971;42:454-455.

105. Clancy M, Steel HH: The effect of an incomplete intertrochanteric osteotomy on Legg-Calvé-Perthes disease. *J Bone Joint Surg Am* 1985;67:213-216.

106. Lee DY, Seong SC, Choi IH, Chung CY, Chang BS: Changes of blood flow of the femoral head after subtrochanteric osteotomy in Legg-Perthes' disease: A serial scintigraphic study. *J Pediatr Orthop* 1992;12:731-734.

107. Kitakoji T, Hattori T, Iwata H: Femoral varus osteotomy in Legg-Calvé-Perthes disease: Points at operation to prevent residual problems. *J Pediatr Orthop* 1999;19:76-81.

108. Edgren W: Coxa plana: A clinical and radiological investigation with particular reference to the importance of the metaphyseal changes for the final shape of the proximal part of the femur. *Acta Orthop Scand Suppl* 1965;84:1-129.

109. Gage JR, Cary JM: The effects of trochanteric epiphyseodesis on growth of the proximal end of the femur following necrosis of the capital femoral epiphysis. *J Bone Joint Surg Am* 1980;62:785-794.

110. Stevens PM, Coleman SS: Coxa breva: Its pathogenesis and a rationale for its management. *J Pediatr Orthop* 1985;5:515-521.

111. Mirovsky Y, Axer A, Hendel D: Residual shortening after osteotomy for Perthes' disease: A comparative study. *J Bone Joint Surg Br* 1984;66:184-188.

112. Betz RR, Kumar SJ, Palmer CT, MacEwen GD: Chiari pelvic osteotomy in children and young adults. *J Bone Joint Surg Am* 1988;70:182-191.

113. Dimitriou JK, Leonidou O, Pettas N: Acetabulum augmentation for Legg-Calvé-Perthes disease: 12 children (14 hips) followed for 4 years. *Acta Orthop Scand Suppl* 1997;275:103-105.

114. Klisic P, Bauer R, Bensahel H, Grill F: Chiari's pelvic osteotomy in the treatment of Legg-Calvé-Perthes disease. *Bull Hosp Jt Dis Orthop Inst* 1985;45:111-118.

115. Ippolito E, Tudisco C, Farsetti P: The long-term prognosis of unilateral Perthes' disease. *J Bone Joint Surg Br* 1987;69:243-250.

116. Reinker KA: Early diagnosis and treatment of hinge abduction in Legg-Perthes disease. *J Pediatr Orthop* 1996;16:3-9.

117. Greis PE, Ward WT, Rodosky M, Rudert MJ, Stanitski C: A clinical and comparative biomechanical evaluation of proximal femoral osteotomy fixation in children. *Orthopedics* 1993;16:273-279.

118. Hau R, Dickens DR, Nattrass GR, O'Sullivan M, Torode IP, Graham HK: Which implant for proximal femoral osteotomy in children? A comparison of the AO (ASIF) 90 degree fixed-angle blade plate and the Richards intermediate hip screw. *J Pediatr Orthop* 2000;20:336-343.

119. Beauchesne R, Miller F, Moseley C: Proximal femoral osteotomy using the AO fixed-angle blade plate. *J Pediatr Orthop* 1992;12:735-740.

120. Hansson G, Wallin J: External rotational positioning of the leg after intertrochanteric combined varus-derotational osteotomy in Perthes' disease. *Arch Orthop Trauma Surg* 1997;116:108-111.

121. Kruse RW, Guille JT, Bowen JR: Shelf arthroplasty in patients who have Legg-Calvé-Perthes disease: A study of long-term results. *J Bone Joint Surg Am* 1991;73:1338-1347.

122. Killian JT, Niemann KM: Preoperative skeletal traction in Legg-Perthes disease. *South Med J* 1985;78:928-932.

123. Bennett JT, Mazurek RT, Cash JD: Chiari's osteotomy in the treatment of Perthes' disease. *J Bone Joint Surg Br* 1991;73:225-228.

124. Barer M: Role of innominate osteotomy in the treatment of children with Legg-Perthes disease. *Clin Orthop* 1978;135:82-89.

125. Dekker M, van Rens TH, Slooff TJ: Abstract: Salter's pelvic osteotomy in the treatment of Perthes' disease. *J Bone Joint Surg Br* 1981;63:282.

126. Ingman AM, Paterson DC, Sutherland AD: A comparison between innominate osteotomy and hip spica in the treatment of Legg-Perthes disease. *Clin Orthop* 1982;163:141-147.

127. Maxted MJ, Jackson RK: Innominate osteotomy in Perthes' disease: A radiological survey of results. *J Bone Joint Surg Br* 1985;67:399-401.

128. Robinson HJ Jr, Putter H, Sigmond MB, O'Connor S, Murray KR: Innominate osteotomy in Perthes disease. *J Pediatr Orthop* 1988;8:426-435.

129. Salter RB: Legg-Perthes Disease: Part V. Treatment by innominate osteotomy. *Instr Course Lect* 1973;22:309-316.

130. Salter RB: Legg-Perthes Disease: The scientific basis for the methods of treatment and their indications. *Clin Orthop* 1980;150:8-11.

131. Salter RB, Brown LW: Abstract: Legg-Perthes disease: The long-term results of innominate osteotomy for children with a poor prognosis. *J Bone Joint Surg Br* 1988;70:335.

132. Sponseller PD, Desai SS, Millis MB: Comparison of femoral and innominate osteotomies for the treatment of Legg-Calvé-Perthes disease. *J Bone Joint Surg Am* 1988;70:1131-1139.

133. Sutherland DH, Greenfield R: Double innominate osteotomy. *J Bone Joint Surg Am* 1977;59:1082-1091.

134. Steel HH: Triple osteotomy of the innominate bone. *J Bone Joint Surg Am* 1973;55:343-350.

135. Staheli LT, Chew DE: Slotted acetabular augmentation in childhood and adolescence. *J Pediatr Orthop* 1992;12:569-580.

136. van der Heyden AM, van Tongerloo RB: Abstract: Shelf operation in Perthes' disease. *J Bone Joint Surg Br* 1981;63:282.

137. Bailey TE Jr, Hall JE: Chiari medial displacement osteotomy. *J Pediatr Orthop* 1985;5:635-641.

138. Chiari K: Ergebnisse mit der Beckenosteotomie als Pfannendachplastik. *Z Orthop* 1955;87:14-26.

139. Chiari K: Medial displacement osteotomy of the pelvis. *Clin Orthop* 1974;98:55-71.

140. Klisic PJ: Treatment of Perthes disease in older children. *J Bone and Joint Surg Br* 1983;65:419-427.

141. Schepers A, von Bormann PF, Craig JJ: Abstract: Coxa magna in Perthes' disease: Treatment by chiari pelvic osteotomy. *J Bone Joint Surg Br* 1978;60:297.

142. Chakirgil GS, Isitman AT, Ceten I: Double osteotomy operation in the surgical treatment of coxa plana disease. *Orthopedics* 1985;8:1495-1504.

143. Salter RB: Innominate osteotomy in the treatment of congenital dislocation and subluxation of the hip. *J Bone Joint Surg Br* 1961;43:518-539.

144. Salter RB, Thompson GH: The role of innominate osteotomy in young adults, in Sledge CB (ed): *The Hip. Proceedings of the Seventh Open Scientific Meeting of the Hip Society.* St Louis, MO, CV Mosby, 1979, pp 278-312.

145. Rab GT: Containment of the hip: A theoretical comparison of osteotomies. *Clin Orthop* 1981;154:191-196.

146. Moberg A, Hansson G, Kaniklides C: Results after femoral and innominate osteotomy in Legg-Calvé-Perthes disease. *Clin Orthop* 1997;334:257-264.

147. Park BM, Kim HW, Park SK: Innominate osteotomy for the treatment of Legg-Calvé-Perthes disease. *Yonsei Med J* 1996;37:200-208.

148. Salter RB: Legg-Perthes Disease: Relevant research and its application to treatment, in Leach RE, Hoaglund FT, Riseborough EJ (eds): *Controversies in Orthopaedic Surgery.* Philadelphia, PA, WB Saunders, 1982, pp 289-298.

149. Canale ST, D'Anca AF, Cotler JM, Snedden HE: Innominate osteotomy in Legg-Calvé-Perthes disease. *J Bone Joint Surg Am* 1972;54:25-40.

150. Cotler JM, Donahue J: Innominate osteotomy in the treatment of Legg-Calvé-Perthes disease. *Clin Orthop* 1980;150:95-102.

151. Huang MJ, Huang SC: Surgical treatment of severe Perthes disease: Comparison of triple osteotomy and shelf augmentation. *J Formos Med Assoc* 1999;98:183-189.

152. Daly K, Bruce C, Catterall A: Lateral shelf acetabuloplasty in Perthes disease: A review of the end of growth. *J Bone Joint Surg Br* 1999;81:380-384.

153. Van Der Geest IC, Kooijman MA, Spruit M, Anderson PG, De Smet PM: Shelf acetabuloplasty for Perthes' disease: 12-year follow-up. *Acta Orthop Belg* 2001;67:126-131.

154. Gill AB: Plastic construction of an acetabulum in congenital dislocation of the hip: The Shelf operation. *J Bone Joint Surg* 1935;17:48-59.

155. Kamhi E, MacEwen GD: Treatment of Legg-Calvé-Perthes disease: Prognostic value of Catterall's Classification. *J Bone Joint Surg Am* 1975;57:651-654.

156. Koyama K, Higuchi F, Inoue A: Modified Chiari osteotomy for arthrosis after Perthes disease: 14 hips followed for 2-12 years. *Acta Orthop Scand* 1998;69:129-132.

157. Vukasinovic Z, Slavkovic S, Milickovic S, Siqeca A: Combined Salter innominate osteotomy with femoral shortening versus other methods of treatment for Legg-Calvé-Perthes disease. *J Pediatr Orthop* 2000;9:28-33.

158. Ratliff AHC: Pseudocoxalgia: A study of late results in the adult. *J Bone Joint Surg Br* 1956;38:498-512.

159. Thompson GH, Salter RB: Legg-Calvé-Perthes disease: Current concepts and controversies. *Orthop Clin North Am* 1987;18:617-635.

160. Loder RT, Farley FA, Herring JA, Schork MA, Shyr Y: Bone age determination in children with Legg-Calvé-Perthes disease: A comparison of two methods. *J Pediatr Orthop* 1995;15:90-94.

Developmental Hip Dysplasia and Dislocation: Part I

Stuart L. Weinstein, MD
Scott J. Mubarak, MD
Dennis R. Wenger, MD

Abstract

A thorough knowledge of the normal growth and development of the hip, the causes of abnormal development, and the structural and functional changes that result from developmental hip dysplasia and dislocation provide needed information for treating these conditions. Ultrasonography, newborn screening, and radiographic evaluation are important diagnostic tools.

The ability to make intelligent decisions regarding treatment of developmental hip dysplasia or dislocation requires a thorough understanding of the factors responsible for normal growth and development of the hip joint, the pathoanatomy of the condition, and its natural history.

Normal Growth and Development of the Hip

For normal growth and development of the hip joint to occur, there must be a genetically determined balance of growth of the acetabular and triradiate cartilages and a well-located and centered femoral head. The components of the hip joint—the femoral head and the acetabulum—develop from the same primitive mesenchymal cells. During about the seventh week of intrauterine life, a cleft develops, defining the future femoral head and acetabulum. By the 11th intrauterine week, the hip joint is fully formed, and this is the first time at which a dislocation may occur.[1]

At birth, there is a single chondroepiphysis of the proximal end of the femur. Between the fourth and seventh months of life, the proximal femoral ossification center appears. This osseous centrum continues to enlarge, along with its cartilaginous anlage, until adult life, when only a thin layer of articular cartilage remains. The proximal part of the femur and the trochanter enlarge by appositional cartilage-cell proliferation.[2] The three main growth areas in the proximal part of the femur are the physeal plate, the growth plate of the greater trochanter, and the femoral neck isthmus (Figure 1). It is the normal growth of these three physes

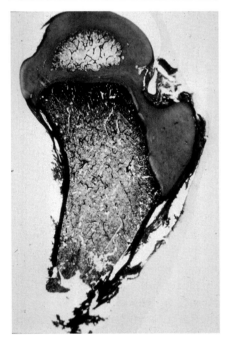

Figure 1 The proximal part of the femur of the infant has three physeal plates: the growth plate of the greater trochanter, the proximal femoral physeal plate, and the growth plate of the femoral neck isthmus connecting the other two plates. (Reproduced with permission from Weinstein SL: Developmental hip dysplasia and dislocation, in Morrissy RT, Weinstein SL (eds): *Lovell and Winter's Pediatric Orthopaedics*, ed 5. Philadelphia, PA, Lippincott Williams & Wilkins, 2001, vol 2, pp 905-956.)

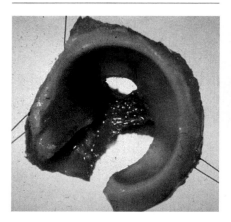

Figure 2 The normal acetabular cartilage complex of a 1-day-old infant. The ilium, ischium, and pubis have been removed with a curet. This lateral view shows the cup-shaped acetabulum. (Reproduced with permission from Ponseti IV: Growth and development of the acetabulum in the normal child: Anatomic, histological, and radiographic studies. *J Bone Joint Surg Am* 1978;60;586-599.)

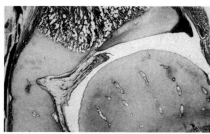

Figure 3 Coronal section through the center of the acetabulum in a full-term infant. Note the fibrocartilaginous edge of the acetabulum, the labrum, at the peripheral edge of the acetabular cartilage. The hip capsule inserts just above the labrum. (Reproduced with permission from Weinstein SL: Developmental hip dysplasia and dislocation, in Morrissy RT, Weinstein SL (eds): *Lovell and Winter's Pediatric Orthopaedics*, ed 5. Philadelphia, PA, Lipincott Williams & Wilkins, 2001, vol 2, pp 905-956.)

that determines adult proximal femoral configuration. Disturbances in growth in any of these three growth plates, by whatever mechanism, alter the shape of the proximal part of the femur. The growth of the proximal part of the femur is also affected by muscle pull, the forces transmitted across the hip joint by weight bearing, normal joint nutrition, circulation, and muscle tone.[3,4] Any alterations in these factors may cause profound changes in the development of the proximal part of the femur.[5] The proximal femoral physeal plate contributes approximately 30% of the growth of the overall length of the femur. Any disruption to the blood supply or damage to the proximal physeal plate results in a varus deformity caused by the continued growth of the trochanter and the growth plate along the femoral neck.[6] Partial physeal arrest patterns may be caused by damage to portions of the proximal femoral physeal plate.

With respect to acetabular development, the acetabular cartilage complex is a three-dimensional structure, interposed between the ilium above, the ischium below, and the pubis in front.[7] The outer two thirds is called the acetabular cartilage and the medial one third, composed of a portion of the ilium, portions of the triradiate cartilage, and a portion of the ischium, is referred to as the nonarticular medial wall (Figure 2). The acetabular cartilage is very cellular hyaline cartilage. Articular cartilage covers the acetabular cartilage on the side that articulates with the femoral head, and on the opposite side is a growth plate with its degenerating cells facing toward the ilium. The lateral portion of the acetabular cartilage is homologous with other epiphyseal cartilages of the skeleton. At the periphery of the acetabular cartilage is the fibrocartilaginous structure known as the labrum. The capsule inserts just above the labrum (Figure 3).

The triradiate cartilage is the con-joined physeal plate of the three pelvic bones. Each side of each limb of the triradiate cartilage has a growth plate. Interstitial growth in the triradiate cartilage causes the acetabulum to expand during growth, determining the acetabular diameter. Differential rates of growth of the triradiate cartilage recently have been defined.[8]

Experimental studies[9] have demonstrated that the development of the acetabulum depends on the geometric pattern within during growth. The concave shape of the hip joint is determined by the presence of a spherical femoral head. This principle is important to remember as a predictor of acetabular shape in the dislocated hip or in a hip in which the proximal femoral growth centers are injured, resulting in deformity. In addition to the presence of a spherical femoral head, several factors determine acetabular depth. These include interstitial growth within the acetabular cartilage, appositional growth under the perichondrium, and growth of adjacent bones (the ilium, ischium, and pubis). Because most of the acetabular shape is determined by the age of 8 years, this is the watershed age for prognosis of many pediatric hip disorders, depending also on other factors including gender and skeletal maturity. Acetabular depth is further enhanced during the adolescent growth spurt by the development of three secondary ossification centers: the acetabular epiphysis, which is the secondary center of ossification of the ilium; the os acetabulum, which is the secondary ossification center of the pubis; and the third, unnamed, secondary ossification center of the ischium. Surgical interventions at the periphery of the acetabulum in the area of the groove of Ranvier or in the area of the development of the secondary centers of ossification have a profound potential to cause growth disturbances leading to dysplasia in adulthood.[10]

One would ideally like to see normal architecture radiographically at maturity, which includes a well-developed teardrop and an intact Shenton line, a downsloping sourcil, and a well-developed Gothic arch (Figure 4).

Pathoanatomy of Developmental Hip Dysplasia and Dislocation

In the normal hip at birth, there is a tight fit between the femoral head and the acetabulum. The femoral head is held in the acetabulum by the surface tension created by the synovial fluid. In postmortem specimens, even after the capsule is sectioned, it is very difficult to dislocate a normal infant's hip. In developmental hip dysplasia or dislocation, however, this tight fit is lost and the femoral head can be made to glide in and out of the acetabulum with a palpable sensation, which feels almost as if the head is gliding in and out over a ridge; this is known as the Ortolani sign.[7,11,12]

The majority of the abnormalities in developmental hip dysplasia or dislocation are on the acetabular side. Changes on the femoral side are secondary to anteversion and pressure changes on the head from the acetabulum or ilium associated with the subluxation or dislocation. With growth and development, however, acetabular growth is affected by the primary disease (abnormal acetabular cartilage either primary or secondary to pressure changes from the femoral head and neck) and any growth alterations incurred from secondary acetabular procedures. Proximal femoral anatomic abnormalities are generally secondary to growth disturbances incurred from treatment.

At birth, the pathologic findings in developmental hip dysplasia or dislocation range from mild capsular laxity to severe dysplastic changes.[13] The typical dysplastic hip has a ridge in the superior-posterior and inferior aspects of the acetabulum. This ridge, or neolimbus, as described by Ortolani is composed of very cellular hyaline cartilage.[13] It is over this ridge that the femoral head glides in and out of the acetabulum, producing the palpable sensation known as the Ortolani sign. In most newborns with developmental hip dysplasia or dislocation, the labrum is everted. There is empiric evidence (such as the 95% success rate of devices like a Pavlik harness) that these pathologic changes are reversible.

Epidemiology and Diagnosis

The etiology of developmental hip dysplasia or dislocation is multifactorial, involving both genetic and intrauterine environmental factors. The overwhelming majority of cases are detectable at birth.[14,15] Despite newborn screening programs, some cases are missed, however. The at-risk group of patients includes those with any combination of the following risk factors: breech delivery, oligohydramnios, female gender, first born, positive family history or ethnic background (eg, Native American), persistent hip asymmetry (eg, abduction of one hip and adduction of the other), torticollis, and lower-limb deformity.[10]

The terminology for developmental hip dysplasia or dislocation is somewhat confusing. The term dysplasia tends to be used for any hip with a positive Ortolani sign (ie, a hip that can be provoked to dislocate or one that is dislocated and can be relocated into the acetabulum). The term dislocation is reserved for any

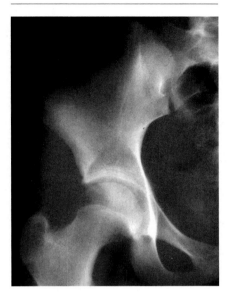

Figure 4 The ideal normal radiographic appearance of the hip at maturity. Note the intact Shenton line (the continuous arch described by the obturator foramen and the femoral neck), a well-developed teardrop figure (the medial floor of the acetabulum), a downsloping sourcil (French for eyebrow [the radiodense arc of the acetabulum above the femoral head]), and a well-developed Gothic arch. (The Gothic arch consists of two groups of trabeculae at the edge of the sourcil. The lateral one extends craniomedially, and the medial one extends craniolaterally. They meet above the sourcil to form an arch.)

hip with a negative Ortolani sign (for example, an unreducible hip) that is associated with secondary adaptive changes of shortening, decreased abduction, and asymmetry of the folds.

Another diagnostic test, the Barlow maneuver, is often referred to as the click of exit. The Barlow maneuver is a provocative maneuver in which the hip is flexed and adducted and the femoral head is felt to exit the acetabulum partially or completely over a ridge of the acetabulum.[16] Many physicians refer to the Ortolani sign as the click of entry, which is caused when the hip is abducted, the trochanter is elevated, and the femoral head glides back into the acetabulum. Some physicians make treatment decisions on the basis of whether they believe that the Ortolani sign is positive instead of on the basis of whether the Barlow sign is positive because they think that a hip with a positive Barlow sign is more stable. In many centers, these classic diagnostic tests have been replaced by ultrasonography, which is used routinely in Europe but rarely as a screening tool in the United States.

If the diagnosis is missed at birth, the natural history of developmental hip dysplasia or dislocation can follow one of four scenarios: the hip can become normal, it can go on to subluxation or partial contact, it can go on to complete dislocation, or it can remain located but retain dysplastic features.[17,18] Because it is not possible to predict the outcome of developmental hip dysplasia or dislocation detected in the newborn and because the risk of complications of treatment by "experts" with a device such as a Pavlik harness is so low, instability of a newborn hip is always treated to ensure the highest rate of normal outcomes.

If the diagnosis of developmental hip dysplasia or dislocation is not made shortly after birth, the obstacles to reduction are different, the risks of treatment are greater, and the results of treatment are considerably less predictable. The physical findings in cases of late diagnosis are limb shortening; asymmetry of the gluteal, thigh, or labial folds; apparent shortening of the femur (the Galeazzi sign); and limited hip abduction, the most reliable late diagnostic sign. A child with bilateral involvement may have a waddling gait and hyperlordosis.[10]

When developmental hip dyspla-sia or dislocation is diagnosed late, the extra-articular obstacles to reduction include the adductor longus and the iliopsoas. The intra-articular obstacles to reduction, in order of decreasing importance, are the antero-medial aspect of the joint capsule, the ligamentum teres, the transverse acetabular ligament, and the neolim-bus (which is rarely an obstacle to reduction).[19] With increasing age at detection (particularly beyond 6 months of age), the obstacles to reduction become increasingly difficult to overcome with nonsurgical methods, and restoration of normal acetabular development is less likely.[20-22]

Much of the older literature describes the limbus as an obstacle to reduction. The definition of the limbus is a hypertrophied labrum. A true limbus is a pathologic structure.[23] In the authors' opinion, a true limbus occurs only in antenatal tera-tologic dislocations or after a failed closed reduction in which the tissue was forced into the acetabulum.[13,24] This is important because the peripheral acetabular tissue in developmental hip dysplasia or dislocation may ossify differently from that in a normal patient. Accessory centers of ossification at the periphery of the acetabular cartilage may appear in as many as two thirds of patients with developmental hip dysplasia or dislocation (Figure 5, A), and they may appear up to 2 to 3 years after reduction.[13,25-27] These accessory centers rarely occur in normal patients (prevalence, 3.5%) and rarely before the age of 11 years. They should be looked for continually after closed or open treatment of developmental hip dysplasia or dislocation, as they must be taken into consideration in the assessment of acetabular development. These accessory centers of ossification are probably the result of damage to the peripheral acetabular cartilage that occurs secondary to pressure from the dislocated femoral head and/or neck pushing against the peripheral acetabular cartilage. This peripheral acetabular tissue, or neolimbus, is rarely an obstacle to reduction and should never be excised.[19,28] Excision will lead to acetabular dysplasia. The apparent acetabular dysplasia in developmental hip dysplasia or dislocation is not a true deficiency but is a failure of ossification of the acetabulum. In young patients, this deficiency is usually anterior. However, in older patients, the deficiency may be anterior, posterior, or global.[29]

The ligamentum teres may be an obstacle to reduction because of its shear bulk and may require removal to obtain a reduction. The transverse acetabular ligament hypertrophies and narrows the inferior aspect of the acetabulum and makes reduction difficult unless it is excised. The most important intra-articular obstacle to reduction is the anteromedial aspect of the joint capsule, which is markedly thickened in dislocated hips and becomes increasingly difficult to overcome the longer that the hip remains dislocated.[10,19]

Natural History in Untreated Patients

The natural history of untreated complete dislocations depends on two factors: bilaterality and the development or lack of development of a false acetabulum.[20,30] Patients with bilateral untreated high dislocation without a false acetabulum have a good range of motion and no pain. However, hyperlordosis and low-back pain develop over time. If the completely dislocated femoral head articulates with the ilium and the patient has a false acetabulum, secondary degenerative arthritis will develop in the false acetabulum. Whether a patient with an untreated unilateral complete dislocation has pain depends on the development or lack of development of a false acetabulum. Other associated problems include limb-length inequality, which can be major (up to 10 cm); ipsilateral valgus knee deformity with attenuation of the medial collateral ligament; degenerative changes in the lateral knee compartment; gait disturbance; and secondary scoliosis.

When discussing the natural history of untreated dysplasia and subluxation in adults, one must first define the terms. Dysplasia has an anatomic definition, which is inadequate development of the femoral head and/or acetabulum. The radiographic definition is determined by the presence or absence of an intact Shenton line. Radiographically, a patient with dysplasia has anatomic abnormalities of the femoral head and/or acetabulum (anatomic dysplasia) with an intact Shenton line, whereas a patient with subluxation has anatomic abnormalities of the femoral head and/or acetabulum (anatomic dysplasia) and a disrupted Shenton line. The natural history of hip subluxation is clear; degenerative joint disease will develop in all patients, usually in the third or fourth decade of life. The natural history of untreated dysplasia in adults is more difficult to predict because physical signs are usually absent and patients only present with dysplasia as an incidental finding on radiographs or if they have symptoms. There is, however, good evidence to support the fact that dysplasia, particularly in females, leads to degenerative joint disease in adults.[31-33]

The information that has been gleaned regarding the natural history of untreated dysplasia and subluxation in adults can be extrapolated to resid-

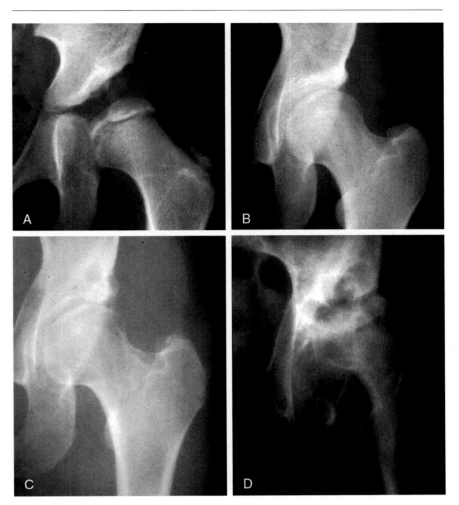

Figure 5 AP radiographs made after closed reduction of a developmental dislocation of the hip that had been performed when the patient was 2 years and 4 months of age. **A,** Thirty-nine months after reduction, when the patient was 5 years and 7 months of age, the accessory centers of ossification were visible in the acetabular cartilage. **B,** Fifteen years after reduction, when the patient was 17 years of age, the Shenton line was intact and there was mild acetabular dysplasia. **C,** Forty-two years after reduction, when the patient was 44 years of age, degenerative changes were present. **D,** Fifty-one years after reduction, when the patient was 53 years of age, the hip was subluxated and had severe degenerative changes (Iowa hip rating, 48 of 100 points). The patient subsequently underwent total hip replacement. (Reproduced with permission from Malvitz TA, Weinstein SL: Closed reduction for congenital dysplasia of the hip: Functional and radiographic results after an average of thirty years. *J Bone Joint Surg Am* 1994;76;1777-1792.)

uals of dysplasia and subluxation after treatment. In a 31-year follow-up study of 152 hips treated with closed reduction, it was evident that the number of subluxations increased over time, as dysplastic hips went on to subluxation and degenerative joint disease developed[22] (Figure 5).

The reason for degenerative changes in dysplastic hips is probably mechanical and is probably related to increased contact stress with time. There is a clear association between excessive contact stress and late de-

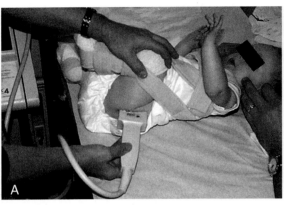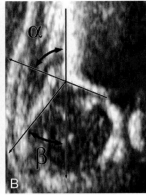

Figure 6 A, For ultrasonography of the hip in a neonate, the hip is positioned in flexion and the transducer is placed in the coronal position to view the acetabulum. Then the hip is stressed to evaluate laxity. Graf's measurements or Harcke's grading of laxity can be performed on this coronal view. **B,** Graf's measurements include the alpha angle (α), measuring the osseous development of the acetabulum, and the beta angle (β), measuring the cartilaginous development of the acetabulum.

generative joint diseases in other mechanical disorders (genu varum and genu valgum). In a recently published study, this same association between dysplastic hips and the development of degenerative joint disease was found at the time of long-term follow-up.[34,35]

The principles of treatment of developmental hip dysplasia or dislocation include obtaining a reduction and maintaining that reduction to provide an optimum environment for acetabular and femoral head development. Intervention to alter an adverse natural history, residual subluxation, and/or residual dysplasia must be considered. The only way to ensure a normal hip in adult life is to detect the disorder at birth.

Management of Developmental Hip Dysplasia or Dislocation

Ultrasonography

The clinical diagnosis of an unstable hip in a newborn can be difficult to make. The physician must have experience, patience, and a relaxed infant to establish this diagnosis. Hip sonography helps to confirm the diagnosis and to identify more subtle forms of the disorder. Almost all newborn infants with dislocatable or dislocated hips can be treated successfully as outpatients when a high-quality Pavlik harness is correctly applied.

Use of ultrasonography to examine hips in neonates was introduced and developed by R. Graf, a pediatric orthopaedist from Austria, in 1980.[36] The method was popularized in the United States by H. Theodore Harcke, a radiologist, in 1984.[37] Harcke's group introduced real-time ultrasonography to evaluate the child's hip in both the coronal and the transverse plane. The ultrasound transducer functions as both a transmitter and receiver of acoustic energy. A high-resolution 5.0-MHz linear transducer is a good standard for most age groups.

Graf's technique initially used a single image with static measurement of the developing acetabulum.[36] Two angles are measured: the alpha angle, measuring the osseous development of the acetabulum, and

the beta angle, measuring the cartilaginous development of the acetabulum (Figure 6). Harcke used real-time sonography to evaluate hip stability. He graded the hips on the basis of the clinical parameters of stability, laxity with stress, subluxation, and dislocation.[37] The problems with the two techniques are that Graf's angular measurements may have weak interrater reliability and Harcke's technique is subjective, with much experience needed to grade the laxity. In 1993, Harcke, Graf, and Clark merged their methods and proposed a dynamic standard minimum examination[38] that included the following positions for the transducer and hip: coronal/neutral, coronal/flexion both at rest and with stress, and transverse/flexion both at rest and with stress. One of the authors (SJM) simplified this technique to include only the flexion position in both the coronal and the transverse view, with and without stress. Most newborns have a hip flexion contracture, which does not allow a neutral view, and later evaluations are usually performed with the infant in the Pavlik harness with the hips flexed (Figure 7).

Ultrasonography is the only diagnostic test that allows real-time evaluation and a three-dimensional view of a neonate's hip.[37,39] The capital femoral epiphysis begins to ossify between the second and eighth months of life, and it develops earlier in females. It is readily seen on ultrasonography.

Newborn Screening

In many centers in Europe, particularly in Austria and Scandinavia, generalized screening of all newborns has been undertaken in a routine fashion. In England and France, selective screening similar to that being performed in the United States is now being used.[38,40] In the United States, it was found that the logistics of screening all newborns, the cost associated with overtreatment of the many children with lax hips, and the still occasionally missed diagnoses in neonates in whom dysplasia later developed dissuaded most centers from carrying out generalized screening. The newborn's hips should be examined clinically at birth, and then the at-risk groups (described above) should be selectively screened with ultrasonography at 4 to 6 weeks of age.

Radiographic Evaluation

Radiographic evaluation to check for hip dysplasia or dislocation in newborns has a high false-negative rate and is seldom diagnostic; however, radiographs often are ordered when the clinical diagnosis is uncertain in the hope that they will clarify the problem. They are difficult to interpret as the hip may or may not be dislocated at the time of the radiographic examination. After the infant reaches 3 to 4 months of age, radiographs become more helpful, demonstrating acetabular dysplasia and hip subluxation. In infants older than 3 months, hips can be classified, according to the appearance on AP and frog-leg lateral radiographs as (1) normal, (2) having acetabular dysplasia (without subluxation), (3) subluxated with associated acetabular dysplasia, or (4) dislocated.

References

1. Watanabe RS: Embryology of the human hip. *Clin Orthop* 1974;98:8-26.

2. Siffert RS: Patterns of deformity of the developing hip. *Clin Orthop* 1981;160:14-29.

3. Gage JR, Cary JM: The effects of trochanteric epiphyseodesis on growth of the proximal end of the femur following necrosis of the capital femoral epiphysis. *J Bone Joint Surg Am* 1980;62:785-794.

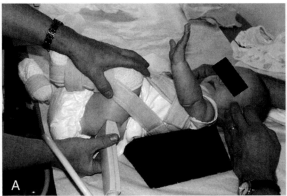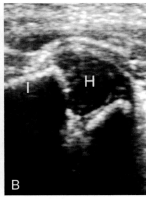

Figure 7 A, Technique for obtaining the transverse view with the hip maintained in flexion. The greater trochanter and the capital femoral epiphysis relative to the ischium are seen on this view. When the hip is stressed in this position, laxity, subluxation, or dislocation can be ascertained quite readily. This is a very important view for validating reduction and final stabilization of the hip. **B,** Transverse view showing the femoral head (H) and its relationship to the acetabulum and ischium (I).

4. Osborne D, Effmann E, Broda K, Harrelson J: The development of the upper end of the femur, with special reference to its internal architecture. *Radiology* 1980;137:71-76.

5. Strayer LM Jr: The embryology of the human hip joint. *Yale J Biol Med* 1943;16:13-26.

6. Iwersen LJ, Kalen V, Eberle C: Relative trochanteric overgrowth after ischemic necrosis in congenital dislocation of the hip. *J Pediatr Orthop* 1989;9:381-385.

7. Ponseti IV: Growth and development of the acetabulum in the normal child: Anatomical, histological, and roentgenographic studies. *J Bone Joint Surg Am* 1978;60:575-585.

8. Portinaro NM, Murray DW, Benson MK: Microanatomy of the acetabular cavity and its relation to growth. *J Bone Joint Surg Br* 2001;83:377-383.

9. Coleman CR, Slager RF, Smith WS: The effect of environmental influence on acetabular development. *Surg Forum* 1958;9:775-780.

10. Weinstein SL: Developmental hip dysplasia and dislocation, in Morrissy RT, Weinstein SL (eds): *Lovell and Winter's Pediatric Orthopaedics,* ed 5. Philadelphia, PA, Lippincott Williams & Wilkins, 2001, vol 2, pp 905-956.

11. Ortolani M: Congenital hip dysplasia in the light of early and very early diagnosis. *Clin Orthop* 1976;119:6-10.

12. Le Damany P: *La Luxation Congenitale de la Hanche: Etudes d'Anatomie Comparee d'Anthropogenie Normale et Pathologique, Deductions Therapeutiques.* Paris, France, Feliz Alcan, 1912.

13. Ponseti IV: Morphology of the acetabulum in congenital dislocation of the hip: Gross, histological and roentgenographic studies. *J Bone Joint Surg Am* 1978;60:586-599.

14. Hadlow V: Neonatal screening for congenital dislocation of the hip: A prospective 21-year survey. *J Bone Joint Surg Br* 1988;70:740-743.

15. Hansson G, Nachemson A, Palmen K: Screening of children with congenital dislocation of the hip joint on the maternity wards in Sweden. *J Pediatr Orthop* 1983;3:271-279.

16. Barlow TG: Early diagnosis and treatment of congenital dislocation of the hip. *J Bone Joint Surg Br* 1962;44:292-301.

17. Coleman SS: Congenital dysplasia of the hip in the Navajo infant. *Clin Orthop* 1968;56:179-193.

18. Yamamuro T, Doi H: Diagnosis and treatment of congenital dislocation of the hip in newborns. *J Jpn Orthop Assoc* 1965;39:492.

19. Ishii Y, Weinstein SL, Ponseti IV: Correlation between arthrograms and operative findings in congenital dislocation of the hip. *Clin Orthop* 1980;153:138-145.

20. Weinstein SL: Natural history of congenital hip dislocation (CDH) and hip dysplasia. *Clin Orthop* 1987;225:62-76.

21. Weinstein SL: Congenital hip dislocation: Long-range problems, residual signs, and symptoms after successful treatment. *Clin Orthop* 1992;281:69-74.

22. Malvitz TA, Weinstein SL: Closed reduction for congenital dysplasia of the hip: Functional and radiographic results after an average of thirty years. *J Bone Joint Surg Am* 1994;76:1777-1792.

23. Leveuf J: Results of open reduction of "true" congenital luxation of the hip. *J Bone Joint Surg Am* 1948;30:875-882.

24. Weinstein SL, Ponseti IV: Congenital dislocation of the hip. *J Bone Joint Surg Am* 1979;61:119-124.

25. Harris NH, Lloyd-Roberts GC, Gallien R: Acetabular development in congenital dislocation of the hip: With special reference to the indications for acetabuloplasty and pelvic or femoral realignment osteotomy. *J Bone Joint Surg Br* 1975;57:46-52.

26. Lindstrom JR, Ponseti IV, Wenger DR: Acetabular development after reduction in congenital dislocation of the hip. *J Bone Joint Surg Am* 1979;61:112-118.

27. Harris NH: Acetabular growth potential in congenital dislocation of the hip and some factors upon which it may depend. *Clin Orthop* 1976;119:99-106.

28. Morcuende JA, Meyer MD, Dolan LA, Weinstein SL: Long-term outcome after open reduction through an anteromedial approach for congenital dislocation of the hip. *J Bone Joint Surg Am* 1997;79:810-817.

29. Millis MB, Murphy SB: Use of computed tomographic reconstruction in planning osteotomies of the hip. *Clin Orthop* 1992;274:154-159.

30. Wedge JH, Wasylenko MJ: The natural history of congenital dislocation of the hip: A critical review. *Clin Orthop* 1978;137:154-162.

31. Schwend RM, Pratt WB, Fultz J: Untreated acetabular dysplasia of the hip in the Navajo: A 34 year case series followup. *Clin Orthop* 1999;364:108-116.

32. Cooperman DR, Wallensten R, Stulberg SD: Acetabular dysplasia in the adult. *Clin Orthop* 1983;175:79-85.

33. Harris WH: Etiology of osteoarthritis of the hip. *Clin Orthop* 1986;213:20-33.

34. Hadley NA, Brown TD, Weinstein SL: The effects of contact pressure elevations and aseptic necrosis on the long-term outcome of congenital hip dislocation. *J Orthop Res* 1990;8:504-513.

35. Maxian TA, Brown TD, Weinstein SL: Chronic stress tolerance levels for human articular cartilage: Two nonuniform contact models applied to long-term follow-up of CDH. *J Biomech* 1995;28:159-166.

36. Graf R: The diagnosis of congenital hip-joint dislocation by the ultrasonic Combound treatment. *Arch Orthop Trauma Surg* 1980;97:117-133.

37. Harcke HT, Grissom LE: Infant hip sonography: Current concepts. *Semin Ultrasound CT MR* 1994;15:256-263.

38. Wientroub S, Grill F: Ultrasonography in developmental dysplasia of the hip. *J Bone Joint Surg Am* 2000;82:1004-1018.

39. Harcke HT, Kumar SJ: The role of ultrasound in the diagnosis and management of congenital dislocation and dysplasia of the hip. *J Bone Joint Surg Am* 1991;73:622-628.

40. Rosendahl K, Markestad T, Lie RT: Ultrasound screening for developmental dysplasia of the hip in the neonate: The effect on treatment rate and prevalence of late cases. *Pediatrics* 1994;94:47-52.

Developmental Hip Dysplasia and Dislocation: Part II

Stuart L. Weinstein, MD
Scott J. Mubarak, MD
Dennis R. Wenger, MD

Abstract

Both nonsurgical and surgical options are available for the treatment of developmental hip dysplasia and dislocation. The advantages, pitfalls, and techniques for using the Pavlik harness should be thoroughly examined before treatment. Other closed and open treatments are aimed at concentric reduction and prevention of residual subluxation and dysplasia. Early diagnosis and treatment lead to the best long-term results for these conditions.

In chapter 4, the basic information underlying decisions regarding treatment of developmental hip dysplasia and dislocation was defined. In this chapter the nonsurgical and surgical management of these conditions will be discussed.

Pavlik Harness

Treatment of the Newborn

The Pavlik harness is used for all degrees of hip dysplasia in otherwise normal newborns. This device has evolved as the clear method of choice for treatment of infants with developmental hip dysplasia or dislocation and has become accepted as the standard of treatment worldwide.[1-13] Although other braces are available,[14] they do not offer the flexibility of use and do not efficiently maintain the hips in the physiologic position of flexion and abduction.

In the 1950s, Arnold Pavlik of Czechoslovakia, wrote five articles on hip dysplasia, his harness, its principles, and his results [15-22](Figure 1). He reported on 1,912 patients, with an 85% rate of good results for dislocated hips and a 2.8% rate of osteonecrosis.

The Pavlik harness consists of a chest strap, shoulder straps, and anterior and posterior stirrup straps that maintain the hips in flexion and abduction while restricting extension and adduction (Figure 2). The kicking motion allowed in the "human position" stretches contracted hip adductors, promotes spontaneous reduction of dislocated hips, and promotes acetabular development. This device should be used to treat newborns with dislocatable or dislocated hips. Infants between 1 and 9 months of age with hip dysplasia, subluxation, or dislocation also are readily managed with the Pavlik harness.

Abduction diapers should be used only for at-risk hips or hips that are identified as unstable in the newborn nursery during the period before definitive treatment with a Pavlik harness can be initiated in the office setting.

Use of the Pavlik harness is contraindicated when there is major muscle imbalance, as in myelomeningocele (L2 to L4 functional level); major stiffness, as in arthrogryposis; or ligamentous laxity, as in Ehlers-Danlos syndrome. Usually, use of the harness should not be initiated for children older than 10 months.[23] Occasionally, a child who starts wearing the harness at 7 or 8 months of age will continue to wear it until 10 to 12 months of age, depending on the child's size. The Pavlik harness also is contraindicated in a family situation in which consistent and careful use cannot be guaranteed.[23]

Treatment of the Infant With Acetabular Dysplasia With or Without Hip Subluxation

The Pavlik harness can be used for infants with limited hip abduction

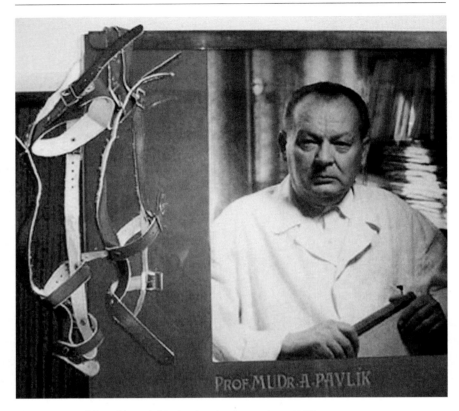

Figure 1 Arnold Pavlik with his leather harness, circa 1955.

and documented acetabular dysplasia with or without subluxation. Following application of the harness, as described, the contracted hip adductors usually stretch, allowing a full range of adduction within 1 to 2 weeks.

In contrast to the newborn with complete dislocation, the infant with dysplasia should be removed from the harness daily for baths. Otherwise, the harness should be worn for 23 hours daily until the findings of clinical and radiographic examination are normal.[23] To achieve this goal, the harness must be worn for a minimum of 3 months by children 3 months of age or younger, whereas children 4 months of age or older usually must wear the harness for approximately double their age. The harness usually is worn part time during the last 2 months. Once the

child approaches the walking age, an alternative form of bracing such as a plastic hip abduction brace will be necessary (Figure 3).

Treatment of Dislocation

A newborn should be placed in a Pavlik harness as soon as the diagnosis of dislocation is made (Figure 4). It is recommended that a newborn with a true dislocation wear the harness full time for several weeks until the dislocatable hip has stabilized in the acetabulum.

Ultrasonography is extremely useful during the early treatment of a patient with developmental hip dislocation. After initially applying the Pavlik harness, one can grade the likelihood of success by evaluating the relationship of the femoral head to the acetabulum.[24,25] The infant should be followed on a weekly basis

with ultrasonography to verify reduction and then stabilization. If the hip continues to demonstrate a positive Ortolani sign, the ultrasound allows viewing of this laxity and determination of whether there has been an improvement or a deterioration in the stability. Studies have shown that monitoring with ultrasonography can markedly decrease the total number of radiographs that have to be made. Furthermore, it greatly increases the chance of successful reduction and stabilization of the hip as it provides evidence of reduction without the need to take the patient to the operating room for arthrographic evaluation.

With the patient followed weekly with ultrasonography and appropriate adjustment of the harness, hip stability usually is achieved by 1 to 3 weeks after initiation of treatment. Once the hip is stable, usually at the 1-week mark, the harness can be removed for one half hour daily for bathing the child and cleaning the harness.

The harness is worn until the findings of the clinical, ultrasound, and radiographic examinations are normal. Radiographs are made with the infant out of the harness at about 3 to 4 months of age. As acetabular development continues, harness wear is gradually limited over the last month to nighttime and naptimes. Infants with a dislocated hip treated at birth wear the harness for an average of 3 months full time and 1 month part time.

The initial ultrasound study made with the patient wearing the harness should document adequate flexion and direction of the femoral head toward the triradiate cartilage.[24,25] If there is still uncertainty about the position of the femoral head despite the ultrasound and radiographs, arthrography should be performed

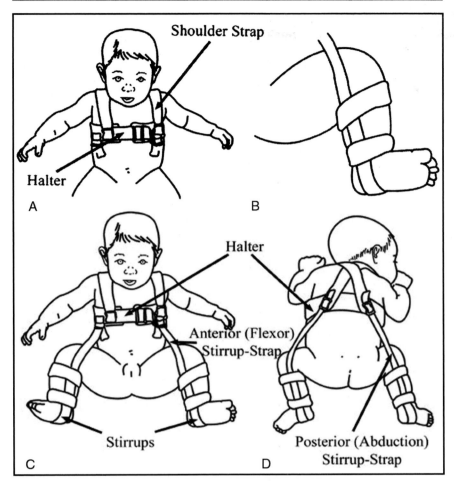

Figure 2 The four steps for application of the Pavlik harness. **A,** The chest halter is applied. The shoulder straps on the halter should cross in the back to prevent them from sliding over and down the child's shoulders. **B,** The leg stirrup straps are applied. The strap for the proximal part of the leg should be located just distal to the popliteal fossa. This strap stabilizes and controls the knee and, when properly positioned, prevents bowstringing of the anterior and posterior stirrup straps. With bowstringing, tightening of the posterior stirrup straps often produces internal rotation and adduction of the hip. **C,** The anterior stirrup straps are attached to the chest halter. The attachment for the anterior (flexor) stirrup straps should be located at the anterior axillary line. If these straps are placed too far medially, tightening them will cause not only flexion but also adduction of the hip. **D,** The posterior (abduction) stirrup straps should be attached over the scapula. The position should be set to hold the hip in 90° of flexion with the posterior straps limiting adduction to prevent dislocation.

with the patient under general anesthesia to evaluate the reduction.

Within 3 weeks following harness application, clinical and ultrasound examinations should confirm hip reduction (Figure 4). Then, if the parents are thought to be reliable and conscientious concerning the care of the child, follow-up can be performed every 4 to 6 weeks. Use of the harness (or, subsequently, an abduction brace) is continued until the hip radiographs show normal findings.

If the hip remains unstable in the Pavlik harness at 3 weeks, use of a hip abduction brace may be tried. This works quite well to stabilize a "loose" hip. Once the hip is stabilized, a return to the Pavlik harness is recommended. If the hip is still not reduced after 3 weeks, the traditional approach is pursued; this includes traction followed by adductor tenotomy, closed reduction and arthrographic assessment under general anesthesia, and spica cast application. Occasionally, open reduction is required.

Results and Pitfalls of Pavlik Harness Use

The reported rate of success of treatment of acetabular dysplasia and subluxation with the Pavlik harness is extremely good.[3,4,9] One of the authors (SJM) had similar success in his experience with treating more than 600 hips in patients ranging from newborn to 9 months of age. Some children must wear the harness for a prolonged period because of delayed acetabular development and severe ligamentous laxity.

At the Children's Hospital San Diego, the success rate of treatment of newborns with an unstable hip (a positive Ortolani sign) is 95%. Use of the Pavlik harness for the treatment of complete dislocation in older infants (more than 1 month of age) leads to successful reduction in about 85% of cases. In children 6 to 9 months of age, this success rate drops further.[23]

In older infants, the most common problem, failure of reduction,[9,13,23] often occurs because the adduction contracture that limits hip abduction prevents reduction of the femoral head. A contracted iliopsoas and constricted hip capsule and/or infolded labrum may also prevent reduction. Obtaining reduction appears to be more difficult in patients with particularly lax ligaments.

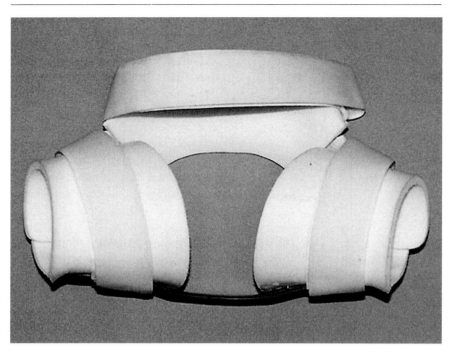

Figure 3 A plastic hip abduction brace can be used to stabilize a newborn's hip or can be used for older children when they begin to walk.

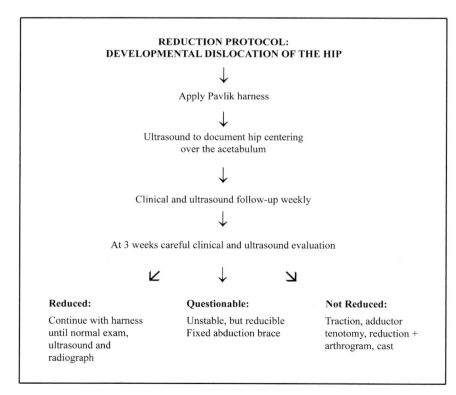

Figure 4 Protocol for reduction of developmental dislocation of the hip.

Mere application of the Pavlik harness does not guarantee reduction in an infant with developmental hip dysplasia or dislocation. Other factors include appropriate indications, selection of a high quality harness, correct application of the harness, and confirmation of concentric reduction by ultrasonography.

Use of the Pavlik harness requires attention to detail; complications can occur (Table 1). Excessive hip flexion can produce an inferior dislocation.[23] Once the femoral head is directed toward the triradiate cartilage, this complication usually can be avoided by relaxing both of the hip flexor stirrup straps and, occasionally, the abductor stirrup straps. Prolonged excessive hip flexion (> 120°) also may cause a femoral nerve palsy.[23] Careful monitoring of femoral nerve function is essential.

The most serious, and fortunately the rarest, complication is osteonecrosis.[13,24-26] The reported prevalence has been higher when the harness has been used to treat complete dislocation of the hip as opposed to subluxation or acetabular dysplasia. Although Pavlik reported osteonecrosis in 2.8% of 632 dislocated hips, the complication developed only in hips requiring manual reduction as well as cast reduction after failure of spontaneous reduction in the harness.[15-22] Current thinking would suggest that the cast, rather than the harness, was the cause of the necrosis in Pavlik's original patients. In a multicenter study of 4,046 hips, Tonnis[27] reported a 15% rate of osteonecrosis, whereas others have reported rates ranging from 4% to 27%.[3,7] In one of those studies,[7] a series of hospitalized patients with developmental hip dysplasia or dislocation were attended by a well-intentioned nursing staff who over tightened the abduction strap to obtain reduction, a step that

Table 1
Problems With Use of a Pavlik Harness and Solutions

Problems	Solutions
Delayed acetabular development as a result of tight adductor, soft-tissue interposition, or neuromuscular disorder	Prolonged harness wear; arthrogram and examination under anesthesia should be considered
Failure of reduction as a result of excessive soft-tissue interposition/ligament laxity	Weekly ultrasound; fixed abduction brace
Inferior dislocation of hip	Decrease flexion to 90° to 110°
Femoral neuropathy	Decrease flexion to 90° to 110°
Osteonecrosis	Decrease abduction
Poor harness construction or fit	Careful evaluation of the harness; change sizes as necessary
Poor compliance	Better parent education regarding developmental hip dysplasia or dislocation and harness use

obviously should be avoided.

The prevalence of osteonecrosis has been found to be negligible when the harness straps are properly adjusted. Kalamchi and MacFarlane,[9] Ramsey and associates,[13] and others[1,2,8] reported no cases of osteonecrosis with use of the harness for the treatment of developmental hip dysplasia or dislocation.

Other pitfalls include a poorly designed harness, patients with developmental delay (hypotonia), or parents who do not fully cooperate with harness use.[23] In addition, some infants who appear to be normal may have a neuromuscular or collagen disorder that will delay the child's and hip's development. Careful attention to the infant's developmental milestones will help the physician to recognize this pitfall.

Parents play a key role in the successful use of the harness; they must be educated about both the disease process (the developmental hip dysplasia or dislocation) and the proper use of the harness. Thorough education of the parents by the orthopaedist and the office staff greatly increases the chance of success.

Abduction Orthosis

An abduction orthosis (Figure 3) should be considered as an alternative to the Pavlik harness for infants more than 9 months of age who require continued abduction positioning because of acetabular dysplasia and/or subluxation. This device maintains abduction while allowing walking, and it is more acceptable for the larger child. An abduction orthosis can be used for patients up to 2.5 years of age. After about 18 months of age, it is usually used only at night, depending on the radiographic appearance of the hip.

Skin Traction Followed by Closed Reduction

Skin traction followed by closed or open reduction is the recommended treatment of older infants with a dislocated hip for which attempted reduction with the Pavlik harness has failed or for children older than 9 months.[1,24,28] This sequence of treatment decreases muscular contractures and allows a safer, gentle closed reduction. The skin traction can be performed at home with the proper set-up.[26,29]

After 2 to 3 weeks of skin traction,

an adductor tenotomy is performed with the child under general anesthesia, closed reduction is attempted, arthrography is performed through a medial approach, and a spica cast is applied. The cast is applied with the hip held in 100° of flexion and 40° to 50° of abduction—the so-called human position (Figure 5).

Preliminary traction is not used to treat children older than 2 years with developmental dislocation of the hip. Such patients are treated with primary femoral shortening, open reduction, capsulorrhaphy, and pelvic osteotomy as described below.

The overall goals in the management of infants with developmental dislocation of the hip are early diagnosis, safe and effective reduction of the hip, minimal inconvenience for the child and family, decreased cost by avoiding prolonged hospitalization, and decreased risks by avoiding anesthesia and spica casts. The results indicate that these goals can best be achieved by understanding Pavlik's method (the correct use of his harness) and using ultrasonography to aid in diagnosis and management.

Surgical Treatment of Developmental Hip Dislocation

Surgical reduction is required for children between the ages of 6 and 18 months when treatment with a Pavlik harness and/or closed reduction attempts have failed. Before attempting the surgical reduction, the surgeon must decide whether traction should be used. We rarely use traction.[30,31] Usually, the decision to perform an open reduction must be made in the operating room following arthrography and failed closed reduction. In this setting, the treating surgeon needs to assess his or her own experience and skills in performing open reduction and also

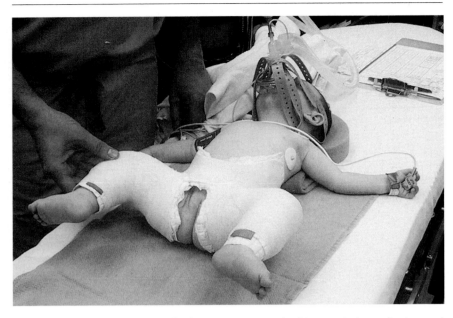

Figure 5 An infant in a cast in the human position. The hips are in hyperflexion and moderate abduction. This provides maximum stability following closed reduction or following a procedure such as the Ludloff operation in which no capsulorrhaphy can be performed.

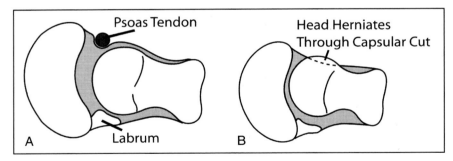

Figure 6 Cross-sectional depiction of the hip in an infant before (**A**) and after (**B**) a Ludloff procedure. Before the Ludloff procedure, the femoral head is lateralized as a result of capsular constriction. After the Ludloff procedure, lengthening the psoas tendon and opening of the capsule has allowed the femoral head to reduce.

whether he or she believes that prior traction will aid in achieving the reduction. Ideally, the surgeon who performs the closed reduction will have the required skills to proceed with an open procedure during the same anesthesia session.

Anteromedial Compared With Anterior Open Reduction (in Children 6 to 24 Months of Age)

In this young age group, either the anteromedial or the anterior approach can be used to reduce the hip. The authors prefer the Mau anteromedial variation of the Ludloff approach.[32] Clear anteromedial exposure allows lengthening of the psoas tendon and opening of the constricted capsule, especially the capsule with an hourglass constriction seen in most dislocated hips (Figure 6), as well as release of the constricted transverse acetabular ligament at the acetabular base. The femoral head can then be safely reduced. Care must be taken to avoid the femoral circumflex vessels with this approach. Also, capsulorrhaphy cannot be performed easily through this approach. Thus, stability is provided by application of the spica cast with the child in the "human position" (as described in the section on closed reduction). Problems with the anteromedial open reduction include redislocation (even in the spica cast), late osteonecrosis,[33] and residual dysplasia. It should be noted that many surgeons and centers have little experience with the anteromedial variation of the Ludloff approach to the hip in an infant. Because the approach, handling of the tissues, and application of the hip spica cast are so demanding, less experienced surgeons should probably choose an anterior open reduction, even in this very young age group. Most surgeons have greater experience with this approach and, furthermore, a capsulorrhaphy can be performed through it. This allows the hip spica to be applied in the relative hip-extended position (Salter), which makes transition to weight bearing easier once the cast is removed (Figure 7).

The hip spica cast in the human position (used with the Ludloff approach) ideally centers the hip for acetabular growth but has associated risks, including that of an increased rate of osteonecrosis.[33] This form of osteonecrosis is usually mild and may be caused by posterolateral labral pressure on the delicate vessels that ascend the femoral neck. Also, this position of hip hyperflexion is maintained for 3 to 4 months, and the required transition to full hip extension for walking (after cast removal) may stress the capsule and may be a cause of residual dysplasia.

For these reasons, most pediatric orthopaedic surgeons use the anteromedial approach primarily in children younger than 1 year. The technique for anterior open reduction will be described in the section below, along with a description of the femoral shortening osteotomy. Anterior open reduction can also be used alone in a child who is younger than 18 months. The technique is identical to that used in the older child.

Surgical Approach to the Older Child (2 Years and Older)

Although open reduction, including femoral shortening, was initially described for children older than 3 to 4 years,[34] we now commonly treat any child older than 2 years with this method.[35] This technique avoids the need for prolonged preliminary traction and has proved to be as effective in younger children as it is in 3- to 4-year-old children. The prevalence of osteonecrosis (10%) in very young children[36] was similar to the prevalence (9%) described in older children.[35] The approach requires treatment in a referral center. Clearly, some surgeons will prefer a more traditional approach of extensive preliminary traction with less comprehensive surgery. The comprehensive single-stage approach to reduction in the older child, which includes capsulorrhaphy, femoral derotational shortening, and acetabuloplasty, will be described.

Open Reduction Including Femoral Shortening and Acetabuloplasty

The pathologic anatomy of the completely dislocated hip was described in chapter 47.[37] The goal of a one-stage reduction is to safely reduce the dislocated hip and to surgically recreate normal anatomy (as closely as possible) that will maintain the re-

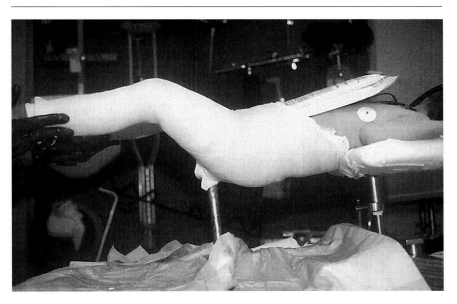

Figure 7 Lateral view of a child in a one and one-half hip spica cast following anterior open reduction of developmental hip dysplasia or dislocation. This relatively hip-extended position can be used following capsulorrhaphy and places the femur in a good position to begin weight bearing once the cast is removed.

duction and allow rapid development of normal hip function.

The patient is placed on a radiolucent operating table in a supine (but 30° oblique) position with a sandbag under the chest but not under the hip as that prevents good skin preparation and good image-intensifier views. Although a sweeping, single anterolateral hip and thigh incision can be used for both the hip reduction and the femoral shortening in very young children, we have found that the resulting scar is likely to spread and may become unsightly. We prefer to use an anterolateral (Salter) incision and a separate lateral longitudinal incision over the femur for the femoral shortening. With femoral shortening, an adductor tenotomy is unnecessary because tension is reduced in all muscle groups, including the adductors.

Capsule Exposure After the skin incision is made, the lateral femoral cutaneous nerve is identified and the interval between the sartorius and

tensor fascia muscles is developed. The iliac crest apophyseal cartilage is then carefully split to allow subsequent anatomic repair. The iliac crest is stripped subperiosteally, first laterally and then medially.

Laterally, the subperiosteal stripping must be carried as distally as possible. In patients with a false acetabulum, the periosteum of the ilium and the distorted hip capsule have condensed into a single layer that must be stripped from the wing of the ilium and the false acetabulum (when present) and down to the level of the true origin of the capsule.

The direct and reflected heads of the rectus femoris tendon are identified, transected, and retracted distally. A plane is developed just above the hip capsule, and the capsule is then dissected from the attached overlying abductors. Clearing the space above the hip capsule as far posteriorly as possible and then connecting it to the already widely opened subperiosteal space on the

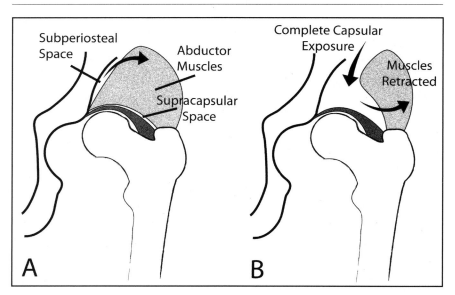

Figure 8 Diagrams illustrating the technique for anterior exposure of a dislocated hip. **A**, The abductor muscles are stripped from the lateral wing of the ilium, and a space above the hip capsule is developed. **B**, With further retraction and dissection, a complete capsular exposure is performed. This includes exposing the anterosuperior and posterior portions of the capsule.

lateral wall of the pelvis provides exposure for the capsulorrhaphy (Figure 8). This cut should extend far posteriorly, providing complete exposure of the displaced hip capsule to a point posterior to the true acetabulum.

Next, the hip is flexed to relax the psoas muscle and to allow a longitudinal incision of the fascia on its deep surface at the pelvic brim. To facilitate exposure of the underlying tendon, the psoas muscle is rotated with a blunt right-angle retractor. A gallbladder-type, right-angle hemostat is placed around only the tendon, allowing the creation of an intramuscular tenotomy. Caution should be used with this maneuver because the femoral nerve, which lies on the anterior surface of the psoas muscle, can easily be mistaken for the psoas tendon.

Capsulotomy Figure 9 illustrates a method for capsulotomy and subsequent corrective capsulorrhaphy. The widely exposed capsule is opened with a scalpel in a T-fashion, with the first cut made parallel to the acetabular rim and a few millimeters below the labrum. This cut is extended posteriorly to a point behind the femoral head. Then, a second capsular cut is made at a right angle to the first and in alignment with the femoral neck. The length of this perpendicular cut determines the size of the triangle of the redundant superolateral capsule that will be excised in preparation for capsular repair. With use of the ligamentum teres as a guide, the capsule is opened distally and medially to the depths of the true acetabulum. Next, the ligamentum teres is transected from the femoral head and, with a Kocher clamp attached to its medial stump, is followed distally and medially to its insertion into the transverse acetabular ligament at the base of the true acetabulum. The transverse ligament is sectioned, and the remains of the ligamentum teres along with any asso-

ciated adipose tissue in the acetabular base are removed. Complete antero-inferior freeing of the constricted capsule provides adequate space for subsequent complete reduction of the femoral head. Often, additional portions of the medial-inferior aspect of the capsule need to be excised.

Femoral Shortening A separate lateral incision is made, beginning at the tip of the greater trochanter and extending distally to a point that provides adequate exposure for femoral shortening. In younger children, this may be nearly to the midpart of the femoral shaft. This longer incision allows careful palpation of the entire greater trochanter. Palpation of the greater trochanteric apophysis, the calcar of the femoral neck, and the lesser trochanter provides landmarks for accurate placement of the initial guidepin and chisel, minimizing image-intensifier exposure. To prepare for derotation, the existing femoral anteversion is estimated by grasping the proximal part of the tibia with the knee flexed to 90°. The anterior aspect of the femoral neck is palpated within the lateral incision to allow an accurate estimation of anteversion.

Anteversion can also be determined by prior CT analysis; however, this is usually not necessary in a patient with no previous treatment in whom the femoral neck can be palpated intraoperatively. In developmental dislocation of the hip, the femur is usually anteverted 40° to 60° compared with the normal 10° to 20°. The neck-shaft angle is usually nearly normal (130° to 140°) and should not be altered with the femoral shortening. Only femoral derotation and shortening are required.

To avoid the production of varus, the initial guide pin is introduced transversely at the distal extent of the greater trochanteric apophysis, and the inserting chisel for the bladeplate is placed parallel to and immediately below the pin. To quantitate the degree of anteversion correction more accurately, a second transverse guide pin is placed in the distal part of the femur just above the femoral condyles (Figure 10). This pin is introduced at a right angle to the femur in the frontal plane but, in cross section, it forms an angular difference in the transverse plane that represents the degree of anteversion correction to be achieved.

A power saw is used to perform the initial osteotomy, 1 cm below and parallel to the inserting chisel. The bone ends are allowed to overlap with the femoral head reduced into the true acetabulum, which allows the surgeon to estimate the degree of shortening required to provide a pressure-free reduction (Figure 11). The femoral shortening osteotomy is then performed with removal of a 1.5- to 2.5-cm segment, as determined by the amount of overlap present with the hip reduced. The osteotomy site is fixed with an appropriately sized blade plate.

Under special circumstances, the surgeon may need to perform femoral shortening in a child whose femur is too small for the AO infant blade plate. In such cases, the four-hole AO mandibular plate is placed anteriorly, bridging the shortening osteotomy at the intertrochanteric level. This plate allows dynamic compression and secure fixation.[36]

Capsulorrhaphy At this point, the femoral head can be easily reduced, and capsular excision and repair can proceed. The Salter-type capsulorrhaphy requires excision of the redundant superolateral and posterior pouch of capsule to minimize the chance of redislocation. Proper excision and repair leaves no space into

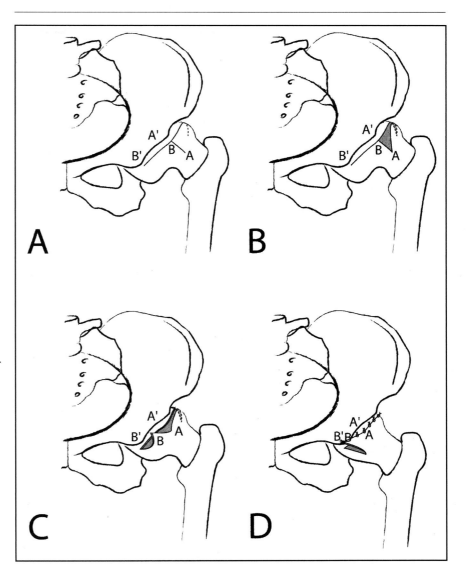

Figure 9 Diagram demonstrating the Salter-type capsulorrhaphy. **A,** Outline of the planned cut in the anterior and superior capsular area. **B,** Excision of the superolateral and posterior segment of redundant capsule (gray shaded area). **C,** Internal rotation of the capsule after the hip has been reduced. Point A, which was on the anterior aspect of the neck, is now rotated to point A', which represents a point just distal to the anterior-inferior iliac spine. The inferior capsular flap (B) is rotated medially and sutured to the periosteum of the pubis (B'). **D,** Careful suturing is done with nonabsorbable sutures, which provides the quality of a hernia repair.

which the head could redislocate.[33]

The T-shaped capsular incision-done previously produced two triangular flaps. The superolateral flap should be excised. As shown in Figure 9, Point A on the capsule, which is the distal extent of the incision parallel to the femoral neck, should be pulled proximally and medially by hip flexion and internal rotation. This maintains the femur in internal rotation and stabilizes the reduction. Point A is sutured to point A', which is on the acetabular rim just distal to the anterior inferior iliac spine. Point B, the corner of the inferomedial

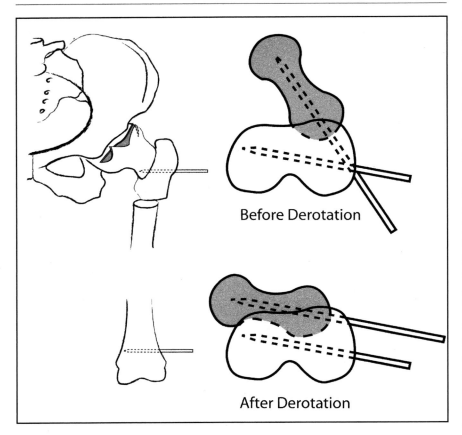

Before Derotation

After Derotation

Figure 10 A method for planning the derotational shortening femoral osteotomy. Smooth pins are placed in the greater trochanteric area and in the distal femoral condyles at an angle equal to the planned degree of anteversion correction. After derotation, the pins are parallel in the transverse plane.

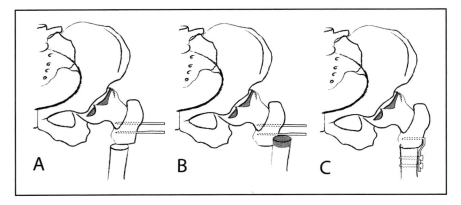

A   B   C

Figure 11 Sequence of the derotational femoral shortening osteotomy. **A,** A subtrochanteric cut is made after the guide pin and AO chisel have been inserted properly. **B,** Overlap method to determine the amount to shorten the femur. The femoral head is reduced in the socket for this assessment. **C,** Internal fixation with an appropriate blade plate.

flap, is sewed to the periosteum of the pubis (B'). Occasionally, this inferior medial flap needs to be excised. The repair is performed with use of interrupted, nonabsorbable sutures in a secure manner similar to that used for a hernia repair. The capsular sutures are usually not tied until the acetabuloplasty (described below) has been performed.

Acetabuloplasty Salter's two landmark publications[37,38] provide an excellent description of the acetabuloplasty. We now perform this procedure in all patients treated with primary open reduction and femoral shortening. We still use Salter's procedure in most patients, although Dega and Pemberton modifications can be used also. The virtue of the traditional Salter procedure is that it redirects the acetabulum, thus immediately improving anterolateral coverage of the femoral head (Figure 12). With other types of acetabuloplasty (especially the Pemberton acetabuloplasty), there is some risk of decreasing acetabular size because the technique includes bending through the triradiate cartilage. Because the acetabulum is already smaller than normal in patients with developmental hip dysplasia or dislocation,[39] one should avoid selecting an acetabuloplasty that may make it even smaller.

In the past, we elected to not perform an acetabuloplasty in younger children[40] (younger than 2 to 3 years) However, subsequent experience has shown this to be an incorrect approach because many of the children later required an acetabuloplasty. We find it far easier to perform the acetabuloplasty at the time of the initial open reduction.

Cast Immobilization After the single-stage hip reduction is complete, suction drainage tubes are placed in each wound and the wounds are closed, ending with a

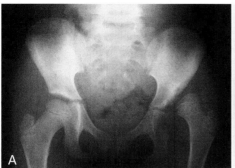
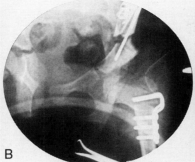
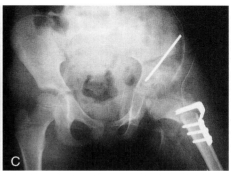

Figure 12 Primary open reduction and derotational femoral shortening together with a Salter innominate osteotomy in a 6-year-old child. **A,** A preoperative radiograph showing a complete dislocation of the left hip. **B,** A radiograph made immediately after derotational femoral shortening and fixation with a blade plate as well as a Salter innominate osteotomy to improve anterolateral coverage of the femoral head. **C,** A radiograph made 6 months postoperatively. The hip remained stable and well reduced.

cosmetic subcuticular suture. The child is placed in a hip spica cast with the hip flexed and abducted 30° (Figure 7).

The hip spica cast is maintained for 6 weeks and then is changed (as a day-surgery procedure with the patient under general anesthesia) to a second, more loosely fitting hip spica cast, which is worn for another 4 to 6 weeks. A Petrie cast can be used for the second cast; however, in young children (especially those who are overweight), such a cast produces excessive stress at the osteotomy site. Therefore, a loosely fitting second hip spica cast is preferred. The second cast is removed 10 weeks after surgery, and no subsequent bracing is required in the typical case.

Summary

Certain patients treated with the one-stage surgical method still have residual hip dysplasia at an older age, which may require another surgical procedure. Surgical correction of residual dysplasia is not covered in this chapter.

Combining primary open reduction, femoral shortening, capsulorrhaphy, and acetabuloplasty in a single operation allows predictable treatment of congenital dislocation of the hip in older children without the time and expense of preliminary traction. In addition to the osseous abnormalities of congenital hip dislocation, the complex pathologic anatomy of the hypertrophied capsule and associated soft tissue must be recognized and corrected. When it is well performed, the one-stage procedure recreates normal hip anatomy (as well as possible) with maintenance of reduction that allows rapid development of normal hip function.

References

1. Erlacher PJ: Early treatment of dysplasia of the hip. *J Int Coll Surg* 1962;38:348-354.

2. Fried A, Seelenfreund M: The treatment of congenital dislocation of the hip by the Pavlik strap brace. *Bull Hosp Joint Dis* 1969;30:153-163.

3. Grill F, Bensahel H, Canadell J, Dungl P, Matasovic T, Vizkelety T: The Pavlik harness in the treatment of congenital dislocating hip: Report on a multicenter study of the European Paediatric Orthopaedic Society. *J Pediatr Orthop* 1988;8:1-8.

4. Guille JT, Pizzutillo PD, MacEwen GD: Development dysplasia of the hip from birth to six months. *J Am Acad Orthop Surg* 2000;8:232-242.

5. Hangen DH, Kasser JR, Emans JB, Millis MB: The Pavlik harness and developmental dysplasia of the hip: Has ultrasound changed treatment patterns? *J Pediatr Orthop* 1995;15:729-735.

6. Hensinger RN: Congenital dislocation of the hip. *Clin Symp* 1979;31:1-31.

7. Iwasaki K: Treatment of congenital dislocation of the hip by the Pavlik harness: Mechanism of reduction and usage. *J Bone Joint Surg Am* 1983;65:760-767.

8. Johnson AH, Aadalen RJ, Eilers VE, Winter RB: Treatment of congenital hip dislocation and dysplasia with the Pavlik harness. *Clin Orthop* 1981;155:25-29.

9. Kalamchi A, MacFarlane R III: The Pavlik harness: Results in patients over three months of age. *J Pediatr Orthop* 1982;2:3-8.

10. McKinnon B, Bosse MJ, Browning WH: Congenital dysplasia of the hip: The lax (subluxatable) newborn hip. *J Pediatr Orthop* 1984;4:422-426.

11. Mubarak SJ, Leach J, Wenger DR: Management of congenital dislocation of the hip in the infant. *Contemp Orthop* 1987;15:29-44.

12. Rachbauer F, Sterzinger W, Klestil T, Krismer M, Frischhut B: Acetabular development following early treatment of hip dysplasia by Pavlik harness. *Arch Orthop Trauma Surg* 1994;113:281-284.

13. Ramsey PL, Lasser S, MacEwen GD: Congenital dislocation of the hip: Use of the Pavlik harness in the child during the first six months of life. *J Bone Joint Surg Am* 1976;58:1000-1004.

14. von Rosen S: Diagnosis and treatment of congenital dislocation of the hip joint in the new-born. *J Bone Joint Surg Br* 1962;44:284-291.

15. Pavlik A: Trmeny jako pomucka pri leceni vrozenych dysplasii kycli u deti. *Lek, listy.* 1950;5:81-85.

16. Pavlik A: Novy smer v lecemi vrozenych vykloubeni kycli u deti do prvniho roku aktivnim pohybem s pomoci trmenu. *Acta Chir Orthop Traum Cech* 1953;20:93-100.

17. Pavlik A: Kotazce funkcniho leceni vrozeneho vymknuti kycli u kojencu. *Acta Chir Orthop Traum Czech* 1955;22:33-40.

18. Pavlik A: Die funktionelle Behandlungsmethode mittels Reimenbügel als Prinzip der konservativen therapie bei angeborenen Huftgelenksverrenkungen der Säuglinge. *Z Orthop Ihre Grenzgeb* 1957;89:341-352.

19. Pavlik A: Kotazce Puvodnosti leceni vrozenych kycelnich dysplasii aktivinim phybem ve tmenech. *Acta Chir Orthop Traum Czech* 1959;26:5-6.

20. Pavlik A: Stirrups as an aid in the treatment of congenital dysplasias of the hip in children: By Arnold Pavlik, 1950. *J Pediatr Orthop* 1989;9:157-159.

21. Pavlik A: The functional method of treatment using a harness with stirrups as the primary method of conservative therapy for infants with congenital dislocation of the hip: 1957. *Clin Orthop* 1992;281:4-10.

22. Pavlik A: To the question of originality of treatment of congenital hip dysplasias by active movement in the stirrups: 1959. *J Pediatr Orthop B* 2001;10:165-168.

23. Mubarak S, Garfin S, Vance R, McKinnon B, Sutherland D: Pitfalls in the use of the Pavlik harness for treatment of congenital dysplasia, subluxation, and dislocation of the hip. *J Bone Joint Surg Am* 1981;63:1239-1248.

24. Suzuki S: Reduction of CDH by the Pavlik harness: Spontaneous reduction observed by ultrasound. *J Bone Joint Surg Br* 1994;76:460-462.

25. Gage JR, Winter RB: Avascular necrosis of the capital femoral epiphysis as a complication of closed reduction of congenital dislocation of the hip: A critical review of twenty years' experience at Gillette Children's Hospital. *J Bone Joint Surg Am* 1972;54:373-388.

26. Joseph K, MacEwen GD, Boos ML: Home traction in the management of congenital dislocation of the hip. *Clin Orthop* 1982;165:83-90.

27. Tonnis D: An evaluation of conservative and operative methods in the treatment of congenital hip dislocation. *Clin Orthop* 1976;119:76-88.

28. Putti V: Early treatment of congenital dislocation of the hip. *J Bone Joint Surg.* 1933;15:16-21.

29. Mubarak SJ, Beck LR, Sutherland D: Home traction in the management of congenital dislocation of the hips. *J Pediatr Orthop* 1986;6:721-723.

30. Quinn RH, Renshaw TS, DeLuca PA: Preliminary traction in the treatment of developmental dislocation of the hip. *J Pediatr Orthop* 1994;14:636-642.

31. Weinstein SL: Traction in developmental dislocation of the hip: Is its use justified? *Clin Orthop* 1997;338:79-85.

32. Mau H, Dorr WM, Henkel L, Lutsche J: Open reduction of congenital dislocation of the hip by Ludloff's method. *J Bone Joint Surg Am* 1971;53:1281-1288.

33. Morceunde JA, Meyer MD, Dolan LA, Weinstein SL: Long-term outcome after open reduction through an anteromedial approach for congenital dislocation of the hip. *J Bone Joint Surg Am* 1997;79: 810-817.

34. Klisic P, Jankovic L: Combined procedure of open reduction and shortening of the femur in treatment of congenital dislocation of the hips in older children. *Clin Orthop* 1976;119:60-69.

35. Galpin RD, Roach JW, Wenger DR, Herring JA, Birch JG: One-stage treatment of congenital dislocation of the hip in older children, including femoral shortening. *J Bone Joint Surg Am* 1989;71:734-741.

36. Wenger DR, Lee CS, Kolman B: Derotational femoral shortening for developmental dislocation of the hip: Special indications and results in the child younger than 2 years. *J Pediatr Orthop* 1995;15:768-779.

37. Salter RB: Innominate osteotomy in the treatment of congenital dislocation and subluxation of the hip. *J Bone Joint Surg Br* 1961;43:518-539.

38. Salter RB, Dubos JP: The first fifteen year's personal experience with innominate osteotomy in the treatment of congenital dislocation and subluxation of the hip. *Clin Orthop* 1974;98:72-103.

39. Ponseti IV: Morphology of the acetabulum in congenital dislocation of the hip: Gross, histological and roentgenographic studies. *J Bone Joint Surg Am* 1978;60:586-599.

40. Wenger DR: Congenital hip dislocation: techniques for primary open reduction including femoral shortening. *Instr Course Lect* 1989;38:343-354.

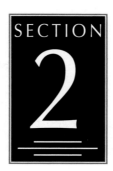

SECTION 2

Congenital Clubfoot

Congenital Clubfoot

The way in which idiopathic clubfoot is treated in the United States and around the world has changed substantially in the past 10 years. In contrast to the rest of surgical evolution, treatment of clubfoot has shifted away from the more invasive posteromedial release toward the minimally invasive Ponseti method. The two articles in this section shed some insight into this change.

Cummings and associates provide a strong, well-crafted review of all aspects of congenital clubfoot. Their article is a good general reference that summarizes current information on genetics, histology, vascular anatomy, radiology, and classification systems. They briefly review the nonsurgical methods of Kite and Ponseti, comparing and contrasting the two. Two of the authors have close connections to the Kite-Lovell school of treatment and to the Ponseti school, which allows for unusually keen insights.

Most of the article, however, is spent detailing the nuances of the open surgical approaches. As more practitioners eschew surgery in favor of the Ponseti approach,

there is a real danger that the next generation of pediatric orthopaedic surgeons will lack the skills for performing these delicate and highly technical posteromedial release surgeries. Many young pediatric orthopaedists may learn this operation from reading descriptions of the procedure rather than from seeing the actual surgery in their residency and fellowship training programs.

The article is an excellent and concise resource for any pediatric orthopaedic surgeon who treats clubfoot. It provides an especially well-organized approach to the surgical treatment of residual deformity, such as forefoot adduction, cavus, heel valgus or varus, dorsal bunion, and dynamic forefoot supination. In addition, the bibliography of 120 articles is comprehensive.

The article by Frederick Dietz is more modest in its goals but no less important for the pediatric orthopaedist treating clubfoot. The author is in the unique position of being both a trainee and partner in practice with Dr. Ponseti and has perhaps the keenest insight into the idiopathic clubfoot outside

of Dr. Ponseti himself. The article addresses management when a relapse develops in a patient treated with the Ponseti method, principally casting, anterior tibialis tendon transfer, and Achilles tendon lengthening.

Various clinical presentations and specific treatment recommendations for children of different ages also are discussed in great detail. This information will be of great value to the new generation of surgeons who use the Ponseti method. These surgeons will have to struggle with a relapse rate that ranges from 1% in the brace-compliant patient to 89% in the noncompliant patient. Dietz cites some intriguing research from Huang and associates that may result in a change in accepted age for anterior tibialis tendon transfer from the current recommendation of 2.5 years of age to 6 to 12 months.

Although these articles are helpful, newer information about clubfoot management has become available since their publication. In this brave new era of nonsurgical management of clubfoot, the role that extensive open surgery (posteromedial release) will play remains to be seen. Neither article addresses some of the newer information coming out of India and Brazil that show efficacy of the Ponseti method in neglected cases of clubfoot in which children present at walking age and older.

The limits of the Ponseti technique also remain unknown. Although many centers have reproduced Dr. Ponseti's short-term results, long-term functional outcome studies done outside of Iowa are needed that compare patients treated with Ponseti method with those who are treated with posteromedial release surgery. The Ponseti method also is used to treat syndromic and teratologic feet, despite the fact that the original description was for idiopathic feet. A novel use of the Taylor spatial frame to recapitulate the Ponseti sequence has been described. I believe that a renaissance of the Ponseti method is upon us and that a veritable cornucopia of new research will soon follow.

John E. Herzenberg, MD, FRCSC
Head of Pediatric Orthopaedics,
  Sinai Hospital of Baltimore
Co-Director, International Center
  for Limb Lengthening
Rubin Institute for Advanced
  Orthopedics
Baltimore, Maryland

Congenital Clubfoot

R. Jay Cummings, MD,
Richard S. Davidson, MD,
Peter F. Armstrong, MD, FRCSC, FAAP
Wallace B. Lehman, MD

Etiology

Genetic Factors

The incidence of clubfoot varies widely with respect to race and sex and increases with the number of affected relatives, suggesting that the etiology is at least partly influenced by genetic factors.[1] The incidence among different races ranges from 0.39 per 1,000 among the Chinese population to 1.2 per 1,000 among Caucasians to 6.8 per 1,000 among Polynesians.[2,3] Lochmiller and associates[4] recently reported a male-to-female ratio of 2.5:1. Siblings of affected individuals have up to a thirtyfold increase in the risk of clubfoot deformity. Clubfoot affects both siblings in 32.5% of monozygotic twins but only 2.9% of dizygotic twins.[5] Lochmiller and associates[4] reported that 24.4% of affected individuals have a family history of idiopathic talipes equinovarus.

Histologic Anomalies

Almost every tissue in the clubfoot has been described as being abnormal.[6] Ultrastructural muscle abnormalities were identified by Isaacs and associates.[7] Handelsman and Badalamente[8] demonstrated an increase in type I:II muscle fiber ratio from the normal 1:2 to 7:1, suggesting a possible link to a primary nerve abnormality. Conversely, Bill and Versfeld[9] were unable to demonstrate neuropathic or myopathic changes in untreated clubfeet with electromyographic studies.

A primary germ plasm defect of bone resulting in deformity of the talus and navicular was suggested by Irani and Sherman in 1963.[10] Defects in the cartilage of clubfeet were demonstrated by Shapiro and Glimcher.[11] Ionasescu and associates[12] identified increased collagen synthesis in clubfeet. Ippolito[13] demonstrated deformity of the talus, with medial angulation of the neck and medial tilting and rotation of the body of the talus. Together with medial tilting and rotation of the calcaneus, these deformities accounted for the varus deformity of the hindfoot, which in turn accounted for the supination of the forefoot. In a study by Davidson and associates, MRI studies demonstrated plantar flexion and varus angular deformity of the talus, calcaneus, and cuboid in the infant's clubfoot (R Davidson, MD, M Hahn, MD, A Hubbard, MD, Amsterdam, The Netherlands, unpublished data, 1996).

Ippolito and Ponseti[6] proposed a theory of retraction fibrosis of the distal muscles of the calf and the supporting connective tissues. In a more recent anatomic and histologic study, Ippolito[13] demonstrated increased fibrosis of muscle tissue in four aborted fetuses with clubfoot. Dietz and associates[14] identified a reduction in cell number and cytoplasm in the posterior tibial tendon sheath compared with that in the anterior tibial tendon sheath, suggesting a regional growth disturbance. Zimny and associates,[15] in an electron microscopic study of the fascia from the medial and lateral sides of clubfeet, suggested that myofibroblasts might contribute to contracture and deformity.

Sano and associates[16] performed immunohistochemical analyses and electron microscopic studies of 41 biopsy specimens from the clubfeet of patients 6 to 30 months old. Contractile proteins and a gradation of cells from fibroblasts to myofibroblasts were observed. The authors suggested that this pattern showed similarities to a healing process and that the presence of the proteins and cells indicated a cause both for the clubfoot deformity and for the common recurrence of the deformity after surgery.

Vascular Anomalies

Hootnick and associates[17] and Sodre and associates[18] observed that the majority of clubfoot deformities were associated with hypoplasia or absence of the anterior tibial artery. Hootnick and associates[17] suggested that vascular dysplasia might have a causal relationship to the clubfoot deformity. Muir and associates[19] found a substantially greater prevalence of the absence of the dorsalis pedis pulse in the parents of children with clubfoot.

Anomalous Muscles

Turco[3] identified anomalous muscles in about 15% of his patients with clubfoot. Porter[20] recently described an anomalous flexor muscle in the calf of five children with clubfoot. He also observed that patients with this anomalous muscle had a greater frequency of first-degree relatives with clubfoot. Chotigavanichaya and associates[21] reported a patient in whom clubfoot was corrected only after release of an accessory soleus muscle.

Intrauterine Factors

Hippocrates suggested that the foot is held in a position of equinovarus by external uterine compression and oligohydramnios.[3] However, Turco[3] suggested that it is unlikely that such increased pressure would repeatedly produce the same deformity, especially when there is sufficient room in the uterus at the time that a clubfoot forms (in the first trimester). In a review of the literature and of his own patients, Turco observed as many left as right clubfeet, despite the asymmetrical positioning of the fetus in the womb. This finding suggests that positioning is not a factor.

Bohm[22] described four stages of fetal development of the foot and suggested the possibility that clubfoot represents an interruption in the development of the normal foot. However, medial displacement of the navicular, which is common in clubfoot, is not seen at any stage in the normally developing foot. Kawashima and Uhthoff[23] studied the anatomy of the human foot from the 8th to the 21st intrauterine week in 147 specimens. Their results suggested that the normal foot appears to be similar to a clubfoot during the ninth week of gestation. They suggested that an interruption in development might be responsible for the deformity.

In recent studies of the complications of amniocentesis, an association has been observed between clubfoot and early amniocentesis (before the 11th week). Farrell and associates[24] reported that the rate of clubfoot after amniocentesis was 1.1%, approximately 10 times higher than the rate of 0.1% associated with all live births. The risk of bilateral deformity was noted to be about the same as that in the general population of patients with clubfoot. When early amniocentesis was associated with an amniotic fluid leak, the risk of clubfoot deformity increased to 15% from 1.1% when leakage did not occur. Farrell and associates[24] postulated that some event during early amniocentesis with fluid leakage stops the development of the foot at a time when the foot is in the clubfoot position. They observed that persistent oligohydramnios was not seen on subsequent ultrasound studies. Farrell and associates also postulated that altered pressure from the leak could alter the developmental process. The CEMAT (Canadian Early and Mid-Trimester Amniocentesis Trial) Group[24] did not find the same association with clubfoot and suggested that the amount of fluid removed at the time of amniocentesis might be responsible for the difference between their findings and those of Farrell and associates.

Robertson and Corbett[25] retrospectively reviewed the medical records of 330 children born with an uncomplicated clubfoot deformity and found that the mean month of conception of these children was June, a finding at variance with the peak months of conception for the overall population of the United States for the same period. They theorized that an intrauterine enterovirus infection with peak rates in the summer and fall could cause anterior horn-cell lesions at the appropriate stage of fetal development, leading to a deformity such as congenital clubfoot.

Physical Examination

It is important to examine the entire body of a patient with clubfoot. Associated anomalies of the upper extremities, back, and legs, as well as abnormal reflexes, can provide information about the etiology of the deformity and the likelihood of successful treatment.

A standardized examination of the clubfoot should be performed initially and after each interval of treatment with manipulation and a cast. A reference point, usually the knee in 90° of flexion, must be chosen for the examination of the foot. Torsional alignment, varus and valgus, and the overall size and shape of the leg, ankle, and foot should be assessed. Torsion is difficult to assess clinically in a patient with clubfoot because the medial malleolus is obscured by the navicular. The congenital clubfoot is generally shorter and wider than the normal foot. Transverse plantar creases or clefts at the midfoot and at the posterior part of the ankle should be noted.[26] Atrophy of the calf is an expected component of clubfoot, particularly in an older child with severe or residual deformity.

Equinus must be assessed with the knee both in extension and in flexion. The true contracture of the gastrocnemius-soleus muscle complex, which crosses the knee, is indicated by the equinus measured with the knee extended. The difference between the equinus measured with the knee flexed and that measured with it extended indicates the amount of stiffness in the ankle joint. The posterior aspect of the calcaneus must be palpated carefully when the equinus is measured because the bone may be pulled proximally away from the heel pad (Fig. 1).

The varus or valgus position of the heel at rest and in the position of best correction should be measured. Flexibility of the subtalar joint is difficult to measure but may give an indication about stiffness.

The lateral border of the foot should be held in the position of maximum correction and measured. Persistent varus, particularly after a trial of cast immobilization, may indicate varus deformity at the calcaneocuboid joint (medialization of the ossification center of the cuboid as

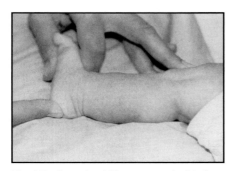

Fig. 1 Equinus should be measured with the knee extended, the subtalar rotation corrected, and the heel in neutral (as much valgus as possible). Although the heel pad may appear to be well positioned, the calcaneus may remain in equinus. Notice how the examiner's finger presses in the heel pad to the calcaneus in equinus position.

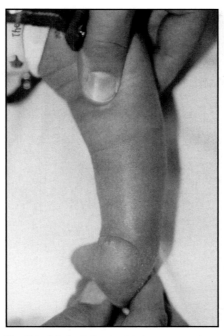

Fig. 2 In this foot, the heel is in varus position but the forefoot is well aligned with the heel. There is no supination of the forefoot on the hindfoot.

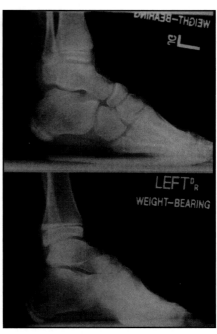

Fig. 3 Two radiographs of the same foot. **Top,** The x-ray beam is focused on the midfoot to demonstrate the talonavicular joint and the midtarsal bones. Note that the fibula is positioned posterior to the tibia and that the talar dome appears flattened. **Bottom,** The x-ray beam is focused on the hindfoot to demonstrate Kite's angle. Note that the fibula overlaps the posterior half of the tibia and that the talar dome is round and high.

described by Simons[27]) or varus deformity of the metatarsals.

The talar head should be palpated dorsolaterally at the midfoot. The talar head usually is lined up with the patella, although in plantar flexion. Manipulation to reduce the forefoot onto the talar head indicates the amount of midfoot stiffness.

Forefoot supination should be noted. All deformities should be assessed in relation to the next most proximal segment—ie, the forefoot on the midfoot, the midfoot on the hindfoot, and the hindfoot on the ankle. If the hindfoot is in 30° of varus and the forefoot (the line of the toes) is angulated 30° in relation to the tibia (Fig. 2), then the deformity is hindfoot varus and there is no forefoot supination. Errors in this assessment may lead the surgeon to overcorrect the forefoot in a cast or to surgically create a pronation deformity.[28]

Palpation of the lateral column with the foot in dorsiflexion can demonstrate overcorrection of the midfoot (iatrogenic rocker-bottom foot).

Radiographic Examination

Although radiographic examination has been used to demonstrate the deformities of the tarsal bones in clubfeet, the images are hard to reproduce, evaluate, and measure. There are several reasons for this: (1) It is difficult to position the foot, particularly when it is very stiff and deformed, in a standard fashion in the x-ray beam. (2) The ossific nuclei do not represent the true shape of the mostly cartilaginous tarsal bones (R Davidson, MD, M Hahn, MD, A Hubbard, MD, Amsterdam, The Netherlands, unpublished data, 1996). (3) In the first year of life, only the talus, calcaneus, and metatarsals may be ossified (the cuboid is ossified at 6 months; the cuneiforms, after 1 year; and the navicular, after 3 years and even later).[29] (4) Rotation distorts the measured angles and makes the talar dome appear flattened (Fig. 3). (5) Failure to hold the foot in the position of best correction makes the foot look worse than it is on the radiograph.

To optimize the radiographic studies, the foot should be held in the position of best correction with weight bearing or, if an infant is being examined, with simulated weight bearing. Because the AP and lateral talocalcaneal angles (Kite's angles[30]) are the most commonly measured angles, the x-ray beam should be focused on the hindfoot (about 30° from the vertical for the AP radiograph, and the lateral radiograph should be transmalleolar with the fibula overlapping the posterior half of the tibia, to avoid rotational distortion) (Fig. 3).

For an older child, it may be useful to focus the x-ray beam on the midfoot because this view allows assessment of dorsolateral subluxation and narrowing of the talonavicular joint. Lateral dorsiflexion and plantar flexion radiographs may be useful to assess ankle motion and hypermobility in the midfoot.

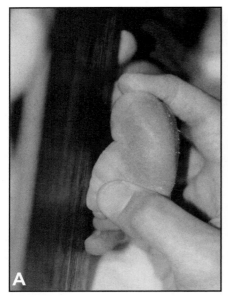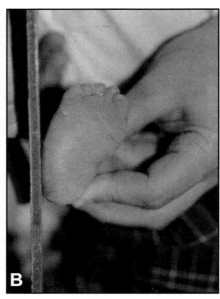

Fig. 4 A clubfoot is bean shaped. **A,** When the radiographic plate is placed against the medial part of the foot, the x-ray beam focuses on the midfoot with the hindfoot rotated, causing increased valgus measurement. **B,** The radiographic plate should be placed against the lateral aspect of the hindfoot so that the x-ray beam is perpendicular to the hindfoot.

Common Radiographic Measurements

Three measurements should be made on the AP radiograph:[30-32] (1) the AP talocalcaneal angle (usually less than 20° in a clubfoot), (2) the talar–first metatarsal angle (up to about 30° of valgus in a normal foot and mild-to-severe varus in a clubfoot), and (3) medial displacement of the cuboid ossification center on the axis of the calcaneus.[33-35] This apparent displacement may represent angular deformity of the calcaneus or medial subluxation of the cuboid on the calcaneus.

To make the lateral radiograph, the foot should be held in maximum dorsiflexion with lateral rotation but without pronation. The x-ray beam should be focused on the hindfoot. The foot should be positioned with the radiographic plate placed laterally against the posterior half of the foot. The clubfoot is bean shaped, and placement of the radiographic plate medially forces the foot to be rotated laterally in the x-ray beam (Fig. 4). Two measurements should be made: (1) the talocalcaneal angle (typically less than 25° in a clubfoot) and (2) the talar–first metatarsal angle. Plantar flexion of the forefoot on the hindfoot indicates contracted plantar soft tissues or midtarsal bone deformity (a triangular navicular).

Classification and Evaluation

Simons[27,32] distinguishes classification from evaluation. Classification involves typing the foot by etiology, such as neurologic, teratologic, or idiopathic. Evaluation involves measuring the foot—ie, the size, shape, range of motion of the joints, and radiographic angles. Both classification and evaluation are important to the understanding of comparative outcome studies and to the successful treatment of each clubfoot.

Clubfeet have been evaluated in many ways, yet there is little agreement on a standard and reproducible method. Cummings and Lovell[35] evaluated 85 parameters of history, physical examination, radiographs, and function in an interobserver study and found only 12 parameters that were reproducible at the 80% level. Watts[36] noted poor reproducibility in the interpretation and measurement of clubfoot radiographs. Flynn and associates[37] studied interobserver reliability in the evaluation of 55 feet with the use of two clubfoot grading systems described by Pirani and associates and by Dimeglio and associates. They found very good reliability after an initial learning curve but observed a lower correlation when therapists' scores were included.

Dimeglio and associates[38] divided clubfeet into four groups with use of a 20-point scale. Points were apportioned according to motion, with 4 points each for equinus, varus of the heel, internal torsion, and adduction. In addition, 1 point each was added for the presence of a posterior crease, a medial crease, cavus, and poor muscle condition. The points were then converted into four grades, each with implications for the success of treatment. Grade I indicated that the clubfoot was mild or postural, not requiring surgery; grade II, that there was considerable reducibility; grade III, that the clubfoot was resistant but partially reducible; and grade IV, that it was teratologic. They recommended that grade I feet be excluded from statistical analysis because they tended to improve results artificially. After excluding grade I feet from their own series, they found that 30% of the remaining deformities were grade II, 61% were grade III, and 9% were grade IV.

Other investigators have developed systems, some employing 100-point scales, for the classification and assessment of function in childhood and adulthood.[39-43] The reproducibility and reliability of these systems have not been established.

Nonsurgical Treatment

The first written record of clubfoot treatment is in the works of Hippocrates from around 400 BC. Hippocrates recommended gentle manipulation of the foot, followed by splinting.[44] The first advance in nonsurgical treatment occurred in 1836, when Guerin introduced the plaster-of-Paris cast.[45] Around the turn of the 20th century, devices such as the Thomas wrench, which allowed the foot to be "corrected" more rapidly through forceful manipulation, were introduced.[46] In 1932, Dr. Hiram Kite,[47] recognizing that forceful manipulation and extensive surgical releases were harmful, recommended a return to gentle manipulation and cast immobilization for the nonsurgical treatment of congenital clubfoot.

Principles of Nonsurgical Treatment
Stretching and Manipulation

The basis on which nonsurgical techniques rest is the correction of deformity through the production of plastic (permanent) deformation (lengthening) of the shortened ligaments and tendons in the involved foot. Serial manipulation and cast immobilization rely on the viscoelastic nature of connective tissue to produce plastic deformation through a process known as stress relaxation. Deformity is corrected as much as possible with gentle stretching, which places the shortened tissues under tension. As the foot is held in the maximally corrected position by the cast, the tension in the shortened tissues decreases over time. When the tension decreases sufficiently, more correction can be obtained by repeating the process.

Most, but not all, advocates of nonsurgical treatment of congenital clubfoot commence manipulative treatment with stretching of the foot. The specific viscoelastic properties of the tissues of the congenital clubfoot relative to those of other connective tissues do not appear to have been studied. Therefore, the duration for which the foot needs to be stretched, the amount of force that needs to be applied, and whether the force should be applied continuously or inter-

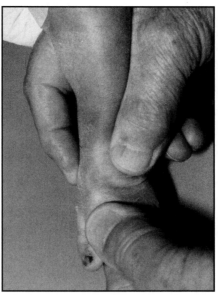

Fig. 5 The Kite and Lovell technique for reduction of the talonavicular joint, using the index finger to gently push the navicular onto the head of the talus.

mittently are unknown. Consequently, there is controversy regarding how much preliminary stretching of the foot should occur before manipulative correction of the deformity is attempted. However, all authors, seem to agree that treatment should be started as early as possible.

There are almost as many techniques for the manipulative treatment of congenital clubfoot as there are authors who write about congenital clubfoot. Many authors have reported success rates of less than 50% for nonsurgical treatment. The two methods that seem to be the most widely performed and that have the highest reported long-term success rates are the Kite and Lovell technique[48] and the Ponseti technique.[49]

The Kite and Lovell technique starts with stretching of the foot through longitudinal traction applied to the foot. Ponseti did not describe the use of preliminary stretching. In both the Kite and Lovell technique and the Ponseti technique, the manipulation starts with reduction of the talonavicular joint. In both

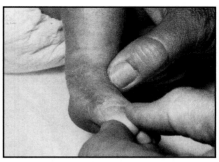

Fig. 6 The Ponseti technique of reduction of the talonavicular joint by pulling the forefoot laterally relative to the hindfoot. Note that the forefoot is aligned with the heel through supination of the forefoot relative to the leg.

techniques, a thumb is placed laterally in the sinus tarsi over the head of the talus. In the Kite and Lovell technique, the navicular is gently pushed onto the head of the talus with the index finger of the same hand (Fig. 5). In the Ponseti technique, the other hand is used to pull the forefoot, and the navicular along with it, laterally onto the head of the talus. Ponseti considered it very important to keep the forefoot supinated during this maneuver (in truth, the forefoot is kept in line with the hindfoot, which is initially in varus) (Fig. 6). Ponseti believed that failing to do so, or pronating the forefoot relative to the hindfoot, produces a cavus deformity. In the Kite and Lovell technique, a slipper cast is applied after the talonavicular joint is reduced. As the cast dries, the foot is molded on Plexiglas, with simultaneous pushing of the heel out of varus and flattening of the foot to prevent cavus.

The lateral pulling of the forefoot relative to the hindfoot in the Ponseti technique also corrects the forefoot adduction. The Kite and Lovell technique corrects forefoot adduction by abducting the forefoot on the hindfoot as the slipper cast dries. In this maneuver, a finger is placed laterally over the distal end of the calcaneus to act as a fulcrum. Ponseti termed this maneuver "Kite's error," con-

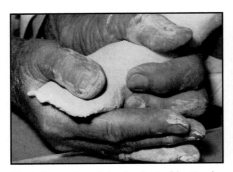

Fig. 7 Correction of the forefoot adduction by abducting the forefoot with counterpressure applied at the calcaneocuboid joint.

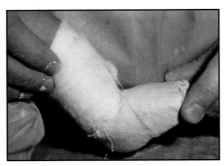

Fig. 8 The slipper cast is used to externally rotate the foot, correcting internal rotation or medial spin of the calcaneus beneath the talus.

tending that any force applied laterally to the distal part of the calcaneus to correct forefoot adduction prevents the distal end of the calcaneus from moving laterally as the calcaneus is externally rotated out from under the talus (Fig. 7). Kite and Lovell actually used the slipper cast to externally rotate the calcaneus and forefoot as a unit from beneath the talus (Fig. 8). In both techniques, the cast is then extended to the thigh while the foot is held in external rotation.

In both the Kite and Lovell technique and the Ponseti technique, no effort is made to correct equinus until forefoot adduction and heel varus are corrected because an attempt to correct equinus before correction of the other deformities leads to a rocker-bottom deformity. According to Ponseti,[49] when equinus persisted after the forefoot and hindfoot were corrected, a tenotomy of the Achilles tendon was performed percutaneously with the use of local anesthesia in the cast room, and then application of the cast was continued. Kite and Lovell preferred wedging the cast when equinus could not be corrected after the forefoot adduction and heel varus were corrected.[48]

Ponseti[49] reported that 89% of the feet in his study had a good or excellent result at 30-year follow-up. However, Achilles tenotomies were required in 70% of his patients. Ponseti reported a 50% rate of recurrence requiring addi-

tional cast treatment. Deformities that recurred frequently required lengthening of the Achilles tendon and transfer of the anterior tibial tendon to maintain correction.[49] Ponseti now reports that the recurrence rate in his patients is far lower (IV Ponseti, MD, personal communication, 2001). Kite and Lovell reported that up to 95% of feet can be completely corrected without any surgery. However, the average duration of cast treatment with their technique is 22 months compared with 2 to 4 months with the Ponseti technique (WW Lovell, MD, personal communication, 1998).

While the most common way to maintain the position of the foot after manipulation is with a plaster cast, other methods have been used. Shaw,[50] among others, favored the use of adhesive tape and reported a success rate of 70% with his technique.

How often the cycle of manipulation and immobilization is repeated varies. Most physicians change the cast and remanipulate the foot at weekly intervals. More rapid correction has been achieved with more frequent (daily) cast changes and manipulation.

After the foot has been corrected (usually as determined on radiographs), it is held in the corrected position for some period of time. The initial holding device is usually a cast, and after 2 to 4 weeks of

such treatment, the patient is frequently managed with braces. Kite used a Phelps splint, which was worn until the age of 10 years. Ponseti recommended that a Denis Browne bar be worn until the age of 2 to 4 years. Currently many surgeons discontinue splinting after the child is able to walk independently.

Newer Methods of Nonsurgical Treatment

For some time, there has been an interest in nonsurgical methods that emphasize motion and minimize immobilization. In 1937, Denis Browne[51] introduced a technique, modified in 1942 by Thomson,[52] in which the child's own "physiologic motions" were used to correct the foot through a dynamic mechanism. The technique consisted of the application of corrective shoes that were then attached to a bar. The attachment of the shoes to the bar allowed progressive external rotation of the feet. While the feet were in this apparatus, the constant kicking by the infant stretched the contracted tissues, thereby correcting the deformity. Recently, Yamamoto and Furuya[53] reported on a series of 91 clubfeet treated with a modified Denis Browne splint. Sixty feet were corrected without surgery, and good or excellent correction was maintained at an average of 6 years 3 months after treatment.

Bensahel and associates[54,55] developed a nonsurgical technique involving manipulation of the foot by a physical therapist. Each manipulative session lasts 30 minutes and is followed by taping of the foot to a wooden splint. This treatment is performed daily for up to 8 months. Bensahel and associates reported that 48% of their patients had a good result.

Dimeglio and associates[56] described what would seem to be the ultimate stretching treatment for congenital clubfoot, continuous passive motion. As with the method of Bensahel and associates, the foot is manipulated by a physical therapist for 30 minutes. After the manipulation, the foot is placed in a machine that performs stretching (continuous passive motion). Treatment is usually started at about 2 weeks of age. The machine is adjusted daily on the basis of an examination of the foot. The foot is maintained in the machine for up to 8 hours each day. After each session, a splint is applied to hold the foot in the maximally corrected position until the next day. Dimeglio and associates[56] reported that, in a series of 216 feet, 45 had to be excluded because the children's parents were "noncompliant" and 68% of the remaining feet were deemed to have a successful result. It is important to note that "success" did not necessarily mean that no surgery was required. Treatment was deemed to be successful when the required surgery proved to be less extensive than that predicted to be necessary on the basis of the examination of the foot before treatment was started. It was possible to avoid surgery on the lateral side of the foot in 32% of the feet that required surgery.

Johnston and Richards[57] recently reported their results with what they termed the French method. In their study, 48 feet were treated with a regimen of stretching exercises. A continuous passive motion machine was not used. Thirty-six feet were successfully treated without surgery, nine required minimal surgery, and three required a comprehensive soft-tissue release. In a follow-up study, Richards and associates found the French technique to be more effective than traditional manipulation and immobilization in a short-leg cast (BS Richards II, MD, CE Johnston II, MD, H Wilson, MD, Vancouver, BC, Canada, unpublished data, 2000). Ponseti, commenting on the later study, noted that short-leg casts, used by Richards and associates, were in his experience less effective than long-leg casts.

An interesting adjunct to the French technique, as described by Johnston and Richards, has recently been reported. Delgado and associates[58] injected botulinum toxin type A (Botox; Allergan, Irvine, CA) into the gastrocnemius-soleus and posterior tibial muscles of three infants with congenital clubfoot that had been incompletely corrected by the French method. After the injections, additional correction was obtained with continued nonsurgical treatment. The rationale for the use of Botox appears to be that a reduction of tone in the most contracted muscles might facilitate their lengthening by manipulative stretching. Determining whether such pharmacologic intervention is useful will require additional study.

Another process that can be used to produce plastic deformation of soft tissues is known as creep. Creep occurs when tendons and ligaments elongate as a result of a continuous stretching. Creep can be produced by dynamic splinting, which has been found to be helpful when used in conjunction with serial manipulation and cast treatment.[59] We have been unable to find reports on the use of dynamic splinting as a primary nonsurgical treatment modality. Skin irritation and, on occasion, skin breakdown may limit the usefulness of this technique.

Surgical Treatment

Despite our best efforts, some clubfeet cannot be completely corrected with nonsurgical treatment. In such feet, soft-tissue release is clearly indicated.

Preoperative Assessment

All clubfeet are not the same. Therefore, it is important to assess the foot carefully to determine the components of the deformity that remain. Once that has been done, the surgeon must think about which anatomic structures contribute to each component of the deformity. Obviously, those are the structures that need to be addressed at the time of surgery. A foot in which all components of the deformity are still present likely requires a full pos-teromedial plantar lateral release. If the clinical examination indicates a flexible forefoot and midfoot with a straight lateral border and a palpable interval between the tuberosity of the navicular and the medial malleolus but a persistent equinus, then a posterior release may be all that is needed.

Radiographic assessment of the foot complements the clinical examination. Radiographs can be used to determine the relationship between the talus and the calcaneus in both the AP and lateral planes. The radiographs reveal whether there is subluxation of the talonavicular joint and the calcaneocuboid joint and whether the foot has a cavus component. The lateral radiograph can reveal the degree of persistent equinus in the ankle. We believe very strongly in the "à la carte" approach to the clubfoot as described by Bensahel and associates[60]—ie, do only what is necessary to get a good correction of the foot.

Age

Most surgeons have one of two opinions concerning the optimum age at which surgery should be performed. Advocates of "early" treatment perform the surgery when the patient is between 3 and 6 months old.[61] They argue that there is a great deal of growth in the foot and therefore a lot of remodeling potential during the first year of life. In contrast, advocates of "late" treatment prefer to wait until the child is 9 to 12 months old.[62] They believe that, because the components of the foot are larger, the pathoanatomy is more obvious, and the surgery is easier to perform. Also, because the child is by then old enough to walk, early weight bearing may help prevent the recurrence of deformity. Simons[63] recommended that the size of the foot rather than the age of the patient be used to determine the optimum time to perform the surgery. He stated that the foot should be 8 cm long or longer at the time of surgery.

Incisions

Incisions fall into one of three categories: the Turco oblique or hockey-stick posteromedial type of incision;[3] the circumferential incision, more commonly referred to as the Cincinnati incision;[64] and the two-incision or Carroll approach.[65] Each has its limitations. The Turco incision crosses the skin creases on the medial side of the foot and ankle. It is certainly more difficult to reach the posterolateral structures, such as the talofibular and calcaneofibular ligaments, through this incision. The origin of the plantar fascia also may be a challenge to expose and release. The Cincinnati incision has the potential for creating problems with the skin edges. It also has been criticized for its limited exposure of the Achilles tendon. The criticism of the Carroll approach is that it can limit the correction of the equinus and/or varus deformity because of the posteromedial skin tether. We prefer the Cincinnati incision.

Medial Plantar Release

The abductor hallucis muscle is the guide for the initial part of the procedure. As long as the surgeon cuts on top of the muscle, no vital structures will be damaged. It should be followed proximally to its origin from the calcaneus. As it is exposed proximally, some thickened fascia that crosses the muscle in a vertical direction may be encountered. The fascia is divided, and the abductor hallucis is released from the calcaneus. The part of the origin that passes between the medial and lateral neurovascular bundles and attaches to the sustentaculum tali also must be released. The muscle is then reflected distally. The motor branch from the medial plantar nerve can be cut without important consequences. Dividing the laciniate ligament then exposes the medial plantar neurovascular bundle. Careful dissection is continued distally to the forefoot. An artery and two small veins cross the nerve in the midfoot. They can be cauterized and divided. The

lateral plantar bundle is then identified. The main calcaneal branch is the most posterior structure. The bundle is protected by a 0.25-inch (0.64-cm) Penrose drain. The interval between the vein and the calcaneal branch is a safe area in which to approach the origin of the plantar fascia and the short toe flexors. Their origins are divided across the plantar aspect. Obviously, this release is done only when the deformity is thought to have a cavus component.[63]

The next structures to be identified are the tendons of the flexor digitorum longus and flexor hallucis longus. They are followed distally past the master knot of Henry and proximally above the ankle joint. As the flexor hallucis longus passes under the sustentaculum tali, there is a thick retinaculum to be divided. McKay[66] described preservation of the sheaths of these tendons. The dissection continues on the plantar aspect of the foot. The tendon of the peroneus longus is identified and is carefully released from its sheath as far as the lateral border of the foot. This tendon passes around the lateral border at the level of the calcaneocuboid joint. It must be carefully protected. Many surgeons make the mistake of looking for the calcaneocuboid joint too distally. Care must be taken because it is very easy to create a joint by cutting through cartilage. Once the joint definitely has been identified, it should be released medially and plantarly. A thin elevator such as a Freer elevator then can be used to fenestrate the lateral part of the capsule. The medial part of the capsule and the spring ligament are divided, which also helps to identify the medial-inferior portion of the talonavicular joint. By lifting the tendons and bundle, the medial portion of the talocalcaneal capsule can be identified and released. Care must be taken not to start the release too far posteriorly, where the ankle and subtalar joints are close together, because it is easy to mistake the subtalar joint for the ankle joint. The risk is that the deep deltoid ligament could be

divided completely. Care also should be taken not to damage the sustentaculum tali.

The tendon of the tibialis posterior muscle is then identified above the ankle joint. The sheath is carefully divided longitudinally. Some of the retinaculum is preserved as a bridge distally. A Z-plasty of the tendon is carried out, and the distal stump is pulled through the retinacular bridge. Finding the talonavicular joint can be somewhat challenging. It is critical to remember that the plane of this joint is parallel to the medial aspect of the talar neck. The inferior portion may be approached first. Distraction of the joint by pulling on the insertion of the tibialis posterior helps in the release. The dorsal structures, such as the tibialis anterior muscle, the extensor tendons, and the neurovascular structures, must be protected. As the capsule is released dorsally, care must be taken not to divide the deep deltoid ligament and to avoid the dorsum of the neck of the talus. Both of these areas contain important blood supplies to the talus. The talonavicular joint capsule should be fully divided dorsally, medially, and plantarly. The Freer elevator can be used to fenestrate the lateral aspect of the capsule. Carroll[67] also suggested division of the slips of the tibialis posterior that run forward to attach to the undersurfaces of the cuneiforms and the bases of the second, third, and fourth metatarsals. The medial plantar release should then be complete (Fig. 9).

Posterior Release

As the posterior part of the skin incision is made, it is important not to cut too deeply. The Achilles tendon is exposed as far proximally as possible. A Z-plasty is performed, detaching the medial end distally, to reduce the tendency of the tendon to pull the heel into varus. McKay[66] preferred to lengthen the Achilles tendon with a coronal Z-plasty.

The structures that pass behind the medial malleolus already have been iden-

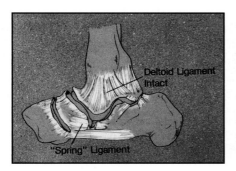

Fig. 9 The medial plantar release.

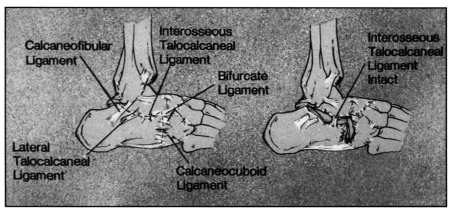

Fig. 10 The lateral release.

tified and protected. The lateral structures now need to be dissected. The sural nerve is found and protected. The peroneal tendons are exposed, and the sheath is divided distally, beginning at the tip of the lateral malleolus. The sheath should not be divided proximal to that level, if possible, to prevent later subluxation of the tendons anterior to the lateral malleolus. The talocalcaneal joint is opened first. The release already has been performed medially and is now continued posteriorly and laterally. With retraction of the lateral structures, the calcaneofibular ligament is divided. This is an important part of the procedure because this ligament tethers the calcaneus to the fibula. It would be impossible to rotate the calcaneus into the corrected position without this release. The lateral capsular release is continued as far as can be seen from the posterior perspective. Then the ankle joint is carefully approached. If the ankle is in substantial equinus, not much of the posterior part of the talar body is between the calcaneus and the tibial plafond. Care must be taken not to enter the distal tibial physis while looking for the ankle joint. The ankle joint capsule is released from the posteromedial corner of the body of the talus to the posterolateral corner. It is easy to mistake the lateral surface of the talus for the posterior surface and therefore carry out an extensive lateral release rather than a posterior release. The posterior talofibular ligament should be divided. Some

authors also have recommended the release of the posterior tibiofibular ligament to allow more room for the body of the talus when it is brought out of equinus.[48]

Lateral Release

The releases described allow for excellent correction of the deformity in many feet. In some feet, however, there will still be difficulty in rotating the calcaneus outwardly relative to the talus. In these cases, a more extensive lateral release needs to be performed (Fig. 10). During this dissection, the sural nerve and peroneal tendons are protected. Capsulotomies of the talonavicular and calcaneocuboid joints should be performed, if necessary. Also, as much of the interosseous ligament as necessary can be divided to spin the calcaneus on the talus. We usually try to preserve at least the medial portion of this ligament.

Reduction and Fixation

The talus should be inwardly rotated slightly, and the navicular should be reduced on the head of the talus. When the navicular is properly reduced, the medial tuberosity should be prominent. If it is flush with the medial aspect of the talar head and neck, it is overreduced laterally. It should, however, be flush with the dorsum of the talar head. According

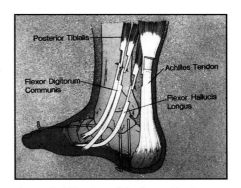

Fig. 11 Stabilization of the foot with pins.

to Simons,[63] the pin should be placed centrally in the head and drilled in a retrograde fashion until it emerges at the posterolateral ridge of the talus. The navicular is reduced, and the pin is then driven across the joint. In the sagittal plane, the pin should be in line with the first metatarsal. Often this is the only pin necessary to maintain the reduction. The calcaneus needs to be rotated such that the tuberosity moves medially away from the fibula. The cuboid needs to be reduced on the end of the calcaneus, and pinning may be required to stabilize this reduction. If the interosseous ligament has been completely released, the subtalar joint needs to be stabilized (Fig. 11). The pin is placed through the plantar surface of the calcaneus, across the subtalar joint and into the talus. It should not pass into the ankle joint. Care should be taken to ensure that the calcaneus is not tipped into varus or valgus.

Intraoperative Assessment

Once the reduction and pinning have been completed, the degree of tightness of the toe flexors should be assessed. If the toes cannot be brought easily to the neutral position, the flexor digitorum longus and/or the flexor hallucis longus should be lengthened. The position of the foot should be checked with the knee in 90° of flexion. It must be plantigrade without a varus, valgus, supination, or pronation deformity. The thigh-foot axis should be outwardly rotated 0° to 20°.

There is a difference of opinion about the value of intraoperative radiographs. Some surgeons use them, and others believe that radiographs are not necessary if the foot is carefully positioned and clinically assessed at the end of the procedure.[48] If there are any doubts about the quality of the reduction on clinical examination, radiographs can help determine the site of the problem. If the reduction is not satisfactory, the pins must be removed and the foot repositioned.

The distal stump of the tibialis posterior tendon is then pulled back under the bridge of the retinaculum. It is sutured under some tension to help to prevent the tendency for an overcorrected planovalgus foot to develop. If the flexor hallucis longus and flexor digitorum longus tendons have been lengthened, they are repaired without tension. The Achilles tendon is repaired with the ankle in 10° of plantar flexion so that there is some tension on it when the foot is in the neutral position.

Wound Closure

Some surgeons allow the foot to return to an equinovarus position and close the skin completely. A manipulation is planned for 1 to 3 weeks postoperatively to bring the foot up into the neutral position. Other surgeons position the foot in the neutral position, approximate the skin medially

and laterally, and leave a skin gap posteriorly. Gaps as large as 2 to 3 cm have been left with good healing and minimal scarring.[69] The wound is dressed, and some form of immobilization, which varies from a soft dressing to a full above-the-knee cast, is applied. Some surgeons bivalve the cast, and others do not.

Postoperative Management

We use either a continuous epidural block, begun after intubation, or a "one-shot" caudal block at the end of the procedure. We have been impressed with the comfort provided to the child, and, at the time of writing, there have not been any complications attributable to these blocks. At 1 week postoperatively, the child is sedated, the postoperative dressing is removed, and the wounds are inspected. The foot is held in the neutral, plantigrade position, and a cast is applied. The knee is held at 90° of flexion, the foot is outwardly rotated, and the cast is extended above the knee. The cast is worn for 4 to 6 weeks, after which the child returns to the clinic, the pin or pins are removed, and an ankle-foot orthosis is fitted. The orthosis is worn for 6 months, and the foot is then reevaluated.

Revision Surgery

The objective of clubfoot surgery is to obtain a complete and lasting correction with one operation. However, about 25% (range, 13% to 50%) of the feet have a recurrence.[69,70] The most common persistent deformities are forefoot adduction and supination. However, varus, equinus, cavus, and overcorrection of the heel all have been reported following clubfoot surgery.[71] Recurrence of one or more components of the clubfoot deformity may result from an incomplete correction, failure to maintain correction, tarsal bone remodeling, abnormal scar formation with tethering of tendons, and tarsal coalition that was either iatrogenic or missed during the surgical procedure.[70]

Preoperative Evaluation

A rating system has been developed to determine the need for revision surgery. S cores of less than 60 points (of a possible total of 100 points) indicate the need for revision (Fig. 12). The preoperative radiographic evaluation includes AP and lateral radiographs of the foot in maximum dorsiflexion, as previously described.[31,32] In addition, when the previously described radiographic angles are measured, the radiographs should be reviewed for other changes, including subluxation of the tarsal navicular, flattening of the trochlear surface of the talus, and shortening of the calcaneus. Once the clinical and radiographic evaluations are complete, attention is turned to correction of the residual deformity. An algorithm has been developed as a guide for the choice of which procedure or procedures to perform (Table 1).[72]

Treatment of Residual Deformity
Residual Forefoot Adduction

Residual adduction is usually found at the midfoot and occasionally at the forefoot. In patients younger than 2 years, forefoot adduction is treated with repeat complete soft-tissue releases.[73] In patients 2 to 4 years old, osteotomies are not recommended because of the immaturity of the foot. Excision of the calcaneocuboid joint cartilage or cuboid enucleation is a better option. These procedures must be combined with a medial soft-tissue release. Cuboid decancellation preserves the articular surface of the cuboid surface proximally and distally, while "crushing" of the bone shortens the lateral column and corrects adduction.[3]

For patients older than 4 years, many procedures have been described, including excision of the distal part of the calcaneus,[74] fusion of the calcaneocuboid joint,[75] opening wedge osteotomy of the first cuneiform, metatarsal osteotomies, and tarsometatarsal capsulotomies.[76] Lichtblau[77] in 1973 described a medial soft-tissue release and an osteotomy of the distal end of the calcaneus in which 1 cm of the distal lateral border and 2 mm of the distal medial border are removed. He claimed that the resected calcaneal articular surface was replaced by fibrocartilage, and he demonstrated mobility at the calcaneocuboid joint up to 6 years after surgery.

Evans[75] in 1961 described a procedure consisting of posteromedial releases in conjunction with lateral calcaneocuboid wedge resection and fusion. The procedure is not recommended for children younger than 4 years because of possible overcorrection. The correction of adduction occurs at the level of the midfoot, not distal to the navicular.[75,78,79] Accurate reduction of the navicular on the talus is essential because the position of the navicular is permanently stabilized by the procedure.[80] Only a narrow wedge from the calcaneocuboid joint should be removed; otherwise, overcorrection into valgus may occur.[75,78,79] The operation decreases growth of the lateral column of the foot. Satisfactory long-term functional results have been documented in 60% to 80% of the patients managed with the procedure.[75,78]

Fowler and associates[81] in 1959 described an opening wedge osteotomy of the medial cuneiform, and Hofmann and associates[82] in 1984 reported on this procedure for the treatment of residual adduction in clubfoot. The Fowler procedure includes an opening wedge osteotomy of the medial cuneiform, a radical plantar release, and a transfer of the tibialis anterior tendon to the dorsum of the first metatarsal. This procedure is reserved for children older than 8 years because a well-ossified first cuneiform is a prerequisite.[81] Supination of the midfoot is not addressed, and the degree of correction is limited by the intact lateral column complex of the calcaneocuboid joint.

McHale and Lenhart[83] described a procedure for an adducted forefoot and a supinated midfoot with hindfoot varus.

Functional Rating System for Clubfoot Surgery

Date: _____

Patient: _____

Date of Birth: _____

Sex: Male / Female   MR #: _____

Clubfoot Side/Type:
Right _____   Left _____

FIRST SURGICAL INTERVENTION
Date: _____

By: _____

Type of Surgery: _____

Special Findings: _____

REVISION SURGERY
Date: _____

By: _____

Type of Surgery: _____

Special Findings: _____

TOTAL SCORE: _____

Points	Rating
85 – 100	Excellent
70 – 84	Good
60 – 69	Fair
≤59	Poor

*   Arc starting from neutral 90 °
**   The *talocalcaneal index* is the sum of the talocalcaneal angles measured on lateral and anteroposterior radiographs.

Category	Points
1. Ankle motion (passive)	
*Arc from neutral >20°	15
Arc from neutral >10°	5
Arc from neutral 0-5°	0
2. Subtalar Joint Motion (passive motion)	
>15°	10
<15°	5
Stiff	0
3. Position of Heel When Standing	
0°-5° Valgus	10
>5° Valgus	5
Varus	0
4. Forefoot (appearance)	
Neutral	10
<5° Adduction/Abduction	5
>5° Adduction/Abduction	0
5. Gait	
Normal heel-toe gait	10
Cannot heel walk	6
Cannot toe walk	6
Flatfoot gait	5
6. Radiographic Measurement	
**Talocalcaneal Index	
≥40°	5
<40°	0
Talar-First Metatarsal Angle	
≤10°	5
>10°	0
7. Shoes	
Regular (no complaints)	5
Regular (with complaints)	3
Orthopaedic Shoes/Inserts/Braces	0
8. Function	
Not limited	15
Occasionally limited	8
Usually limited	0
9. Pain	
Never	10
Occasionally	5
Usually	0
10. Flexor Tendons	
Full function	5
Partial function	2
No function	0

Fig. 12 Functional rating system for clubfoot surgery.

The procedure combines an opening wedge osteotomy of the medial cuneiform with a closing wedge osteotomy of the cuboid, treating both residual forefoot adduction and midfoot supination. The authors showed in a cadaver model that a cuboid osteotomy is necessary for correction of midfoot supination. Although hindfoot varus is not addressed, the procedure has gained popularity and good results have been reported.[84]

Köse and associates[85] in 1999 described transmidtarsal osteotomy. The procedure involves an opening wedge osteotomy of the medial cuneiform and dorsal, truncated wedge osteotomies of the middle and lateral cuneiforms. Osteotomy of the middle and lateral cuneiforms allows better correction of rotational and cavus deformities. Again, the procedure requires well-formed tarsal bones and is most appropriate for patients older than 6 years.

Metatarsal osteotomies were described first by Steytler and Van der Walt[86] in 1966 and are indicated when the adduction deformity originates distal to the navicular. Care must be taken to avoid injury to the physis of the first metatarsal by osteotomy or by periosteal stripping;

Table 1
Algorithm for Surgical Reintervention in Clubfeet

Age of Patient at Time of Revision	Step	Method of Treatment
6 mo to 2 yr	1	Revision soft-tissue clubfoot release
	2	If prominent plantar crease, add plantar release
	3	If forefoot adductus is not corrected, add capsulotomies (navicular-first cuneiform or first cuneiform-first metatarsal), as needed
2 to 4 yr	4	If forefoot adductus is not fully corrected after steps 1, 2, and 3, add excision of cartilage of calcaneocuboid joint or decancellation of cuboid
4 to 8 yr	5	If forefoot adductus is not fully corrected after steps 1 through 4, add one of the following steps
	5A	Fusion of calcaneocuboid joint (Dillwyn Evans procedure)
	5B	Excision of distal part of calcaneus (Lichtblau procedure)
	5C	Cuboid decancellation
	5D	Opening wedge osteotomy of first cuneiform
	5E	Tarsometatarsal capsulotomies*
	5F	Metatarsal osteotomies (for patients > 5 yr old)
	6	If patient has overactive tibialis anterior tendon and weak peroneals, add tibialis anterior tendon transfer
	7	If varus angulation of heel remains uncorrected, add osteotomy of heel (Dwyer procedure)
8 to 10 yr†	8	Midtarsal osteotomy for persistent cavus
	9	Distraction osteogenesis (Ilizarov) as only procedure
>10 yr	10	Triple arthrodesis as only procedure

*Not recommended by authors of reports in the literature or by us.
†Note that in patients ≤ 10 years old, it is possible to start with steps 1 and 2, then proceed according to the deformity that remains—that is, proceed to step 7 if there is a deformity of the calcaneus or proceed to step 5A, 5B, 5C, or 5F if there is forefoot adductus.

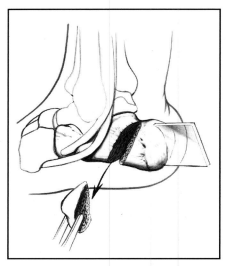

Fig. 13 Lateral closing wedge calcaneal osteotomy, as described by Dwyer.[89]

otherwise, shortening of the first metatarsal will result.[87] Heyman and associates[76] described release of the tarsometatarsal joints for correction of resistant metatarsus adductus or for treating residual clubfoot adduction deformity. Through a dorsal incision, complete capsulotomies and ligament releases were performed. Because of reports of frequent postoperative stiffness and pain, this procedure is not recommended.

Residual Cavus

Inadequate plantar release and muscle imbalance are both possible causes of residual cavus deformity. Soft-tissue release should be adequate in patients younger than 2 years. Steindler[88] in 1920 described release of the plantar fascia from its insertion at the calcaneus. Rigid cavus in children older than 8 years may require osteotomy of the tarsal bones or the calcaneus.[89] The Japas V-osteotomy, recommended for patients older than 6 years, allows correction at the midfoot without shortening the foot.[90] The Akron midtarsal osteotomy also allows correction at the midfoot but uses a so-called dome-type osteotomy to allow dorsoplantar and varus-valgus control.[91] A more distal osteotomy, at the level of the tarsometatarsal joints, was proposed by Jahss.[84] The wedge osteotomy of the tarsometatarsal joints is not intended for patients who have not reached skeletal maturity and requires normal vascular

and skin conditions. Arthrodesis at the hindfoot-midfoot region also has been described.[89]

Residual Varus or Valgus Angulation of the Heel

Dwyer[89] described a calcaneal osteotomy with either an opening or a closing wedge to treat varus and cavus angulation of the heel. Dwyer's lateral closing wedge osteotomy is recommended for children older than 4 years. The osteotomy does not correct the deformity at its apex, which is usually at the level of the midfoot (Fig. 13).

The extra-articular Grice procedure, originally developed for paralytic or spastic foot deformity, can be used to treat valgus angulation of the heel in younger patients because it does not interfere with subsequent growth.[92-94] It has been successful for flexible feet in children 4 to 10 years old. Rigid, overcorrected feet may require repeat soft-tissue releases, as well.[94]

Salvage Procedures

Triple arthrodesis has been used in children older than 10 years and is considered a salvage procedure (Fig. 14).[95] In a study of 15 patients with clubfoot deformity treated with this procedure, Adelaar and associates[96] noted that 11 had a good result and 2 each had a fair and a poor result. Angus and Cowell[97] noted that 65% of 26 feet with a rigid equinus foot deformity had a poor result at an average of 13 years after triple arthrodesis.

Wei and associates[98] and Fogel and associates[99] reported on limited talonavicular arthrodesis in patients who had had previous clubfoot surgery and had talonavicular osteoarthritis with dorsolateral subluxation and pain. The patients in the study by Wei and associates[98] were an average of 11 years old at the time of the surgery. Unlike adults who have undergone talonavicular arthrodesis, children have been noted to retain some subtalar motion. Fifteen of 16 patients reported satisfaction with the procedure after an average follow-up of 4 years.[98]

The Ilizarov apparatus has been combined with various osteotomies to provide distraction osteogenesis for the correction of residual deformity in the clubfoot and other foot deformities.[100,101] Equinus, varus angulation of the hindfoot, midfoot adductus, and cavus all may be addressed with the use of a circular frame and Kirschner wires. However, the potential complications are numerous.[100,101] Paley[101] reported that treatment of 25 various foot deformities with the Ilizarov apparatus resulted in 20 minor and major complications in 18 feet. The patient must understand that the final functional outcome will be a stiff but cosmetically improved plantigrade foot.

Dynamic Forefoot Supination
Transfer of the tibialis anterior tendon has a role in the treatment of a supple recurrent clubfoot (Fig. 15). Garceau[102] and Garceau and Palmer[103] mentioned several prerequisites for successful transfer of the tibialis anterior tendon for the treatment of recurrent varus and adductus. The patient must be younger than 6 years and have a passively correctable

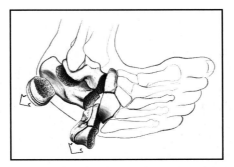

Fig. 14 Triple arthrodesis wedges removed for treatment of residual varus and forefoot adduction.

deformity, weak peroneals confirmed by electromyography, and no active abduction or eversion. Stiff joints or strong peroneals are contraindications. Gartland and Surgent[104] noted that recurrence after primary correction is more likely to respond to tibialis posterior transfer.

Residual Toeing-in
Two alternatives for a patient with a recurrent clubfoot with residual toeing-in are supramalleolar tibial osteotomy and talocalcaneal osteotomy. Hjelmstedt and Sahlstedt[105-107] recommended talocalcaneal wedge osteotomy through the talar neck and reported that 60% of 36 feet managed with the procedure had a good result, 20% had a fair result, and 20% had a poor result. Lloyd-Roberts and associates[108] and Swann and associates[109] reported on a supramalleolar tibial osteotomy with apex posterior angulation and medial rotation to correct equinus and adductus primarily. Neither of these osteotomy procedures is in wide use.

Dorsal Bunion
Dorsal bunion refers to a plantar flexion contracture of the first metatarsophalangeal joint with a dorsiflexion contracture of the first tarsometatarsal joint. It can be the result of imbalance between weak Achilles and peroneus longus tendons and strong flexor hallucis longus and tibialis anterior tendons. One proce-

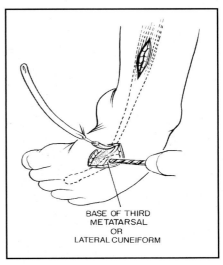

Fig. 15 Transfer of the tibialis anterior tendon to the base of the third metatarsal or lateral cuneiform.

dure described for its correction is the "reverse Jones" procedure,[110] which involves transfer of the flexor hallucis longus to the head of the first metatarsal. If necessary, a plantar flexion first metatarsal osteotomy and capsulorrhaphy can be included.

The Overcorrected Foot
Valgus position of the hindfoot and pronation of the forefoot characterize the overcorrected clubfoot deformity. Multiple factors may produce this deformity, including the release of the interosseous ligament at the subtalar joint and division of the deep deltoid ligament. The forefoot may be corrected nonsurgically by stretching and bracing and surgically by metatarsal and midfoot osteotomies. Treatment of the overcorrected clubfoot includes the use of orthoses for flexible deformity in children younger than 4 years and repeat soft-tissue release for rigid deformity. Subtalar or triple arthrodesis is recommended for a child older than 10 years. Combination medial and lateral column osteotomies of the calcaneus, cuboid, and cuneiforms also have been described.[111-114]

Skin Problems

Frequently, severe recurrent clubfoot deformities are associated with difficulty in skin closure. This problem is especially true of posteromedial wounds. Options to address the problem include tissue expanders;[115-117] free muscle flaps;[118] and partial wound closure, which allows secondary healing to close a wound to decrease the risk of necrosis.[119] Free muscle flaps such as gracilis flaps require microvascular techniques, but no debulking is required because shrinkage is expected. Other techniques that may assist in wound closure are lateral skin release and Z-plasty of the skin.[116]

Summary

Although the etiology of congenital clubfoot remains unknown, reproducible pretreatment grading now seems possible. However, the lack of an agreed-on and reproducible posttreatment evaluation system still hinders outcome studies of the treatment of clubfoot.

The literature from about 1970 to 1990[3,66,120] contains enthusiastic reports on the correction of congenital clubfoot through extensive surgical release procedures. Over time, we have come to recognize the complications of such surgery, including recurrence, overcorrection, stiffness, and pain (WJ Shaughnessy, MD, P Dechet, MD, HB Kitaoka, MD, Vancouver, BC, Canada, unpublished data, 2000). Perhaps because of these findings, there is a renewed interest in nonsurgical techniques for the correction of congenital clubfoot. Recent studies have documented the effectiveness of the two leading techniques involving serial manipulation and cast treatment. The Ponseti technique[49] appears to be effective and requires only a reasonable amount of time out of the lives of the patient and his or her parents. The technique frequently includes some minimally invasive surgery. The Kite and Lovell technique[48] requires minimally invasive surgery less often but is more time consuming.

French investigators and others have introduced new ideas that may reduce the need to immobilize the foot. The French approach requires fairly extensive physical therapy and demands substantial parental time and attention.[56] It is not yet clear that the French technique is more successful in obviating the need for surgery than is expertly applied serial manipulation and cast immobilization. It also has not been proved that the long-term results of the French technique are better than those of serial manipulation and cast immobilization. It is probably that unless the French technique is found to substantially decrease the need for surgery, it will prove to be less cost effective than serial manipulation and cast immobilization.

It is likely that a small number of clubfeet will require surgery even after expertly applied nonsurgical treatment. However, it is hoped that such surgery will be less extensive than procedures commonly performed in the recent past.

References

1. Wynne-Davies R: Family studies and the cause of congenital club foot: Talipes equinovarus, talipes calcaneo-valgus, and metatarsus varus. *J Bone Joint Surg Br* 1964;46:445-463.

2. Shimizu N, Hamada S, Mitta M, Hiroshima K, Ono K: Etiological considerations of congenital clubfoot deformity, in Simons GW (ed): *The Clubfoot: The Present and a View of the Future*. New York, NY, Springer-Verlag, 1994, pp 31-38.

3. Turco VJ: Surgical correction of the resistant club foot: One-stage posteromedial release with internal fixation: A preliminary report. *J Bone Joint Surg Am* 1971;53:477-497.

4. Lochmiller C, Johnston D, Scott A, Risman M, Hecht JT: Genetic epidemiology study of idiopathic talipes equinovarus. *Am J Med Genet* 1998;79:90-96.

5. The foot and leg, in Tachdjian MO (ed): *Pediatric Orthopedics*, ed 2. Philadelphia, PA, WB Saunders, 1990, pp 2405-3012.

6. Ippolito E, Ponseti IV: Congenital club foot in the human fetus: A histological study. *J Bone Joint Surg Am* 1980;62:8-22.

7. Isaacs H, Handelsman JE, Badenhorst M, Pickering A: The muscles in club foot: A histological histochemical and electron microscopic study. *J Bone Joint Surg Br* 1977;59:465-472.

8. Handelsman JE, Badalamente MA: Neuro-muscular studies in clubfoot. *J Pediatr Orthop* 1981;1:23-32.

9. Bill PL, Versfeld GA: Congenital clubfoot: An electromyographic study. *J Pediatr Orthop* 1982;2:139-142.

10. Irani RN, Sherman MS: The pathological anatomy of club foot. *J Bone Joint Surg Am* 1963;45:45-52.

11. Shapiro F, Glimcher MJ: Gross and histological abnormalities of the talus in congenital club foot. *J Bone Joint Surg Am* 1979;61:522-530.

12. Ionasescu V, Maynard JA, Ponseti IV, Zellweger H: The role of collagen in the pathogenesis of idiopathic clubfoot: Biochemical and electron microscopic correlations. *Helv Paediatr Acta* 1974;29:305-314.

13. Ippolito E: Update on pathologic anatomy of clubfoot. *J Pediatr Orthop B* 1995;4:17-24.

14. Dietz FR, Ponseti IV, Buckwalter JA: Morphometric study of clubfoot tendon sheaths. *J Pediatr Orthop* 1983;3:311-318.

15. Zimny ML, Willig SJ, Roberts JM, D'Ambrosia RD: An electron microscopic study of the fascia from the medial and lateral sides of clubfoot. *J Pediatr Orthop* 1985;5:577-581.

16. Sano H, Uhthoff HK, Jarvis JG, Mansingh A, Wenckebach GF: Pathogenesis of soft-tissue contracture in club foot. *J Bone Joint Surg Br* 1998;80:641-644.

17. Hootnick DR, Levinsohn EM, Crider RJ, Packard DS Jr: Congenital arterial malformations associated with clubfoot: A report of two cases. *Clin Orthop* 1982;167:160-163.

18. Sodre H, Bruschini S, Mestriner LA, et al: Arterial abnormalities in talipes equinovarus as assessed by angiography and the Doppler technique. *J Pediatr Orthop* 1990;10:101-104.

19. Muir L, Laliotis N, Kutty S, Klenerman L: Absence of the dorsalis pedis pulse in the parents of children with club foot. *J Bone Joint Surg Br* 1995;77:114-116.

20. Porter RW: An anomalous muscle in children with congenital talipes. *Clin Anat* 1996;9:25-27.

21. Chotigavanichaya C, Scaduto AA, Jadhav A, Otsuka NY: Accessory soleus muscle as a cause of resistance to correction in congenital club foot: A case report. *Foot Ankle Int* 2000;21:948-950.

22. Böhm M: The embryologic origin of club-foot. *J Bone Joint Surg* 1929;11:229-259.

23. Kawashima T, Uhthoff HK: Development of the foot in prenatal life in relation to idiopathic club foot. *J Pediatr Orthop* 1990;10:232-237.

24. Farrell SA, Summers AM, Dallaire L, Singer J, Johnson JA, Wilson RD: Club foot, an adverse outcome of early amniocentesis: Disruption or deformation? CEMAT: Canadian Early and Mid-Trimester Amniocentesis Trial. *J Med Genet* 1999;36:843-846.

25. Robertson WW Jr, Corbett D: Congenital clubfoot: Month of conception. *Clin Orthop* 1997;338:14-18.

26. Carroll NC: Pathoanatomy and surgical treatment of the resistant clubfoot. *Instr Course Lect* 1988;37:93-106.

27. Simons GW: Calcaneocuboid joint deformity in talipes equinovarus: An overview and

update. *J Pediatr Orthop B* 1995;4:25-35.

28. Ponseti IV (ed): *Congenital Clubfoot: Fundamentals of Treatment.* Oxford, England, Oxford University Press, 1996, p 55.

29. Howard CB, Benson MK: The ossific nuclei and the cartilage anlage of the talus and calcaneum. *J Bone Joint Surg Br* 1992;74:620-623.

30. Kite JH: Non-operative treatment of congenital clubfeet: A review of one hundred cases. *South Med J* 1930;23:337-345.

31. Simons GW: Analytical radiography of club feet. *J Bone Joint Surg Br* 1977;59:485-489.

32. Simons GW: A standardized method for the radiographic evaluation of clubfeet. *Clin Orthop* 1978;135:107-118.

33. McKay DW: New concept of and approach to clubfoot treatment: Section III. Evaluation and results. *J Pediatr Orthop* 1983;3:141-148.

34. Vanderwilde R, Staheli LT, Chew DE, Malagon V: Measurements on radiographs of the foot in normal infants and children. *J Bone Joint Surg Am* 1988;70:407-415.

35. Cummings RJ, Lovell WW: Operative treatment of congenital idiopathic club foot. *J Bone Joint Surg Am* 1988;70:1108-1112.

36. Watts H: Reproducability of reading club foot x-rays. *Orthop Trans* 1991;15:105.

37. Flynn JM, Donohoe M, Mackenzie WG: An independent assessment of two clubfoot-classification systems. *J Pediatr Orthop* 1998;18:323-327.

38. Dimeglio A, Bensahel H, Souchet P, Mazeau P, Bonnet F: Classification of clubfoot. *J Pediatr Orthop B* 1995;4:129-136.

39. Bensahel H, Catterall A, Dimeglio A: Practical applications in idiopathic clubfoot: A retrospective multicentric study in EPOS. *J Pediatr Orthop* 1990;10:186-188.

40. Bensahel H, Dimeglio A, Souchet P: Final evaluation of clubfoot. *J Pediatr Orthop B* 1995;4:137-141.

41. Berenshtein SS: Classification of congenital clubfoot. [Russian] *Ortop Travmatol Protez* 1983;5:32-35.

42. Catterall A: A method of assessment of the clubfoot deformity. *Clin Orthop* 1991;264:48-53.

43. Goldner JL: Congenital talipes equinovarus. *Foot Ankle* 1981;2:123-125.

44. Withington ET (trans): *Hippocrates.* Loeb Classical Library. London, England, Heinemann, 1927, vol 3.

45. Guerin M: Division of the tendon Achilles in clubfoot. *Lancet* 1935;2:648.

46. Preston ET, Fell TW: Congenital idiopathic clubfoot. *Clin Orthop* 1977;122:102-109.

47. Kite JH: The treatment of congenital clubfeet: A study of the results in two hundred cases. *JAMA* 1932;99:1156-1162.

48. Kite JH (ed): *The Clubfoot.* New York, NY, Grune and Stratton, 1964.

49. Ponseti IV: Treatment of congenital club foot. *J Bone Joint Surg Am* 1992;74:448-454.

50. Shaw NE: The early management of clubfoot. *Clin Orthop* 1972;84:39-43.

51. Browne D: Modern methods of treatment of club-foot. *Br Med J* 1937;2:570-572.

52. Thomson SA: Treatment of congenital talipes equinovarus with a modification of the Denis Browne method and splint. *J Bone Joint Surg* 1942;24:291-298.

53. Yamamoto H, Furuya K: Treatment of congenital club foot with a modified Denis Browne splint. *J Bone Joint Surg Br* 1990;72:460-463.

54. Bensahel H, Guillaume A, Czukonyi Z, Desgrippes Y: Results of physical therapy for idiopathic clubfoot: A long-term follow-up study. *J Pediatr Orthop* 1990;10:189-192.

55. Bensahel H, Guillaume A, Czukonyi Z, Themar-Noel C: The intimacy of clubfoot: The ways of functional treatment. *J Pediatr Orthop B* 1994;3:155-160.

56. Dimeglio A, Bonnet F, Mazeau P, De Rosa V: Orthopaedic treatment and passive motion machine: Consequences for the surgical treatment of clubfoot. *J Pediatr Orthop B* 1996;5:173-180.

57. Johnston WH, Richards BS: Abstract: Non-operative treatment of clubfoot: The French technique. *Proceedings of the 1999 Annual Meeting, Pediatric Orthopaedic Society of North America.* Lake Buena Vista, FL, Pediatric Orthopaedic Society of North America, 1999, p 25.

58. Delgado MR, Wilson H, Johnston C, Richards S, Karol L: A preliminary report of the use of botulinum toxin type A in infants with clubfoot: Four case studies. *J Pediatr Orthop* 2000; 20:533-538.

59. Reimann I, Lyquist E: Dynamic splint used in the treatment of club foot. *Acta Orthop Scand* 1969;40:817-824.

60. Bensahel H, Csukonyi Z, Desgrippes Y, Chaumien JP: Surgery in residual clubfoot: One-stage medioposterior release "a la carte." *J Pediatr Orthop* 1987;7:145-148.

61. Osterman K, Merikanto J: Critical aspects of neonatal surgery in clubfoot. *J Pediatr Orthop B* 1996;5:55-56.

62. Turco VJ: Resistant congenital club foot: One-stage posteromedial release with internal fixation: A follow-up report of a fifteen-year experience. *J Bone Joint Surg Am* 1979;61:805-814.

63. Simons GW: Complete subtalar release in club feet: Part II. Comparison with less extensive procedures. *J Bone Joint Surg Am* 1985; 67:1056-1065.

64. Crawford AH, Marxen JL, Osterfeld DL: The Cincinnati incision: A comprehensive approach for surgical procedures of the foot and ankle in childhood. *J Bone Joint Surg Am* 1982;64:1355-1358.

65. Henry AK: *Extensile Exposure,* ed 2. Baltimore, MD, Williams and Wilkins, 1970.

66. McKay DW: New concept of and approach to clubfoot treatment: II. Correction of the clubfoot. *J Pediatr Orthop* 1983;3:10-21.

67. Carroll NC: Controversies in the surgical

management of clubfoot. *Instr Course Lect* 1996;45:331-337.

68. Mountney J, Khan T, Davies AG, Smith TW: Scar quality from partial or complete wound closure using the Cincinnati incision for clubfoot surgery. *J Pediatr Orthop B* 1998;7:223-225.

69. Crawford AH, Gupta AK: Clubfoot controversies: Complications and causes for failure. *Instr Course Lect* 1996;45:339-346.

70. Vizkelety T, Szepesi K: Reoperation in treatment of clubfoot. *J Pediatr Orthop* 1989;9:144-147.

71. Tarraf YN, Carroll NC: Analysis of the components of residual deformity in clubfeet presenting for reoperation. *J Pediatr Orthop* 1992;12: 207-216.

72. Lehman WB, Atar D, Grant AD, Strongwater AM: Re-do clubfoot: Surgical approach and long-term results. *Bull NY Acad Med* 1990;66: 601-617.

73. Lichtblau S: Section of the abductor hallucis tendon for correction of metatarsus varus deformity. *Clin Orthop* 1975;110:227-232.

74. Toohey JS, Campbell P: Distal calcaneal osteotomy in resistant talipes equinovarus. *Clin Orthop* 1985;197:224-230.

75. Evans D: Relapsed club foot. *J Bone Joint Surg Br* 1961;43:722-733.

76. Heyman CH, Herndon CH, Strong JM: Mobilization of the tarsometatarsal and inter-metatarsal joints for the correction of resistant adduction of the fore part of the foot in congenital club-foot or congenital metatarsus varus. *J Bone Joint Surg Am* 1958;40:299-310.

77. Lichtblau S: A medial and lateral release operation for club foot: A preliminary report. *J Bone Joint Surg Am* 1973;55:1377-1384.

78. Addison A, Fixsen JA, Lloyd-Roberts GC: A review of the Dillwyn Evans type collateral operation in severe club feet. *J Bone Joint Surg Br* 1983;65:12-14.

79. Graham GP, Dent CM: Dillwyn Evans operation for relapsed club foot: Long-term results. *J Bone Joint Surg Br* 1992;74:445-448.

80. Abrams RC: Relapsed club foot: The early results of an evaluation of Dillwyn Evans' operation. *J Bone Joint Surg Am* 1969;51:270-282.

81. Fowler SB, Brooks AL, Parrish TF: The cavovarus foot. *J Bone Joint Surg Am* 1959;41:757.

82. Hofmann AA, Constine RM, McBride GG, Coleman SS: Osteotomy of the first cuneiform as treatment of residual adduction of the fore part of the foot in club foot. *J Bone Joint Surg Am* 1984;66:985-990.

83. McHale KA, Lenhart MK: Treatment of residual clubfoot deformity—the "bean-shaped" foot—by opening wedge medial cuneiform osteotomy and closing wedge cuboid osteotomy: Clinical review and cadaver correlations. *J Pediatr Orthop* 1991;11:374-381.

84. Jahss MH: Tarsometatarsal truncated-wedge arthrodesis for pes cavus and equinovarus deformity of the fore part of the foot. *J Bone Joint Surg Am* 1980;62:713-722.

85. Köse N, Günal I, Gökturk E, Seber S: Treatment of severe residual clubfoot deformity by trans-midtarsal osteotomy. *J Pediatr Orthop B* 1999;8:251-256.

86. Steytler JC, Van der Walt ID: Correction of resistant adduction of the forefoot in congenital clubfoot and congenital metatarsus varus by metatarsal osteotomy. *Br J Surg* 1966; 53:558-560.

87. Holden D, Siff S, Butler J, Cain T: Shortening of the first metatarsal as a complication of metatarsal osteotomies. *J Bone Joint Surg Am* 1984;66:582-587.

88. Steindler A: Stripping of the os calcis. *J Orthop Surg* 1920;2:8-12.

89. Dwyer FC: Osteotomy of the calcaneum for pes cavus. *J Bone Joint Surg Br* 1959;41:80-86.

90. Japas LM: Surgical treatment of pes cavus by tarsal V-osteotomy: Preliminary report. *J Bone Joint Surg Am* 1968;50:927-944.

91. Wilcox PG, Weiner DS: The Akron midtarsal dome osteotomy in the treatment of rigid pes cavus: A preliminary review. *J Pediatr Orthop* 1985;5:333-338.

92. Grice DS: Further experience with extra-articular arthrodesis of the subtalar joint. *J Bone Joint Surg Am* 1955;37:246-259, 365.

93. Grice DS: An extra-articular arthrodesis of the subastragalar joint for correction of paralytic flat feet in children. *J Bone Joint Surg Am* 1952;34:927-940.

94. Scott SM, Janes PC, Stevens PM: Grice subtalar arthrodesis followed to skeletal maturity. *J Pediatr Orthop* 1988;8:176-183.

95. Galindo MJ, Siff SJ, Butler JE, Cain TE: Triple arthrodesis in young children: A salvage procedure after failed releases in severely affected feet. *Foot Ankle* 1987;7:319-325.

96. Adelaar RS, Dannelly EA, Meunier PA, Stelling FH, Goldner JL, Colvard DF: A long term study of triple arthrodesis in children. *Orthop Clin North Am* 1976;7:895-908.

97. Angus PD, Cowell HR: Triple arthrodesis: A critical long-term review. *J Bone Joint Surg Br* 1986;68:260-265.

98. Wei SY, Sullivan RJ, Davidson RS: Talo-navicular arthrodesis for residual midfoot deformities of a previously corrected clubfoot. *Foot Ankle Int* 2000;21:482-485.

99. Fogel GR, Katoh Y, Rand JA, Chao EY: Talonavicular arthrodesis for isolated arthrosis: 9.5-year results and gait analysis. *Foot Ankle* 1982;3:105-113.

100. Lehman WB, Grant AD, Atar D: The use of distraction osteogenesis (Ilizarov) in complex foot deformities, in Jahss MH (ed): *Disorders of the Foot and Ankle: Medical and Surgical Management*, ed 2. Philadelphia, PA, WB Saunders, 1991, pp 2735-2744.

101. Paley D: The correction of complex foot deformities using Ilizarov's distraction osteotomies. *Clin Orthop* 1993;293:97-111.

102. Garceau GJ: Anterior tibial tendon transfer for recurrent clubfoot. *Clin Orthop* 1972;84:61-65.

103. Garceau GJ, Palmer RM: Transfer of the anterior tibial tendon for recurrent club foot: A long-term follow-up. *J Bone Joint Surg Am* 1967;49:207-231.

104. Gartland JJ, Surgent RE: Posterior tibial transplant in the surgical treatment of recurrent clubfoot. *Clin Orthop* 1972;84:66-70.

105. Hjelmstedt A, Sahlstedt B: Talo-calcaneal osteotomy and soft-tissue procedures in the treatment of clubfeet: I. Indications, principles and technique. *Acta Orthop Scand* 1980;51:335-347.

106. Hjelmstedt A, Sahlstedt B: Talo-calcaneal osteotomy and soft-tissue procedures in the treatment of clubfeet: II. Results in 36 surgically treated feet. *Acta Orthop Scand* 1980; 51:349-357.

107. Hjelmstedt A, Sahlstedt B: Role of talocalcaneal osteotomy in clubfoot surgery: Results in 31 surgically treated feet. *J Pediatr Orthop* 1990; 10:193-197.

108. Lloyd-Roberts GC, Swann M, Catterall A: Medial rotational osteotomy for severe residual deformity in club foot: A preliminary report on a new method of treatment. *J Bone Joint Surg Br* 1974;56:37-43.

109. Swann M, Lloyd-Roberts GC, Catterall A: The anatomy of uncorrected club feet: A study of rotation deformity. *J Bone Joint Surg Br* 1969; 51:263-269.

110. Kuo KN, Jansen LD: Rotatory dorsal subluxation of the navicular: A complication of clubfoot surgery. *J Pediatr Orthop* 1998;18:770-774.

111. Rathjen KE, Mubarak SJ: Calcaneal-cuboidcuneiform osteotomy for the correction of valgus foot deformities in children. *J Pediatr Orthop* 1998;18:775-782.

112. Mosca VS: Calcaneal lengthening for valgus deformity of the hindfoot: Results in children who had severe, symptomatic flatfoot and skewfoot. *J Bone Joint Surg Am* 1995;77:500-512.

113. Evans D: Calcaneo-valgus deformity. *J Bone Joint Surg Br* 1975;57:270-278.

114. Phillips GE: A review of elongation of os calcis for flat feet. *J Bone Joint Surg Br* 1983;65:15-18.

115. Atar D, Grant AD, Silver L, Lehman WB, Strongwater AM: The use of a tissue expander in club-foot surgery: A case report and review. *J Bone Joint Surg Br* 1990;72:574-577.

116. Lehman WB, Atar D: Complications in the management of talipes equinovarus, in Drennan JC (ed): *The Child's Foot and Ankle*. New York, NY, Raven Press, 1992, pp 135-153.

117. Grant AD, Atar D, Lehman WB, Strongwater AM: The use of tissue expanders in clubfoot surgery, in Simons GW (ed): *The Clubfoot: The Present and a View of the Future*. New York, NY, Springer-Verlag, 1994, pp 235-241.

118. Haasbeek JF, Zuker RM, Wright JG: Free gracilis muscle transfer for coverage of severe foot deformities. *J Pediatr Orthop* 1995;15:608-612.

119. Ferlic RJ, Breed AL, Mann DC, Cherney JJ: Partial wound closure after surgical correction of equinovarus foot deformity. *J Pediatr Orthop* 1997;17:486-489.

120. Simons GW: Complete subtalar release in club feet: Part I. A preliminary report. *J Bone Joint Surg Am* 1985;67:1044-1055.

Treatment of a Recurrent Clubfoot Deformity After Initial Correction With the Ponseti Technique

Frederick R. Dietz, MD

Abstract

Early recognition and appropriate treatment of recurrent deformity (relapse) is an important component of the Ponseti technique of clubfoot correction. After correction of a clubfoot deformity by the Ponseti technique, relapse usually involves equinus and varus of the hindfoot. Cavus and adductus rarely recur to a clinically significant degree. Clubfoot recurs most frequently and quickly while the foot is rapidly growing—during the first several years of life. Recurrence of deformity will almost always occur, even after complete correction with the Ponseti technique, if appropriate bracing is not used.

Treatment of clubfoot relapse in infants and toddlers is identical to the original correction maneuver. In a patient approximately 2.5 years of age, a relapse can be treated with anterior tibial tendon transfer to the third cuneiform with or without Achilles tendon lengthening. The indication for anterior tibial tendon transfer is the presence of dynamic supination during gait. After tendon transfer, bracing is no longer required because the eversion force of the transferred tendon maintains the correction. In a long-term follow-up study of patients treated by the Ponseti technique, the necessity for anterior tibial tendon transfer did not compromise the outcome with respect to level of pain and functional limitations. Because anterior tibial tendon transfer is joint sparing, the foot retains maximal strength and suppleness. Good long-term results can be anticipated despite clubfoot relapse.

Recurrence of deformity or relapse is the development of one or more of the original deformities of equinus, varus, adduction, and cavus after full correction of an idiopathic clubfoot. After correction of clubfoot by the Ponseti technique, relapse usually involves equinus and varus of the hindfoot.[1] Cavus and adductus rarely recur to a clinically significant degree. Worsening of incompletely corrected foot deformities is expected; appropriate initial treatment achieves full and complete correction. The cause of a relapse in a foot that had been completely corrected by the Ponseti technique is unknown, but would logically result from the same pathology that initially caused clubfoot. Unfortunately, this pathology remains incompletely understood despite more than a century of investigation.

One striking characteristic of clubfoot is its tendency to recur most frequently and most quickly while the foot is rapidly growing—during the first several years of life. Relapses are most common in the first through third years of life. Relapse is less common after age 3 years, rare after age 5 years, and almost never occurs in patients older than 7 years of age. These findings suggest that the pathologic process is most active during the most rapid growing period of the foot or is in some way dependent on rapid growth to create the deformity. Identifying genes that may predispose some people to clubfoot appears to be the most promising avenue for discovering the causes of idiopathic clubfoot.

Bracing

Almost all clubfeet will relapse after full correction if appropriate bracing is not used. Simple abduction bracing can prevent most relapses. Because part-time bracing used during sleeping hours can prevent relapse, it is believed that the pathologic process must be subtle. However, the pathology is also persistent because bracing is required for 3 to 4 years to prevent most relapses. A study by

Morcuende and associates[2] clearly showed the importance of using a foot abduction orthosis to prevent relapse after clubfoot correction. The authors reviewed the outcomes of 157 patients (256 feet) who were treated between 1991 and 2001 using the Ponseti method. Seventeen patients (11%) had a relapse. They found that 2 of 140 patients (approximately 1%) whose parents reported compliance with the bracing regimen had a relapse, compared with the occurrence of a relapse in 15 of 17 patients (89%) whose parents were not compliant with the bracing regimen. Dobbs and associates[3] evaluated recurrence risk in 51 consecutive infants with 86 idiopathic clubfeet and found that brace wear compliance was the factor that was most strongly related to relapse with an odds ratio of 183 ($P < 0.00001$).

Neither study found a correlation between the initial severity of the deformity, place of prior treatment, number of casts required for initial correction, or patient age at initiation of treatment. Therefore, ensuring parent and patient compliance with the bracing regimen is the most effective method for avoiding relapse. The author's approach to achieving this goal is to emphasize the importance of the brace at every office visit, especially at the prenatal visit and during every cast change; to state with conviction that if the brace is not used the clubfoot deformity will return and that further casting and even surgical intervention will then be necessary; and to recommend the use of the brace whenever the child is put in the crib or bed to sleep. Children are much less likely to resist brace wear if the brace is used in a completely consistent manner. Most children will become unwilling to wear the brace sometime between 3 and 4 years of age. Because this is past the peak time for relapse, discontinued use of the brace is acceptable. If the patient and the family are not resistant to brace wear, the author recommends use of the brace until the child is 5 years old because relapse after that age is extremely rare.

Presentation of Relapse

Clubfoot relapses will occur and are more effectively and easily treated if recognized promptly. Most relapses that occur before walking age are attributable to failure to wear the abduction foot orthosis. The parents will often describe a history of difficulty in applying the braces as prescribed. As a relapse occurs, bracing becomes more difficult. Equinus recurs first and makes it difficult to place the patient's heel completely "down" into the heel of the orthotic shoe. Therefore, the heel slips up and often completely out of the shoe. The parents report having to reposition the foot in the shoe multiple times or that the brace is not on the patient's foot in the morning. Physical examination will show less dorsiflexion than on previous examinations. If the foot cannot be dorsiflexed past neutral, and usually at least 5° to 10°, treatment for a relapse should begin.

Treatment

Treatment for recurrent clubfoot is identical to the original corrective maneuver. The foot is abducted using the head of the talus as the fulcrum. In most feet, in which complete correction had been obtained, the foot will again abduct and dorsiflex into full correction. Two or three castings are usually required and are applied at 2-week intervals in these older infants. If the foot corrects except for the equinus, a percutaneous Achilles tenotomy should be repeated. The upper patient age limit for a percutaneous Achilles tenotomy as opposed to an open Achilles tendon lengthening has not been established. The author has performed a percutaneous tenotomy in an 18-month-old patient, although traditionally open lengthening has been performed in patients older than 1 year of age.

Clubfoot relapse in children of walking age who are younger than 2.5 years of age will usually have the same history and static physical findings. In addition, the treating physician can observe the recurrent equinus and varus during gait. Most commonly, relapse in patients in this age group consists of recurrent equinus with or without recurrent varus. Mild adductus may be present in a small percentage of such patients. Recurrence of cavus is rare. Treatment is needed for these patients because the relapse will not "walk itself out." Treatment consists of manipulation and casting, which can be challenging in children of walking age if they are uncooperative. With patience, correction can be regained in most children. Occasionally, the patient's history will reveal no difficulties with brace wear and the static examination will show a fully corrected foot; however, the child ambulates in a supinated position. These feet should be treated with abduction/dorsiflexion manipulation and two or three castings at 2-week intervals. These feet have an incomplete reduction of the navicular resulting in a supinating force of the anterior tibial tendon. Because patients younger than 2.5 years of age are too young for an anterior tibial tendon transfer to the third cuneiform, manipulation and casting are appropriate. In the author's experience, most feet that relapse after walking age will require an anterior tibial tendon transfer when the patient is old enough for the procedure. This situation probably occurs because families who were noncompliant with brace wear after the initial treatment for clubfoot remain noncompliant with brace wear even after treatment for the first relapse.

Relapses in infants or toddlers may occur more than once. Each time a relapse is identified, it is treated in the same manner. Abduction manipulation is performed. The foot usually will dorsiflex as the calcaneus moves into a more valgus position. If equinus is persistent, the Achilles tendon must be relengthened, either percutaneously or by an open lengthening, depending on the age of the child.

Tendon Transfer

When a patient is approximately 2.5 years of age, a relapse can be treated by anterior tibial tendon transfer to the third cuneiform with or without Achilles tendon lengthening. At age 2.5 years, the ossific nucleus of the third cuneiform is sufficiently large that the anterior tibial tendon can be transferred into the ossific nucleus, ensuring tendon healing to bone and avoiding damage to the growth cartilage of the third cuneiform.

The necessity of anchoring the transferred tendon into bone has been questioned. Huang and associates[4] reported on anterior tibial tendon transfer as the principal corrective procedure after initial manipulation and casting in 159 feet in 111 patients. Sixty-seven transfers were made to the third cuneiform, 88 transfers were made to the medial cuboid, and 2 were made to the second cuneiform. Additional procedures consisted mainly of percutaneous or open lengthening of the Achilles tendon. Thirty-three transfers were performed on 6- to 12-

month-old patients and 35 procedures were done on children 1 to 3 years of age. All patients in this study were at least 13 years of age at follow-up. No complications with tendon pullout or cuneiform growth disturbance from anchoring the anterior tibial tendon into the cartilage anlagen of the cuneiform were found (L Zhao, MD, personal communication, 2000). Huang and associates reported 91.8% good and excellent results using a rating system that combined satisfaction, function, and anatomic criteria. Outcomes were best when surgery was performed before the children were 5 years old. Huang and associates[4] concluded that the optimal time for tendon transfer was when patients were between 6 and 12 months old.

The author has not used anterior tendon transfer into the cartilage of the third cuneiform because of concerns regarding tendon pull-out, growth disturbance, or overcorrection of deformity. The approach of using an anterior tibial tendon transfer to treat infants is intriguing, especially as an alternative to repeated casting for patients who are noncompliant with brace wear.

At the author's institution, an anterior tibial tendon transfer is not performed until the ossific nucleus of the third cuneiform is large enough to accept the entire tendon. Based on the results of a 30-year follow-up study[5] on Ponseti's early patients, tendon transfer is a recommended procedure. In this study, 45 patients with 71 clubfeet who were an average of 34 years old at follow-up answered questions about pain and function to measure outcome satisfaction. These patients were compared with a control group of patients who had no congenital foot deformity. Fifty-three percent of the feet with clubfoot deformity had

undergone anterior tibial tendon transfer and had outcomes, with respect to pain and function, that were comparable with feet that did not require the transfer. Outcomes were not significantly different in the control group without clubfoot. The high percentage of feet requiring anterior tibial tendon transfer in this cohort study resulted from Ponseti's developing recognition of the importance of overcorrection of the deformity and the necessity of abduction bracing of the feet for a prolonged period of time (IV Ponsetti, MD, Iowa City, IA, personal communication).

The indication for anterior tibial tendon transfer is the presence of dynamic supination during gait. The entire foot supinates during the swing phase and is supinated to some degree in the stance phase such that weight bearing is placed excessively on the lateral border of the foot. This condition usually results from an incomplete correction of the medial displacement of the navicular, which may occur in severe clubfoot deformities despite optimal manipulation and casting. As with all tendon transfers, the deformity observed during gait must be passively correctable. If the equinus and varus are not passively correctable, two or three manipulation and casting sessions are necessary until the static deformity is completely corrected. If 10° of dorsiflexion is not obtained, Achilles tendon lengthening should be performed at the time of anterior tibial tendon transfer. After tendon transfer, bracing is no longer required because the eversion force of the transferred tendon maintains the correction.

Techniques for Anterior Tendon Transfer

To perform an anterior tendon transfer (Figure 1), a 3- to 4-cm incision is made over the medial as-

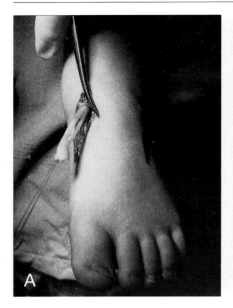
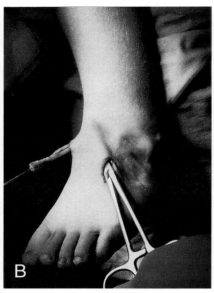
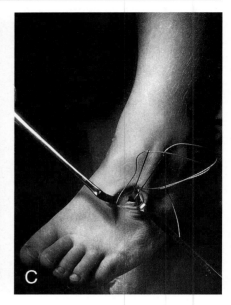

Figure 1　**A,** The anterior tibial tendon is released from its insertion on the base of the first metatarsal and freed of all peritendinous attachments proximally to the extensor retinaculum of the ankle. **B,** The third cuneiform is identified through a small, separate lateral incision. A large hemostat is passed subcutaneously from the lateral wound into the medial wound, thereby creating a tunnel for the redirection of the anterior tibial tendon. **C,** The anterior tibial tendon is anchored into a drill hole in the ossific nucleus of the third cuneiform.

pect of the foot in line with the anterior tibial tendon. The tendon is released from its insertion on the base of the first metatarsal maintaining maximum length. Attachments to the tendon that would tether it during transfer are released up to the inferior ankle retinaculum using scissors. A Bunnell stitch is placed in the tendon using a heavy nonabsorbable suture. A second 3-cm incision is made over the third cuneiform. In younger children (age 2.5 to 5 years), the author uses Fluoro-Scan (FluoroScan Imaging Systems, Northbrook, IL) and a Keith needle to identify the center of the ossific nucleus of the third cuneiform. A hand drill is used to make a hole larger than the tendon (so no binding of the tendon in the bone tunnel will occur) in the center of the ossific nucleus. A large hemostat is introduced through the incision over the third cuneiform. The hemostat is pushed under the subcutaneous tis-

sue in a proximal-medial direction to the center of the inferior ankle retinaculum. The hemostat is then directed medially into the wound over the anterior tibial tendon. The sutures in the tendon are grasped and the tendon is brought into the wound over the third cuneiform. The tendon is drawn into the bone tunnel using Keith needles and the suture is tied over a padded button on the sole of the foot. The foot should lie with the calcaneus in neutral varus-valgus and should lie in 10° or less of plantar flexion. If 10° to 15° of dorsiflexion were not present prior to surgery, Achilles tendon lengthening should be performed before the anterior tibial tendon transfer is sutured. The author performs a coronal Z-lengthening with the tendon cuts performed anteriorly in the distal tendon and posteriorly in the proximal tendon. This technique ensures that there is no raw tendon surface distally where

the tendon is most subcutaneous and therefore avoids the risk of scarring of the tendon to the overlying tissues. An above-knee cast is placed with the knee flexed 90° to ensure that weight bearing does not occur for 6 weeks. For children younger than 5 years of age, the cast and button are removed at 6 weeks and unrestricted weight bearing is permitted. Older children have the cast changed at 6 weeks. The button and suture are removed and a below-knee walking cast is applied for 3 weeks to ensure complete healing of the transferred tendon to the bone.

Summary

To prevent clubfoot relapse it is important to encourage compliance with brace wear. Even with proper compliance, relapses will occur and should be recognized early for optimal outcomes. A small amount of heel varus or equinus will not resolve spontaneously. Treatment should be done with repeat manipulations and castings. In children older than 2.5 years of age with dynamic supination, treatment is performed by an anterior tibial tendon transfer to the third cuneiform with Achilles tendon lengthening as needed. Because this approach is joint sparing, the foot retains maximal strength and suppleness. Good long-term results can be anticipated despite the occurrence of clubfoot relapse.

References

1. Ponseti IV: *Congenital Clubfoot: Fundamentals of Treatment.* New York, NY, Oxford University Press, 1996.

2. Morcuende JA, Dolan L, Dietz FR, Ponseti IV: Radical reduction in the rate of extensive corrective surgery for clubfoot using the Ponseti Method. *Pediatrics* 2004;113:376-380.

3. Dobbs MB, Rudzki JR, Purcell DB, et al: Factors predictive of outcome after use of the Ponseti method for treatment of idiopathic clubfeet. *J Bone Joint Surg Am* 2004;86-A:22-27.

4. Huang YT, Lei W, Zhao L, et al: The treatment of congenital club foot by operation to correct deformity and achieve dynamic muscle balance. *J Bone Joint Surg Br* 1999;81:858-862.

5. Cooper DM, Dietz FR: Treatment of idiopathic clubfoot: A thirty-year follow-up note. *J Bone Joint Surg Am* 1995;77:1477-1489.

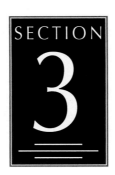

SECTION 3

Musculoskeletal Trauma and Infection

Musculoskeletal Trauma and Infection

In this age of specialization, the general orthopaedic surgeon usually refers all pediatric orthopaedic problems to a local pediatric orthopaedist. Because most general pediatric conditions can be evaluated and treated on an elective basis, any delay from the time of diagnosis until the initiation of treatment usually does not compromise the final outcome. However, acute conditions, such as musculoskeletal trauma and infections, often require prompt treatment that may require urgent management by the general orthopaedist. This collection of articles provides an excellent review on the current management of these acute conditions.

Much has changed in the management of pediatric fractures in the past 50 years. Walter Blount, who is considered by many to be the father of pediatric fracture management, once stated that the surgical management of fractures in children was "a sign of impetuousness and should be avoided." In the 1950s when his classic text was written, the surgical incisions were large and the fixation methods not very secure. Today, minimally invasive techniques that provide secure fixation are available. Likewise, nonsurgical techniques used in the past required either long periods of hospitalization or immobilization. This is a philosophy that is no longer currently acceptable in pediatric orthopaedics because of the increased emphasis on rapid return to normal physical activity. That is not to say that most pediatric trauma should be treated surgically. In fact, the contrary is true. The authors in this section have done an outstanding job of identifying which traumatic conditions are best managed by the newer surgical procedures available.

In the first of two articles on management of pediatric fractures, Flynn and associates offer clear guidelines for surgical intervention of upper extremity pediatric fractures. Their treatment methods, however, are not necessarily universally accepted, especially for treatment of fractures of the distal radial metaphysis. The first area of controversy lies in the debate over the type of cast to use following fracture reduction. The use of a long arm cast has not been proved to increase the stability of the reduction. In fact, recent postreduction studies comparing the use of long arm casts with short arm casts report that the use of short arm casts alone was equally effective in maintaining the reduction. Care is needed when applying the short arm cast to ensure that the proper cast index has been achieved.

The second area in which there may be some disagreement is with the routine use of percutaneous pin fixation for fractures of the distal radial metaphysis. My experience and that of others is that if a properly applied short arm cast is utilized, an adequate reduction is usually maintained. Thus, use of percutaneous pin fixation should be limited to only those diaphyseal fractures in which a stable reduction cannot be obtained and maintained with a properly applied short arm cast. Other indications for percutaneous pin fixation include an open fracture, fractures with severe swelling, a fracture in an obese patient, or the presence of ipsilateral fractures.

The authors laud the merits of percutaneous intramedullary nail fixation for certain radial and ulnar diaphyseal fractures and recommend the routine use of a long arm cast following this type of stabilization. They also leave the cut end of the nail outside the skin. Experience has shown that leaving the nail cut outside the skin often leads to the need for premature removal of the nails, which increases the risk of refracture. The AO technique recommends stabilizing both bones, burying the tips of the nails next to the cortex, and immobilizing the arm with only a splint so that motion can begin as soon as it can be tolerated. This appears to be a more physiologic approach.

The authors also point out that compartment syndrome can commonly occur following diaphyseal radial and ulnar fractures. Emphasizing this point is excellent because most surgeons associate compartment syndrome primarily with supracondylar fractures. In their discussion of compartment syndromes associated with both diaphyseal forearm and supracondylar fractures, there needs to be emphasis on the clinical manifestations. The use of technology alone, such as measuring compartment pressures in determining the presence of absence of a compartment syndrome, is dangerous. These technical devices are not infallible.

The use of multiple lateral pins for stabilization of type III supracondylar fractures has now been well studied and accepted. This change from the original medial-lateral configuration has greatly reduced the incidence of iatrogenic neurapraxia.

Another change from tradition mentioned in this article is that the indications for surgical intervention of medial epicondylar fractures may be better determined by function rather than the amount of fragment displacement.

In their second article, Flynn and associates describe how long bone fractures in the lower extremity are now being managed more often surgically and justifiably so. There is very little disagreement regarding the surgical indications for managing long bone fractures in the lower extremity. The use of intramedullary nail fixation has greatly facilitated a rapid return to functional activities. The authors do an excellent job of defining the indications and techniques and are wise to express caution in the use of rigid intramedullary nail fixation systems in the skeletally immature patient because of the risk of osteonecrosis of the femoral head. That condition will create a lifetime disability.

They emphasize that with improved imaging techniques, many extra-articular fractures about the knee can be managed with percutaneous screw fixation. One new approach to the fractures of the anterior tibial spine has been the use of the arthroscope to obtain a reduction. This technique has substantially decreased the morbidity associated with this injury.

The use of flexible intramedullary nails for simple tibial shaft fractures has become more widely accepted, which has decreased the need for external fixation devices. The authors emphasize the necessity of obtaining CT for distal tibia physeal fractures. The increased use of this imaging technique has greatly increased our understanding of the structure of these fracture patterns. In many cases, it also it has enabled us to reduce and stabilize the fragment percutaneously.

Tepper and Ireland outline in great detail the management of the two principal physeal fractures about the knee. They emphasize the fairly high frequency in which physeal arrest can occur with these fractures and provide excellent guidelines for its management. They warn that even though the primary failure has occurred in the osseous tissues, concurrent failure of the ligamentous structures also is a possibility. As a result, the integrity of the surrounding soft tissues must be thoroughly assessed. The judicious use of the arthroscope has allowed for minimally invasive management of many intra-articular fractures. The authors also offer guidelines regarding which lesions can be effectively managed arthroscopically.

The next article by Moti and Micheli provides an excellent description of the management of lesions involving the nonosseous intra-articular structures of the knee. Their article is especially valuable in this collection because most of the arthroscopic literature focuses on sport injuries in adults. The current guidelines for addressing unique conditions in the pediatric patient, such a discoid meniscus, are an especially valuable resource.

Musculoskeletal infections in children, if not promptly recognized and treated appropriately, can result in long-term deformities and compromised function. McCarthy and associates have constructed one of the best organized, most complete summaries of the management of musculoskeletal infections in the present literature. These authors provide excellent guidelines for recognizing and appropriately managing these infections.

In the past, the diagnosis was confirmed only after the development of the classic bony changes associated with acute hematogenous osteomyelitis. The authors point out that deep soft-tissue swelling is one of the key early changes. Although imaging studies that help define the location and nature of the pathology of acute osteomyelitis are well described, the authors emphasize that the most important part of the diagnostic process is identifying the offending organism through aspiration of the affected bone. The organism also can be obtained often from the initial blood cultures.

Treatment consisting of 6 weeks of intravenous antibiotics is no longer standard. The authors emphasize that treatment must be individualized, based on the patient's age, duration of the infection, organism involved, and the bone affected. The use of the erythrocyte sedimentation rate to gauge the response to treatment has been replaced with the C-reactive protein, which gives a more accurate indication of whether the antibiotic is effective against the causative organism.

One of the outstanding aspects of this article is a summary of the characteristics of the unusual forms of osteomyelitis and the approach to making a definitive diagnosis of osteomyelitis in unusual anatomic locations. This information serves as an excellent resource for anyone confronted with a patient who has an atypical clinical picture or unusual location for osteomyelitis. This information, which previously has been scattered throughout the medical literature, is beautifully summarized in one article.

The authors also provide an excellent summary of the diagnosis and management of the musculoskeletal soft-tissue infections, including guidelines for treatment and a complete discussion of less common soft-tissue infections such as Lyme disease and herpetic whitlow.

These articles are an excellent resource for all orthopaedic surgeons who manage acute musculoskeletal conditions in children. The articles are complete and clearly delineate the current accepted methods of treatment. I predict that many orthopaedic surgeons will consider these articles as their "Bible" when confronted with these acute pediatric conditions.

Kaye E. Wilkins, DVM, MD
Professor of Orthopaedics and
  Pediatrics
University of Texas Health Science
  Center at San Antonio
San Antonio, Texas

The Surgical Management of Pediatric Fractures of the Upper Extremity

John M. Flynn, MD
John F. Sarwark, MD
Peter M. Waters, MD
Donald S. Bae, MD,
Laura Powers Lemke, MD

Abstract

The vast majority of pediatric fractures of the upper extremity can and should be treated with closed reduction, immobilization, and close follow-up. However, there is an ongoing debate in the orthopaedic community regarding the exact role of surgical management in the treatment of pediatric fractures. In the past 2 decades, surgical management of certain fractures (eg, percutaneous pinning of displaced supracondylar fractures) has provided better results than closed management. Surgical management is clearly indicated for certain injuries, such as those requiring anatomic realignment of the physis or articular surface. Increasingly, however, surgical management is being used to maintain optimal alignment or to allow early motion. In many such cases, both nonsurgical and surgical methods have yielded good results and have vocal advocates. Certain technical advances, such as flexible intramedullary fixation and bioreabsorbable implants, have further increased enthusiasm for surgical management of pediatric fractures.

The goal of this chapter is to describe current concepts in the surgical management of selected pediatric fractures of the upper extremity. The focus is on specific indications, techniques, and potential complications in managing fractures of the forearm and elbow in children. The full scope of pediatric fracture management is a subject for textbooks. For introductory information and descriptions of techniques of successful nonsurgical management, the reader is directed to comprehensive sources.[1,2]

Wrist and Forearm Fractures

Forearm fractures are among the most common orthopaedic injuries in children, accounting for 30% to 50% of all pediatric fractures.[3,4] Historically, almost all forearm fractures in skeletally immature patients were treated nonsurgically. Recent information regarding functional outcomes, however, has challenged many of the traditional tenets of forearm fracture care. Furthermore, with the advent of newer technology, instrumentation, and techniques of fracture fixation, the treatment options have expanded.[5]

Distal Radial Fractures

Because of their proximity to the distal radial physis, distal radial fractures have tremendous remodeling potential.[6-8] As a result, substantial residual angulation and displacement can be accepted with the expectation of correction and continued growth. Up to 20° to 25° of angulation in the sagittal plane can be accepted in patients younger than 12 years. Up to 10° to 15° of sagittal angulation and up to 10° of radial deviation can be accepted in patients older than 12 years, depending upon their degree of skeletal maturity.

These criteria provide a framework for determining how much angulation and displacement may be corrected by remodeling and, thus, which fractures may be treated with nonsurgical means. An additional important consideration, however, is fracture instability, which is usually proportional to the amount of initial fracture displacement. If there is substantial fracture instability, surgical fixation should be considered to ensure healing in an anatomic position and the best possible functional result.

Closed reduction of a bicortical fracture of the distal radial metaphysis is performed when there is unacceptable angulation or displacement. Immobilization in an above-the-elbow cast is continued for 3 to 4 weeks, after which time a below-the-elbow cast is worn until healing, which usually occurs by 4 to 6 weeks after injury. If reduction is lost within the first 3 weeks, remanipulation with or without surgical fixation should be considered.

Recently, there has been interest in expanding the indications for percutaneous pin fixation to include substantially displaced fractures of the distal radial metaphysis. Studies by Gibbons and associates[9] and Proctor and associates[10] revealed that reduction is lost after closed treatment in 28% to 91% of patients. In a recent prospective, randomized study of 34 patients with a displaced distal radial fracture treated with either cast immobilization alone or percutaneous pinning,[11] cast immobilization was associated with a 30% prevalence of loss of reduction requiring repeat manipulation or another type of intervention. Percutaneous pinning provided stable, anatomic reductions without the need for additional treatment; however, there was a similar rate of complications, as a result of pin-track infection, irritation of the radial sensory nerve, or irritation of an extensor tendon. There were no instances of tendon disruption, permanent nerve injury, or growth arrest. Also, there were no major differences in clinical, radiographic, or cost-of-treatment outcomes between these two groups at the time of final follow-up. The decision to use a cast or percutaneous pinning depends on the surgeon's preference and should be based on a thorough understanding of the risks and benefits associated with each procedure.

Fractures of the distal radial physis are accorded special consideration. Displaced Salter-Harris type I and II fractures[12] are usually treated with closed reduction and immobilization in an above-the-elbow cast for 4 to 6 weeks. Reduction maneuvers should be performed gently with the patient under conscious sedation or general anesthesia. Multiple attempts at closed reduction should be avoided, as up to one fourth of patients undergoing multiple reduction attempts subsequently have growth arrest.[13] Manipulation should not be attempted after 7 to 10 days. In these sit-

uations, close clinical and radiographic follow-up is recommended, and corrective osteotomies may be considered if deformity does not remodel.[14] Closed reduction with percutaneous pinning is recommended for unstable injuries, injuries associated with severe swelling or neurovascular compromise (eg, acute carpal tunnel syndrome), and injuries associated with an ipsilateral displaced supracondylar fracture of the humerus.

Diaphyseal Fractures of the Forearm

In general, diaphyseal fractures can be divided into three categories on the basis of the pattern of injury: plastic deformation, greenstick, and complete diaphyseal fractures. Plastic deformation, or "traumatic bowing," occurs when forces applied to the skeletally immature radius or ulna exceed the limits of elastic deformation but fall short of the bone's ultimate strength. If left uncorrected, plastic deformation may limit rotation of the forearm.[15] Although some authorities have used 20° of angulation as a guideline for closed reduction, it is generally believed that any acute fracture that limits forearm rotation should be reduced. Reduction requires prolonged three-point bending, with pressure over the apex of the deformity, counteracted by opposite forces proximal and distal to the apex. Reductions require general anesthesia because often forces as high as 30 kg must be maintained for several minutes to achieve adequate correction of the deformity.[16]

Greenstick fractures are diaphyseal injuries characterized by complete fracture of the convex cortex and plastic deformation of the opposite, concave cortex. Closed reduction and immobilization in an above-the-elbow cast is recommended for any acute injury with obvious deformity and more than 15° to 20° of angulation. For apex-dorsal fractures, the distal segment is supinated, and volarly directed pressure is applied to the fracture site. Conversely, for apex-volar

injuries, the wrist is pronated, and a dorsally directed pressure is applied. These guidelines are often referred to as the "rule of thumbs," as the thumb is rotated toward the apex of the deformity during the reduction maneuver.[6] Immobilization is then achieved with a well-molded, above-the-elbow cast.

Several principles guide decision making with regard to the treatment of complete diaphyseal fractures of the forearm in children. Residual deformity may result in loss of forearm rotation and a poor functional outcome. While alignment of the ulna primarily influences the cosmetic appearance of the forearm, radial alignment determines forearm rotation.[17] Patients with less than 1 year of skeletal growth remaining have limited remodeling potential and thus should be treated as adults. Many of these fractures are treated with open reduction and internal fixation.[18] In general, 15° to 20° of midshaft angulation is considered acceptable in children younger than 8 years,[7,19] whereas only 10° of angulation should be accepted in older children.[20,21] In children younger than 8 years, bayonet apposition may remodel and may be acceptable if rotation and angulation are adequately corrected.[20]

Previous reports have suggested that up to 30° of rotational malalignment and loss of forearm rotation can be tolerated with minimal functional loss.[20] However, because rotational malalignment does not remodel, maximal correction of malrotation should be attained in the acute treatment of pediatric fractures of the forearm.

Given these principles, angulation of up to 20° is acceptable in children younger than 8 years, but no more than 10° is acceptable in older children. Cast immobilization should be applied with three-point contact and an interosseous mold. The forearm is immobilized in neutral rotation or slight supination to limit loss of supination. Although guidelines regarding age and acceptable parameters of alignment are helpful, the most important issue in the treatment of diaphyseal fractures is fracture stability. The indications for surgical treatment include instability, unacceptable alignment, an open fracture, a fracture associated with vascular injury, or a refracture with displacement.

Intramedullary Fixation

Intramedullary fixation with closed or open reduction is ideal for unstable transverse fractures.[20,22-24] Intramedullary devices provide an internal splint, maintaining both length and alignment. When intramedullary fixation is applied with a gentle curve throughout the entire length of the radius and ulna, three-point contact may be established, adding stability to the reduction. Theoretically, by providing longitudinal and angular stability while still allowing some compression and distraction, intramedullary fixation stimulates abundant fracture callus formation. Rotation is not completely controlled. Because these devices do not provide rigid fixation, postoperative cast immobilization is required.

The technique of intramedullary fixation of diaphyseal fractures of the forearm has been well described.[20,22-24] The choice of implant depends largely on the size of the fracture fragments and thus the age of the patient. Kirschner wires may be used in younger patients, and flexible titanium intramedullary rods can be used in older children and adolescents. Fluoroscopy is necessary to determine the largest caliber implant that will pass through the diaphyseal isthmus of the affected bone.

Because the ulna is subcutaneous, easily manipulated, and relatively straight, it is usually reduced and fixed first. A small longitudinal incision is made over the olecranon process, and dissection is carried down through the subcutaneous tissue and triceps insertion to the bone. A small drill is used to create an entry hole for insertion of the intramedullary rod. After fracture reduction, the rod is passed

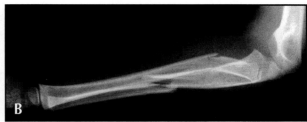
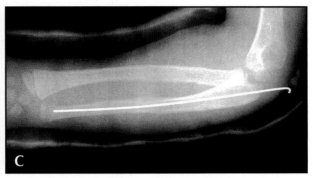
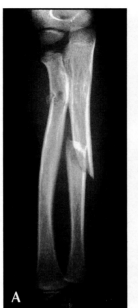

Fig. 1 A diaphyseal fracture of the forearm. AP **(A)** and lateral **(B)** radiographs showing a diaphyseal fracture of the forearm with unacceptable angulation of the radius. Satisfactory closed reduction of both bones could not be maintained simultaneously. **C,** Closed reduction of the radius could be maintained after the ulna was stabilized with a single intramedullary Kirschner wire placed percutaneously.

in an antegrade fashion through the medullary canal and across the fracture site to within 2 cm of the distal physis. The proximal tip of the rod may be cut above the level of the skin, allowing for easier removal. After intramedullary fixation of the ulna, the radial fracture is reduced. If a stable anatomic reduction can be obtained, single-bone fixation is sufficient[20] (Fig. 1).

If the reduction of the radius is unstable after ulnar fixation, a dorsal radial incision is made just proximal to the Lister tubercle. Dissection is carried out between the second and third dorsal extensor compartments to cortical bone. After fluoroscopic confirmation that the approach has been made proximal to the distal radial physis, a small drill hole is made in the dorsal surface. Directing the drill hole slightly proximal and volar allows easier passage of the intramedullary rod through the radial diaphysis. A 20° bend in the rod also results in easier

passage. The extensor pollicis longus tendon must be protected during drilling and rod passage. After the rod has been placed across the fracture site and reduction has been confirmed with fluoroscopy, the distal end is bent and cut above the skin. The extremity is then placed in a well-padded long arm cast.

Plate Fixation

Patients with a comminuted fracture or less than 1 year of skeletal growth remaining are candidates for plate and screw fixation with use of standard techniques.[25] Standard 3.5-mm dynamic compression, pelvic reconstruction, or single or double-stacked semitubular plates may be used, depending on the size of the bones to be fixed. Excellent results have been reported with use of these techniques.[25]

There continues to be controversy regarding the need for removal of the plate. Theoretical concerns about retained plates include late infection, metallic cor-

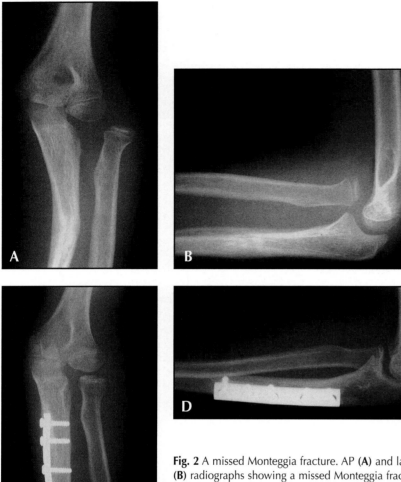

Fig. 2 A missed Monteggia fracture. AP **(A)** and lateral **(B)** radiographs showing a missed Monteggia fracture with lateral angulation of the ulna. AP **(C)** and lateral **(D)** radiographs made after an open reduction of the radial head and an ulnar osteotomy stabilized with plate osteosynthesis.

convex radial head and a hypoplastic capitellum—or an acute, traumatic Monteggia fracture-dislocation.

Treatment of Monteggia lesions is based on the age of the patient, the pattern of the injury, the time from the initial injury, and the stability of the fracture. A child with an acute incomplete fracture or plastic deformation of the ulna can be managed with closed reduction followed by immobilization in an above-the-elbow cast. The limb should be immobilized with supination of the forearm, and 90° to 110° of elbow flexion is recommended, although elbow extension may be necessary for type II (posterior) Monteggia fractures. When there is a complete ulnar fracture, surgical stabilization of the ulna is recommended to reduce the risk of redisplacement. Transverse or short oblique fractures can be treated with intramedullary fixation of the ulna, whereas long oblique, segmental, or comminuted injuries are best treated with open reduction and ulnar plate fixation.[29]

Monteggia fracture-dislocations are frequently missed on initial presentation. Closed reduction and cast immobilization or internal fixation can be attempted when the fracture is seen within 2 to 3 weeks after the injury. However, those seen more than 3 to 4 weeks after the injury may require open reduction with repair or reconstruction of the annular ligament and/or ulnar corrective osteotomy[30] (Fig. 2).

Complications of Pediatric Fractures of the Forearm

Nonunion is an extremely rare complication after a pediatric fracture of the forearm. Open fractures with soft-tissue loss, vascular insufficiency, and/or infectious complications are more likely to have delayed healing or nonunion.[31] In these situations, restoration of vascularity and soft-tissue coverage, eradication of infection, and rigid internal fixation, with bone grafting when indicated, usually result in satisfactory healing. Malunion of a fore-

rosion, stress-shielding of the bone under the plate, increased risk of adjacent fracture due to a stress-riser effect of the plate, and difficulty with subsequent plate removal after long-term osseous overgrowth. Currently, the orthopaedic literature provides no definitive evidence for or against routine plate removal. The risks of refracture and neurovascular injury during plate removal, however, have been well described.[26,27]

Monteggia Fracture-Dislocations

Monteggia fracture-dislocation refers to a fracture of the ulna with an associated radiocapitellar dislocation.[28] Although originally described in association with a fracture of the proximal third of the ulna, the term is commonly used to describe any ulnar fracture associated with a radiocapitellar dislocation. In a normal forearm, a line drawn along the axis of the radius through the radial head should bisect the capitellum on every radiographic view. A Monteggia injury is present when this radiographic relationship is disrupted in the setting of an ulnar fracture. Care should be taken not to mistake a chronic, congenitally dislocated radial head—characterized by a small,

arm fracture may result in loss of rotation, although this may not interfere with the activities of daily living of an adult. Normal forearm supination has been reported to be 80° to 120°, and normal forearm pronation has been estimated to be 50° to 80°.[21] Patients with a malunited forearm fracture, limited forearm rotation, and major functional compromise may be candidates for corrective osteotomy with internal fixation.[32] There is evidence suggesting that the functional outcomes of these corrective procedures are more favorable when they are performed within a year after the original injury.

Management of pediatric fractures of the forearm is sometimes complicated by compartment syndrome. In a recent review of 34 cases of compartment syndrome, 10 were associated with a fracture of the forearm or the distal part of the radius.[33] Early diagnosis and prompt surgical decompression are critical to prevent long-term complications. The absence of neurovascular deficits may be misleading; in fact, often the first indication of an impending compartment syndrome is an increased need for analgesia.[33] The compartment pressures should be measured in any child with a swollen, injured forearm and increasing pain or pain with passive movement of the fingers. Pressures of greater than 30 mm Hg support the diagnosis of compartment syndrome. Once the diagnosis has been established, fasciotomy should be performed immediately.

Neurologic and vascular injuries are uncommon with closed fractures of the forearm. The majority of nerve injuries are neurapraxias that resolve without the need for surgical treatment. Certain neurovascular deficits have been associated with particular fracture patterns. The posterior interosseous nerve may be injured in a Monteggia fracture-dislocation, particularly a Bado type III (lateral) injury.[34] Injury of the anterior interosseous nerve has been described in association with displaced fractures of the

proximal part of the radius and Galeazzi fracture-dislocations.

Refracture is a well-described complication of pediatric fractures of the forearm; it occurs in as many as 5% of patients.[35] Children are at highest risk for refracture immediately after cessation of cast immobilization or after removal of internal fixation. Diaphyseal fractures are more likely to be followed by a refracture than are metaphyseal fractures. The risk of refracture is inversely proportional to the duration of cast immobilization. For this reason, it is recommended that patients avoid high-risk activities and wear protective, removable wrist splints immediately after discontinuation of cast immobilization or elective removal of hardware.

An average of 6 mm of overgrowth may occur after a forearm fracture, but it is usually of little functional or cosmetic consequence. More troubling is the complication of growth arrest, which may occur after 1% to 7% of fractures of the distal radial physis.[13] Substantial physeal arrest may lead to abnormal wrist mechanics, ulnar overgrowth with ulnocarpal impaction, tears of the triangular fibrocartilage complex, and instability of the distal radioulnar joint. Management of distal physeal arrest depends on the pattern of arrest, degree of deformity, and amount of skeletal growth remaining. Physeal bar resections, completion epiphyseodeses, and/or corrective osteotomies may be considered for symptomatic patients with progressive deformity.[14]

Elbow Fractures

Elbow fractures are common in children. Diagnosis may be challenging. Physical examination of a grossly swollen elbow in an uncooperative child is difficult. Also, a large portion of a child's elbow is unossified, making radiographic interpretation sometimes difficult. Acute and long-term complications of pediatric elbow fractures can be severe. Therefore, an understanding of the anatomy of the immature elbow as well as up-to-date techniques in

fracture management provide the best chances for successful outcomes.

Supracondylar Fractures of the Humerus

Supracondylar fracture of the humerus is the most common pediatric elbow fracture. The peak age of occurrence is between 3 and 8 years. Ninety-eight percent of supracondylar fractures are the extension type, caused by a fall on an outstretched hand with hyperextension of the elbow. On the basis of radiographic evaluation, Gartland classified hyperextension injuries as type I (nondisplaced), type II (displaced with posterior cortical contact), or type III (completely displaced).[36] Although the reliability of the classification has recently been demonstrated, treatment should not be based solely on fracture classification.[37] Type I fractures are immobilized with the elbow flexed 90°. Type II fractures are characterized by a disrupted anterior cortex but an intact posterior cortex. The distal fragment is posteriorly angulated and can be rotated. If the fragments are seen to be in acceptable alignment on AP and lateral radiographs, a long arm cast can be used for 3 weeks. The position on the lateral radiograph is considered satisfactory if the anterior humeral line passes through the capitellar ossification center. If angulation is seen on the AP radiograph, especially one obtained for a medially impacted, varus type injury, closed reduction and percutaneous pinning is indicated. Percutaneous pinning may also be used for type II fractures that reduce well but are unstable.

Type III fractures demonstrate complete loss of contact of the anterior and posterior cortices. This fracture pattern requires closed reduction and percutaneous pinning, or open reduction if the fracture is irreducible.[38] These fractures have the greatest risk of being associated with neurovascular injury. Skin or skeletal traction is rarely used because they have been associated with a higher complication rate.[39]

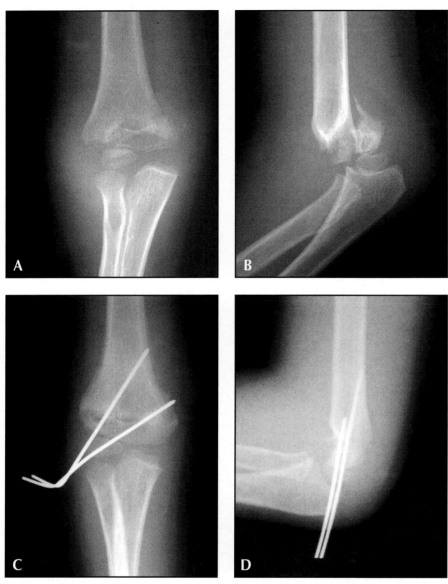

Fig. 3 Type III supracondylar fracture of the humerus. AP **(A)** and lateral **(B)** radiographs showing a closed type III supracondylar fracture of the humerus. The child had a normal neurovascular examination. AP **(C)** and lateral **(D)** radiographs made 3 weeks after closed reduction and percutaneous pinning. Note that the two lateral pins were placed in a divergent configuration to obtain optimal fixation of the distal piece. After the two pins were placed, the fracture stability was tested with use of intraoperative fluoroscopic imaging. No motion was noted with elbow extension or arm rotation. Because the fracture was found to be stable, no medial pin was necessary. A perfect anatomic reduction was maintained. (Courtesy of David Skaggs, MD.)

medially displaced fractures and supination for laterally displaced fractures.[38] Use of a 0.062-in (1.57-mm) Kirschner wire is recommended for patients who are 6 years old and younger, and a 0.078-in (1.98-mm) Kirschner wire is recommended for those older than 6 years.[38] The optimal pin configuration is controversial. Although crossed pins provide good stability, a recent study suggested that two properly placed lateral pins confer enough stability to prevent redisplacement.[41] A medial pin places the ulnar nerve at risk. Pins are left protruding percutaneously and are bent to 90° for ease of removal. Postoperative immobilization should include a well-padded posterior splint or cast.[38] There is a trend for experienced surgeons to place two bicortical lateral pins, test stability, and then add a medial pin if there is persistent rotational instability[41,42] (Fig. 3).

Flexion-type injuries account for 2% of supracondylar fractures. If there is excessive flexion, closed reduction and percutaneous pinning is recommended. Open reduction may be required because closed reduction is difficult.[38,43]

Vascular complications are most common with type III injuries.[44] The brachial artery is injured in 0.5% of patients. When radial and ulnar pulses are not palpable, a viable (pink) hand must be differentiated from a nonviable (white) hand, which is an orthopaedic emergency. When an extremity is pulseless, the first step is to reduce the fracture. After reduction, if the hand has good capillary refill and a pulse is documented with Doppler examination, pin fixation and observation are appropriate. If pulses are not detectable with the Doppler examination and the color of the hand or capillary refill is abnormal, exploration of the brachial artery is indicated.[45] Arteriography is not mandatory because the site of injury is known.[46] If the extremity becomes pulseless after closed reduction, open exploration is indicated. The brachial artery is explored after closed reduction

Reductions are performed with the patient under general anesthesia. The degree of urgency is dictated by swelling, vascular status, and skin integrity. A recent study suggested that delay of definitive treatment is acceptable if the hand is perfused and the findings of the neurologic examination are normal.[40] The technique of closed reduction consists of (1) longitudinal traction, (2) correction of medial or lateral displacement, (3) elbow flexion, and (4) pronation for

and percutaneous pinning of the fracture so that the elbow can be extended without risk of fracture displacement.

Observation is recommended for at least 24 hours after treatment of an acute fracture. If compartment syndrome is suspected, the splint should be removed. If the symptoms resolve, observation is appropriate. If the symptoms persist, compartment pressures should be measured. If the forearm compartment pressures measure more than 30 mm Hg or symptoms of compartment syndrome persist, fasciotomies are indicated.

Neurologic injury occurs in association with 7% to 11% of fractures.[47] The specific nerve that is injured may depend on the direction of the initial displacement of the fracture.[48] Thirty-five percent to 45% of the neurologic injuries involve the radial nerve, and they are most common when the distal fragment is displaced posteromedially. Thirty-two percent to 40% of the neurologic injuries involve the median nerve or anterior interosseous nerve, and those injuries are most common with posterolaterally displaced fractures.[49] A neurologic injury that occurs at the time of fracture can be observed to see if recovery occurs for 3 to 6 months. Exploration is indicated when nerve entrapment occurs at the time of reduction.[43] When a medial pin is used, it should be placed with the elbow flexed less than 90°, or by making a 1-cm incision medially to protect the ulnar nerve behind the medial epicondyle when the elbow is swollen.[41]

Cubitus varus is a cosmetic problem that occurs in 5% to 10% of patients with a supracondylar humeral fracture. It is the result of malunion caused by improper reduction in the coronal plane or by late displacement. Functional impairment is rare. Late open reduction or fracture manipulation after 21 days can increase the risk of myositis ossificans and is not recommended. Distal humeral osteotomy can be performed later for correction of cubitus varus.

Fractures of the Lateral Condyle of the Humerus

A fracture of the lateral condyle of the humerus generally results from a varus stress to the extended elbow and supinated forearm. Milch[50] classified these fractures according to the location of the fracture line through the distal part of the humerus. With a Milch type I fracture, the fracture line is lateral to the trochlear groove. With a Milch type II fracture, the line is medial to the trochlear groove and, therefore, because of loss of trochlear abutment, the ulna and radius are often displaced laterally. Because the full extent of the fracture line can be difficult to perceive on preoperative plain radiographs, the Milch classification may be wrong for more than 50% of fractures.[51]

The stability of the lateral condyle has been classified into three stages of displacement: type I is displaced less than 2 mm, type II is displaced 2 to 4 mm, and type III is completely displaced.[52] Treatment of type I fractures is controversial. Splinting with close follow-up is acceptable. Late displacement, with an increased risk of nonunion, has been reported in up to 10% of patients.[38] Standard treatment for fractures with 2 mm or more of displacement is reduction and internal fixation[51] (Fig. 4). Open reduction is performed through the interval of the brachioradialis and the triceps. It is very important to preserve the posterior soft-tissue attachment to the lateral condyle because it provides the primary blood supply to the capitellum. After anatomic reduction, the fracture is stabilized with 0.062-in (1.57-mm) Kirschner wires. Traditionally, Kirschner wires have been left in place for 6 weeks; however, a recent study suggested that results are equally good with only 3 weeks of pin fixation.[53]

Nonunion can occur when a fracture is not recognized or when it undergoes late displacement. Cubitus valgus deformity can occur as a result of nonunion or malunion.[54] Treatment is dictated by

the position of the nonunion.[55] Reconstruction can be done when fracture fragments are within 1 cm of the joint or when there is a large metaphyseal fragment. The blood supply to the lateral condyle should be carefully preserved. If the fragment is displaced more than 1 cm, observation may be preferable. Tardy ulnar nerve palsy can occur with nonunion or malunion of the lateral condyle. Anterior transposition of the ulnar nerve should be performed early if symptoms develop.

Osteonecrosis may result from the injury itself, but it is more likely caused by extensive surgical soft-tissue dissection posteriorly at the time of fracture fixation.

Growth arrest can occur in the area where the fracture crosses the distal humeral physis. This causes a fishtail deformity appearance on radiographs but is generally not symptomatic.[38]

Fractures of the Medial Epicondyle of the Humerus

Fractures of the medial epicondyle of the humerus account for 11% of pediatric elbow fractures and occur most commonly in children between the ages of 9 and 14 years.[38] Up to 50% of these fractures are associated with an elbow dislocation.[56] Minimally displaced fractures can be treated with splinting in 90° of flexion. Active range-of-motion exercises can begin within 2 weeks. A 35-year follow-up study of 56 unreduced medial epicondylar fractures demonstrated adequate function and range of motion after treatment with immobilization alone.[57] Pseudarthrosis occurred in 55% of the patients, but symptoms did not differ between that group and those with osseous healing.[57] We are not aware of any study defining the exact amount of displacement for which surgical treatment yields better results than nonsurgical treatment. The only absolute indications for surgical treatment are irreducible incarceration of the fragment within the

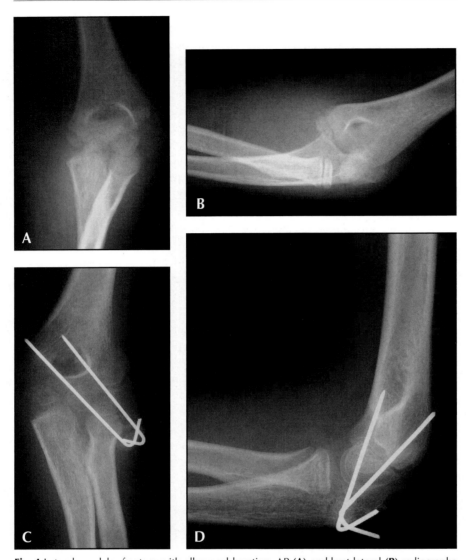

Fig. 4 Lateral condylar fracture with elbow subluxation. AP **(A)** and best lateral **(B)** radiographs showing a type II lateral condylar fracture with elbow subluxation in an 11-year-old patient. AP **(C)** and lateral **(D)** radiographs made 4 weeks after surgery, showing abundant callus laterally and maintenance of anatomic reduction. The pins were pulled at this time.

band suture, which avoids the need for later wire removal.[59] Epiphyseal (apophyseal) fracture separation is less common than is metaphyseal injury, but it occurs through a similar mechanism. Such fractures are most often treated nonsurgically. Apophyseal fracture may require surgical fixation if there is loss of motion, wide displacement, or persistent pain.[59]

Fractures of the Radial Neck

Fractures of the radial neck may occur through the physis (in young children) or through the metaphysis at the insertion of the annular ligament (usually in children between the ages of 8 and 12 years). Diagnosis can be difficult if there is a cartilaginous epiphysis. Arthrography, MRI, or ultrasonography may be necessary to define the injury.

Treatment is dictated by the amount of initial displacement and angulation and by the patient's age. Closed reduction is always attempted first. The reduction is acceptable when there is less than 4 mm of translation and less than 30° to 60° of angulation.[60] When the reduction is not acceptable, percutaneous Kirschner-wire manipulation is often successful.[61] If closed or percutaneous reduction is unsuccessful, open reduction is indicated. At the time of open reduction, the annular ligament and other soft-tissue attachments should be preserved. An oblique Kirschner wire placed through the head fragment and into the metaphysis as well as supplemental cast immobilization can maintain the reduction. Transcapitellar fixation is associated with a risk of pin breakage. Excision is never indicated in children because even a necrotic radial head that is devoid of soft tissue has some potential for healing and is an ideal biologic spacer.[43]

The most important complications are osteonecrosis and loss of motion, particularly pronation and supination, of the radial head. Complications are most common after open reduction. However,

elbow joint or an open fracture. When a fragment is incarcerated, closed reduction can be attempted by creating a valgus stress on the minimally flexed elbow and supinated forearm. If this maneuver is unsuccessful, open reduction and internal fixation is indicated. Children who are expected to place a great deal of valgus stress on the elbow (such as gymnasts and pitchers) are usually treated with internal fixation.[58]

Fractures of the Olecranon Process of the Ulna

Fracture of the proximal part of the ulna is relatively uncommon and can occur at any age. Metaphyseal fractures are often minimally displaced and can be treated closed. If there is more than 3 mm of intra-articular displacement, open reduction and internal fixation is indicated.[59] Fixation after open reduction is most commonly done with use of a tension

whether these complications are caused by the severity of the injury or by the dissection during the open reduction is still a subject of controversy. In one study with up to 20 years of follow-up, all conservatively treated fractures with up to 50° of angulation had satisfactory remodeling.[62] Thirty-one of the 38 patients had residual deformity of the radial head, but only 4 had a loss of function.

Fractures of the Distal Humeral Epiphysis

Fracture-separation of the distal humeral epiphysis is rare. It is usually a Salter-Harris type II injury. DeLee and associates[63] described three types based on the shape of the Thurston Holland fragment and the age of the patient. The injury is most common in children 2 to 3 years old. It is difficult to diagnose because the only ossified structure about the elbow in children of this age is the capitellum. If the diagnosis is uncertain, ultrasonography, MRI, or arthrography may be necessary.[38]

Treatment options include open or closed reduction with pinning, closed reduction without pinning, and cast immobilization without reduction.[64] We recommend closed reduction with pinning, given the early risk of loss of reduction and later problems with cubitus varus and osteonecrosis of the medial humeral condyle.[65]

T-Condylar and Supracondylar Fractures

T-condylar fractures of the distal part of the humerus are rare in children. They most often occur by the same mechanism that causes supracondylar fractures but with higher energy. It has been postulated that the olecranon acts as a wedge, splitting the trochlea.[66] If the T-condylar component is not displaced, the fracture can be treated in the same manner as a supracondylar fracture. If the intra-articular fracture is displaced more than 2 to 3 mm, then open reduction is required.[38] Treatment depends on the age of the

child and the displacement of the fracture. In very young children, Kirschner wires can be used to fix the condylar fragments to each other and to the humeral shaft. Treatment of adolescents is similar to that of adults: internal fixation is performed with a posterior plate on the medial side and a lateral plate on the lateral side. The approach can be posteromedial (Bryan-Morrey approach), through an olecranon osteotomy, or triceps-splitting. Because intra-articular comminution is rare in children and adolescents, it is rarely necessary to perform an olecranon osteotomy for direct visualization of the trochlear articular surface.

Ulnar and radial neuropathies have been reported with these injuries. When ulnar neuropathy is present, the nerve can be transposed or decompressed at the time of surgery. In one report, the nerve palsy resolved within 1 year.[66] Care should be taken with pin placement after closed reduction.

Alternative Methods of Fixation

Traditional pin fixation with Kirschner wires was discussed throughout this chapter. However, the use of absorbable pins for fixation of fractures in children has also been reported. In one study of 71 patients with various types of fractures (predominantly humeral fractures), the results after use of absorbable pins were deemed satisfactory; however, 3 patients with a supracondylar fracture had pin breakage and fracture displacement.[67]

Summary

Surgical treatment is rarely necessary in pediatric wrist and forearm fractures. Very unstable metaphyseal fractures in older children, especially if there is an ipsilateral injury, open injury, or severe swelling, may be best managed with percutaneous pin fixation. Intramedullary fixation of one or both bones is a valuable technique for managing unstable pediatric diaphyseal forearm fractures. Plates used to treat these fractures should be

smaller than the diameter of the bone; a 2.7-mm plate is ideal in many instances. Monteggia fracture-dislocations can be difficult injuries to treat by casting alone. When there is a complete ulna fracture, surgical stabilization of the ulna is valuable to reduce the risk of redisplacment. Transverse or short oblique ulna fractures can be treated with intramedullary fixation of the ulna, whereas more unstable fractures are best treated with ulnar plating. A Monteggia fracture-dislocation that has not been satisfactorily managed in the first 3 to 4 weeks after injury may require open reduction with repair or reconstruction of the angular ligament, and/or ulnar corrective osteotomy. Most type II and III supracondylar humerus fractures should be treated with closed reduction and pinning. Two divergent lateral pins often provide satisfactory fixation. If the supracondylar fracture remains unstable, then a third lateral pin or a medial pin can be added. When the radial pulse cannot be palpated after a supracondylar humerus fracture, the fracture should be reduced and pinned, and hand vascularity should be reassessed. If the hand is well perfused, careful observation is warranted. If the hand remains ischemic, exploration of the brachial artery is indicated. Medial epicondyle fractures are often associated with elbow dislocation. In such injuries, and in widely displaced fractures in athletes, internal fixation of the fracture allows early motion and a lower risk of nonunion. Lateral condyle fractures that are more than 2 mm displaced should be reduced and pinned. Many such fractures require open reduction for anatomic positioning. Radial neck fractures reduced to a position of less than 4 mm of translation and less than 30° of angulation can be treated with immobilization alone. The radial head of a child should not be excised. T-condylar fractures in teenagers can usually be satisfactorily exposed using a posterior medial (Bryan-Morrey) approach without olecranon osteotomy.

Medial and lateral plate fixation, as in adults, is usually required.

References

1. Wilkins KE: Operative management of children's fractures: Is it a sign of impetuousness or do the children really benefit? *J Pediatr Orthop* 1998;18:1-3.

2. Graham TJ, Waters PM, Price CT, et al: Upper extremity, in Beaty JH, Kasser JR (eds): *Rockwood and Wilkins' Fractures in Children*, ed 5. Philadelphia, PA, Lippincott-Williams & Wilkins; 2001, p 267-806.

3. Jones IE, Cannan R, Goulding A: Distal forearm fractures in New Zealand children: Annual rates in a geographically defined area. *N Z Med J* 2000;113:443-445.

4. Worlock P, Stower M: Fracture patterns in Nottingham children. *J Pediatr Orthop* 1986;6:656-660.

5. Cheng JC, Ng BK, Ying SY, Lam PK: A 10-year study of the changes in the pattern and treatment of 6,493 fractures. *J Pediatr Orthop* 1999;19:344-350.

6. Blount WP, Shaefer AA, Johnson JH: Fractures of the forearm in children. *JAMA* 1942;120:111-116.

7. Fuller DJ, McCullough CJ: Malunited fractures of the forearm in children. *J Bone Joint Surg Br* 1982;64:364-367.

8. Hogstrom H, Nilsson BE, Willner S: Correction with growth following diaphyseal forearm fracture. *Acta Orthop Scand* 1976;47:299-303.

9. Gibbons CL, Woods DA, Pailthorpe C, Carr AJ, Worlock P: The management of isolated distal radius fractures in children. *J Pediatr Orthop* 1994;14:207-210.

10. Proctor MT, Moore DJ, Paterson JM: Redisplacement after manipulation of distal radius fractures in children. *J Bone Joint Surg Br* 1993;75:453-454.

11. Miller BS, Waters PM, Taylor B: A prospective, randomized study of displaced pediatric metaphyseal distal radius fractures: Cast immobilization versus percutaneous pin fixation, in *67th Annual Meeting Proceedings of the American Academy of Orthopaedic Surgeons*. Rosemont, IL, American Academy of Orthopaedic Surgeons, 2000, p 501.

12. Sutter RB, Harris WR: Injuries involving the epiphyseal plate. *J Bone Joint Surg Am* 1963;45:587-622.

13. Lee BS, Esterhai JL Jr, Das M: Fracture of the distal radial epiphysis: Characteristics and surgical treatment of premature, post-traumatic epiphyseal closure. *Clin Orthop* 1984;185:90-96.

14. Hove LM, Engesaeter LB: Corrective osteotomies after injuries of the distal radial physis in children. *J Hand Surg Br* 1997;22:699-704.

15. Borden S IV: Traumatic bowing of the forearm in children. *J Bone Joint Surg Am* 1974;56:611-616.

16. Sanders WE, Heckman JD: Traumatic plastic deformation of the radius and ulna: A closed method of correction of deformity. *Clin Orthop* 1984;188:58-67.

17. Tynan MC, Fornalski S, McMahon PJ, Utkan A, Green SA, Lee TQ: The effects of ulnar axial malalignment on supination and pronation. *J Bone Joint Surg Am* 2000;82:1726-1731.

18. Ortega R, Loder RT, Louis DS: Open reduction and internal fixation of forearm fractures in children. *J Pediatr Orthop* 1996;16:651-654.

19. Vittas D, Larsen E, Torp-Pedersen S: Angular remodeling of midshaft forearm fractures in children. *Clin Orthop* 1991;265:261-264.

20. Price CT, Scott DS, Kurzner ME, Flynn JC: Malunited forearm fractures in children. *J Pediatr Orthop* 1990;10:705-712.

21. Daruwalla JS: A study of radioulnar movements following fractures of the forearm in children. *Clin Orthop* 1979;139:114-120.

22. Flynn JM, Waters PM: Single-bone fixation of both-bone forearm fractures. *J Pediatr Orthop* 1996;16:655-699.

23. Shoemaker SD, Comstock CP, Mubarak SJ, Wenger DR, Chambers HG: Intramedullary Kirschner wire fixation of open or unstable forearm fractures in children. *J Pediatr Orthop* 1999;19:329-337.

24. Van der Reis WL, Otsuka NY, Moroz P, Mah J: Intramedullary nailing versus plate fixation for unstable forearm fractures in children. *J Pediatr Orthop* 1998;18:9-13.

25. Wyrsch B, Mencio GA, Green NE: Open reduction and internal fixation of pediatric forearm fractures. *J Pediatr Orthop* 1996;16:644-650.

26. Bednar DA, Grandwilewski W: Complications of forearm-plate removal. *Can J Surg* 1992;35:428-431.

27. Deluca PA, Lindsey RW, Ruwe PA: Refracture of bones of the forearm after the removal of compression plates. *J Bone Joint Surg Am* 1988;70:1372-1376.

28. Bado JL: The Monteggia lesion. *Clin Orthop* 1967;50:71-86.

29. Ring D, Waters PM. Operative fixation of Monteggia fractures in children. *J Bone Joint Surg Br* 1996;78:734-739.

30. Rodgers WB, Waters PM, Hall JE: Chronic Monteggia lesions in children: Complications and results of reconstruction. *J Bone Joint Surg Am* 1996;78:1322-1329.

31. Haasbeek JF, Cole WG: Open fractures of the arm in children. *J Bone Joint Surg Br* 1995;77:576-581.

32. Trousdale RT, Linscheid RL: Operative treatment of malunited fractures of the forearm. *J Bone Joint Surg Am* 1995;77:894-902.

33. Bae DS, Kadiyala RK, Waters PM: Acute compartment syndrome in children: Contemporary diagnosis, treatment, and outcome. *J Pediatr Orthop* 2001;21:680-688.

34. Bader JL: The Monteggia lesion. *Clin Orthop* 1967;50:71-86.

35. Schwarz N, Pienaar S, Schwarz AF, Jelen M, Styhler W, Mayr J: Refracture of the forearm in children. *J Bone Joint Surg Br* 1996;78:740-744.

36. Gartland JJ: Management of supracondylar fractures of the humerus in children. *Surg Gynecol Obstet* 1959;109:145-154.

37. Barton KL, Kaminsky CK, Green DW, Shean CJ, Kautz SM, Skaggs DL: Reliability of a modified Gartland classification of supracondylar humerus fractures. *J Pediatr Orthop* 2001;21:27-30.

38. Beaty JH, Kasser JR. Fractures about the elbow. *Instr Course Lect* 1995;44:199-215.

39. Rodriguez Merchan EC: Supracondylar fractures of the humerus in children: Treatment by overhead skeletal traction. *Orthop Rev* 1992;21:475-482.

40. Green NE: Overnight delay in the reduction of supracondylar fractures of the humerus in children. *J Bone Joint Surg Am* 2001;83:321-322.

41. Skaggs DL, Hale JM, Bassett J, Kaminsky C, Kay RM, Tolo VT: Operative treatment of supracondylar fractures of the humerus in children: The consequences of pin placement. *J Bone Joint Surg Am* 2001;83:735-740.

42. Gordon JE, Patton CM, Luhmann SJ, Bassett GS, Schoenecker PL: Fracture stability after pinning of displaced supracondylar distal humerus fractures in children. *J Pediatr Orthop* 2001;21:313-318.

43. Wilkins KE, Beaty JH, Chamber HG, Toniolo RM, Sanders JO, Curtis RJ: Fractures and dislocations of the elbow region, in Rockwood CA Jr, Wilkins KE, Beaty JH (eds): *Fractures in Children*, ed 4. Philadelphia, PA, Lippincott-Raven, 1996, pp 653-904.

44. Lyons ST, Quinn M, Stanitski CL: Neurovascular injuries in type III humeral supracondylar fractures in children. *Clin Orthop* 2000;376:62-67.

45. Sabharwal S, Tredwell SJ, Beauchamp RD, et al: Management of pulseless pink hand in pediatric supracondylar fractures of humerus. *J Pediatr Orthop* 1997;17:303-310.

46. Shaw BA, Kasser JR, Emans JB, Rand FF: Management of vascular injuries in displaced supracondylar humerus fractures without arteriography. *J Orthop Trauma* 1990;4:25-29.

47. Brown IC, Zinar DM: Traumatic and iatrogenic neurological complications after supracondylar humerus fractures in children. *J Pediatr Orthop* 1995;15:440-443.

48. Kiyoshige Y: Critical displacement of neural injuries in supracondylar humeral fractures in children. *J Pediatr Orthop* 1999;19:816-817.

49. Cramer KE, Green NE, Devito DP: Incidence of anterior interosseous nerve palsy in supracondylar humerus fractures in children. *J Pediatr Orthop* 1993;13:502-505.

50. Milch H: Fractures and fracture-dislocations of the humeral condyles. *J Trauma* 1964;4:592-607.

51. Mirsky EC, Karas EH, Weiner LS: Lateral condyle fractures in children: Evaluation of classification and treatment. *J Orthop Trauma* 1997;11:117-120.

52. Jakob R, Fowles JV, Rang M, Kassab MT: Observations concerning fractures of the lateral humeral condyle in children. *J Bone Joint Surg* 1975;57:430-436.

53. Thomas DP, Howard AW, Cole WG, Hedden DM: Three weeks of Kirschner wire fixation for displaced lateral condylar fractures of the humerus in children. *J Pediatr Orthop* 2001;21:565-569.

54. Flynn JC: Nonunion of slightly displaced fractures of the lateral humeral condyle in children: an update. *J Pediatr Orthop* 1989;9:691-696.

55. Shimada K, Masada K, Tada K, Yamamoto T: Osteosynthesis for the treatment of non-union of the lateral humeral condyle in children. *J Bone Joint Surg Am* 1997;79:234-240.

56. Wilson NI, Ingram R, Rymaszewski L, Miller JH: Treatment of fractures of the medial epicondyle of the humerus. *Injury* 1988;19:342-344.

57. Josefsson PO, Danielsson LG: Epicondylar elbow fracture in children: 35-year follow-up of 56 unreduced cases. *Acta Orthop Scand* 1986;57:313-315.

58. Case SL, Hennrikus WL: Surgical treatment of displaced medial epicondyle fractures in adolescent athletes. *Am J Sports Med* 1997;25:682-686.

59. Gaddy BC, Strecker WB, Schoenecker PL: Surgical treatment of displaced olecranon fractures in children. *J Pediatr Orthop* 1997;17: 321-324.

60. Evans MC, Graham HK: Radial neck fractures in children: A management algorithm. *J Pediatr Orthop B* 1999;8:93-99.

61. Gonzalez-Herranz P, Alvarez-Romera A, Burgos J, Rapariz JM, Hevia E: Displaced radial neck fractures in children treated by closed intramedullary pinning (Metaizeau technique). *J Pediatr Orthop* 1997;17:325-331.

62. Vocke AK, Von Laer L: Displaced fractures of the radial neck in children: Long-term results and prognosis of conservative treatment. *J Pediatr Orthop Br* 1998;7:217-222.

63. DeLee JC, Wilkins KE, Rogers LF, Rockwood CA: Fracture-separation of the distal humeral epiphysis. *J Bone Joint Surg Am* 1980;62:46-51.

64. Skaggs DL: Elbow fractures in children: diagnosis and management. *J Am Acad Orthop Surg* 1997;5:303-312.

65. Oh CW, Park BC, Ihn JC, Kyung HS: Fracture separation of the distal humeral epiphysis in children younger than three years old. *J Pediatr Orthop* 2000;20:173-176.

66. Re PR, Waters PM, Hresko T: T-condylar fractures of the distal humerus in children and adolescents. *J Pediatr Orthop* 1999;19:313-318.

67. Bostman O, Makela EA, Sodergard J, Hirvensalo E, Tormala P, Rokkanen P: Absorbable polyglycolide pins in internal fixation of fractures in children. *J Pediatr Orthop* 1993;13:242-245.

The Surgical Management of Pediatric Fractures of the Lower Extremity

John M. Flynn, MD
David L. Skaggs, MD
Paul D. Sponseller, MD
Theodore J. Ganley, MD
Robert M. Kay, MD
Khristinn Kellie Leitch, MD, FRCSC

Abstract

The majority of pediatric fractures of the lower extremity can and should be treated with closed reduction, immobilization, and close follow-up. However, there is an ongoing debate in the orthopaedic community regarding the exact role of surgical management in the treatment of pediatric fractures. In the past 2 decades, surgical management of certain fractures provided markedly better results than closed management. In certain cases, such as those requiring anatomic realignment of the physis or articular surface, there are clear indications for surgical management. Increasingly, however, surgical management is being used to maintain optimal alignment, to allow early motion, or to facilitate mobilization of children with a lower extremity fracture. For many types of fractures, both nonsurgical and surgical methods have yielded good results and have vocal advocates. Certain technical advances, such as the use of flexible intramedullary fixation and bioreabsorbable implants, have further increased enthusiasm for surgical management of pediatric fractures of the lower extremity.

The goal of this chapter is to describe current concepts in the surgical management of selected pediatric fractures of the lower extremity. The focus is on specific indications, techniques, and potential complications of the management of selected fractures of the femur, knee, tibia, and ankle in children. The full scope of pediatric fracture management is a subject for textbooks. For introductory information and descriptions of techniques of successful nonsurgical management, the reader is directed to comprehensive sources.[1,2]

Femoral Shaft Fractures

A femoral fracture is the most common major pediatric injury treated by orthopaedic surgeons. Although the majority heal without long-term sequelae, the most frequent and expensive complications in the field of orthopaedics result from the closed treatment of pediatric femoral fractures.[3] Thus, the occasional unsatisfactory outcome maintains focus on evolving treatment recommendations.

A spica cast applied early is a very effective treatment for most children who are younger than age 6 years. A skeletally mature teenager is best managed as an adult, with an antegrade interlocked intramedullary nail. It is the group in between (ie, skeletally immature school-aged children and adolescents) who present the most difficult challenges in decision making. For generations, such children were managed with a period of traction followed by application of a spica cast. In the past 2 decades, there has been a strong trend toward treatment methods that allow rapid mobilization. Most orthopaedic surgeons recognize the adverse impact of prolonged hospitalization and spica cast immobilization on children and their families.[4] In many cases, both parents work outside the home; thus, the burden of home tutoring, nursing care, and transportation can be substantial. These social factors, along with the increasing emphasis toward minimizing hospital stay and complications, have generated enthusiasm for internal and external fixation of pediatric femoral fractures, despite the fact that the combination of traction and cast immobilization yields good results.

Surgical Decision Making

Indications for surgical management of pediatric femoral fractures are based on a sound understanding of remodeling after fracture union. Remodeling potential is greatest in children younger than age 10 years, in fractures near the physis, and in deformities in the plane of joint motion. Substantial remodeling of malrotation has not been documented,[5] to our knowledge. Remodeling occurs most rapidly in the 2 years following injury, although some additional improvement may occur for several years. Angular deformity is tolerated better near the hip than near the knee. As a general guideline, acceptable fracture alignment at union in children who are 2 to 10 years old is up to 15° of varus or valgus angulation, up to 20° of anterior or posterior angulation, and up to 30° of malrotation.

Shortening and overgrowth have been studied extensively.[6-8] Overgrowth may vary with the age of the child, the fracture pattern and location, the amount of shortening,[6] and possibly the treatment method. In children between the ages of 2 and 10 years, overgrowth averages 0.9 cm, with a range of 0.4 to 2.5 cm.[8] On the basis of published data, shortening at union should be no more than 1.5 to 2.0 cm in children younger than 10 years. In older children, no more than 1.0 cm of shortening is recommended.

In addition to remodeling, several other factors should be considered by the surgeon before he or she decides on a management plan. Fracture pattern, stability, and location are important factors in the determination of the suitability of certain treatment options. For example, flexible nails are less suitable for fractures that are spiral, comminuted, or very proximal or distal in the femur. Relative contraindications to traction and cast immobilization for children older than 6 years include obesity, multiple injuries, major head injury, floating knee injury, and a very distal fracture that compromises placement of traction pins. As a group, adolescents are best treated surgically,[9,10] as the complication rate of nonsurgical management of these patients is

30%. After consideration of all of these factors and the unique socioeconomic characteristics of the child and family, the surgeon can present possible treatment options, describing the risks and benefits of each as outlined below.

External Fixation

External fixation can be thought of as a form of "portable traction" for a pediatric femoral fracture. It is an excellent method for restoring the length of the limb and achieving satisfactory alignment without long incisions, exposure of the fracture site, major blood loss, or the risk of physeal injury or osteonecrosis.[11,12] With relatively quick application of widely available and familiar equipment, external fixation offers a valuable solution for several difficult problems: open fractures or fractures associated with severe soft-tissue injury, children with multiple trauma or head injury, or fracture patterns not amenable to flexible intramedullary nailing.

In recent years, enthusiasm for the use of external fixation as the principal treatment method for children age 6 to 16 years has waned because of frequently reported complications[13,14] and increasing evidence supporting the benefits of flexible intramedullary fixation.[15] Problems with family acceptance of the fixator, pin site irritation or infection, knee stiffness, and unsightly scars on the thigh are familiar to surgeons who use fixators for other disorders. However, reports of delayed union and refracture[13,14] after the removal of external fixators raised concern that the devices may cause stress-shielding of the fracture site and prevent the development of satisfactory fracture callus, especially if the fixator is not effectively dynamized. While flexible nailing is ideal for the treatment of midshaft transverse fractures, external fixation is better for highly comminuted fractures, or for long spiral fractures that have a larger surface for callus formation. External fixation also works well for frac-

tures at the distal diaphyseal-metaphyseal junction (Fig. 1), where callus formation is good but proximity to the insertion site makes flexible nailing unsuitable. Thus, when the fracture pattern has been considered in the decision making, external fixators complement flexible intramedullary nailing well.

An external fixator can be applied with the patient on either a radiolucent bed or a fracture table. We prefer a fracture table because it allows correction of length, rotation, and most angulation before the start of the procedure. Regardless of the type of fixator that is used, the size of the device and the constraints on pin placement (due to the location of the fracture and the proximity to the trochanter or distal physis) must be considered during careful preoperative planning. After predrilling at each site, the most proximal and distal pins are placed first, both perpendicular to the long axis of the shaft. The two central pins are then placed; spacing them farther from the fracture and closer to the first two pins decreases the stiffness of the frame (and thus stress-shielding). After final radiographs have been made, any skin tented by the pins is released and a sterile dressing is applied. Pin site care with diluted hydrogen peroxide is begun on the second postoperative day and continued until the pin entry sites heal. Showering and washing the sites with soap and water are then encouraged. Usually, weight bearing as tolerated is allowed, and the frame is dynamized once callus is visible. Once the callus is mature (ie, at least three cortices with bridging callus are seen on AP and lateral radiographs, at 2 to 4 months[13]), the fixator is removed and the fracture and pin sites are protected by allowing only partial weight bearing in a brace or knee immobilizer for several weeks.

Flexible Intramedullary Nail Fixation

Flexible intramedullary nail fixation can be thought of as an internal splint that

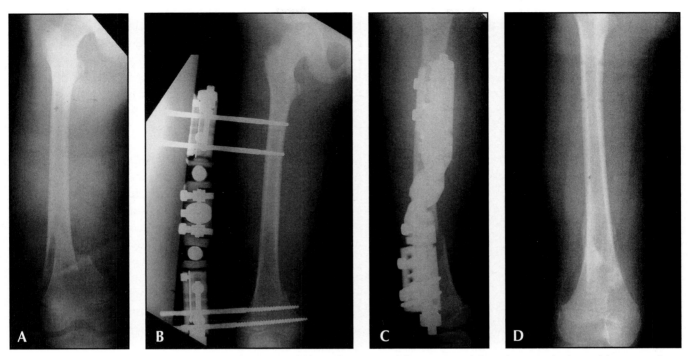

Fig. 1 Distal femoral fracture. **A,** AP radiograph of a 13-year-old boy who was struck by an automobile and sustained a femoral fracture at the junction of the distal metaphysis and the diaphysis. The fracture was deemed too distal for titanium elastic nail fixation. The proximal femoral physis was open. AP **(B)** and lateral **(C)** radiographs made immediately after reduction and external fixation. Alignment is satisfactory. **D,** AP radiograph made 10 weeks after injury, immediately after removal of the external fixator. A long leg cast was then applied to protect the fracture site and the pinholes, and weight bearing as tolerated was begun.

maintains length and alignment but permits sufficient motion at the fracture site to generate excellent callus formation.[16] Because flexible intramedullary nailing allows rapid mobilization of children with little risk of osteonecrosis, physeal injury, or refracture, there has been a recent surge in its popularity. However, this method is certainly not a new way to treat pediatric femoral fractures—excellent results have been reported over the past 2 decades for both Ender nails[17,18] and titanium elastic nails.[16,19] Currently, flexible intramedullary nailing is the pediatric orthopaedist's treatment of choice for skeletally immature children older than 6 years of age with a transverse fracture in the middle 60% of the femoral diaphysis.[20] More proximal and distal fractures and those with comminution or a spiral pattern are less amenable to flexible nailing; in such cases, the intra-

medullary fixation may be supplemented with a cast or brace. In the only published randomized trial that we know of comparing the two methods, Bar-On and associates[15] reported better results with flexible intramedullary nailing than with external fixation.

Although both Ender nails and titanium elastic nails provide flexible intramedullary fixation, the techniques have important differences. Ender nails are stainless steel and stiffer than titanium elastic nails. Stability with Ender nails is achieved by both the bend placed in the nail and stacking of the nails to increase "canal fill." The titanium nail technique involves balancing the forces of two opposing implants (Fig. 2), as described by its French developers.[19,21] The entry sites, nail sizes, and nail lengths should be symmetric; stacking is not part of the titanium nail fixation strategy. The most persis-

tently reported complication is soft-tissue irritation by the extraosseous portion of the nail tip at the site of its insertion.[16,19]

Preoperative planning includes measurement of the narrowest diameter of the femoral canal and multiplying by 0.4 to determine nail size; for example, if the minimum canal diameter is 10 mm, two 4.0-mm nails are used. Like external fixation, the procedure can be performed with the patient on a radiolucent table. However, we prefer to use a fracture table, with the "well" leg abducted out of the way and an optimal reduction achieved prior to preparation and draping. The nails should enter the bone about 2.5 cm proximal to the distal femoral physis. An incision is made from this point and extended distally approximately 2 to 3 cm. Great care is taken to avoid any deep dissection in the area of the distal femoral physis. An appropriately

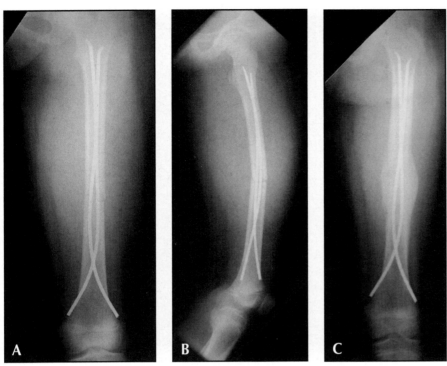

Fig. 2 Titanium elastic nail fixation for a midshaft femoral fracture. AP **(A)** and lateral **(B)** radiographs made in the operating room immediately following closed reduction and internal fixation of a midshaft femoral fracture in an 8-year-old girl who was struck by an automobile. Note that the nails were bent to establish cortical contact at the level of the fracture. Note also that, to avoid soft-tissue irritation, only a small extraosseous portion of the nail was left distally. **C,** Three months after surgery, anatomic alignment was maintained and there was abundant callus at the fracture site. The child began walking independently about 3 weeks after surgery.

sized drill bit (eg, a 4.5-mm drill bit for 4.0-mm nails) is used to broach the cortex of the femur, at the same distance from the physis on the medial and lateral sides. The drill should be angled obliquely within the medullary canal and aimed proximally to create a sharply angled distal-to-proximal track for the nail to follow. The nails are then bent with a gentle contour such that the apex of the convexity will be at the level of the fracture. Both nails are tapped up to the fracture site. The nail that will improve the alignment is advanced first across the fracture site and into the proximal fragment. The second nail is then passed into the proximal fragment. Often, it is helpful to rotate the nail tip up to 180° to facilitate passage. The nails are then tapped distal to proximal until the proximal tip of the

nail that entered laterally is at the level of the greater trochanteric apophysis and the tip of the nail that entered medially is at the same level near the medial aspect of the femoral neck. After the nails are fully inserted, each is backed out slightly, cut at the skin, and then tapped back in so that only 1 to 1.5 cm of the nail lies in the soft tissues. The nail can be bent slightly away from the femur to facilitate later removal, but it should not be bent sharply as this will cause soft-tissue irritation.[22]

Once fixation is complete, traction is released and the fracture can be gently impacted by manipulation so that it is not fixed in distraction. Normal rotation is ensured before the patient leaves the operating room. Postoperative immobilization is chosen on the basis of the fracture pattern. After fixation of stable trans-

verse fractures, a knee immobilizer is used with partial weight bearing. Immobilization is discontinued once callus is noted at the fracture site (at about 6 weeks in most cases). Nail removal is offered once the fracture line is no longer visible, usually at 6 to 12 months after injury.

Rigid Intramedullary Nail Fixation
Rigid, antegrade intramedullary nail fixation offers maximum stability and load-sharing. As it is in adults, it is the treatment of choice for displaced femoral shaft fractures in skeletally mature adolescents. A number of investigators have reported attempts to extend the indications for rigid antegrade nails to children with open proximal femoral physes.[23-26] Although the results have been good, there has also been an increasing number of reports of osteonecrosis of the femoral head.[20,26] The standard technique for antegrade int ramedullary nail fixation is well known and effective. Recommendations for use of the technique in adolescents stipulate an entry site through the tip of the greater trochanter, with avoidance of the piriformis fossa and damage to the blood supply of the femoral head. However, a recent survey of pediatric orthopaedists documented 14 cases of osteonecrosis, including several in which a "proper lateral technique" had been used.[20] Until better nail designs allow introduction of the nail without the risk of osteonecrosis, other options are recommended for skeletally immature adolescents.

Open Reduction and Plate Fixation
Plate fixation is an effective treatment for pediatric femoral fractures.[27-29] Advantages include the familiarity of the technique and widely available equipment as well as rigid fixation in anatomic alignment that allows rapid mobilization. However, the large incision, greater blood loss, refractures, hardware failure,[27,28] and issues regarding hardware removal limit the

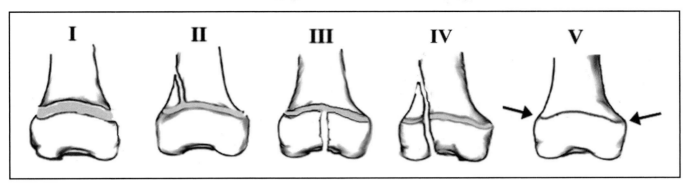

Fig. 3 Salter-Harris classification.

indications when better methods are available. The narrow indications include multiple injuries in a child younger than age 12 years and a child needing concomitant repair of the femoral artery. Some surgeons use plates for very proximal or distal fractures, for which there is no other treatment that would allow rapid mobilization. Specific technical recommendations include the use of 4.5-mm dynamic compression plates, with fixation of at least six cortices on each side of the fracture. Newer recommendations for plate fixation[30] include the use of longer plates but fewer screws, and indirect reduction with less soft-tissue stripping. We are not aware of any published studies on children treated with these newer techniques. After surgery, 6 to 8 weeks of protected weight bearing is common.

Fractures About the Knee

Fractures about the knee have important implications for growth. They also necessitate accurate reduction, because even minor angulation at the knee produces visible deformity. Even in children, stiffness and articular degeneration may follow if cartilage or muscle damage has occurred.[31] Finally, the surgeon should remember that ligament injuries may coexist with physeal fractures about the knee.[32]

The knee joint capsule and collateral ligaments originate just distal to the distal

femoral physis, concentrating any regional stress on this vulnerable growth cartilage. Injuries of the distal part of the femur are approximately twice as common as those of the proximal part of the tibia.[33] The distal femoral physis has a complex, undulating shape, forming four depressions into which four matching mamillary processes of the distal femoral metaphysis fit. This shape provides some degree of resistance to shear. However, it also may decrease the odds of a "clean" cleavage plane along the physis and therefore increase the risk of focal damage to the physis.[34] The proximal tibial epiphysis is spanned by and protected by the collateral ligaments. The physis is continuous with that of the tibial tubercle, which becomes visible radiographically in preadolescence. The neurovascular structures are at particular risk with proximal tibial injuries because of three sites of tethering: the popliteal artery at its trifurcation, the peroneal nerve at the proximal part of the fibula, and the tibial nerve at the proximal interosseous membrane. The results of a neurovascular examination should be documented, but an arteriogram is not routinely needed for patients with a displaced fracture if the distal pulses and capillary filling are normal.

Distal Femoral Epiphyseal Injuries

Because there is no eponymic classification system for these injuries, description

of a given injury should take into account the direction and degree of displacement, physeal injury pattern, and age of the patient.[31] Stress radiographs have been used to diagnose undisplaced physeal fractures. The diagnosis of occult fracture can provide an explanation for swelling about the knee in some injured adolescents.[35] The pattern of physeal injury does not predict the risk of growth disturbance in this region as well as does the pattern of injuries to other physes. Although growth disturbance in young patients with this injury is less common, its implications are far greater. CT with reconstruction is helpful to assess some complex Salter-Harris type IV fractures[36] (Fig. 3). The most predominant displacement—valgus or hyperextension—influences the method of reduction and immobilization. In addition, a hyperextension pattern is associated with a greater risk of neurovascular injury. More displaced fractures are more unstable, even after reduction.

Closed treatment is appropriate for all undisplaced fractures. Closed reduction should also be attempted for all minimally to moderately displaced Salter-Harris type I and II fractures. Fractures with greater displacement, especially those with a hyperextension pattern, are associated with an increased risk of redisplacement so percutaneous fixation is recommended.[37] An additional factor in this decision is the shape of the thigh. A

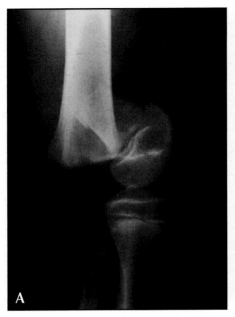
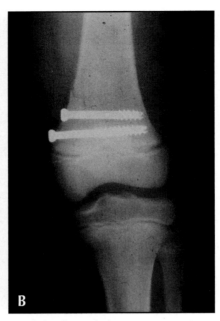

Fig. 4 Salter-Harris type II distal femoral fracture. **A,** Lateral radiograph showing an extension-type Salter-Harris type II distal femoral fracture. **B,** AP radiograph made after internal fixation with two cannulated interfragmentary screws.

large thigh girth makes cast immobilization more difficult. For fractures that do not reduce easily in the emergency department or that appear to be unstable, closed or open reduction followed by internal fixation is preferred. Percutaneous screws are preferred for fixation if they can be inserted without crossing the physis. Salter-Harris type II fractures can be stabilized by fixation across the Thurston-Holland metaphyseal spike if it is large enough (Fig. 4). If metaphyseal stability cannot be obtained, Salter-Harris type I and II fractures can be fixed with one or two smooth Steinmann pins from the epiphysis to the metaphysis. It is our preference to leave these pins buried under the skin and to remove them later. If the pins are left outside of the skin, they can cause much irritation and may even lead to septic arthritis. Salter-Harris type III and IV fractures can be fixed with intraepiphyseal screws.[35]

Complex, displaced transphyseal fractures, which may result from crushing or sharp injuries, require open ana-tomic reduction and internal fixation. Alignment can be difficult to assess because, once the fragments are reassembled, only the periphery of the growth plate can be seen. Secondary clues to alignment, such as the articular surface and metaphyseal fracture line, should be used. Use of cannulated screws helps to place the fixation away from both the joint surface and the growth plate in small epiphyses (Fig. 5).

Growth should be assessed carefully at about 6 months after injury, on radiographs coned and centered on the physis, by looking at the appearance of the physis as well as Park-Harris[38] growth lines parallel to it. The distance to these lines should be greater than the distance of the lines from the adjacent proximal tibial physis, which grows more slowly. MRI with gradient echo sequence will show the physis provided that there is no implant in the region. Long radiographs of both limbs, demonstrating length and angulation, can be used to assess a growth disturbance if more time has passed since

the fracture. If an injury to the growth plate is identified, options include bar resection, completion of the epiphysiodesis, contralateral epiphysiodesis, and corrective osteotomy with or without lengthening.

Stiffness may develop if there is a substantial associated injury to the quadriceps or the articular surface. In those situations, optimal internal fixation to allow early motion provides the best results. If loss of motion is severe despite conservative therapy, one should avoid the temptation to manipulate the knee in a child with open physes; separation may occur through the growth plate instead of movement at the joint.[39] Quadriceps-plasty and/or lysis of adhesions is safer if a plateau of motion has been reached. Injury to nerves or vessels occurs in about 1% to 3% of these fractures.

Proximal Tibial Epiphyseal Injuries
Injuries to the proximal tibial epiphysis are uncommon. They are most often the result of force applied to the planted leg.[40] Displacement is similar to that of fractures of the distal part of the femur; it is usually in the direction of hyperextension or valgus. Neurovascular injury is associated with up to 10% of these fractures, especially those with an apex-posterior angulation.[41]

The circulation should be carefully assessed, and an intraoperative arteri-ogram should be made when the vascular supply is compromised. A compartment syndrome should be ruled out clinically. Fractures that can be reduced by closed methods can usually be held in alignment with a long leg cast. If the fracture is displaced, the cast should be bivalved and the patient should be observed overnight for vascular complications. Because of the shape of the epiphysis, the Salter-Harris type III pattern of injury is rare in the proximal part of the tibia, except as a pattern of tibial tubercle avulsion. Unstable fractures of any pattern and all displaced type IV fractures should be

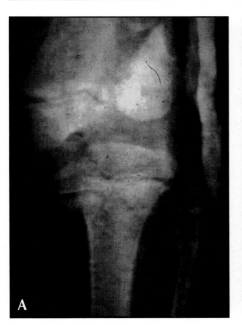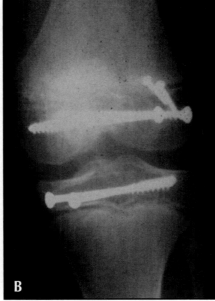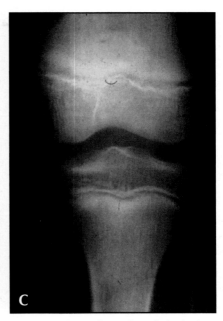

Fig. 5 Comminuted intra-articular fracture of the distal part of the femur and proximal part of the tibia. **A,** AP radiograph, made with the limb in a splint, showing a Salter-Harris type IV fracture of the distal part of the femur and the proximal part of the tibia. **B,** AP radiograph made after internal fixation with multiple interfragmentary screws. **C,** AP radiograph made after removal of the screws. There is no evidence of growth arrest at this time. The articular surfaces are positioned anatomically.

reduced and stabilized with internal fixation such as smooth Steinmann pins.[42]

Tibial Spine Avulsion

Tibial spine avulsions occur both during sports and as a result of trauma. Because the tibial spine has less resistance to tensile stress than does the anterior cruciate ligament, the bone usually fails before the ligament in young children.[43] However, there is substantial overlap between the two injuries. Tears of the anterior cruciate ligament are now recognized more frequently in preadolescents. In addition, the ligament usually stretches in patients who sustain a tibial spine avulsion, leading to mild residual laxity even after anatomic reduction of the tibial spine. Although most patients have some residual laxity, it is rarely symptomatic.[44,45]

Meyers and McKeever classified these fractures into three types: undisplaced (type I), hinged (type II), and completely displaced (type III).[46] Type I fractures are treated in a long leg cast.

Type II fractures can usually be reduced with extension of the knee and held in a cast for 6 weeks. While some authors advise attempting to reduce type III fractures by extending the knee, these fractures usually are irreducible or unstable. Open or arthroscopic reduction and internal fixation is the most effective treatment. The surgeon should be alert for meniscal entrapment under the cartilaginous flaps of the tibial spine.[47] Internal fixation may be achieved with use of peripheral sutures, a transepiphyseal pull-out suture, or, if the patient is near maturity, an infraepiphyseal screw.[48,49] A block to extension of the knee may occur if the fragment heals with excessive proximal displacement.

Tibial Tubercle Avulsion

Tibial tubercle avulsions occur through the physis of the tubercle. The injury varies in the degree of propagation proximally.[50] Ogden and associates[51] classified the injuries into three types. All types of

tibial tubercle avulsion are due to the pull of the quadriceps against the fixed knee and usually occur during jumping or landing. These injuries should be distinguished from the Osgood-Schlatter lesion, which is a chronic stress avulsion of the insertion of the patellar tendon into the superficial surface of the tubercle. Preexisting symptoms of an Osgood-Schlatter lesion have been reported in patients with acute tibial tubercle avulsion.[52] Small, undisplaced avulsions may be treated with a cast in extension. If the fracture is displaced, the tubercle should be replaced anatomically.[53] Interposed periosteal fragments should be removed. Small (type I) avulsion fragments may be anchored with use of Krackow tendon-holding sutures in the patellar tendon, anchored into bone around a screw or buried wire. Large (type II and III) avulsion fragments may be held with screws into the metaphysis. Growth disturbance is not usually a problem in children older than age 11 years.[54] Most of these injuries occur in children who are near skeletal maturity. If the child is more than 3 years from skeletal maturity, smooth pins and tension sutures should be used.

Most of these injuries heal uneventfully. Genu recurvatum may develop following the rare tubercle fracture that occurs before the age of 11 years. Compartment syndrome has been reported in association with type III fractures, presumably as a result of bleeding from the anterior tibial recurrent artery.[55]

Patellar Fractures

Patellar fractures are rare in children, presumably because of their decreased body mass and increased resistance to impact.[56] One unique feature in this age group is the relatively thick layer of unossified cartilage (the patella is completely cartilaginous until about the age of 4 years).[57] Therefore, a small rim of bone avulsed from the inferior pole of the patella in a young child represents a large cartilaginous and soft-tissue injury. This pattern has been termed a "sleeve fracture."[58] Treatment of an undisplaced patellar fracture in a cylinder cast for 6 weeks is advised. There is usually no problem with regaining motion. Open reduction and internal fixation with a tension band technique is recommended for fractures displaced more than 2 to 3 mm.

Tibial Shaft and Ankle Fractures
Proximal Tibial Metaphyseal Fractures

Fractures involving the proximal tibial metaphysis in children commonly occur between the ages of 2 and 8 years.[59] Occasionally, soft-tissue interposition blocks the reduction and the soft tissue must be removed from the fracture site. Fractures that cannot be reduced may require an open reduction.[60,61] A valgus deformity of the tibia may occur after these fractures. Monitoring healing with serial radiographs is recommended. The child's parents should be informed that post-traumatic valgus deformity can occur after

any form of treatment and its development is unpredictable.[62,63] Spontaneous correction of the valgus deformity can be expected up to 3 years following the injury. In the unusual case in which sufficient correction does not occur, two options are available for correction of the tibial valgus: proximal tibial hemiepiphysiodesis or proximal tibial osteotomy.

Tibial Shaft Fractures

Diaphyseal fractures of the tibia are the most common lower extremity fractures in children. Following a reduction, the limits of acceptable positioning are 10 mm of shortening; less than 10° of varus, valgus, or recurvatum; and no malrotation.[59] If these criteria cannot be met with closed reduction, surgical treatment is indicated. When a patient has a fracture of the distal part of the tibia or fibula, the foot can be left in equinus in the cast for the first 4 to 6 weeks, until callus forms. This is often necessary to prevent recurvatum at the fracture site. Unlike adults, children rarely have permanent stiffness about the ankle under this scenario.

The most common indication for surgical management of a tibial shaft fracture is soft-tissue injury, whether it is caused by an open fracture, compartment syndrome, or injury to the soft tissue alone. A second indication for rigid fracture immobilization is polytrauma. Rigid fracture immobilization allows mobilization and easier nursing care.

If a closed reduction of a tibial shaft fracture cannot be maintained, percutaneous pinning may be indicated. Although the pinning alone does not provide rigid fixation, when it is supplemented with cast immobilization it can be used successfully to treat many unstable tibial fractures. The technique is particularly valuable for open fractures.[64] After closed reduction with the patient under general anesthesia, two or more percutaneous Kirschner wires are placed across the fracture site. A long leg cast is applied to supplement stability. Once sufficient cal-

lus is seen on radiographs, the pins are removed and the cast is converted to a short leg cast. The total time in the cast is usually between 6 and 12 weeks.

Severe soft-tissue injury is the primary indication for external fixation of pediatric tibial fractures. The complications associated with external fixators are pin track infections, neurovascular injury on pin insertion, refracture after removal of the device, delayed union, and nonunion. While the application of these devices is quick and straightforward, their downside is stress-shielding that may slow healing. Preoperative planning should include consideration of the optimum pin placement to allow future wound management. The fixator should not protrude medially such that it hinders the contralateral lower limb during walking and other activities. The fixator is applied with a closed technique with use of fluoroscopy for pin placement. The use of 4-mm half-pins is recommended for smaller children, whereas 5- or 6-mm pins can be used in larger children. Usually, two bicortical pins placed proximal and distal to the fracture site are sufficient. Each of these pins must be at least 1 cm away from the physis and the fracture site. For fractures adjacent to the physes, one may consider using a thin wire external fixator or Kirschner wire fixation. An equinus contracture may develop in a child whose ankle is left in equinus when the fracture is associated with severe soft-tissue injury. In order to hold the ankle in a neutral position, the fixator can incorporate the foot with a pin in the first metatarsal. If fracture stability and the soft tissues allow it, partial to full weight bearing is permitted immediately after placement of the fixation device.

Because of the lower refracture rate and decreased time to fracture union associated with flexible intramedullary nail fixation, that method has become a good alternative to external fixation when skeletal fixation is indicated for a noncomminuted tibial shaft fracture in a

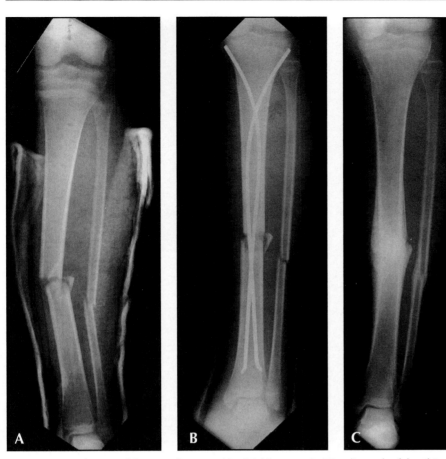

Fig. 6 Titanium elastic nail fixation of an unstable tibial fracture. **A,** AP radiograph of the tibia and fibula of a 13-year-old girl who was struck by an automobile. The injury was closed but unstable. Both the proximal and the distal tibial physes were open. **B,** AP radiograph made immediately after internal fixation with titanium elastic nails. Note that the reduction is anatomic but the nails cross just distal to the fracture site, compromising stability. The patient was treated in a patellar tendon-bearing cast. **C,** AP radiograph made 6 months after injury and after removal of the nails. The fracture was well healed, but the tibia was in approximately 5° of varus.

child (Fig. 6). Indications include soft-tissue injury, polytrauma, and an inability to maintain a good reduction with a cast. Contraindications include severe comminution and shortening. The nail size should be chosen so that the nail fills approximately 40% of the canal isthmus. Two small incisions are made, one medial and one lateral, at the level of the proximal metaphysis. The nails may be inserted distally for proximal fractures. Drill holes are made at least 2 cm from the physis. A proximal entry site must be posterior to the apophysis of the tibial tubercle, or growth disturbance and recurvatum may result. Nails are bent to a gentle c-shape and are inserted under image guidance to reach within 1 cm of the distal tibial physis. If the fibula is intact, a single larger nail may provide adequate fixation. A cast or fracture brace may be applied to facilitate early walking by patients with a stable fracture pattern. When a child has an unstable fracture, weight bearing should be delayed until callus is present.

The Floating Knee

The literature suggests that the clinical course of a floating knee in a child is most

affected by the child's age. Specifically, children under the age of 10 years are at a higher risk for tibial malunion and limb-length discrepancy.[65] McBryde and Blake reported high rates of delayed union (20%) and malunion (30%) in children treated with closed reduction of both fractures.[66] In order to improve these outcomes, fixation of at least one fracture has been advocated.[67]

Distal Tibial and Ankle Fractures

Salter-Harris type I and II fractures account for approximately 15% and 40% of fractures of the distal tibial physis, respectively.[68] These fractures can almost always be treated closed, except in the rare instance in which soft-tissue interposition prevents reduction. Acceptable alignment of displaced fractures in children with at least 2 years of growth remaining consists of no more than 15° of plantar tilt for posteriorly displaced fractures, no more than 10° of valgus for laterally displaced fractures, and no varus for medially displaced fractures. In children with less than 2 years of growth remaining, the amount of acceptable angulation is reduced to less than 5° in all planes.[69] When necessary, operative treatment consists of removal of the interposed soft tissue and application of smooth Kirschner wire fixation, followed by application of a long leg cast.

Unlike Salter-Harris type I and II fractures, types III and IV frequently require surgery. In one series, a growth disturbance developed in only 1 of 20 patients with a Salter-Harris type III or IV fracture treated with accurate open reduction and internal fixation in contrast to 5 of 9 patients with a similar fracture treated with closed reduction.[68] Medial malleolar fractures may have a Salter-Harris type III or IV pattern. Displaced fractures usually require surgical reduction and fixation in order to prevent growth disturbance. Visualization of the joint surface is a useful way to ensure anatomic reduction. This is accom-

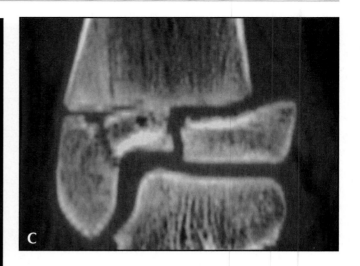

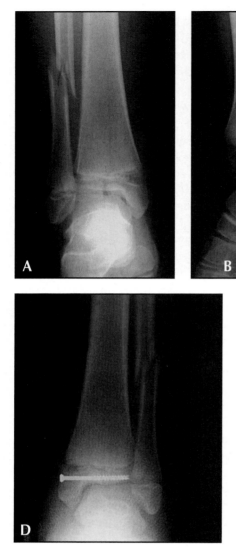

Fig. 7 Comminuted intra-articular fracture of the distal tibial physis. A, AP radiograph showing a comminuted distal tibial plafond fracture in a 14-year-old boy following a motor-vehicle accident. B, Lateral radiograph showing some posterior translation with fibular angulation. C, CT scan with reconstruction revealing the true extent of the fracture with comminution and intra-articular displacement. D, AP radiograph of the distal parts of the tibia and fibula, made immediately after open reduction and internal fixation of the fracture with a cannulated 4.5-mm screw. For optimal compression, the screw thread should not span the fracture site as it does in this case.

plished through a small (2-cm) oblique incision along the anterior border of the medial malleolus. Arthroscopic visualization has also been used. The fracture is stabilized with fixation placed parallel to the physis with 3.5- or 4.0-mm cannulated screws. Because the distal part of the tibia is dome-shaped, with the central portion more proximal than the anterior and posterior lips, it may be difficult to interpret the position of the screws on an anteroposterior radiograph. Thus, a lateral radiograph is essential to ensure that the screws are not violating the joint or the physis.

Tillaux fractures are Salter-Harris type III fractures of the anterolateral portion of the distal part of the tibia resulting from an epiphyseal avulsion at the site of the attachment of the anteroinferior tibiofibular ligament. The anterolateral location results from the direction of closure of the distal tibial physis (which initially occurs centrally, then medially, and finally laterally). The true extent of this fracture may not be appreciated on plain radiographs. A CT scan with sagittal reconstruction aids in the evaluation of the full extent of articular involvement. Tillaux fractures occur in adolescents in

whom the physes are partially closed, and thus there is no concern about future growth disturbance. Treatment is directed at obtaining and maintaining reduction of the distal articular surface of the tibia. Fractures with less than 2 mm of displacement can be treated with a long leg cast for 4 weeks, followed by a short leg cast for an additional 2 weeks. Following reduction, plain radiographs and CT scans confirm the adequacy of reduction. Fractures with 2 to 5 mm of displacement but no articular step-off represent a gray zone between open and closed treatment. In such cases, we often treat larger fragments surgically and smaller fragments nonsurgically. For open treatment, fixation with percutaneous 4.0-mm cannulated screws or wires, often facilitated by direct visualization of the joint surface, may be used. Schlesinger and Wedge[70] also described percutaneous manipulation of the displaced Tillaux fracture with a Steinmann pin followed by percutaneous fracture fixation.

Triplane fractures are complex Salter-Harris type IV fractures that have components in the sagittal, coronal, and transverse planes. As with Tillaux fractures, they occur in adolescents during closure of the distal tibial physis. Triplane fractures are easily underappreciated on plain radiographs. After a fracture line is seen on an AP or mortise radiograph, careful evaluation of the ankle on a lateral radiograph often reveals a posterior metaphyseal fracture. CT scans are valuable for assessing fracture alignment (Fig. 7). An articular step-off of more than 2 mm or a fracture gap of more than 2 to 4 mm is an indication for open reduction. A closed reduction by application of traction to the leg, with the patient under conscious sedation, may be successful for the treatment of a two-part triplane fracture, but such reduction is less often successful for three- or four-part fractures. Ertl and associates[71] showed that 2 mm or more of residual intra-articular displacement compromises the results of treatment. They reported marked deterioration of results over time, with 7 of 15 patients having residual symptoms after 3 to 13 years of follow-up. In a study reported in 1978 in which 12 of 14 children with a triplane fracture were treated with closed reduction, 4 children had radiographic evidence of physeal closure; however, none had more than 5 mm of shortening or substantial angular deformity.[71] Open reduction is generally carried out through an anterior approach, which may be medial or lateral depending on the fracture pattern. Depending on the fracture configuration, either the metaphyseal or the epiphyseal fragment may be fixed initially. Articular congruity must be restored. Most often, fixation can be achieved in both the metaphysis and the epiphysis. As this fracture occurs in adolescents during closure of the physis, fixation may cross the physis if necessary.

Open injuries at the level of the ankle joint are relatively uncommon and often involve a large amount of soft-tissue injury. Children struck by automobiles or injured by lawnmowers may have severe soft-tissue injuries. Because there is very little soft tissue in this region, coverage and reconstruction are very challenging. The growth plate injury is often not fully appreciated in the setting of severe soft-tissue injuries, although growth disturbance commonly follows such injuries. All open injuries are treated with irrigation, débridement, and appropriate stabilization. For most fractures, stabilization is accomplished with external fixation spanning the ankle joint.

Summary

Although the majority of pediatric femur fractures heal without long-term sequelae, closed treatment can result in frequent and expensive complications. A spica cast is usually the best treatment for children younger than age 6 years. However, over the past 10 years, there has been a strong trend to manage most pediatric femur fractures in children age 6 to 16 years with internal or external fixation. However, flexible intramedullary nailing, either by titanium elastic nails or stainless steel Ender nails, is currently the most popular method for managing fractures in children age 6 to 14 years. Rigid intramedullary nailing is generally reserved for those children with a closed proximal femoral physis because of the risk of osteonecrosis in the skeletally immature population. Newer nails, designed for the trochanteric entry site, may be a promising solution for the teenager with open physes. Plating was previously reserved for open fractures, vascular injuries, or fractures for which no other method was satisfactory. Recently, submuscular plating has been considered, but currently there are little data in the literature to support its widespread use. In fractures about the knee in children, reduction should be anatomic, realigning the articular surface and physis. Distal femoral epiphyseal injuries should be treated with internal fixation if there is displacement; cast treatment along risks late displacement and angulation close to the knee. Irreducible tibial spine avulsion fractures are now usually managed successfully with arthroscopic-assisted reduction and internal fixation with sutures, pins, or a screw. Tibial shaft fractures that can be reduced to less than 10° of varus, valgus, or recurvatum and less than 10 mm of shortening are best treated with cast immobilization. External fixation is a valuable tool to manage open tibial fractures. To avoid delayed union or nonunion, the external fixator construct should be planned to minimize stress shielding. Physeal fractures of the distal tibia may require open reduction and internal fixation if there is more than 2 mm of articular displacement or unacceptable plantar, valgus, or varus title. A CT scan, after an attempt at closed reduction, is valuable in assessing residual displacment and possible need for open reduction.

References

1. Wilkins KE: Operative management of children's fractures: Is it a sign of impetuousness or do the children really benefit? *J Pediatr Orthop* 1998;18:1-3.

2. Canale ST, Beaty JH, Blasier RD, et al: Lower extremity, in Beaty JH, Kasser JR (eds): *Rockwood and Wilkins' Fractures in Children*, ed 5. Philadelphia, PA, Lippincott-Williams & Wilkins, 2001, pp 881-1222.

3. Wilkins KE, Beaty JH, Chamber HG, Toniolo RM, Sanders JO, Curtis RJ: Fractures and dislocations of the elbow region, in Rockwood CA Jr, Wilkins KE, Beaty JH (eds): *Fractures in Children*, ed 4. Philadelphia, PA, Lippincott-Raven, 1996, pp 653-904.

4. Hughes BF, Sponseller PD, Thompson JD: Pediatric femur fractures: Effects of spica cast

treatment on family and community. *J Pediatr Orthop* 1995;15:457-460.

5. Davids JR: Rotational deformity and remodeling after fracture of the femur in children. *Clin Orthop* 1994;302:27-35.

6. Kohan L, Cumming WJ: Femoral shaft fractures in children: The effect of initial shortening on subsequent limb overgrowth. *Aust N Z J Surg* 1982;52:141-144.

7. Wallace ME, Hoffman EB: Remodelling of angular deformity after femoral shaft fractures in children. *J Bone Joint Surg Br* 1992;74:765-769.

8. Shapiro F: Fractures of the femoral shaft in children: The overgrowth phenomenon. *Acta Orthop Scand* 1981;52:649-655.

9. Reeves RB, Ballard RI, Hughes JL: Internal fixation versus traction and casting of adolescent femoral shaft fractures. *J Pediatr Orthop* 1990;10:592-595.

10. Herndon WA, Mahnken RF, Yngve DA, Sullivan JA: Management of femoral shaft fractures in the adolescent. *J Pediatr Orthop* 1989;9:29-32.

11. Blasier RD, Aronson J, Tursky EA: External fixation of pediatric femur fractures. *J Pediatr Orthop* 1997;17:342-346.

12. Aronson J, Tursky EA: External fixation of femur fractures in children. *J Pediatr Orthop* 1992;12:157-63.

13. Skaggs DL, Leet AI, Money MD, Shaw BA, Hale JM, Tolo VT: Secondary fractures associated with external fixation in pediatric femur fractures. *J Pediatr Orthop* 1999;19:582-586.

14. Probe R, Lindsey RW, Hadley NA, Barnes DA: Refracture of adolescent femoral shaft fractures: A complication of external fixation: A report of two cases. *J Pediatr Orthop* 1993;13:102-105.

15. Bar-On E, Sagiv S, Porat S: External fixation or flexible intramedullary nailing for femoral shaft fractures in children: A prospective, randomised study. *J Bone Joint Surg Br* 1997;79:975-978.

16. Flynn JM, Hresko T, Reynolds RA, Blasier RD, Davidson R, Kasser J: Titanium elastic nails for pediatric femur fractures: A multicenter study of early results with analysis of complications. *J Pediatr Orthop* 2001;21:4-8.

17. Heinrich SD, Drvaric DM, Darr K, MacEwen GD: The operative stabilization of pediatric diaphyseal femur fractures with flexible intramedullary nails: A prospective analysis. *J Pediatr Orthop* 1994;14:501-507.

18. Cramer KE, Tornetta P III, Spero CR, Alter S, Miraliakbar H, Teefey J: Ender rod fixation of femoral shaft fractures in children. *Clin Orthop* 2000;376:119-123.

19. Ligier JN, Metaizeau JP, Prevot J, Lascombes P: Elastic stable intramedullary nailing of femoral shaft fractures in children. *J Bone Joint Surg Br* 1988;70:74-77.

20. Sanders JO, Browne RH, Mooney JF, et al: Treatment of femoral fractures in children by pediatric orthopedists: Results of a 1998 survey. *J Pediatr Orthop* 2001;21:436-41.

21. Ligier JN, Metaizeau JP, Prevot J, Lascombes P: Elastic stable intramedullary pinning of long bone shaft fractures in children. *Z Kinderchir* 1985;40:209-212.

22. Flynn JM, Luedtke L, Ganley TJ, Pill SG: Titanium elastic nails for pediatric femur fractures: Lessons from the learning curve. *Am J Orthop* 2002;31:71-74.

23. Stans AA, Morrissy RT, Renwick SE: Femoral shaft fracture treatment in patients age 6 to 16 years. *J Pediatr Orthop* 1999;19:222-228.

24. Buford D Jr, Christensen K, Weatherall P: Intramedullary nailing of femoral fractures in adolescents. *Clin Orthop* 1998;350:85-89.

25. Thometz JG, Lamdan R: Osteonecrosis of the femoral head after intramedullary nailing of a fracture of the femoral shaft in an adolescent: A case report. *J Bone Joint Surg Am* 1995;77:1423-1426.

26. Beaty JH, Austin SM, Warner WC, Canale ST, Nichols L: Interlocking intramedullary nailing of femoral-shaft fractures in adolescents: Preliminary results and complications. *J Pediatr Orthop* 1994;14:178-183.

27. Fyodorov I, Sturm PF, Robertson WW Jr: Compression-plate fixation of femoral shaft fractures in children aged 8 to 12 years. *J Pediatr Orthop* 1999;19:578-581.

28. Kregor PJ, Song KM, Routt ML Jr, Sangeorzan BJ, Liddell RM, Hansen ST Jr: Plate fixation of femoral shaft fractures in multiply injured children. *J Bone Joint Surg Am* 1993;75:1774-1780.

29. Ward WT, Levy J, Kaye A: Compression plating for child and adolescent femur fractures. *J Pediatr Orthop* 1992;12:626-632.

30. Rozbruch SR, Muller U, Gautier E, Ganz R: The evolution of femoral shaft plating technique. *Clin Orthop* 1998;354:195-208.

31. Beaty JH, Kasser JR: Fractures about the elbow. *Instr Course Lect* 1995;44:199-215.

32. Bertin KC, Goble EM: Ligament injuries associated with physeal fractures about the knee. *Clin Orthop* 1983;177:188-195.

33. Mann DC, Rajmaira S: Distribution of physeal and nonphyseal fractures in 2,650 long-bone fractures in children aged 0-16 years. *J Pediatr Orthop* 1990;10:713-716.

34. Riseborough EJ, Barrett IR, Shapiro F: Growth disturbances following distal femoral physeal fracture-separations. *J Bone Joint Surg Am* 1983;65:885-893.

35. Torg JS, Pavlov H, Morris VB: Salter-Harris type-III fracture of the medial femoral condyle occurring in the adolescent athlete. *J Bone Joint Surg Am* 1981;63:586-591.

36. Rogers LF, Poznanski AK: Imaging of epiphyseal injuries. *Radiology* 1994;191:297-308.

37. Thomson JD, Stricker SJ, Williams MM. Fractures of the distal femoral epiphyseal plate. *J Pediatr Orthop* 1995;15:474-478.

38. Park EA: The imprinting of nutritional disturbances on the growing bone. *Pediatrics* 1964;33:815-862.

39. Simonian PT, Staheli LT: Periarticular fractures after manipulation for knee contractures in children. *J Pediatr Orthop* 1995;15:288-291.

40. Burkhart SS, Peterson HA: Fractures of the proximal tibial epiphysis. *J Bone Joint Surg Am* 1979;61:996-1002.

41. Shelton WR, Canale ST: Fractures of the tibia through the proximal tibial epiphyseal cartilage. *J Bone Joint Surg Am* 1979;61:167-173.

42. Blanks RH, Lester DK, Shaw BA: Flexion-type Salter II fracture of the proximal tibia: Proposed mechanism of injury and two case studies. *Clin Orthop* 1994;301:256-259.

43. Wiley JJ, Baxter MP: Tibial spine fractures in children. *Clin Orthop* 1990;255:54-60.

44. Janarv PM, Westblad P, Johansson C, Hirsch G: Long-term follow-up of anterior tibial spine fractures in children. *J Pediatr Orthop* 1995;15:63-68.

45. Willis RB, Blokker C, Stoll TM, Paterson DC, Galpin RD: Long-term follow-up of anterior tibial eminence fractures. *J Pediatr Orthop* 1993;13:361-364.

46. Meyers MH, McKeever FM: Fracture of the intercondylar eminence of the tibia. *J Bone Joint Surg Am* 1970;52:1677-1684.

47. Burstein DB, Viola A, Fulkerson JP: Entrapment of the medial meniscus in a fracture of the tibial eminence. *Arthroscopy* 1988;4:47-50.

48. Mah JY, Otsuka NY, McLean J: An arthroscopic technique for the reduction and fixation of tibia-eminence fractures. *J Pediatr Orthop* 1996;16:119-121.

49. Zaricznyj B: Avulsion fracture of the tibial eminence: Treatment by open reduction and pinning. *J Bone Joint Surg Am* 1977;59:1111-1114.

50. Christie MJ, Dvonch VM: Tibial tuberosity avulsion fracture in adolescents. *J Pediatr Orthop* 1981;1:391-394.

51. Ogden JA, Tross RB, Murphy MJ: Fractures of the tibial tuberosity in adolescents. *J Bone Joint Surg Am* 1980;62:205-215.

52. Levi JH, Coleman CR: Fracture of the tibial tubercle. *Am J Sports Med* 1976;4:254-263.

53. Hand WL, Hand CR, Dunn AW: Avulsion fractures of the tibial tubercle. *J Bone Joint Surg Am* 1971;53:1579-1583.

54. Gautier E, Ziran BH, Egger B, Slongo T, Jakob RP: Growth disturbances after injuries of the proximal tibial epiphysis. *Arch Orthop Trauma Surg* 1998;118:37-41.

55. Pape JM, Goulet JA, Hensinger RN: Compartment syndrome complicating tibial tubercle avulsion. *Clin Orthop* 1993;295:201-204.

56. Bostrom A: Fracture of the patella: A study of 422 patellar fractures. *Acta Orthop Scand* 1972;143(suppl):1-80.

57. Grogan DP, Carey TP, Leffers D, Ogden JA: Avulsion fractures of the patella. *J Pediatr Orthop* 1990;10:721-730.

58. Houghton GR, Ackroyd CE: Sleeve fractures of the patella in children: A report of three cases. *J Bone Joint Surg Br* 1979;61:165-168.

59. Heinrich SD: Fractures of the shaft of the tibia and fibula, in Beaty JH, Kasser JR (eds): *Rockwood and Wilkins' Fractures in Children*, ed 5. Philadelphia, PA, Lippincott-Williams & Wilkins, 2001, pp 1077-1119.

60. Robert M, Khouri N, Carlioz H, Alain JL: Fractures of the proximal tibial metaphysis in children: Review of a series of 25 cases. *J Pediatr Orthop* 1987;7:444-449.

61. Skak SV: Valgus deformity following proximal tibial metaphyseal fracture in children. *Acta Orthop Scand* 1982;53:141-147.

62. Hensinger RN, Beaty JH, Devito DP, Kasser JR, Loder RT, Rab GT: *Operative Management of Lower Extremity Fractures in Children*. Park Ridge, IL, American Academy of Orthopaedic Surgeons, 1992.

63. Canale ST, Beaty JH: *Operative Pediatric Orthopaedics*, ed 2. St. Louis, MO, Mosby-Year Book, 1995.

64. Cullen MC, Roy DR, Crawford AH, Assenmacher J, Levy MS, Wen D: Open fracture of the tibia in children. *J Bone Joint Surg Am* 1996;78:1039-1047.

65. Bohn WW, Durbin RA: Ipsilateral fractures of the femur and tibia in children and adolescents. *J Bone Joint Surg Am* 1991;73:429-439.

66. McBryde AM Jr, Blake R: The floatingknee: Ipsilateral fractures of the femur and tibia. *J Bone Joint Surg Am* 1974;56:1309.

67. Letts M, Vincent N, Gouw G: The "floating knee" in children. *J Bone Joint Surg Br* 1986;68:442-446.

68. Kay RM, Tang CW: Pediatric foot fractures: evaluation and treatment. *J Am Acad Orthop Surg* 2001;9:308-319.

69. Cummings RJ: Distal tibial and fibular fractures, in Rockwood CA Jr, Wilkins KE, Beaty JH (eds): *Fractures in Children*, ed 4. Philadelphia, PA, Lippincott-Raven, 1996, pp 1377-1428.

70. Schlesinger L, Wedge JH: Percutaneous reduction and fixation of displaced juvenile Tillaux fractures: A new surgical technique. *J Pediatr Orthop* 1993;13:389-391.

71. Ertl JP, Barrack RL, Alexander AH, VanBuecken K: Triplane fracture of the distal tibial epiphysis: Long-term follow-up. *J Bone Joint Surg Am* 1988;70:967-976.

Fracture Patterns and Treatment in the Skeletally Immature Knee

Kenneth B. Tepper, MD
Mary Lloyd Ireland, MD

Abstract

Knee injuries commonly occur in children and adolescents who participate in athletic activities. Open growth plates, apophyses, and chondroepiphyses are unique to the skeletally immature knee and account for the differences in injury patterns observed in children and adults. An understanding of anatomy and classification as related to treatment and outcome of fractures in the skeletally immature knee is important.

Child and adolescent participation in athletic activities has dramatically increased over the last few decades. Injuries sustained during these activities account for 30% to 40% of all injuries to children, and the knee is a common injury site.[1,2] Although the mechanism of injury in the child is similar to that in the adult athlete, the injury patterns seen in children differ from those seen in skeletally mature individuals. The open growth plates, apophyses, and chondroepiphyses are the "weak links" and all are susceptible to injury. Furthermore, children have increased bone plasticity, increased joint hyperelasticity, and articular cartilage softness that contribute to the difference in injury patterns.[3-5] Therefore, for orthopaedists who treat children and adolescents, it is important to have an understanding of the unique fracture patterns and treatments available for injuries of the skeletally immature knee.

Epidemiology

Injury rates among boys and girls differ depending on the athletic activities in which they participate.[6] However, an overall equal distribution has been reported by Castiglia[7] and Sahlin.[8] Among children and adolescents, lower extremity injuries account for 34.5% of total body injuries, the knee is the most commonly injured lower extremity joint and hemarthosis has been reported to be a good indicator of intra-articular pathology.[1,2,9,10] However, physeal fractures about the knee are less common than those involving the upper extremity and the ankle[3,11,12] (Table 1).

Anatomy and Embryology

The structures vulnerable to injury among children and adolescents include the growth plates of the distal femur and proximal tibia, the chondroepiphyses, the apophyses, and the ligamentous struc-

tures. An understanding of the appearance and closure of lower extremity growth plates is necessary for radiographic interpretation of these injuries (Fig.1).

The distal femoral epiphyseal center is the largest and most rapidly growing epiphysis in the lower extremity. It is present at birth in full-term newborns and is the last epiphysis to fuse in the adult. The proximal tibial epiphysis appears between the first and third month of life. The proximal fibula secondary ossification center and the patella are not visible until age 3 to 5 years, at which time ossification begins.[3,13]

The distal femoral physis contributes 1.0 cm of growth per year until maturity. This corresponds to 70% of the length of the femur and 40% of the entire leg (Fig. 2). It fuses with the metaphysis between ages 14 and 16 years in girls and 16 and 18 years in boys. The physis is entirely extra-articular and has an undulating configuration that contributes to its stability.[3,13]

The proximal tibial physis contributes 0.65 cm of growth per year until maturity. This corresponds to 45% of the tibia and 27% of the entire leg (Fig. 2). The ossification center is slightly conical centrally as it extends toward the tibial spines and becomes more prominent in late childhood and early adolescence. Oc-

Table 1
Epiphyseal Fracture Rates: Lower Extremity

| | | Fractures, No. (%) | |
	Ogden[3] (N = 236)	Peterson and associates[11] (N = 128)	Neer and Horowitz[12] (N = 587)
Distal femur	36 (15.2)	18 (14.1)	28 (4.8)
Tibial tuberosity	22 (9.3)		
Proximal tibia	14 (5.9)	6 (4.7)	17 (2.9)
Proximal fibula	4 (1.7)		2 (0.3)
Distal tibia	83 (35.2)	59 (46.1)	238 (40.5)
Distal fibula	18 (7.6)	21 (16.4)	302 (51.4)
Trochanters	19 (8.0)		
Proximal femur	11 (4.7)	7 (5.5)	
Metatarsals	7 (3.0)	6 (4.7)	
Phalanges (toes)	22 (9.3)	11 (8.6)	

(Adapted with permission from Ogden JA: Radiologic aspects, in Ogden JA (ed): *Skeletal Injury in the Child*, ed 2. Philadelphia, PA, WB Saunders, 1990, pp 97-173.)

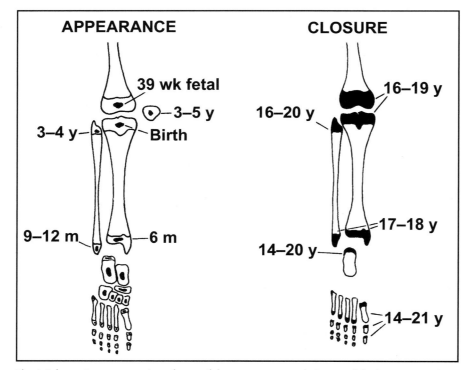

Fig. 1 Schematic representation of ages of the appearance and closure of the lower extremity secondary ossification centers. y = years, wk = weeks, and m = months. (Reproduced with permission from Ogden JA: Radiologic aspects, in Ogden JA (ed): *Skeletal Injury in the Child*, ed 2. Philadelphia, PA, WB Saunders, 1990, pp 65-96.)

casionally, two ossification centers may exist. The articular surface develops with a posterior tilt of 15° to 20°.[3,13]

The tibial tuberosity develops at about 12 to 15 weeks of gestation as an extension of the proximal tibial epiphysis. The tuberosity is well developed by birth and is at the level of the tibial physes. Distal "migration" of the tubercle occurs after birth. Initially, the cartilage underlying the tuberosity is almost completely fibrocartilage and has a modified configuration to resist the tensile stresses imparted by the patellar tendon. The tuberosity develops a secondary ossification center, usually in the most distal region at age 7 to 9 years. The center gradually enlarges and extends toward the secondary ossification center of the tibia, where it will fuse at ages 13 to 15 years in girls and 15 to 19 years in boys. The area under the proximal tibia closes first, starting centrally, and the region under the tuberosity is the last to close and does so in a proximal to distal direction.

The patella ossifies from one central ossicle or as many as six ossicles that will eventually coalesce. The peripheral margins are typically irregular, and there is much normal variability. Ossification is completed by age 10 years. The incidence of bipartite patella is reported to range from 0.2% to 6.0%, is more common in males, and may be unilateral.[3]

The anterior cruciate ligament (ACL) and the posterior cruciate ligament attach to the femoral and tibial chondroepiphyses via a perichondral cuff, which will become the fibrocartilage interface in an adult. The synovial sheath provides blood supply. Notch morphology is variable and is probably determined by genetics as well as by use of the knee.[3]

The medial and lateral collateral ligaments originate from the femoral epiphysis. The deep collateral ligaments attach to the proximal tibial epiphyseal perichondrium. Some of the superficial collateral fibers as well as the pes anserinus attach to the proximal tibial metaphysis.[3]

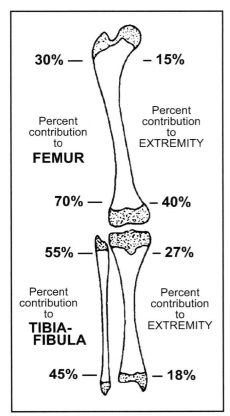

Fig. 2 Diagram of the lower extremity growth plate contributions to individual bone and lower extremity length. (Reproduced with permission from Ogden JA: Radiologic aspects, in Ogden JA (ed): *Skeletal Injury in the Child*, ed 2. Philadelphia, PA, WB Saunders, 1990, pp 65-96.)

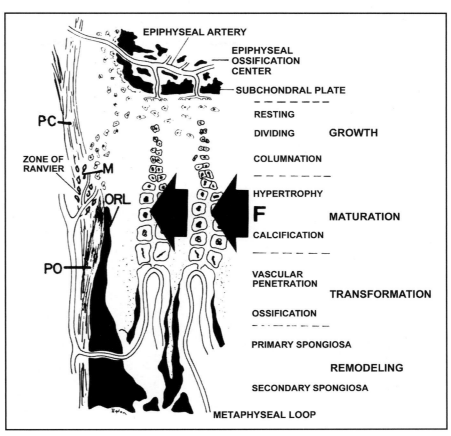

Fig. 3 Depiction of the usual fracture propagation (F, *arrows*) through the growth plate in SH I, II, and III fractures. Note the perichondrium (PC), periosteum (PO), mesenchymal cells (M) and ossification ring of Lacroix (ORL). (Reproduced with permission from Ogden JA: Tibia and fibula, in Ogden JA (ed): *Skeletal Injury in the Child*, ed 2. Philadelphia, PA, WB Saunders, 1990, pp 787-863.)

Fractures

Fracture patterns in children differ from those in adults because open epiphyseal plates are weaker than the surrounding ligamentous structures.[5,14] Fractures usually occur through or near the zone of calcification (Fig. 3) but may vary according to the shape of the physis, the amount of axial compression at the time of injury, and the obliquity of the forces causing the fracture.[15]

Classification

Numerous physeal classification systems exist, but the most commonly used system is that proposed by Salter and Harris[16] (Fig. 4). Salter-Harris I injuries represent epiphysiolysis; the fracture line stays entirely within the physis. In nondisplaced Salter-Harris I injuries, initial radiographs may be normal; however, callus may be present on follow-up radiographs. Salter-Harris II injuries are the most common, and the fracture traverses the growth plate for a variable distance and exits though the metaphysis, producing a metaphyseal fragment. This metaphyseal fragment (Thurston-Holland sign) is produced where the periosteum remains continuous, acting as an intact bridge, which is an advantage in reduction. Salter-Harris III injuries traverse the growth plate and exit through the epiphysis and, hence, into the joint. These are more unusual and may require surgical intervention. Salter-Harris IV injuries are vertical fractures that split the metaphysis, growth plate, and epiphysis. Salter-Harris V injuries represent a compression injury to the growth plate, which is a significant injury to the physis. Frequently, the initial injury may be missed and is retrospectively discovered once growth arrest or deformity occurs.

Fractures involving the tibial eminence are typically classified according to a system described by Meyers and Mc-Keever[17] and tibial tuberosity fractures according to a system described by Watson-Jones[18] and Ogden and associates.[19] These classification systems will be addressed later.

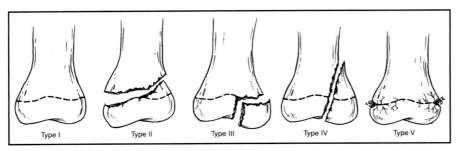

Fig. 4 The Salter-Harris classification of physeal fractures. (Reproduced from Edwards PH Jr, Grana WA: Physeal fractures about the knee. *J Am Acad Orthop Surg* 1995;3:63-69.)

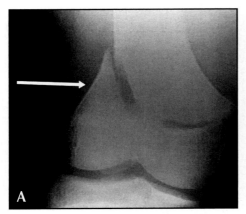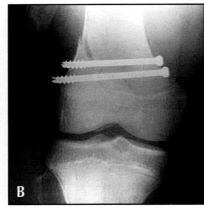

Fig. 5 Salter-Harris II fracture of the distal femur. **A,** The arrow depicts a large metaphyseal Thurston-Holland fragment. **B,** The same after closed reduction and percutaneous fixation with cannulated screws.

Distal Femoral Physeal Fractures

Although fractures involving the distal femoral physis are rare, they are the most common physeal injury about the knee and account for 5% to 15% of all physeal fractures in the lower extremities.[3,11,12,20] An Salter-Harris II fracture with coronal displacement is the most common distal femoral physeal fracture.[3] Historically, these fractures were described as "wagon-wheel" injuries and had a high amputation rate secondary to popliteal vessel injury.[21] The injury usually occurred when a child's leg was caught in the spoke of a moving wheel and the lower leg would forcefully hyperextend, resulting in anterior displacement of the epiphysis. Sports injuries (in children 11 years and older) and being struck by a motor vehicle (in those age 2 to 10 years) have replaced the wagon as the most common causes of injury today.[22] Typically the force causing the injury is medial or lateral, and the popliteal neurovascular structures are preserved.[15]

Physical examination may reveal pain, varying degrees of hemarthrosis, swelling, and deformity. Tenderness is present throughout the physis. Weight bearing is usually not tolerated, and the knee is usually held in flexion and has an apparent ligamentous laxity. A neurovascular examination must be performed and results documented. Radiographs are sufficient to demonstrate the injury and displacement. AP, lateral, and oblique radiographs should be routinely obtained. In Salter-Harris I injuries, only physeal widening may be present; in Salter-Harris V injuries, a decrease in the phy-

seal width may be visualized. The physis is localized at about the same level as the proximal pole of the patella, and tenderness may be the only evidence of a nondisplaced Salter-Harris I fracture. Stress views are not recommended because further physeal injury may occur while obtaining them, and stress view findings will not influence treatment. An MRI is sometimes useful to evaluate a physeal injury without causing further damage to the physis.[23] An arteriogram is indicated when there is concern about vascular compromise.

Treatment is determined by fracture type and displacement. Varus and valgus displacement does not remodel with further growth, and anatomic reduction should be achieved.[24] Nondisplaced Salter-Harris I and Salter-Harris II fractures should be treated with above-knee casts or spica immobilization for a minimum of 6 weeks. Treatment of displaced Salter-Harris I and Salter-Harris II fractures consists of anatomic reduction, either closed or open. This is best accomplished under general anesthesia; the reduction is obtained primarily through traction with minimal manipulation, thereby preventing additional physeal injury. In the rare instance of being unable to obtain an anatomic reduction, open reduction should be considered rather than attempting a forceful reduction, again in the interest of preventing additional physeal injury.

If anatomic reduction can be obtained in a closed fashion, treatment consists of percutaneous fixation. Salter-Harris II fractures with a sufficiently large metaphyseal fragment (Fig. 5) allow for percutaneous cannulated screw fixation of the fragment to the metaphysis and thereby avoid physeal violation. Smooth pins are used for Salter-Harris II fractures with small metaphyseal fragments as well as for Salter-Harris I fractures. The pins should be placed central in the physis, and they should cross in the metaphysis. Hardware is placed using fluoroscopic imaging. If closed reduction cannot be obtained, it is usually the result of the interposition of periosteum, in which instance open reduction will be required.

Salter-Harris III and Salter-Harris IV fractures involve the articular surface. As with other joints, articular displacement of 2 mm requires reduction, which is usually best accomplished in an open procedure. This injury is approached by a longitudinal anterior incision with care being taken not to damage the peripheral physis. Cannulated screws are placed in the epiphysis and parallel to the physis. Additional fixation may be placed in the metaphysis for Salter-Harris IV fractures that have a fragment large enough to accept hardware.

Postoperative immobilization in a cylinder or above-knee cast for a minimum of 4 weeks is mandatory in the child. Toe-touch ambulation and isometric exercises are initiated once symptoms permit. Rapid healing occurs with physeal fractures, which may heal up to twice as fast as non–growth-plate injuries.[3] Frequent radiographic monitoring of fracture reduction should occur in the early postoperative period. Range of motion, strengthening, and return of proprioception are emphasized on cast removal. The estimated time to return to athletic activity is 4 to 6 months, depending on the extent of intra-articular involvement.

Unfortunately, complications following distal femoral physeal injuries are common, and they should be discussed with the patient and the family during the first encounter. Neurovascular compromise must be immediately ruled out. If a vascular injury is present, urgent vascular consultation is recommended. After treatment, angular deformity and limb-length discrepancy occur most commonly; however, in the athletic adolescent, this is rarely a problem because little growth potential remains. Growth arrest typically occurs opposite the metaphyseal fragment produced by the Thurston-Holland sign. Risk factors for complica-

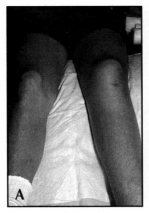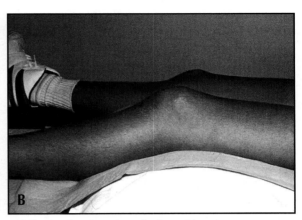

Fig. 6 Typical physical examination following fractures about the knee. Note the hemarthrosis (**A**) and the knee held in flexion (**B**).

tions include younger age at time of injury, displacement greater than half the diameter of the bone, and severity of trauma.[15] Patients should be routinely examined both clinically and radiographically for at least 2 years following injury; the occurrence of osseous bars, limb-length inequalities, and/or angular deformities require additional assessment. Because growth arrest may be seen even in nondisplaced Salter-Harris I fractures, the prognostic implications of the Salter-Harris classification system have been questioned for distal femoral physeal fractures. If more than 2 years of growth remain, osseous bars smaller than half the size of the physis should be resected.[25] Angular deformity may be treated with epiphysiodesis or osteotomy. Although limb-length discrepancy (LLD) less than 2.5 cm is left untreated, LLD between 2.5 and 5.0 cm can be treated with epiphysiodesis, and LLD greater than 5 cm will require limb lengthening or shortening.[26] Ligament injury may occur with a distal femoral physeal injury. Bertin and Goble[27] reported ligamentous instability in 14 of 29 patients; therefore, ligament instability should be carefully evaluated.

Proximal Tibial Physeal Fractures

Proximal tibial physeal fractures account for 3% to 6% of lower extremity physeal injuries and less than 1% of all physeal injuries.[3,11,12,20] The infrequent involvement of the physis in this type of fracture is related to the protected nature of the proximal tibia. The collateral ligaments have attachments that extend distally to the metaphysis, and the proximal fibula provides additional stability by acting as a buttress. Injuries are most common in 11- to 14-year-old boys. The mechanism of injury is typically hyperextension, and most fractures are Salter-Harris I or Salter-Harris II.[28,29]

Physical examination demonstrates pain and point tenderness, and a hemarthrosis may be present (Fig. 6). Weight bearing typically is not possible. Posterior fracture displacement places the neurovascular structures at risk because the popliteal artery is tethered at the level of the tibial epiphyseal. Neurovascular status must be immediately evaluated. Vascular compromise may be subtle and an arteriogram should be obtained if there is any concern about arterial injury.

Diagnostic radiographs will demonstrate displacement and physeal widening, and the abnormality may be mild (Fig. 7) in Salter-Harris I fractures. Oblique radiographs may be helpful in assessing intra-articular involvement.

Treatment for most Salter-Harris I and Salter-Harris II fractures is closed

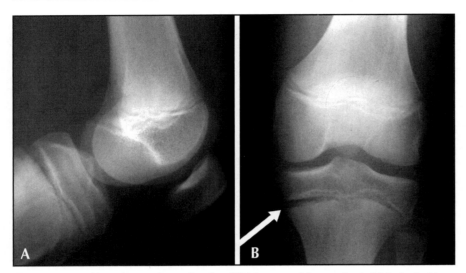

Fig. 7 AP (**A**) and lateral (**B**) radiographs of an SH I fracture of the proximal tibial physis. Note the medial physeal widening (*arrow*).

reduction and cast immobilization. Fixation is not necessary because these fractures are typically stable. Displaced Salter-Harris III and Salter-Harris IV fractures require reduction and percutaneous fixation. Arthroscopic assistance is useful for assessing fracture reduction and evaluating for meniscal entrapment. Above-knee cast immobilization for a minimum of 4 weeks is recommended. The estimated time until return to athletic activity is 3 to 4 months for Salter-Harris I and Salter-Harris II fractures and 4 to 6 months for Salter-Harris III and Salter-Harris IV fractures.

Angular deformities and LLDs in Salter-Harris I and Salter-Harris II fractures are rare. Most deformities are a result of an open Salter-Harris IV injury caused by a lawnmower.[30] Vascular compromise is the most serious complication and should be thoroughly assessed.[29] As with distal femoral physeal fractures, routine clinical and radiographic follow-up is recommended to assess for physeal bar formation or arrest.

Tibial Tuberosity Fractures
Tibial tuberosity fractures are rare. Ehrenborg[31] divided tubercle development into four phases: cartilaginous, apophyseal, epiphyseal, and bony. The apophyseal phase begins between ages 8 and 12 years in girls and 9 and 14 years in boys. The tubercle coalesces with the proximal tibial epiphysis at about age 15 years in girls and 17 years in boys. As the apophysis matures, the fibrocartilaginous precursors transform into columnar cells from a proximal to distal direction. The columnar cells do not resist traction as well as the fibrocartilage, and a severe eccentric or concentric contraction of the extensor mechanism produces a fracture through this vulnerable level of the apophysis.

Athletic activities involving jumping—basketball, for example—are the most common mechanism of injury. Avulsion of the tuberosity is distinct from Osgood-Schlatter disease, which represents a more chronic avulsion of the anterior aspect of the tubercle and the physeal germinal cartilage remains attached to the tuberosity. It has been postulated that Osgood-Schlatter disease may be a predecessor of tubercle avulsion, but no study findings have linked these entities definitively.

The classification system commonly used for tibial tubercle fractures was pro-posed by Watson-Jones[18] and later modified by Ogden and associates[19] (Fig. 8). Type I injuries are superiorly displaced, have a small fragment of the tuberosity avulsed, and the fracture exits through the secondary ossification center. In type II injuries, the fracture exits through the cartilage between the ossification center and the proximal tibial physes. In type III injuries, the fracture continues to propagate proximally through the proximal tibial epiphysis and into the knee joint. Ogden and asociates[19] further modified this classification system with subtypes A and B, which account for comminution of the tubercle.

Physical examination reveals pain, swelling, and tenderness over the tubercle. The knee is held in flexion because of hamstring spasm and hemarthrosis. The extensor mechanism is disrupted in type III and most type II injuries, and the patient cannot extend the knee. A defect may be palpable, and patella alta may be observed.

Diagnostic radiographs should include AP, lateral, and oblique views. Classification, size, and displacement are best visualized on the lateral radiograph. Oblique views are helpful for visualizing intra-articular fracture extension.

Treatment requires restoration of extensor mechanism isometry and joint congruency. Nondisplaced type IA, IB, and IIA fractures are treated with cast immobilization and the knee in full extension for 4 to 6 weeks. Comparison radiographs may help confirm reduction by assessing patellar position. Type IIB, IIIA, and IIIB (Fig. 9) and displaced type IA, IB, and IIA fractures require open reduction and internal fixation. Type III fractures require reduction of the articular surface. Typically, a large periosteal flap is interposed at the fracture site and requires removal to obtain reduction. Fixation methods include using cannulated screws, tension band wiring, and direct suture. Physeal sparing is recommended when the patient is significantly skeletally immature. The periosteal flap should be repaired.

Complications are rare with the appropriate treatment. Growth disturbances do not occur because little growth potential remains in the normal patient following such an injury. The estimated time until return to athletic activity is 3 to 6 months and depends on the amount of intra-articular involvement of the fracture.

Fractures of the Patella

Fractures of the patella are rare in children because the patella has a large ratio of cartilage to bone, increased mobility, and increased tissue resilience.[3] A direct blow, hyperflexion, or sudden contraction of the extensor mechanism are the most common mechanisms of injury. The general principles of adult patella fractures apply to the child. Displacement and extensor mechanism disruption necessitate open reduction and internal fixation.

Patellar sleeve fractures are unique to the adolescent and must be identified.[32] In sleeve fractures, a large cartilaginous portion of the patella and periosteum is pulled from the main body of the patella and a small fragment of the bone is pulled from the patella.

Physical examination will demonstrate pain, hemarthrosis, extensor lag, and patella alta. Diagnostic radiographs underestimate the severity of the injury because only a small portion of bone is visualized. Treatment requires open reduction and internal fixation, with periosteal suturing, tension band wiring, or screw fixation. Cast immobilization for 4 weeks is followed by rehabilitation. Prognosis is good if extensor mechanism length is restored.[33] The estimated time until return to athletic activity is 3 to 4 months.

Tibial Eminence Fractures

Tibial eminence fractures involve a chondroepiphyseal avulsion of the tibial end of the ACL. However, chrondroepiphyseal failure does not necessarily occur

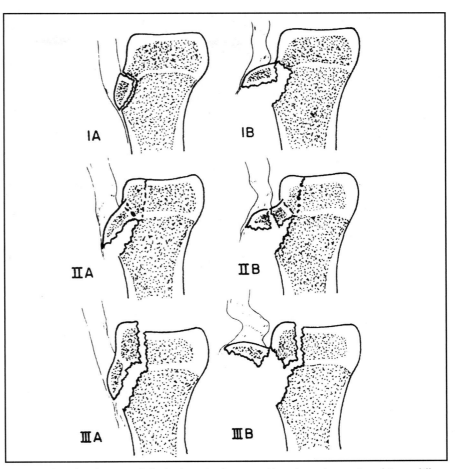

Fig. 8 Ogden classification of tibial tuberosity fractures. Note that subtypes A and B are differentiated by comminution. (Reproduced with permission from Ogden JA: Tibia and fibula, in Ogden JA (ed): *Skeletal Injury to the Child*, ed 2. Philadelphia, PA, WB Saunders, 1990, pp 787-863.

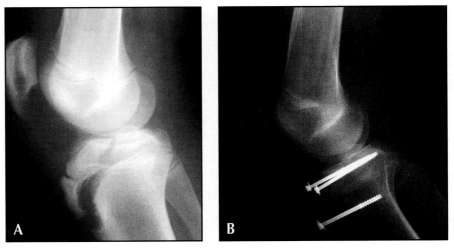

Fig. 9 Tibial tuberosity fracture, **A,** Lateral radiograph of an Ogden type IIIB injury. **B,** The same after open reduction and internal fixation.

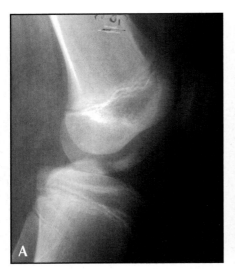
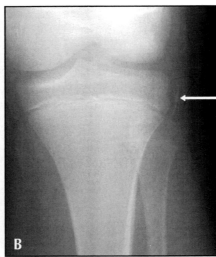
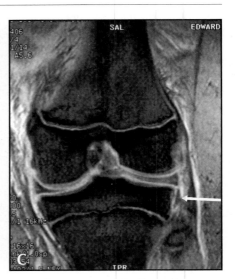

Fig. 10 Tibial eminence fracture. **A,** Lateral radiograph of a Meyers and McKeever type III tibial eminence fracture (*arrow*). Radiographic **(B)** and MRI **(C)** representation of second fracture (*arrows*).

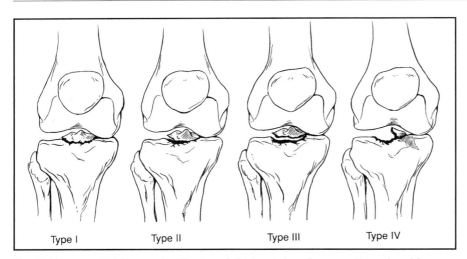

Fig. 11 Meyers and McKeever classification of tibial eminence fractures. (Reproduced from Edwards PH Jr, Grana WA: Physeal fractures about the knee. *J Am Acad Orthop Surg* 1995;3:63-69.)

because of immaturity of the perichondral cuff; rather, it is a function of a high-energy force delivered at a low-load rate. Ligament injury, in contrast, occurs with rapid loading of a low-energy force.[34] Tibial eminence fractures most commonly occur between the ages of 8 and 12 years following a hyperflexion injury during athletic activity or a bicycle accident.[17,35]

Examination may reveal pain, hemarthrosis, anterior laxity, and loss of mo-tion. Loss of motion is a result of hamstring spasm, hemarthrosis, or fracture displacement. A thorough knee examination is mandatory to evaluate for other associated injuries. Diagnostic radiographs include AP, lateral, and notch views. The fracture is best visualized and classified on the lateral radiograph. The notch view will best identify a femoral avulsion.[36] When extension into the medial or lateral compartment is suspected, oblique views should be obtained.[37] A second fracture may be present in conjunction with the tibial eminence fracture (Fig. 10).

The classification system commonly used to identify tibial eminence fractures was proposed by Meyers and McKeever[17] and later modified by Zaricznyj[38] (Fig. 11). Type I fractures are minimally displaced (< 3 mm). In type II fractures, the anterior one third to one half of the avulsed fragment is elevated with an intact posterior hinge. In type III fractures, the fracture fragment is completely displaced from the proximal tibia. In a type III+ fracture, the fragment is rotated 180°. A type IV fracture is comminuted.

With advances in arthroscopy, associated injuries are being recognized more frequently and include entrapment of the medial or lateral meniscus in the fracture and meniscal tears.[39] The fracture may include a substantial portion of the articular surface of the medial or lateral compartment.[40] Injuries to the medial and lateral collateral ligaments and posterior cruciate ligaments rarely occur.[41]

Treatment is determined by displacement and associated injuries. Nondisplaced type I fractures with no other associated injuries are treated with above-knee cast immobilization for 4 to 6 weeks. The position of the knee is controversial, with some physicians contending that full extension allows the femoral condyles or the intercondylar notch to reduce the fracture and others contending that 30° of flexion reduces tension on the ACL. Either position is acceptable, but hyperextension should be avoided. Weekly radiographs to assess fracture reduction should be obtained for the first 2 to 3 weeks.

Type II fractures require reduction. This can be readily accomplished with aspiration of hemarthrosis and intra-articular injection of local anesthetic. If the fracture can be reduced to within 2 mm, the treatment is an above-knee cast for 4 to 6 weeks. A true lateral radiograph is needed to assess the reduction. Again, weekly radiographs for the first 2 to 3 weeks should be obtained to assess fracture reduction. If the fracture cannot be adequately reduced, surgery is indicated, in which case arthroscopic evaluation and treatment may be helpful. Arthroscopy readily assesses blocks to reduction. Most commonly, the medial meniscus is involved and can be elevated from under the fracture. Once reduced, the eminence usually does not require fixation because the posterior hinge remains intact.

Type III, III+, and IV fractures require internal fixation. A medial parapatellar arthrotomy can be performed, but arthroscopic treatment has become an increasingly popular alternative.[42,43] Once the fracture is visualized, hematoma and fibrous tissue are débrided, and other impediments to reduction are addressed, including meniscal pathology.[44] Fracture reduction can be aided with the use of an ACL tibial tunnel guide. If the fragment is large enough (> 1 cm^2), a single 4.0-mm cannulated screw is recommended and placed within the ACL substance to avoid notch impingement.[42] Placement of the screw requires an additional portal just medial to the middle of the patella, and

guidewire placement is facilitated with intraoperative fluoroscopy. For smaller fragments that are not large enough to accept a screw, nonabsorbable suture or wire fixation is recommended and passed through the ACL bone stump and the anterior tibial epiphysis.[44-46]

The proximal tibial growth plate should be avoided with whichever technique is chosen. If fixation is rigid, early range of motion can occur. With suture fixation, above-knee cast immobilization for 4 weeks is recommended before commencing motion. Monitoring of the reduction with weekly radiographs is recommended. Rehabilitation is similar to post-ACL reconstruction protocols, with emphasis on regaining full extension.

Results following tibial eminence fracture are generally good.[44] Increased tibial translation is common, yet instability is rare.[47] Increased translation may be a result of ligament stretching before the occurrence of the eminence fracture.[48,49] Wiley and Baxter[50] noted increased tibial translation following tibial eminence fracture, but instability did not occur. Loss of motion may occur, especially after malunion, and may require arthroscopic release of adhesions and notchplasty.[51] Aggressive manipulation under anesthesia should not be performed to avoid fracturing the distal femoral physis.

Summary

Injuries to the skeletally immature knee differ from injuries in the adult and include injury to the growth plates, chondroepiphyses, and apophyses. The orthopaedic surgeon must recognize these serious injuries and avoid further damage to the physis. With an appropriate understanding of the anatomy and injuries unique to the growing skeleton, common complications such as growth arrest and angular deformity will be minimized.

References

1. Pasque CB, McGinnis DW: Knee, in Sullivan JA, Anderson SJ (eds): *Care of the Young Athlete.* Rosemont, IL, American Academy of

Orthopaedic Surgeons and American Academy of Pediatrics, 2000, pp 377-404.

2. DeHaven KE, Lintner DM: Athletic injuries: Comparison by age, sport, and gender. *Am J Sports Med* 1986;14:218-224.

3. Ogden JA (ed): *Skeletal Injury in the Child,* ed 2. Philadelphia, PA, WB Saunders, 1990.

4. Stanish WD: Lower leg, foot, and ankle injuries in young athletes. *Clin Sports Med* 1995;14: 651-668.

5. Maffulli N, Baxter-Jones AD: Common skeletal injuries in young athletes. *Sports Med* 1995;19:137-149.

6. Tursz A, Crost M: Sports-related injuries in children: A study of their characteristics, frequency, and severity, with comparison to other types of accidental injuries. *Am J Sports Med* 1986;14:294-299.

7. Castiglia PT: Sports injuries in children. *J Pediatr Health Care* 1995;9:32-33.

8. Sahlin Y: Sports accidents in childhood. *Br J Sports Med* 1990;24:40-44.

9. Schmidt B, Höllwarth ME: Sports accidents in children and adolescents. *Z Kinderchir* 1989;44:357-362.

10. Stanitski CL, Harvell JC, Fu F: Observations on acute knee hemarthrosis in children and adolescents. *J Pediatr Orthop* 1993;13:506-510.

11. Peterson HA, Madhok R, Benson JT, Ilstrup DM, Melton LJ III: Physeal fractures: Part I. Epidemiology in Olmsted County, Minnesota, 1979-1988. *J Pediatr Orthop* 1994;14:423-430.

12. Neer CS II, Horwitz BS: Fractures of the proximal humeral epiphysial plate. *Clin Orthop* 1965;41:24-31.

13. Pritchett JW: Longitudinal growth and growth-plate activity in the lower extremity. *Clin Orthop* 1992;275:274-279.

14. Micheli LJ, Fehlandt AF Jr: Overuse injuries to tendons and apophyses in children and adolescents. *Clin Sports Med* 1992;11:713-726.

15. Lombardo SJ, Harvey JP Jr: Fractures of the distal femoral epiphyses: Factors influencing prognosis: A review of thirty-four cases. *J Bone Joint Surg Am* 1977;59:742- 751.

16. Salter RB, Harris WR: Injuries involving the epiphyseal plate. *J Bone Joint Surg Am* 1963;45:587-622.

17. Meyers MH, McKeever FM: Fracture of the intercondylar eminence of the tibia. *J Bone Joint Surg Am* 1970;52:1677-1684.

18. Trickey EL: Injuries of the knee, in Watson-Jones R, Wilson JN (eds): *Fractures and Joint Injuries,* ed 5. Edinburgh, Scotland, Churchill Livingstone, 1976, vol 2, pp 1012-1067.

19. Ogden JA, Tross RB, Murphy MJ: Fractures of the tibial tuberosity in adolescents. *J Bone Joint Surg Am* 1980;62:205-215.

20. Mann DC, Rajmaira S: Distribution of physeal and nonphyseal fractures in 2,650 long-bone fractures in children aged 0-16 years. *J Pediatr Orthop* 1990;10:713-716.

21. Poland J (ed): *Traumatic Separation of the Epiphyses.* London, England, Smith, Elder, 1898.

22. Roberts JM: Abstract: Fracture-separation of the distal femoral epiphysis. *J Bone Joint Surg Am* 1973;55:1324.

23. Close BJ, Strouse PJ: MR of physeal fractures of the adolescent knee. *Pediatr Radiol* 2000;30:756-762.

24. Blount WP (ed): *Fractures in Children.* Huntington, NY, Robert E. Krieger, 1977.

25. Roberts JM: Operative treatment of fractures about the knee. *Orthop Clin North Am* 1990;21:365-379.

26. Menelaus MB: Correction of leg-length discrepancy by epiphysial arrest. *J Bone Joint Surg Br* 1966;48:336-339.

27. Bertin KC, Goble EM: Ligament injuries associated with physeal fractures about the knee. *Clin Orthop* 1983;177:188-195.

28. Aitken AP: Fractures of the proximal tibial epiphysial cartilage. *Clin Orthop* 1965;41:92-97.

29. Burkhart SS, Peterson HA: Fractures of the proximal tibial epiphysis. *J Bone Joint Surg Am* 1979;61:996-1002.

30. Wozasek GE, Moser KD, Haller H, Capousek M: Trauma involving the proximal tibial epiphysis. *Arch Orthop Trauma Surg* 1991;110:301-306.

31. Ehrenborg G: The Osgood-Schlatter lesion: A clinical and experimental study. *Acta Chir Scand Suppl* 1962;288:1-36.

32. Houghton GR, Ackroyd CE: Sleeve fractures of the patella in children: A report of three cases. *J Bone Joint Surg Br* 1979;61:165-168.

33. Dai LY, Zhang WM: Fractures of the patella in children. *Knee Surg Sports Traumatol Arthrosc* 1999;7:243-245.

34. Iobst CA, Stanitski CL: Acute knee injuries. *Clin Sports Med* 2000;19:621-635.

35. Gronkvist H, Hirsch G, Johansson L: Fracture of the anterior tibial spine in children. *J Pediatr Orthop* 1984;4:465-468.

36. Robinson SC, Driscoll SE: Simultaneous osteochondral avulsion of the femoral and tibial insertions of the anterior cruciate ligament: Report of a case in a thirteen-year-old boy. *J Bone Joint Surg Am* 1981;63:1342-1343.

37. Crawford AH: Fractures about the knee in children. *Orthop Clin North Am* 1976;7:639-656.

38. Zaricznyj B: Avulsion fracture of the tibial eminence: Treatment by open reduction and pinning. *J Bone Joint Surg Am* 1977;59:1111-1114.

39. Chandler JT, Miller TK: Tibial eminence fracture with meniscal entrapment. *Arthroscopy* 1995;11:499-502.

40. McLennan JG: Lessons learned after second-look arthroscopy in type III fractures of the tibial spine. *J Pediatr Orthop* 1995;15:59-62.

41. Hayes JM, Masear VR: Avulsion fracture of the tibial eminence associated with severe medial ligamentous injury in an adolescent: A case report and literature review. *Am J Sports Med* 1984;12:330-333.

42. Berg EE: Pediatric tibial eminence fractures: Arthroscopic cannulated screw fixation. *Arthroscopy* 1995;11:328-331.

43. Wall EJ: Tibial eminence fractures in children. *Oper Tech Sports Med* 1998;6:206-212.

44. Mah JY, Adili A, Otsuka NY, Ogilvie R: Follow-up study of arthroscopic reduction and fixation of type III tibial-eminence fractures. *J Pediatr Orthop* 1998;18:475-477.

45. Matthews DE, Geissler WB: Arthroscopic suture fixation of displaced tibial eminence fractures. *Arthroscopy* 1994;10:418-423.

46. Perez Carro L, Garcia Suarez G, Gomez Cimiano F: The arthroscopic knot technique for fracture of the tibia in children. *Arthroscopy* 1994;10:698-699.

47. Willis RB, Blokker C, Stoll TM, Paterson DC, Galpin RD: Long-term follow-up of anterior tibial eminence fractures. *J Pediatr Orthop* 1993;13:361-364.

48. Noyes FR, DeLucas JL, Torvik PJ: Biomechanics of anterior cruciate ligament failure: An analysis of strain-rate sensitivity and mechanisms of failure in primates. *J Bone Joint Surg Am* 1974;56:236-253.

49. Smith JB: Knee instability after fractures of the intercondylar eminence of the tibia. *J Pediatr Orthop* 1984;4:462-464.

50. Wiley JJ, Baxter MP: Tibial spine fractures in children. *Clin Orthop* 1990;255:54-60.

51. Luger EJ, Arbel R, Eichenblat M, Menachem A, Dekel S: Femoral notchplasty in the treatment of malunited intercondylar eminence fractures of the tibia. *Arthroscopy* 1994;10:550-551.

Meniscal and Articular Cartilage Injury in the Skeletally Immature Knee

Arya W. Moti, DO
Lyle J. Micheli, MD

Abstract

Meniscal and articular cartilage injuries in skeletally immature patients appear to be occurring with increased frequency, particularly in athletically active children. The orthopaedic surgeon should understand the principles of diagnosis and management, as well as be aware of current surgical treatment options available.

The orthopaedic surgeon who treats meniscal and articular cartilage injuries in the skeletally immature knee should have a fundamental knowledge of the development, structure, and function of the normal meniscus and articular cartilage. This chapter provides the orthopaedic surgeon with the fundamentals of meniscal and articular cartilage embryology, development, and anatomy, as well as essential guidelines for diagnosis and treatment of meniscal and articular cartilage injuries of the skeletally immature knee. Although the meniscus and articular cartilage share proximity in the knee, they are discussed separately because of differences in anatomy, mechanism of injury, and treatment.

Meniscus

Embryology and Development

Streeter[1] has classically described the first 8 weeks of gestation as occurring in 23 distinct morphologic stages known as horizons. The leg bud first appears during horizon XIII, which correlates to approximately 28 gestational days. The menisci first appear in horizon XXII at about 45 days of gestation. The menisci are well defined by the eighth week and will have obtained an adult form and are well vascularized by the 12th week. Historically, the menisci were once thought to develop as discoid in shape in the fetus and assume an adult form through resorption of the central portion.[2] Later studies, however, have suggested that the menisci are not discoid in shape in the course of normal development.[3,4]

Anatomy

From a histologic perspective, the menisci are composed primarily of type I collagen with many fibroblasts and fibrocartilaginous cells present. These collagen bundles are arranged in a circumferential pattern in the periphery and are oriented in a radial pattern centrally. Circumferential fibers enable the menisci to more effectively disperse the hoop stresses of compressive loads, and radial fibers improve rigidity and prevent longitudinal tearing.[5]

The blood supply to the menisci is derived from superior and inferior medial and lateral geniculate arteries, with the main vascular supply coming from the superior and inferior lateral geniculate arteries.[6] In the adult, the perimeniscal capillary plexus supplies only the peripheral 30% of the meniscus. Typically, only tears within the periphery have adequate blood supply to heal, whereas more centrally located tears do not. At birth, there is an overall decrease in meniscal cellularity and vascularity. There is also a relative increase in the dry weight amount of collagen present.

The gross appearance of the menisci is triangular on cross section. The medial meniscus is typically C-shaped, and the lateral meniscus is more semicircular in shape. The anterior horns of the menisci are attached to each other by the transverse intermeniscal ligament. The deep portion of the medial collateral ligament is intimately associated with the midbody of the medial meniscus. The posterior horn of the lateral meniscus is connected to the medial femoral condyle by two variable meniscofemoral ligaments. The anterior meniscofemoral ligament of Humphrey courses anteriorly and the posterior meniscofemoral ligament of Wrisberg courses posteriorly to the posterior cruciate ligament on the way to attachment to the intercondylar wall.

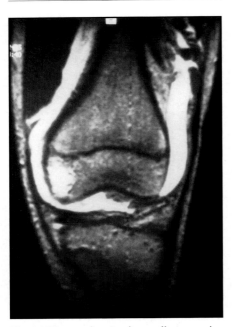

Fig. 1 MRI scan showing large effusion and epiphyseal bruise in a child.

The incidence of discoid lateral meniscus variants has been reported to be as high as 3% to 5% in the United States and 16.6% in Japan.[7] Discoid menisci occur much more frequently on the lateral side of the knee than the medial side. The incidence of discoid medial meniscus variants has been reported to be approximately 0.25%.[4]

Function

The menisci absorb shock and transmit compressive loads across the knee joint. They also increase the conformity of the knee joint by deepening the articular surface of the tibial plateau. In addition, the menisci play a role in joint lubrication and nutrition, and there is evidence that the medial meniscus helps stabilize the anterior cruciate ligament (ACL)–deficient knee.[8]

Meniscal Injury

Meniscal injuries in children do not commonly occur in the first decade of life. As more children begin to participate in athletic activities at an earlier age, the incidence of meniscal injury in this age group may tend to rise. The ability of a meniscal tear to heal depends primarily on the location of the tear. Although there are three classic areas of vascularity in the adult meniscus (the red-red zone, the red-white zone, and the white-white zone), the meniscus in a child may be slightly more vascular until age 10 years, soon after which meniscal anatomy and blood supply assume an adult form. Peripheral capsular detachment is described as a tear within the red-red zone of the meniscus, with adequate vascularity on both sides of the tear. A tear within the red-white zone maintains vascularity on the peripheral side of the tear. A tear within the white-white zone is avascular and will not heal without vascular enhancement. Children have an increased ability to heal meniscal tears because of the increased vascularity of their menisci. Medial meniscal tears are much more common than lateral meniscus tears in the pediatric population, just as they are in adults. Making the diagnosis of these injuries in the pediatric population is dependent on proper history taking and physical examination. Also necessary are appropriate plain radiographs and an MRI scan when indicated.

History The history of a traumatic twisting injury to the knee suggests the possibility of a meniscal injury. Almost one third of patients will present with no history of major trauma, and little or no trauma may be required for a discoid meniscus to tear or become symptomatic. Patients often will complain of pain, swelling, and mechanical symptoms, such as locking and giving way.

Physical Examination Pain with provocative flexion and/or extension is often found. Joint-line tenderness along the compartment involved is a reliable indicator of meniscal pathology. In the acute setting, the presence of an effusion caused by hemarthrosis is usually seen, and chronic effusion can be present as well (Fig. 1). Children with meniscal injuries may have a positive result on a McMurray's test and Apley's compression or distraction test. Pain may also be elicited by having the patient duck walk.

Imaging Studies Radiographs of the skeletally immature patient who has signs and symptoms of meniscal pathology are helpful to rule out other pathologies such as a loose body or an osteochondral lesion. AP, lateral, skyline, and tunnel view radiographs should be obtained. Although these radiographs usually show no evidence of meniscal pathology, obtaining them is a necessary part of the diagnostic workup. Positive radiographic findings in a child with a discoid meniscus can include joint-space widening, cupping of the tibial plateau, and sclerosis of the tibial plateau.

The role of MRI in the evaluation of pediatric knee injuries is somewhat controversial. According to Stanitski,[9] physical examination has a 93.3% sensitivity and 92.3% specificity and an overall clinical accuracy rate of 92.8% in the diagnosis of meniscal injury; MRI has only a 50% sensitivity and a 37.5% accuracy rate. Many false-positive results are caused by the increased hydration of the normal pediatric meniscus. The examiner should be aware of the type I increased signal intensity that is normally seen within the body of the meniscus on T2-weighted imaging, with a decreased signal intensity seen in the same area on T1-weighted imaging. Special attention should be paid to the signal intensity that extends to either (type 2 signal intensity) or both (type 3 signal intensity) articular surfaces (Fig. 2). MRI should be used only as an adjunct to proper patient history and physical examination.

Arthroscopy

Diagnostic arthroscopy has a role in the evaluation and treatment of meniscal injuries in the pediatric population. The child who complains of persistent knee pain and mechanical symptoms is a candidate for diagnostic arthroscopy, even with no evidence of injury on MRI and plain radiographs and once other potential sources of pain, in particular the hip, have been ruled out.

Treatment

Once the diagnosis of a meniscal tear is established, the rationale for treatment is based on the classification of the tear, the presence of other injuries, and the ability of the surgeon to treat the tear. A meniscal tear can be classified based on its morphology, location in relation to blood supply, and size. Morphologically, meniscal tears are described as being vertical, longitudinal, oblique, or radial. A bucket-handle tear is a type of longitudinal tear that has a tendency to displace and cause mechanical blockage (Fig. 3). The most common tear pattern seen is the vertical tear of the medial meniscus. Horizontal tears occur rarely in children. Management options include leaving the tear alone, removing the tear, or repairing the tear.

Leaving the Tear Alone A stable meniscal injury that is within the zone of vascularity, less than 10 mm in length, and less than 3 mm maximally displaceable with a probe may heal without surgical stabilization.

Removing the Tear A tear within the white-white zone will have little or no healing without enhancement of the healing process. A peripherally based radial tear is not amenable to surgical repair. Other types of tears that are usually not reparable include parrot-beak, flap, and double-flap tears. These tears should be treated with partial meniscetomy. Total meniscectomy should be avoided at all costs since long-term follow-up of children treated with meniscectomy has yielded unfavorable results.[10,11]

Repairing the Tear Complete longitudinal, vertical, and bucket-handle tears within the red-red and red-white zones are most amenable to repair. In children, longitudinal tears in the white-white zone should be repaired as well. Surgical

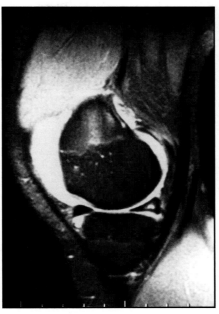

Fig. 2 Sagittal MRI scan showing false-positive type 2 signal in medial meniscus of a child.

enhancement of vascularity at the repair site has been shown to increase the healing of meniscal repair.[12] Vascular ingrowth channels may be created by trephination. Rasping and/or débridement of the tear edges can also enhance healing. The aid of a fibrin clot has also been shown to be beneficial.[13] Meniscal repair has been shown to be more successful when performed in conjunction with ACL reconstruction in adults[14] (Fig. 4).

Meniscal Repair Options

Suture repair is the treatment of choice and the gold standard for meniscal repair in children. It can be performed using an inside-out technique with the aid of cannulas. Suture may also be placed in an outside-in manner with the use of an 18-gauge spinal needle. Great care must be taken to ensure that the peroneal nerve or the saphenous nerve is not harmed when repairing medial or lateral meniscal tears, respectively. The disadvantages of suture repair include the need for a secondary incision, increased surgical time, and increased risk for neurovascular injury.

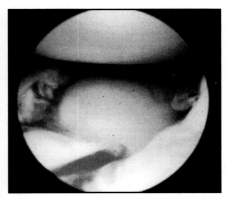

Fig. 3 A bucket handle tear of the medial meniscus is shown.

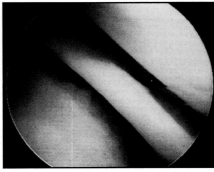

Fig. 4 Vertical "inside-out" suturing of a medial meniscus tear.

All-inside meniscal repair techniques using bioabsorbable implants or suture has become significantly more popular in the past 6 years. In 1996, there were 136,000 meniscal repairs performed in the United States, of which 3.3% were done with an all-inside technique. In the year 2000, there were 200,000 meniscal repairs, of which 43% were performed with an all-inside technique. The decreased risk of nerve injury with the all-inside implants and the relative ease of implantation have made this repair technique attractive to many orthopaedic surgeons. The development of biodegradable implants has significantly increased the number of meniscal repairs performed annually in the United States and has encouraged more orthopaedists to perform meniscus repair.

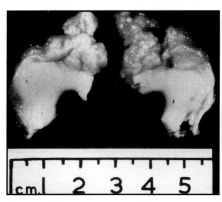

Fig. 5 Pathologic specimen of two type III discoid lateral menisci. Complete removal of this type of discoid lateral menisci is never indicated.

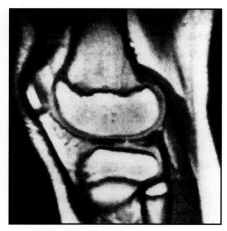

Fig. 6 Sagittal MRI scan showing horizontal cleavage tear of discoid lateral meniscus in a child.

Meniscal repair strength is greatest with the vertical-mattress suture configuration. Suture placed in this manner will take hold of a large bundle of circumferential fibers. The load to failure of vertically placed suture is more than double that of horizontally placed suture.[15] Fixation strengths of bioabsorbable implants are comparable with the strength of horizontally placed suture.[16] Discoid meniscal variants may also require peripheral reattachment. Saucerization of the discoid area can decrease the symptoms associated with the discoid meniscus.[17]

Postoperative Care

Postoperative care following meniscal surgery in the skeletally immature patient should be individualized. For children treated with partial meniscectomy, immediate weight bearing as tolerated without bracing has yielded favorable results.[11] For children who have undergone combined ACL reconstruction and meniscus repair, bracing with flexion limited to 30° and weight bearing as tolerated is recommended. Flexion should be limited so as not to place excessive stresses on the site of meniscus repair.

For the isolated meniscus repair, immediate postoperative bracing with motion restricted from 0° to 30° and

weight bearing as tolerated is recommended. For smaller longitudinal type tears that have been solidly repaired, flexion up to 45° may be permitted. Flexion with weight bearing and, in particular, squatting places significant stresses across the repair site and increases the risk of failure. Bracing may be discontinued after 4 to 6 weeks, and children may gradually be allowed to resume their previous activity levels over the next 6 weeks.

Discoid Meniscus

Discoid meniscus occurs in 3% to 5% of all US children and in 15% to 20% of all Japanese children.[7] The lateral meniscus is affected much more commonly than the medial meniscus, and the condition is bilateral in about 25% of the cases.[4]

Discoid menisci are classified by Watanabe and associates[18] into three types. In the type I discoid meniscus, the meniscus covers the lateral tibial plateau, is discoid in shape, and is stabilized by the coronary and meniscofemoral ligaments. In type II, the meniscus only partially covers the lateral tibial plateau, is discoid in shape, and is still stabilized by the meniscofemoral and coronary ligaments. In type III or the Wrisberg variant, the meniscus is destabilized because of its

lack of a meniscotibial attachment with the coronary ligament, rendering the posterior horn unstable; this type of variant can be normal or discoid in shape (Fig. 5).

The child with a discoid meniscus may be asymptomatic or may present with a popping or snapping knee. Mechanical symptoms, such as catching or locking, may be present as well and reproducible with the McMurray's sign. Standard radiographs should be obtained. Joint-space widening of the affected compartment, as well as squaring of the femoral condyle and cupping the tibial plateau may be seen. In diagnosing discoid meniscus, MRI has a high specificity but a low sensitivity, which means that positive test results suggest a high likelihood of discoid meniscus, with very few false-positive results. On the other hand, low sensitivity suggests a greater incidence of false-negative results with MRI (Fig. 6).

Tear patterns in discoid menisci are usually longitudinal; however, complex tears may occur as well. A discoid meniscus need not be torn to become symptomatic.

Treatment is based on the presence or absence of symptoms as well as the presence or absence of stability at the posterior meniscotibial interface. For patients in whom the discoid meniscus is asymptomatic, stable, and found incidentally, observation is best. For those in whom the type I or II discoid meniscus is not torn but causes symptoms, arthroscopic saucerization should be performed. A stable rim of 6 to 8 mm of meniscus should be left behind after saucerization. For those in whom the type I or II discoid meniscus is torn, saucerization followed by repair with suture when possible is optimal. The type III (Wrisberg) variant should be saucerized as necessary and stabilized to the capsule with suture. Total meniscectomy should be avoided at all costs because it has been demonstrated that complete meniscectomy does not lead to the regeneration of the meniscus.[17]

Articular Cartilage

Embryology and Anatomy

From an embryologic perspective, articular cartilage first develops in the knee during the first trimester. At the time of birth and throughout the remainder of life, the articular cartilage of the knee is organized into four zones: the superficial zone, the transitional zone, the radial zone, and the calcified cartilage zone. The orientations of collagen fibrils characterize these zones, which allow for a gradual transition from a smooth gliding articular surface to anchoring subchondral bone.

From a histologic perspective, articular cartilage is composed primarily of water, chondrocytes, and a collagen matrix. The predominant matrix component is type II collagen; however, several other types (V, VI, IX, X, and XI) are present in variable amounts.

The superficial zone contains fibrils that run parallel to the articular surface. This arrangement of collagen fibrils that are tangential to the gliding surface allows for minimal friction between two articular surfaces. It also maximizes the tensile strength and ability to resist shear forces within this zone. Between the tangentially oriented fibrils of the superficial zone and the radially oriented fibrils of the radial zone lies the transitional zone. The fibrils found in this zone are neither consistently tangential nor consistently radial to the articular surface, but they have been shown to be arranged in a relatively oblique arcade of collagen. Beneath the transitional layer lies the radial zone. The radial orientation of fibrils within this zone increases the ability to resist compressive forces. The zone of calcified cartilage directly overlies subchondral bone. This layer provides an area for the more superficial articular cartilage layers to firmly connect with subchondral bone.

Function

Articular cartilage lines the ends of bones and provides a low-friction surface that allows joint motion with minimal dissipation of mechanical energy and wear within the joint. The presence of synovial fluid further decreases the friction produced when motion occurs within the knee. The histologic organization of articular cartilage yields sufficient tensile and compressive strength to prevent injury, even when forces greater than six times the body weight are transmitted across the knee joint, as can occur during running. The friction produced by the articular surfaces of the knee by joint motion has been described as six times more efficient than the friction produced by the motion of ice on ice. In addition to decreasing mechanical friction, articular cartilage serves to cushion the forces across the knee joint during the gait cycle.

Acute Articular Cartilage Injury

Clinical Presentation Articular cartilage injury may occur in the skeletally immature knee as the result of either an acute traumatic event or repetitive microtrauma/osteochondritis dissecans (OCD). The acute traumatic event may lead to a partial- or even full-thickness articular cartilage injury in the skeletally immature knee. For example, a valgus-type knee injury can disrupt the medial collateral ligament and the ACL and also produce an impaction injury laterally, creating a "nutcracker" lesion in the lateral tibial plateau and lateral femoral condyle. This mechanism will often lead to subchondral bruising in both the lateral femoral condyle and the lateral tibial plateau, which is readily visible on T1- and T2-weighted MRI. Occasionally, this mechanism can result in a full-thickness, focal, articular cartilage defect on the lateral femoral condyle.

Diagnosis and Treatment When encountered, the acute, posttraumatic, full-thickness articular cartilage defect in the skeletally immature knee should be treated surgically, and arthroscopic examination should be performed. All attempts should be made to find the loose frag-

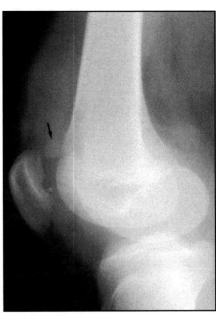

Fig. 7 Lateral radiograph showing osteochondral fragment from patella articular surface (*arrow*).

ment and stabilize it to its crater (Fig. 7). Early diagnosis is necessary to prevent degradation and additional fragmentation of the osteochondral fragments.

In the child, the articular cartilage is anatomically similar to the physis. As in the physis, fracture here occurs through the zone of provisional calcification rather than at the bone-cartilage interface. Consequently, mechanical reattachment usually results in rapid union and healing as opposed to chondral injuries in the adult. For osteochondral fragments, we prefer to replace a fragment as anatomically as possible. We then suture it in place with 6-0 polyglactin 910 sutures (Vicryl, Ethicon Inc, Somerville, NJ). If the fragment is relatively large, fixation is supplemented by polylactic acid pins that are often placed at oblique angles to each other.

Various surgical stabilization methods include fixation with bioabsorbable smooth pins and compression with the Herbert (Zimmer, Warsaw, IN) or Acutrak (Acumed, Inc, Hillsboro, OR) screw.

These methods of fixation enable the surgeon to countersink the head of the fixation mechanism beneath the chondral surface, which allows the child to begin early motion—one of the key tenets for optimal functional outcome. We prefer to use the cannulated Herbert-Whipple screw for surgical stabilization.

With a completely detached fragment that has been present for months, there is often a size mismatch between the loose fragment and the bed from which it dislodged. This is in part caused by swelling of the loose fragment and partial filling in of the crater with fibrocartilage. When a size mismatch is encountered, the loose fragment should be trimmed to fit the bed to which it is to be stabilized. Once the recipient site and the loose fragment are matched in size, surgical stabilization should be performed. Excision of the fragment should be avoided whenever possible. When a fragment requires excision because it is inadequate for surgical stabilization, mircrofracture, subchondral drilling, or any other method that allows for vascular access to the site of injury can yield a bed of fibrocartilage in the area of the articular cartilage defect.

Each method of surgical stabilization is not without its pitfalls, however. Although bioabsorbable pins provide adequate stability for healing of the fragment to occur, are relatively easy to insert, and do not require a second procedure for surgical removal, they provide minimal compression. Intra-articular bioabsorbable implants have also been implicated in chronic synovitis. Although rigid fixation with the Herbert or Acutrak screw allows compression of the fragment to the underlying crater, both of these screws are headless and have the potential to become prominent when fragment resorption or loosening occurs, which can have significant adverse effects on the tibial plateau.[19] Therefore, many surgeons prefer to remove these screws in a second procedure after healing of the fragment has occurred. Finally, although

the recent development of headless, bioabsorbable screws that provide compression shows promise in the treatment of focal articular cartilage defects, the likelihood of intra-articular bioabsorbable fixation leading to synovitis continues to be problematic.

In addition to creating vascular ingrowth channels via microfracture, abrasion, and drillings, newer techniques are available to repair focal articular cartilage defects that are not amenable to fragment stabilization.[20-22] For example, autologous chondrocyte implantation (Carticel, Genzyme Biosurgery, Cambridge, MA) and osteochondral autograft transfer are gaining popularity in both adult and pediatric populations.[23-27] Autologous chondrocyte implantation requires surgical harvesting of a chondral biopsy specimen from the periphery of the site of injury. This specimen is then sent to the laboratory where the chondrocytes are grown. After 6 weeks of growth, the liquid form of the chondrocytes is placed underneath a periosteal patch over the articular cartilage defect. The periosteal patch taken from the tibia must be sewn to the defect and sealed with fibrin to form a watertight seal that prevents extrusion when the chondrocytes are injected into the defect.[23-27] Osteochondral autograft transfer requires harvesting one or more osteochondral plugs from a relatively minimal weight-bearing area of the knee and impacting them into the prepared articular cartilage defect.[28,29]

Articular Cartilage Injury From Repetitive Microtrauma/Osteochondritis Dissecans

The etiology of OCD is still being debated. Hypotheses include hereditary developmental anomalies, ischemia resulting from vascular occlusion, acute trauma, and repetitive microtrauma.[30] The apparent increased prevalence of OCD of the knee in children who participate in athletic activities suggests that repetitive microtrauma is a major etiologic factor.

Whatever the primary event, the common denominator in this type of articular cartilage injury is necrosis of subchondral bone, with the overlying articular cartilage initially being viable and mechanically intact. As the revascularization of this necrotic bone occurs, new bone is laid down on the necrotic elements by a process of "creeping substitution." If most or all of the involved subchondral bone remains avascular, the fragment may become mechanically unstable, and a fracture of the overlying articular cartilage may occur, exposing the underlying necrotic bone to synovial fluid, which may inhibit revascularization and healing. The fragment will eventually loosen and breaks off into the joint as a loose body if healing does not occur or more definitive treatment is not initiated.

Clinical Presentation The usual clinical presentation is pain with activity, which is often poorly localized. Effusion may be present, and, particularly with unstable lesions, mechanical symptoms such as locking or catching may be described. If a loose body has developed, mechanical symptoms and episodic locking may predominate. However, localization of symptoms may depend on the location of the lesion.

When occurring on the inner aspect of the medial femoral condyle (the "classic site"), anterior or central pain may be described as well as an area of tenderness with the knee in a flexed position. In a large multicenter study in Europe, Hefti and associates[30] found that only 51% of reported lesions were located at this "classic site." Patients may present with pain in atypical locations, including the patella, trochlea, lateral femoral condyle or posterior aspect of the medial femoral condyle, and symptoms mirroring patellofemoral disorders; alternatively, patients may be relatively asymptomatic until a loose body forms.

Diagnosis and Treatment As noted, clinical signs and symptoms may vary, suggesting patellofemoral disorders or internal derangement. In a child presenting with nonspecific knee pain, we always obtain the following four-view radiographs: AP, lateral, tunnel or notch, and skyline views. The notch view may demonstrate central or posterior condyle lesions not seen on the AP view, and the skyline and lateral views provide an AP and lateral view of the patella and trochlea. If needed, MRI can provide a more specific determination of the size and extent of the lesion. Additionally, when an effusion is present in a joint or contrast material is added to the joint, the resulting magnetic resonance arthrogram may indicate whether the lesion is closed or open and thereby determine if it is exposed to synovial fluid.[30]

The range of treatment options for an identified lesion includes relative rest and observation, cast or brace immobilization, removal, transarticular drilling, antegrade débridement with replacement and fixation, and retrograde grafting and stabilization. The factors that influence management, whether surgical or nonsurgical, include the age and relative maturity of the patient, the size of the lesion, the location of the lesion, whether the lesion is open or closed, and whether the lesion is mechanically unstable or a loose body.

Hefti and associates[30] classified the OCD lesions they studied as favorable or unfavorable. Favorable lesions, those with a favorable prognosis, had no effusion, were smaller than 20 mm, and demonstrated no evidence of dissection on magnetic resonance arthrogram. Unfavorable lesions, those with an unfavorable prognosis, lacked the foregoing favorable factors, were usually in an atypical location, and occurred in more skeletally mature individuals and/or those who participated in organized sports. Surgical and nonsurgical treatment of favorable lesions had an identical rate of success. However, surgical treatment of unfavorable lesions had a significantly better success rate than nonsurgical treatment.

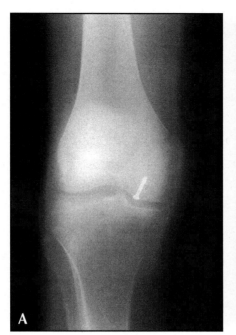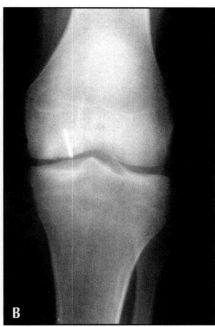

Fig. 8 A and **B,** AP radiographs of an unstable medial femoral OCD treated with compression screw fixation.

Thus, the appropriate initial management of a relatively small closed lesion (< 2 cm) in a skeletally immature child should be relative rest or a period of 6 to 8 weeks of immobilization. Sequential follow-up with radiographs or MRI is essential because clinical signs and symptoms are unreliable measures of healing. Alternatively, arthroscopy may be used to assess the lesion size and stability. If the lesion is stable and closed, particularly in a younger child, transarticular drilling may be attempted. This is done with a fine, smooth Kirschner wire across the articular cartilage and necrotic subchondral bone into the viable bone underneath in an attempt to restore vascular channels from the viable bone to the necrotic bone. Kocher and associates[31] reported an 80% success rate with this technique, but the success rate decreased progressively with increased skeletal maturity.

When the lesion is open or unsable at the time of arthroscopy, particularly in a more skeletally mature child, transarticu-

lar fixation with compression screws may be necessary. In the case of a loose fragment in a lesion smaller than 10 mm, removal and marrow stimulation of the base is usually successful. In the case of larger lesions, particularly in atypical locations that are mechanically unstable, every attempt should be made to débride the site and restore a relatively satisfactory mechanical fit with compression screw fixation (Fig. 8). In cases in which the fragment has been previously discarded or cannot be restored because of excessive fragmentation and mechanical replacement is no longer an option, cartilage repair techniques may be indicated, particularly in larger lesions. We prefer autologous cartilage implantation. Others have reported success with autologous bone plugs or allografts.[23,28,29]

Summary

Meniscal and articular cartilage injuries in the skeletally immature patient appear to be occurring with increased frequency, particularly in athletically active children.

The orthopaedic surgeon should understand the principles of diagnosis and management of these injuries and should be aware of the current treatment options that are available.

References

1. Streeter GL (ed): *Developmental Horizons in Human Embryos: Age Groups XI-XXIII.* Washington, DC, Carnegie Institution of Washington DC, 1951, vol 2.

2. Smillie IS: The congenital discoid meniscus. *J Bone Joint Surg Br* 1948;30:671-682.

3. Clark CR, Ogden JA: Development of the menisci of the human knee joint: Morphological changes and their potential role in childhood meniscal injury. *J Bone Joint Surg Am* 1983;65:538-547.

4. Kaplan EB: Discoid lateral meniscus of the knee joint: Nature, mechanism, and operative treatment. *J Bone Joint Surg Am* 1957;39:77-87.

5. Renstrom P, Johnson RJ: Anatomy and biomechanics of the menisci. *Clin Sports Med* 1990;9:523-538.

6. Arnoczky SP, Warren RF: Microvasculature of the human meniscus. *Am J Sports Med* 1982;10:90-95.

7. Ikeuchi H: Arthroscopic treatment of the discoid lateral meniscus: Techniques and long-term results. *Clin Orthop* 1982;167:19-28.

8. Levy IM, Torzilli PA, Warren RF: The effect of medial meniscectomy on anterior-posterior motion of the knee. *J Bone Joint Surg Am* 1982;64:883-888.

9. Stanitski CL: Correlation of arthroscopic and clinical examination with magnetic resonance imaging findings of injured knees in children and adolescents. *Am J Sports Med* 1998;26:2-6.

10. Manzione M, Pizzutillo PA, Peoples AB, et al: Meniscectomy in children: A long-term follow-up study. *Am J Sports Med* 1983;11:111-115.

11. Medlar RC, Mandiberg JJ and Lyne ED: Meniscectomies in children: Report of long term results (mean, 8.3 years) of 26 children. *Am J Sports Med* 1980;8:87-92.

12. Mintzer CM, Richmond JC, Taylor J: Meniscal repair in the young athlete. *Am J Sports Med* 1998;26:630-633.

13. Henning CE, Lynch MA, Yearout KM, Verquist SW, Stallbaumer RJ, Decker KA: Arthroscopic meniscal repair using an exogenous fibrin clot. *Clin Orthop* 1990;252:64-72.

14. Cannon WD Jr, Vittori JM: The incidence of healing in arthroscopic meniscal repairs in anterior cruciate ligament-reconstructed knee versus stable knees. *Am J Sports Med* 1992;20:176-181.

15. Barber FA, Herbert MA: Meniscal repair devices. *Arthroscopy* 2000;16:613-618.

16. Rimmer MG, Nawana NS, Keene GC, Pearcy MJ: Failure strengths of different meniscal suturing techniques. *Arthroscopy* 1995;11:146-150.

17. Albertsson M, Gillquist J: Discoid lateral menisci: A report of 29 cases. *Arthroscopy* 1988;4:211-214.

18. Watanabe M, Takeda S, Ikeuchi H (eds): *Atlas of Arthroscopy,* ed 3. Tokyo, Japan, Igaku-Shoin, 1979.

19. Thomson NL: Osteochondritis dissecans and osteochondral fragments managed by Herbert compression screw fixation. *Clin Orthop* 1987;224:71-78.

20. Insall J: The Pridie debridement operation for osteoarthritis of the knee. *Clin Orthop* 1974;101:61-67.

21. Johnson LL: Arthroscopic abrasion arthroplasty: Historical and pathologic perspective: Present status. *Arthroscopy* 1986;2:54-69.

22. Pridie KH: Abstract: A method of resurfacing osteoarthritic knee joints. *J Bone Joint Surg Br* 1959;41:618-619.

23. Brittberg M, Lindahl A, Nilsson A, Ohlsson C, Isaksson O, Peterson L: Treatment of deep cartilage defects in the knee with autologous chondrocyte transplantation. *N Engl J Med* 1994;331:889-895.

24. Brittberg M, Tallheden T, Sjogren-Jansson B, Lindahl A, Peterson L: Autologous chondrocytes used for articular cartilage repair: An update. *Clin Orthop* 2001;(suppl 391):S337-S348.

25. Minas T, Peterson L: Advanced techniques in autologous chondrocyte transplantation. *Clin Sports Med* 1999;18:13-44.

26. Peterson L, Brittberg M, Kiviranta I, Akerlund EL, Lindahl A: Autologous chondrocyte transplantation: Biomechanics and long-term durability. *Am J Sports Med* 2002;30:2-12.

27. Peterson L, Minas T, Brittberg M, Nilsson A, Sjogren-Jansson E, Lindahl A: Two- to 9-year outcome after autologous chondrocyte transplantation of the knee. *Clin Orthop* 2000;374:212-234.

28. Hangody L, Kish G, Karpati Z, Eberhart R: Osteochondral plugs: Autogenous osteochondral mosaicplasty for the treatment of focal chondral and osteochondral articular defects. *Op Tech Orthop* 1997;7:312-322.

29. Matsusue Y, Yamamuro T, Hama H: Arthroscopic multiple osteochondral transplantation to the chondral defect in the knee associated with anterior cruciate ligament disruption. *Arthroscopy* 1993;9:318-321.

30. Hefti F, Berguiristain J, Krauspe R, et al: Osteochondritis dissecans: A multicenter study of the European Pediatric Orthopedic Society. *J Pediatr Orthop B* 1999;8:231-245.

31. Kocher MS, Micheli LJ, Yaniv M, Zurakowski D, Ames A, Adrignolo AA: Functional and radiographic outcome of juvenile osteochondritis dissecans of the knee treated with transarticular arthroscopic drilling. *Am J Sports Med* 2001;29:562-526.

Musculoskeletal Infections in Children: Basic Treatment Principles and Recent Advancements

James J. McCarthy, MD
John P. Dormans, MD
Scott H. Kozin, MD
Peter D. Pizzutillo, MD

Abstract

Pediatric musculoskeletal infections are common disorders that can result in significant disability. Because the understanding, diagnosis, and treatment of infections of the bones, joints, and soft tissues have continued to improve over time, it is important for orthopaedic surgeons to have an understanding of the etiology, diagnosis, basic treatment principles, and recent advancements to achieve successful outcomes. Although each infectious process is unique, there are certain treatment principles that apply to all pediatric musculoskeletal infections. These include prevention, a prompt and accurate diagnosis, and timely medical and/or surgical intervention. Continued evaluations are mandatory to assure good long-term outcomes. Because the effects of infection may last beyond the acute episode in pediatric patients, long-term follow-up is needed to assess for late sequelae such as angular deformities and limb-length inequalities.

It has been reported that most bacterial infections of childhood are easily diagnosed, readily treated, and have good outcomes. By contrast, suppurative infections of the skeletal system still present challenges because these illnesses are often difficult to recognize and localize early in the course of illness, and many are difficult to manage medically and surgically. Despite best treatment efforts, however, a substantial portion of those treated are left with disabling sequelae.[1]

Sepsis accounts for 200,000 deaths each year in the United States.[2] One in 5,000 children younger than 13 years will have osteomyelitis, and about twice as many will have septic arthritis (Figure 1). The outcome is poor in 27% of patients with septic arthritis and in nearly 40% of those with involvement of the hip.[1] Unique to the infectious process is the fact that the disease actually changes over time. The incidence of infections, especially gram-positive infections, is rising. Fortunately, physicians are getting better at diagnosis and treatment.

Prior to antibiotic treatment, the mortality rate associated with infection was close to 50%; now it is less than 1%. The *Haemophilus influenzae* type B vaccination has essentially eliminated septic arthritis caused by this organism in immunized patients. New techniques for diagnosis, such as the use of polymerase chain reaction for the detection of bacterial pathogens or ultrasonography, may help make the diagnosis more quickly. Therefore, it is important for orthopaedic surgeons to have an understanding of the etiology, diagnosis, treatment principles, and recent advancements in the management of bone, joint, and soft-tissue infections in children.

Acute Hematogenous Osteomyelitis

Acute hematogenous osteomyelitis in children is an inflammation of bone caused by bacteria that reach the bone through a hematogenous route. No consistent peak incidence in a specific age group has been reported in the literature, although the infection usually occurs in the first decade of life. During the years after the introduction of penicillin (1944 through 1950), the incidence of osteomyelitis decreased. Then, after 1950, the incidence increased with the development of antibiotic-resistant organisms.[3] During the past 15 years, there has been little change in the number of cases per year.[4]

Etiology

Typically, acute hematogenous osteomyelitis in children begins in the metaphyseal venous sinus, where there are vascular loops and terminal branches

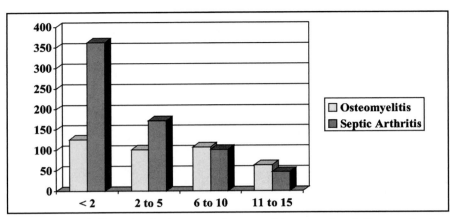

Figure 1 Bar graph illustrating the frequency of osteomyelitis and septic arthritis according to age (years).

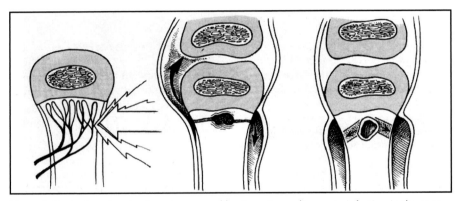

Figure 2 Illustration showing how trauma and bacteremia predispose to infection in the metaphysis, which may track into the joint. (Reproduced from Dormans JP, Drummond DS: Pediatric hematogenous osteomyelitis: New trends in presentation, diagnosis, and treatment. *J Am Acad Orthop Surg* 1994;2:333-341.)

with low oxygen tension and inhibited phagocytosis that is conducive to bacterial growth. The initial bacteremia may occur from a daily event such as tooth brushing, which results in bacteremia 25% of the time,[5] or it may be related to another cause such as trauma or decreased host resistance. Trauma may play a role in up to 30% of the cases of acute hematogenous osteomyelitis. Studies of a rabbit model showed that trauma increased the chance of acute hematogenous osteomyelitis when there was concurrent bacteremia[6,7] (Figure 2).

Thrombosis of the venous sinus and nutrient artery can occur with bacterial proliferation and result in a loss of medullary blood supply, slowing mobilization of infection-fighting cells. By 72 hours, inflammatory processes are well developed, and an exudate forms that can exit the bone through the porous cortex of the metaphysis. In some locations, such as the proximal part of the femur, the metaphysis may be within the joint capsule and result in the coexistence of septic arthritis and osteomyelitis. If the elevated periosteum remains viable, it will produce new bone and, over time, an involucrum will form; the adjoining cortex can become nonviable and become a sequestrum. Acute hematogenous osteo-

myelitis in children is more common in the lower extremity and tends to affect the most rapidly growing ends of the long bones, such as the distal part of the femur and proximal part of the tibia.

Diagnosis

The diagnosis of acute hematogenous osteomyelitis in children is difficult and is still often made late. The most important factors in making the diagnosis are the clinical findings, and a high index of suspicion on the part of the clinician is essential. Unexplained bone pain with fever indicates osteomyelitis until proven otherwise.

The onset of acute hematogenous osteomyelitis is usually sudden, and 30% to 50% of patients with the disease have had a recent or have a concurrent nonmuscular infection. Often, these infants and children appear systemically ill, with localization of the cardinal signs of infection: swelling, redness, warmth, and pain. The patient may have findings of an adjacent sympathetic joint effusion, with joint irritability and a limited range of motion or even pseudoparalysis.

An elevated white blood cell count and erythrocyte sedimentation rate are seen in most of these children, but these tests are not as reliable in the neonate. Blood cultures are positive in 30% to 50% of infants and children. Radiographs do not show osseous changes for 7 to 10 days. Deep soft-tissue swelling is the key finding early in the process.

MRI is the best imaging modality for the diagnosis of acute hematogenous osteomyelitis and is especially useful in the axial skeleton;[8] it is better able to differentiate abnormal bone marrow involvement than bone scans, CT scans, or radiographs.[9] However, MRI lacks the specificity to demonstrate whether the abnormal changes are caused by osteomyelitis.[10]

Another imaging study that may be helpful is the technetium Tc 99m diphosphonate bone scan, a three-phase scan that usually demonstrates increased uptake as a result of alteration in the physiology of involved bone.[11] An abnormal technetium bone scan is nonspecific and may yield false-positive results associated with trauma or tumors. There is a 4% to 20% rate of false-negative results (a lack of increased uptake despite the presence of acute hematogenous osteomyelitis), which may be seen with osteonecrosis or in very early cases. A bone scan is best used to identify multiple or difficult locations (the spine and pelvis).

Early studies showed that technetium scans were unreliable for infants and neonates, as they detected only 50% of foci,[12,13] but high-resolution techniques have improved the sensitivity.[14] Use of technetium scans in neonates is particularly helpful, especially for finding multiple sites of infection. Bone scans (or other diagnostic imaging) should not delay treatment, and aspiration does not produce false-positive results.[15] If needed, the accuracy of technetium scans can be increased by repeating the scan in 48 to 72 hours.[16]

With osteomyelitis, there is an almost immediate increase in uptake on gallium 67 citrate-labeled leukocyte bone scans.[17] These scans are obtained less frequently, primarily because they are more expensive, are associated with more radiation exposure, and take longer to complete (48 to 72 hours). The accuracy of early diagnosis may be increased by following a negative technetium scan with a gallium scan.[18] Indium-labeled leukocyte bone scans[19] require labeling of leukocytes and thus can be performed only at selected facilities. Although indium-labeled leukocyte bone scans are very accurate, their use is limited primarily to difficult diagnostic situations in which other imaging modalities are less ideal, such as chronic osteomyelitis.[19]

CT scans show nonspecific changes early[20] and then demonstrate increased intramedullary density later in the course of the osteomyelitis.[21] The deep soft-

tissue swelling is better defined by CT than by plain radiographs. CT may be valuable for detecting extraosseous deep soft-tissue swelling or abscesses and is useful primarily for the diagnosis of subacute and chronic forms of infection that may be confused with a neoplasm when other imaging modalities (such as MRI) are not practical.

Aspiration is critical for bacteriologic diagnosis and should be done early, even if there is no abscess. The technique involves locating the point of maximum tenderness and swelling (usually in the metaphysis) and then using a 16- or 18-gauge spinal trocar needle to aspirate material extraperiosteally, subperiosteally, and intraosseously. All material should be smeared and cultured, and antibiotics should be started on the basis of the most likely suspected organism while awaiting definitive culture results. Aspiration produces positive results in 60% of patients and biopsy in 90%.

Treatment

The general principles of treatment of acute hematogenous osteomyelitis are similar to those for other infections, with the focus on identifying the organism or organisms and their sensitivities, use of the correct antimicrobial treatment and delivery in sufficient concentrations to kill the organism, and surgical débridement if the infection is refractory to medical treatment or if an abscess is identified.

Staphylococcus aureus is still the predominant infecting organism, with the prevalence ranging from 60% to

90%,[4,22,23] followed by *Streptococcus* (prevalence, 20% to 50%) (Table 1). The rate of streptococcal osteomyelitis has increased in infants; this represents an increase in the incidence of group B *Streptococcus* in neonatal sepsis.[24-26] Gram-negative organisms account for less than 5% of the cases, with *H influenzae* formerly being the predominant gram-negative organism.[4] Salmonella should always be considered in the differential diagnosis of children with sickle cell disease.

Traditionally, intravenous antibiotics have been administered for approximately 3 weeks before switching to oral treatment, but if there is a prompt response to the intravenous antibiotics, then oral medication can be initiated at 5 to 7 days. Ten percent of infants and children do not respond to oral medication and need continued intravenous antibiotic treatment. Typically, the prerequisites for switching to oral medications have been identification of the organism, determination of antibiotic sensitivities and susceptibilities, and confirmation of bactericidal antibiotic levels. Currently, the clinical response to treatment as well as laboratory values (usually the C-reactive protein level) is used to determine whether switching to oral medications is appropriate. The C-reactive protein level rises faster and returns to normal more quickly than does the erythrocyte sedimentation rate and is the laboratory indicator of choice when observing infants and children being treated for osteomyelitis. Historically, the total duration of treatment has been as long as 6 weeks, but now a shorter duration of

Table 1
Organisms Causing Acute Hematogenous Osteomyelitis

	Organism	Antibiotic
Neonates	Group B *Streptococcus*, *S aureus*, gram-negative rods	Cefotaxime or oxacillin and gentamicin
Infants and children	*S aureus* (90%)	Oxacillin
Patients with sickle cell disease	*S aureus* or *Salmonella*	Oxacillin and ampicillin or cefotaxime or chloramphenicol

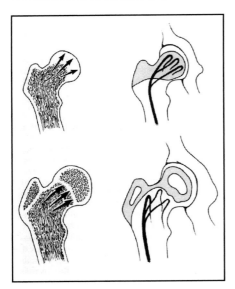

Figure 3 Illustration showing the blood supply and spread of infection in the infant and child. (Reproduced from Dormans JP, Drummond DS: Pediatric hematogenous osteomyelitis: New trends in presentation, diagnosis, and treatment. *J Am Acad Orthop Surg* 1994;2:333-341.)

antibiotic therapy may be adequate. However, there is no established duration, which depends on clinical characteristics such as the site of the infection, amount of destruction, treatment, and response to treatment. For example, a child with femoral osteomyelitis who has considerable destruction of the femur may need 8 to 12 weeks of treatment, whereas a child with early metacarpal osteomyelitis may need only 14 to 21 days and a neonate may need only 7 days.

Most children older than 1 year and with a duration of symptoms of less than 48 hours respond to antibiotic treatment alone (without surgery). If a child does not respond to antibiotics within 36 hours, surgical débridement should be considered.

The primary role of surgery is to evacuate purulent material. If the pus accumulates under the periosteum for any length of time, the periosteum can be destroyed. The periosteum may serve as the only source of osteogenic regenera-

tion of the dead bone. If the bone does not regenerate, a permanent defect may result. Surgery is also very effective in removing sequestra to clear up chronic infections. An appropriate aphorism is "Antibiotics save the life; surgery saves the bone."

The surgical technique for patients with established osteomyelitis includes periosteal incision and removal of all exudate and necrotic bone. The role of drilling the cortex is somewhat controversial. If suction irrigation tubes are used, they should be removed by 48 hours. Placement of long-term intravenous access with the patient under the same anesthetic should be considered.

Other Forms of Osteomyelitis

Several unique forms of osteomyelitis can occur in children. These include neonatal osteomyelitis, subacute hematogenous osteomyelitis, and chronic recurrent multifocal osteomyelitis. It is important to understand the characteristics of these disorders and how they differ from the more common acute hematogenous osteomyelitis.

Neonatal osteomyelitis differs from acute hematogenous osteomyelitis in four ways: (1) the musculoskeletal anatomy of the neonate is unique, and an infection ultimately affects growth of the physis and/or enters the joint in 76% of patients; (2) the organism that causes the infection may differ from that seen with acute hematogenous osteomyelitis; (3) multiple sites are commonly involved (40% of patients); and (4) infants have an immature immune system, and therefore diagnosis can be difficult.

Neonates and young infants with osteomyelitis have a unique anatomy that differs from that of older children with acute hematogenous osteomyelitis (Figure 3). For example, before the epiphyseal ossification centers form in the proximal part of the femur, metaphyseal vessels penetrate directly into the cartilaginous precursor. Infection can destroy

these fragile growth centers[27] and enter the hip joint directly. Transphyseal vessels persist for up to 12 to 18 months. In older children, the physis serves as a mechanical barrier to infection, but in infants, the osseous architecture is more fragile and is very easily injured.[28] The morbidity rate is higher (up to 76%) for neonates.

S aureus is the most common organism in neonates and infants with osteomyelitis, especially in cases associated with invasive procedures.[29] Other organisms are not uncommon and include group B *Streptococcus*, gram-negative organisms (in 10% to 15% of patients), and *Candida albicans*. Staphylococcal infections, which are associated with less purulent exudate, tend to be associated with less morbidity and fewer clinical symptoms. The diagnosis of these infections is often delayed.[30]

Neonates with osteomyelitis have an immature immune system, are less able to produce an inflammatory response, and are susceptible to organisms that are less virulent in older children and adults. The temperature and white blood cell count of neonates with osteomyelitis may be normal, and there may be few findings on physical examination or imaging (including false-negative results on bone scans). Often, these factors delay the diagnosis.

In general, the characteristics of neonatal osteomyelitis vary depending on whether the infection was acquired in the hospital or community. When neonatal osteomyelitis is acquired in the hospital, it is often caused by invasive monitoring devices such as umbilical catheters,[29] fetal monitors,[31] or heel puncture instruments.[32] Neonates more often have multiple sites of infection, and bone scans are often helpful in identifying the multiple locations. Neonates who acquire osteomyelitis after discharge from the hospital are normally not ill and more often have normal development and feeding habits. In these infants, the organism is more commonly group B *Streptococcus* and the osteomyelitis more commonly affects a single site.

Subacute hematogenous osteomyelitis differs from acute hematogenous osteomyelitis in that the child is typically less symptomatic, with less pain and often no fever. Many children with subacute hematogenous osteomyelitis (30% to 40%) have had a trial of antibiotics. The results of laboratory assessments (including blood and tissue cultures) are more commonly normal. Unlike radiographs of patients with acute hematogenous osteomyelitis, radiographs of patients with subacute hematogenous osteomyelitis usually show changes (Figure 4). Nearly all instances of subacute hematogenous osteomyelitis are caused by *S aureus*, but recently some streptococcal infections have been identified. The most important aspect of treating children and adolescents with subacute hematogenous osteomyelitis is ruling out tumors. In addition to cultures of involved tissue, a biopsy is needed, and this is the classic situation for which the mantra "culture all biopsies, and biopsy all cultures" is applied. Treatment consists of administration of appropriate antibiotics and, when the osteomyelitis is chronic (with symptoms for more than 1 month), débridement and removal of any sequestrum may be required.

Subacute hematogenous osteomyelitis can also occur in the epiphyses of the long bones.[33,34] Radiographs usually demonstrate a well-defined lesion, possibly with a sclerotic rim, and chondroblastoma should be considered in the differential diagnosis. Usually, the nidus of epiphyseal osteomyelitis heals with appropriate antibiotic treatment. Physeal damage and involvement of the articular surface are uncommon.

Chronic recurrent multifocal osteomyelitis differs from acute hematogenous osteomyelitis in that there is an insidious onset of bone pain and tenderness. Patients with chronic recurrent multifocal osteomyelitis most often present with only one site of involvement, although other sites develop with time. Chronic recurrent multifocal osteomyelitis may be confused with pyogenic osteomyelitis, but typically no organisms are isolated with the former. Furthermore, chronic recurrent multifocal osteomyelitis does not typically respond to antibiotic treatment. Synovitis, acne, pustulosis, hyperostosis, osteitis (SAPHO) syndrome is not uncommon in children who present with manifestations that are similar to those of chronic recurrent multifocal osteomyelitis as well as with skin lesions, most commonly palmoplantar pustulosis.[35] Radiographs of patients with chronic, recurrent multifocal osteomyelitis often demonstrate eccentric metaphyseal sclerotic lucencies; bone scintigraphy may help to identify additional lesions. Treatment consists of nonsteroidal anti-inflammatory drugs and management of the symptoms. In one series of 12 patients with chronic recurrent multifocal osteomyelitis,[36] five patients had a limb-length inequality of greater than 1.5 cm. Other orthopaedic deformities may also occur. The long-term outcome of treatment of chronic recurrent multifocal osteomyelitis is generally good, although recurrence is common. As many as 26% of patients have active disease at the time of long-term follow-up.[37] Few patients have functional limitations, even without complete resolution of symptoms.[36]

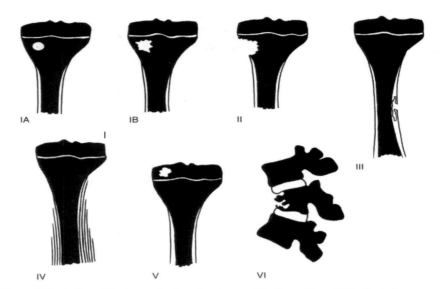

Figure 4 Illustration of the types of subacute osteomyelitis. Types IA and IB indicate lucency; type II, metaphyseal with loss of cortical bone; type III, diaphyseal; type IV, onion skinning; type V, epiphyseal; and type VI, spine. (Reproduced from Dormans JP, Drummond DS: Pediatric hematogenous osteomyelitis: New trends in presentation, diagnosis, and treatment. *J Am Acad Orthop Surg* 1994;2:333-341.)

Acute Hematogenous Osteomyelitis in Unusual or Difficult-to-Diagnose Locations

Acute hematogenous osteomyelitis usually occurs in the metaphyses of long bones, but it can also develop in unusual locations, such as the epiphysis,[38] the pelvis, the calcaneus, the talus, and the metatarsals. Historically, the diagnosis of pelvic and sacroiliac joint infection has been delayed, but newer imaging modalities have made the diagnosis easier. The physical examination findings are variable and may include a positive FABER test (pain with flexion, abduction, and external [lateral] rotation of the hip). Pain may also occur with lateral compression/distraction of the iliac wings and with straight-leg raising or hyperextension of the hip (Gaenslen's sign). The child may have direct tenderness over the sacroiliac joint or may refuse to stand on the limb.

Evaluation should include routine laboratory studies, such as a white blood cell count and measurement of the erythrocyte sedimentation rate. It is also important to rule out other causes for the symptoms, such as noninflammatory arthritis. About half of the patients have positive blood cultures. Stool and urine samples can also be obtained for testing if the diagnosis is still in question.

Radiographs of the area in question and a bone scan may be helpful, but the findings can be negative early in the disease course, and therefore MRI is the most accurate modality for evaluation. CT-guided biopsy may be needed to rule out a psoas abscess.[39]

Aspiration can be performed when the diagnosis is uncertain and when the patient does not respond to more conservative therapy.[40] A bone biopsy can be considered when aspiration does not yield fluid. *S aureus* is the most common organism with involvement of the sacroiliac joint. Treatment is initiated with antibiotics, which is sufficient in most cases. If an abscess is identified, surgical drainage should be considered.[41]

Acute hematogenous osteomyelitis of the calcaneus can also be difficult to diagnose.[42,43] Although foot puncture wounds are common, true calcaneal osteomyelitis is uncommon. Radiographically, there is very little periosteal bone reaction. Most patients respond to antibiotics with or without curettage.

Subacute osteomyelitis of the talus and metatarsals has been reported.[42,44,45] Usually, no systemic signs are reported, so there is often a delay of several months in the diagnosis. Radiographic changes are slow to develop, but radiographs show a lytic lesion. The organism is usually coagulase-negative *Staphylococcus*.

Treatment consists of surgical curettage, antibiotics, and rest.

It is important to remember that several bone tumors can simulate subacute and chronic osteomyelitis. The most common is Ewing's sarcoma,[46,47] but eosinophilic granuloma and leukemia can also present in a fashion that is similar to that of osteomyelitis, and they should be included in the differential diagnosis. Thirty percent of children with leukemia present with bone pain.

Septic Arthritis

Septic arthritis in children can occur in any joint, but the most common and most devastating location is the hip.

Etiology

Septic arthritis can occur from primary seeding of the synovial membrane, secondarily from infection in the adjacent metaphyseal bone or directly from infection in the adjoining epiphysis. In the hip, shoulder, ankle, and elbow, the joint capsule overlaps a portion of the adjoining metaphysis, and if a focus of osteomyelitis breaks through the soft metaphyseal bone, it can directly seed the joint and lead to concurrent septic arthritis. Additionally, in the hip, vessels cross the epiphysis until the age of approximately 18 months, and this provides a direct route for infection to spread from the metaphysis to the hip joint[48] (Figure 3).

Destruction of the articular cartilage begins quickly and is secondary to proteolytic enzymes released from synovial cells. Interleukin-1 triggers the release of proteases from chondrocytes and synoviocytes in response to polymorphonuclear leukocytes and bacteria. Degradation results in loss of proteoglycans at 5 days and of collagen by 9 days. Impairment of the intracapsular vascular supply also plays a role in the articular destruction, with elevation of the intracapsular pressure, thrombosis, and progressive displacement of the femoral head from the acetabulum.[49-53]

Diagnosis

The diagnosis of septic arthritis is based on the clinical findings. Typically, the disease has an acute onset in which the child is irritable, febrile, and anorexic. When the infection is in the lower extremity, the child limps or refuses to bear weight. There is severe pain with attempted passive motion of the hip joint. When the hip is affected, the child typically holds that joint in a position of flexion, abduction, and external rotation as the intracapsular pressure increases. Swelling of the anterior aspect of the thigh is a late sign.[48,54,55] Neonates may display only anorexia, irritability, and lethargy and may not move the affected limb (pseudoparalysis).[27,52]

Laboratory tests include peripheral blood studies, which typically demonstrate a white blood cell count of greater than 12,000/mm³ (> 12.0 × 10⁹/L), with 40% to 60% polymorphonuclear leukocytes, and an erythrocyte sedimentation rate of greater than 50 mm/h. Blood cultures are positive in 30% to 50% of patients. The C-reactive protein level is a very good indicator of disease progression, although it is nonspecific. It is elevated in more than 90% of children with musculoskeletal infection at the time of admission, it peaks 2 days after admission, and it quickly returns to normal after treatment. Measurement of the C-reactive protein level may also be helpful in the identification of septic arthritis in children with underlying acute hematogenous osteomyelitis.[56]

Joint aspiration is essential for the diagnosis and typically reveals a white blood cell count of greater than 50,000/mm³ (> 50.0 × 10⁹/L), with 75% polymorphonuclear leukocytes, but 34% of patients have white blood cell counts of less than 25,000/mm³ (< 25.0 × 10⁹/L). Gram stains of the aspirate are positive in 30% to 50% of patients, and cultures of the aspirate are positive in 50% to 80%. Synovial protein levels that are 40 mg/dL (400 mg/L) and are less than the serum protein levels are consistent with septic arthritis. Lactate levels are typically elevated in the joint fluid in patients with septic arthritis (except in those with gonococcal infection), and the glucose level in the aspirate is lower than the level in the serum. On direct examination, the aspirate may demonstrate gross pus, and the result of the mucin (string) test is poor when infection is present.

Transient synovitis is not uncommon in children, and the primary differential diagnosis is between it and septic arthritis in the hip. With both disorders, young children may present with substantial pain, which can cause crying and can limit motion of the hip dramatically. Also, with both disorders, the child may be carried in or may limp and tends to sit or lie with the lower limb held in flexion and in external rotation. The differential diagnosis between these two disorders is extremely important and can be difficult. Treatment varies dramatically, from open arthrotomy for septic arthritis to simple observation and nonsteroidal anti-inflammatory drugs for transient synovitis. To help examiners make this diagnosis more accurately, Kocher and associates[57] developed four clinical criteria to aid in the assessment of a child with a painful hip; these criteria include non-weight bearing, an erythrocyte sedimentation rate of at least 40 mm/h, fever, and a white blood cell count of greater than 12,000/mm^3 (> 12.0 × 10^9/L). In their study, when all four of the criteria were met, there was a 99% chance that the child had septic arthritis. There was a 93% chance of septic arthritis when three of the four criteria were met, a 40% chance when two criteria were met, and a 3% chance when only one criterion was met. When this paradigm was applied to different populations, the probability of septic arthritis dropped to about 90% when all four predictors were present and 70% when three of the four were present (MS Kochar, MD and associates, unpublished data presented at the Annual

Meeting of the Pediatric Orthopaedic Society of North America, 2003). Despite this decreased sensitivity, the clinical factors identified by these authors are excellent predictors to help guide the differential diagnosis and subsequent treatment.

Imaging may assist in the diagnosis. Plain radiography can reveal subtle signs early in the disease process (capsular distention and joint space widening) and metaphyseal lucency later in the course. Technetium bone scans may show decreased uptake (cold) early in the disease process and increased uptake (hot) later, as a result of a hyperemic response. Gallium and indium-labeled leukocyte scans may be helpful in the diagnosis of atypical cases, but, as mentioned in the previous section, they are difficult to obtain and take 48 to 72 hours to complete.[58]

Ultrasonography is quick and painless and imparts no ionizing radiation. It can detect an effusion in 100% of cases, with a criterion being a capsule-to-bone distance that is more than 2 mm wider than the distance on the contralateral side. This finding is not specific for septic arthritis, but the absence of an effusion makes septic arthritis unlikely. Ultrasonography is also a useful tool for guiding aspiration and confirming needle location.

Treatment

Septic arthritis is a true emergency, and treatment often involves the emergency department as well as the radiology and orthopaedic departments. It is therefore important to have an established algorithm for treatment. Any evaluation of a painful hip must rule out the possibility of septic arthritis, and if septic arthritis is suspected, it must be treated emergently. When concomitant osteomyelitis is suspected, aspiration of the proximal part of the femur should be considered at the time of hip joint aspiration.

The cornerstone of treatment is surgical drainage and irrigation of the hip joint with appropriate constitutional support, including hydration and antibiotics.

A capsular window should be removed to ensure continued drainage, and a drain should be left in place until the volume of the drainage decreases. Arthroscopic treatment of septic arthritis was reported to have an excellent result in 10 patients at 5-year follow-up.[59] If surgery is not followed by a rapid reversal of clinical symptoms and normalization of vital signs, reexploration should be considered.

The antibiotic regimen should be started immediately after aspiration. It should initially be based on the suspected organism and later tailored to the culture results. Intravenous antibiotic therapy should be continued until constitutional signs improve. Switching to oral antibiotics may be considered if no concurrent osteomyelitis is present. Recently, there has been a trend toward decreasing the period of parenteral antibiotic treatment.[60,61] When there is concurrent osteomyelitis, intravenous antibiotic therapy should be continued as described in the preceding section.

The causative organisms vary depending primarily on the age of the patient. Group B *Streptococcus* is most common in healthy neonates (< 28 days old), and *S aureus* is most common in high-risk neonates. Gram-negative bacilli must also be considered as possible infecting organisms. Recommended antibiotic treatment includes oxacillin or cefotaxime, with the addition of gentamicin for a high-risk neonate (Table 2).

S aureus is the most common organism in infants and children up to 3 years of age. Infection with *H influenzae* type B is occurring much less frequently, and it is virtually nonexistent in children immunized with the *H influenzae* type B vaccine.[62] However, 20% to 30% of children with a diagnosis of *H influenzae* type B septic arthritis have concomitant meningitis. *Kingella kingae* infection is being recognized more frequently, primarily in healthy children younger than 4 years, and it is often associated with an upper respiratory infection. To identify

Table 2
Antibiotic Dosages for Children With Musculoskeletal Infections*

Age	Antibiotic and Dosage
< 28 days	Oxacillin: 25 to 50 mg/kg/6 to 12 h Cefotaxime: 50 mg/kg/8 to 12 h Gentamicin: 2.5 mg/kg/8 to 24 h
28 days to 3 years	Cefotaxime: 100 to 200 mg/kg/day in 3 to 4 divided doses Ceftriaxone: 50 to 100 mg/kg/day in 1 to 2 divided doses Penicillin G: 100,000 to 400,000 units/kg/day in 4 to 6 divided doses intravenously
> 3 years	Oxacillin: 100 to 200 mg/kg/day in 4 to 6 divided doses

*These are only guidelines; an infectious disease specialist or pharmacist should be consulted for the appropriate antibiotic dose and frequency

Table 3
Sequelae of Septic Arthritis of the Hip

Partial or complete destruction of the proximal femoral physis

Osteonecrosis of the femoral head

Trochanteric overgrowth

Pseudarthrosis of the femoral neck

Complete dissolution of the femoral neck and head

Progressive limb-length discrepancy

Varus or valgus alignment of the femoral head

Unstable hip articulation

Hip dislocation

Ankylosis of the hip joint

this organism, the culture must be performed in a BACTEC bottle (Becton Dickinson Diagnostic Instrument Systems, Sparks, MD) and needs to be observed for 14 days. This culture technique is 87% sensitive for detecting *K kingae*. Recommended antibiotics for patients who are 28 days to 3 years of age include cefotaxime or ceftriaxone and penicillin for *K kingae* infection.[63,64]

S aureus infection is still common in older children and adolescents, but other organisms such as *Neisseria gonorrhoeae* and *Borrelia burgdorferi* (Lyme disease) must be considered. The recommended antibiotic for *S aureus* infection is oxacillin.

Gonococcal arthritis is usually found in sexually active teenagers or is transmitted to newborns from their mothers dur-

ing birth. It is associated with a rash, tenosynovitis, and migratory polyarthralgia. The knee is the most commonly affected joint. Children with gonococcal disease have often been sexually abused.[65]

The diagnosis of gonococcal arthritis is confirmed by culture, which needs to be performed under special conditions (warm, with a low CO_2 level, and in special culture media [sterile specimens on chocolate blood agar and nonsterile specimens on Thayer-Martin agar]). Treatment is initiated with antibiotics. There is a growing resistance to penicillin and, therefore, a third-generation cephalosporin should be used for the initial treatment. Open drainage is indicated for septic arthritis of the hip, whereas repeated aspirations have been successful for the treatment of other infected joints, such as the knee.

Lyme disease is caused by the spirochete *B burgdorferi*, which is carried by the deer tick. It is typically described as occurring in three stages: stage I is a localized infection (erythema migrans), stage II is early disseminated disease (myocarditis and/or Bell's palsy), and stage III is persistent infection (arthritis). However, the clinical manifestations can be variable, and only 40% of those presenting with Lyme disease have classic Lyme arthritis. Lyme arthritis often presents as an episodic synovitis affecting one to four joints, with asymptomatic intervals, and it is considered to be a great

mimicker in that the presentation can be similar to that of other forms of chronic or even acute arthritis.

The laboratory diagnosis of Lyme disease is made with the use of the enzyme-linked immunosorbent assay test, which is sensitive but not specific; therefore, when the test result is negative, no further diagnostic evaluation is needed. However, when it is positive, a Western blot test is needed to confirm the diagnosis. The results of other laboratory tests, such as the antinuclear antibody, may also be positive (in up to 30% of patients).

Treatment consists of appropriate antibiotics, which reportedly have been associated with few long-term problems in children.[66] Surgical intervention is rarely needed, although synovectomy has been performed for chronic arthritis of the knee.[67]

Several factors place a child with septic arthritis at risk for a poor result. These include prematurity, age younger than 6 months, a delay in treatment of more than 4 days, concurrent osteomyelitis of the femur, and septic dislocation of the hip joint.

Sequelae of septic arthritis of the hip are common, with poor results occurring in as many as 40% of children (Table 3) (Figure 5). Long-term follow-up is critical to identify these possible sequelae. When deciding on treatment options, the physician must consider not only the insult to the hip joint but future growth disturbances and the limb-length inequality or trochanteric overgrowth that may occur. Appropriately timed epiphysiodesis of the contralateral limb may be more appropriate than lengthening of the affected limb, especially with a dysplastic hip joint. Performance of ipsilateral epiphysiodesis of the greater trochanter, in an attempt to maintain the proximal femoral anatomy (the articular trochanteric distance) as close to normal as possible, should be considered.[68] For the more severely dysplastic hip, other treatment options, such as bone grafting for a pseudarthrosis of the femoral neck or a valgus osteotomy of the proximal part of the femur, may be indicated. Arthrodesis or hip joint arthroplasty may be indicated for a painful hip with severe osteoarthrosis.[69-71]

Infections of the Soft Tissues

Infections of the soft tissues are common in children and are usually easily treated, with few residual long-term problems. However, a few soft-tissue infections are not so easily managed, and prompt diagnosis and appropriate treatment are needed. Some of these infections are life-threatening, and many commonly occur in the upper extremity.

Cellulitis

Cellulitis is a common, diffuse inflammation with hyperemia, leukocyte inflammation, and edema but without abscess formation. It is most frequently caused by *Streptococcus* (group A β-hemolytic) and *S aureus*. Treatment includes a trial of oral antibiotics, but intravenous antibiotics may be necessary for resolution of more severe symptoms or for those resistant to oral antibiotics. If an abscess forms, prompt surgical drainage is also indicated.

One of the most common ways in which cellulitis develops is through a puncture wound of the foot, with such injuries responsible for 0.8% of visits to the emergency department by children. Although the most common manifestation of a puncture wound of the foot is cellulitis, usually caused by *S aureus*, a deep infection or another complication will develop in 5% to 10% of patients.[72,73] Puncture wounds may be associated with *Pseudomonas*, especially if the puncturing object passes through an athletic shoe. *Pseudomonas* is part of the normal skin flora and grows well in the moist environment of the shoe. It does not incite much of an inflammatory response, but it has a propensity to infect cartilage.[74]

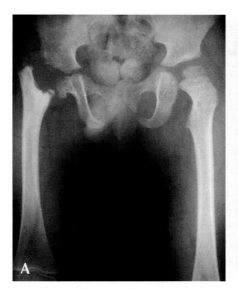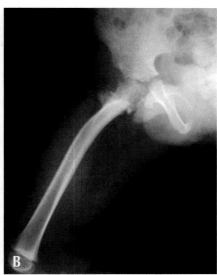

Figure 5 A and **B,** Hip radiographs of a patient after delayed treatment of septic arthritis demonstrate nearly complete destruction of the hip.

Treatment depends on whether the puncture wound is deep or superficial, whether a foreign body is present, whether there is evidence of articular or osseous injury, and the initial response to antibiotic treatment. When there is a superficial puncture wound, superficial débridement should be performed in the emergency department and evidence of a foreign body should be sought. Tetanus toxoid should be administered if indicated. A deep puncture wound should be managed with exploration and débridement in the emergency department, and the wound should be left open. When a foreign body is present, the bone or joint is penetrated, or there are signs of infection at 3 to 5 days after the injury, appropriate antibiotics should be used. If the patient does not respond to antibiotic treatment, formal surgical débridement followed by 3 weeks of culture-specific intravenous antibiotics should be considered, especially when there is a possibility of osteomyelitis.[73,75]

Necrotizing Fasciitis

Necrotizing fasciitis is a life and limb-threatening event. Although it is uncom-mon in children, familiarity with this disorder is crucial because of the deceivingly benign presentation of the infection and the devastating consequences of a missed or delayed diagnosis.[76] The orthopaedic surgeon is typically consulted when the disorder involves an extremity, which is a common location (especially the lower extremity, which is involved in 70% of cases). Necrotizing fasciitis can occur after major or minor trauma or postoperatively.

As the name indicates, necrotizing fasciitis is an infectious process that involves the deep dermis and underlying fascia. It is most frequently polymicrobial, with streptococcal species being the most commonly isolated organism.[77] Physical findings are often subtle initially, and the diagnosis is rarely made at the time of admission. Early in its course, necrotizing fasciitis may present as an area of unremarkable cellulitis that is usually surprisingly tender. It quickly progresses to a more painful and intense cellulitis that advances rapidly. Skin bullae and ecchymoses occur later, often well after the patient has become hemodynamically unstable. There often is a sub-

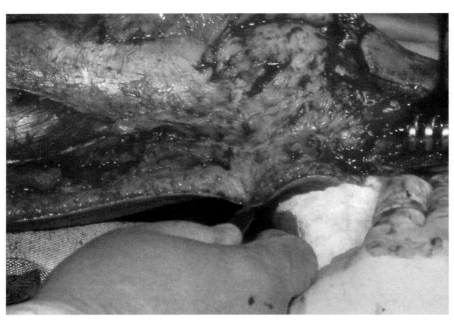

Figure 6 Photograph showing surgical dissection of necrotizing fasciitis.

tle etiology, such as a small laceration or relatively minor surgery. Early administration of intravenous antibiotics, often before the diagnosis, may mask the severity of the infection, increasing the delay in diagnosis and treatment.

Early diagnosis is critical and can be made definitively only with a biopsy, although ultrasound, CT, and MRI have been used to determine if there is inflammation of the fascial layer.[78,79] Use of these modalities should not delay surgical intervention.

Treatment includes emergent surgical débridement of all nonviable tissue, appropriate antibiotics, and supportive care. The skin and fascia are usually involved, but the muscle is spared. At the time of surgery, a grayish necrotic fascia that is less adherent and associated with minimal bleeding is noted, with a foul-smelling "dishwater" type of pus (Figure 6). Extensive débridement with removal of all necrotic fascia is needed. A second débridement 24 hours later may be necessary.

Antibiotics include penicillin, with the addition of an aminoglycoside for penicillinase-resistant *Staphylococcus*. Even

with this aggressive treatment, the mortality rate is as high as 18% for children and can be higher for adults.[76]

Disk Space Infection (Diskitis)

Disk space infections often occur in children. The infection does not propagate from the Batson plexus, as previously proposed, but from arterioles that terminate in the disk. In adults, the disk is avascular; arterioles terminate in the vertebral end plate and, therefore, a primary hematogenous disk infection is not likely.

Signs and symptoms vary and tend to change with age. Seventy-five percent of children limp or will not walk. They may demonstrate the quarter sign (inability to bend over to pick up a quarter) and irritability when the hip is held in extension (log roll test). Abdominal pain is not uncommon, especially in children between the ages of 3 and 9 years (Table 4). Spine tenderness is common in older children.[80] Pain frequently occurs at night, and children are usually not systemically ill.[81]

Laboratory evaluation includes measurement of the erythrocyte sedimenta-

tion rate, which is elevated in 80% to 90% of children. The white blood cell count may be elevated but frequently is normal in children. Blood and stool cultures should be performed if salmonella is suspected.

Imaging studies include radiographs, bone scans, and MRI. Radiographs show disk space narrowing with irregularity of vertebral end plates but preservation of the vertebral body. Destruction of the vertebra may indicate osteomyelitis. These changes may not be seen for 3 weeks. Bone scans are helpful but not specific, and false-negative findings have been reported; therefore, the diagnosis should not be excluded on the basis of a negative bone scan.[82] MRI is becoming the diagnostic modality of choice and may be the most sensitive imaging study.[83]

S aureus is the most frequent infecting organism. Usually neither aspiration nor biopsy is needed, but if one of those procedures is used it is diagnostic in approximately 50% of children. A biopsy should be considered for atypical cases, when there is no response to treatment, or when the diskitis occurs in an adolescent who is suspected of abusing drugs.[81]

Treatment consists of antistaphylococcal intravenous antibiotics, and rapid improvement is usually seen in 3 to 5 days. If there is a good response, intravenous antibiotic therapy is continued for 3 to 4 weeks and then followed by oral antibiotics for another 2 to 3 weeks. The use of a prefabricated orthosis can also be considered. When there is no early response, aspiration or biopsy should be performed, followed by culture-specific antibiotic treatment.

Soft-Tissue Infections Unique to the Hand

A felon is an infection that occurs in the digital pad of the fingertip.[84] The pulp region is a closed compartment that is segregated into even smaller areas by multiple fibrous septa that attach the der-

Table 4
Symptoms of Diskitis

Age (years)	Common Sign
< 3	Positive log roll test, limp
3 to 9	Abdominal pain
> 9	Back pain

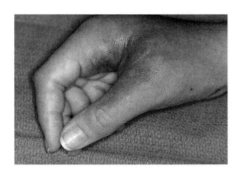

Figure 7 Photograph showing the flexed resting position of the index finger, which is one of the signs of flexor tenosynovitis identified by Kanavel.[87]

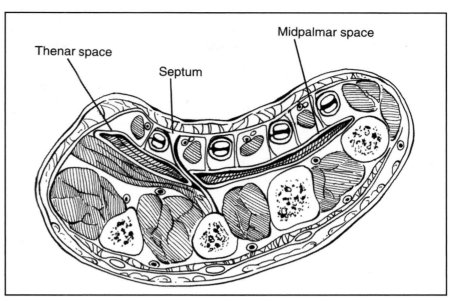

Figure 8 Illustration of a transverse section of the hand demonstrating the septum from the palmar fascia to the third metacarpal, which divides the hand into thenar and midpalmar spaces. (Reproduced with permission from Seiler JG III (ed): American Society for Surgery of the Hand: *Essentials of Hand Surgery*. Philadelphia, PA, Lippincott Williams and Wilkins, 2003, p 9.)

mis to the distal phalanx. Each section contains fat globules, sweat glands, and/or terminal branches of the digital arteries that supply the distal phalanx. Obvious or inconspicuous trauma can penetrate the closed pulp space, deposit bacteria, and lead to abscess formation. Even an innocuous finger stick in the pediatric intensive care unit can lead to formation of a felon. The pus within the fingertip space creates pressure and impairs tissue perfusion. Failure to decompress the abscess can result in contiguous spread to the distal phalanx (osteomyelitis), distal interphalangeal joint (septic arthritis), or flexor tendon sheath (flexor tenosynovitis). A neglected felon may eventually lead to extrusion or osteonecrosis of the distal phalanx. Intense, throbbing pain and extreme tenderness are characteristic findings of a felon. The most common infecting organism is *S aureus*. Treatment consists of surgical drainage and antibiotics. A high lateral incision on the less used side

of the digit (the radial side of the thumb and small finger and the ulnar side of the index, long, and ring fingers) is preferred.[85] A fish mouth type incision should be avoided because it may lead to vascular compromise of the digital pad. The neurovascular bundles must be avoided during surgical drainage.

Flexor tenosynovitis is a bacterial infection of the flexor tendon sheath. The four classic signs have been identified by Kanavel[86] as (1) a flexed resting posture, (2) tenderness over the flexor sheath, (3) fusiform swelling, and (4) pain on passive extension[86,87] (Figure 7). Early infection can be treated with a trial of intravenous antibiotics for 24 hours followed by reassessment. A failure to improve warrants urgent incision and drainage. A delayed diagnosis or an established infection warrants immediate incision and drainage as well.

Deep space infections of the hand are usually the result of penetrating trauma or contiguous spread from neglected

flexor tenosynovitis. The deep spaces are located dorsal to the flexor tendons and palmar to the metacarpals.[86] A septum from the third metacarpal to the palmar skin separates the hand into a thenar and a midpalmar space (Figure 8). The causative organism is usually *S aureus* or *Streptococcus*. Treatment consists of incision and drainage.

Viral hand infections usually are caused by the herpes simplex virus. Herpes infection of the nail bed and/or pulp is termed herpetic whitlow.[87] Herpetic whitlow is one of the more common infections of toddlers' hands. These infections are associated with oral lesions, and sucking of the digits (autoinoculation) is the mode of transmission to the hand in up to 80% of patients.[88] Children typically present with pain, tingling, and vesicular eruptions over an erythematous base. However, young children cannot relate a tingling sensation. Involvement of multiple digits is more common in children than it is in

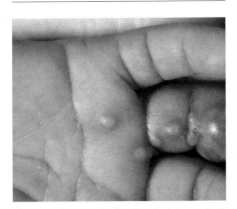

Figure 9 Photograph showing vesicles typical of herpetic infection.

adults. Constitutional symptoms (such as fever, chills, and malaise) are usually absent.[87] The diagnosis is made on the basis of clinical examination, a Tzanck smear, and cultures (with a 1- to 5-day incubation period). Clear vesicles that may become turbid after a few days characterize early herpetic infection (Figure 9). The vesicles gradually undergo crusting over the next few weeks, and complete resolution occurs within 2 to 3 weeks. In children, concomitant bacterial infection by S aureus or Streptococcus can cause blistering dactylitis, which confuses the diagnosis. The Tzanck smear requires unroofing of a vesicle and staining the fluid in search of multinucleated giant cells. The smear identifies multinucleated giant cells only 70% of the time, and viral culture may be required for a definitive diagnosis. Successful treatment depends on a high index of suspicion. Herpetic whitlow is a self-limited process, and surgical treatment is not necessary. Antibiotic therapy is indicated only for bacterial superinfection.[88] The virus avoids immune clearance by harboring in a latent stage within the ganglia of nerves. This shields the virus and allows recurrences. Administration of acyclovir may decrease the duration of the lesions and prevent recurrences.

Human and animal bites in children can lead to serious infection, morbidity,

and even mortality. Misdiagnosis and undertreatment of human bites is still a prevailing problem. Infection can occur after nail biting (usually a paronychia), sucking a bleeding wound, sucking by a toddler, violent tooth injury (clenched-fist injury), or bites during a fight. A clenched-fist injury is often overlooked as a minor accident, only to later result in a major infection. Considerable injury and bacterial inoculation can occur through a small puncture wound. The tooth can easily penetrate the extensor tendon, dorsal joint capsule, and metacarpal head. This passage carries bacteria into the joint and/or metacarpal head. The human mouth is a rich culture medium replete with organisms. One milliliter of saliva may contain up to 100 million organisms and 42 different strains of bacteria.[89] The common isolates are S aureus, Streptococcus, Eikenella corrodens (in one third of patients), and Bacteroides (the most common anaerobe).[90] Treatment begins with immediate recognition of the injury by taking a careful history and performing a physical examination. Early treatment is far superior to late management with regard to outcome, complications, and sequelae. A puncture wound over the metacarpal head should be considered a clenched-fist injury until proven otherwise.[90] The mainstay of treatment is thorough surgical exploration combined with irrigation and débridement. The wound is left open and then reassessed 24 hours after surgery. Antibiotics covering S aureus, Streptococcus, and E corrodens are prescribed. Prophylaxis against tetanus is also part of the treatment regimen.

Dogs cause most animal bites to the hand (9 out of 10). Over 1 million dog bite injuries are treated in the United States each year. More than 50% of the dog bites are inflicted on children younger than 12 years, and about one half of those wounds are of the hand and/or forearm.[91] Even more frightening, approximately a dozen people die each

year from dog bites in the United States, and one third of them are infants younger than 12 months.[91] Similar to the human mouth, the canine oral cavity is full of organisms, including S aureus, viridans streptococci, Pasteurella multocida, and Bacteroides. Treatment principles are similar to those for human bites and include urgent recognition and immediate débridement of all nonviable tissue. Antibiotic coverage must include P multocida. The possibility of rabies is also a consideration, although rabies is rare after dog bites and surveillance of the dog for 10 days is the simplest monitoring method. In contrast, wild animal bites require prophylactic treatment of rabies, as skunks and raccoons are responsible for most cases of rabies.

Cat bites are less common than dog bites, although they commonly result in a deep infection (50% of the time). Cats have needle-sharp canine teeth that drive bacteria deep into tissue. A cat bite over the volar aspect of the finger frequently penetrates the flexor tendon sheath and causes flexor tenosynovitis. Typical causative organisms include P multocida, S aureus, and viridans streptococci. Deep infections can occur secondary to inoculation into the flexor tendon sheath or deep spaces of the hand. Treatment consists of débridement, copious irrigation, and antibiotic coverage. Bites by other domestic animals, such as pet rabbits, hamsters, and guinea pigs, are treated in the same manner as cat bites.

Summary
Musculoskeletal infections in children are common. The etiology can be diverse and the presentation is often variable, making diagnosis difficult. The effects of infection in children may last well beyond the acute episode, and long-term follow-up is needed to assess for late sequelae such as angular deformities and limb-length inequality. Principles of treatment of musculoskeletal infections in children involve prevention, accurate

diagnosis, and prompt intervention (including antibiotic therapy and surgical débridement). Close follow-up is mandatory to ensure a good long-term outcome.

References

1. Nelson JD: Skeletal infections in children. *Adv Pediatr Infect Dis* 1991;6:59-78.

2. Manthous CA: The pathophysiology and management of sepsis. *Res Staff Phys* 2001;47:34-46.

3. Gilmour WN: Acute haematogenous osteomyelitis. *J Bone Joint Surg Br* 1962;44:841-853.

4. Dich VQ, Nelson JD, Haltalin KC: Osteomyelitis in infants and children: A review of 163 cases. *Am J Dis Child* 1975;129:1273-1278.

5. Everett ED, Hirschmann JV: Transient bacteremia and endocarditis prophylaxis: A review. *Medicine (Baltimore)* 1977;56:61-77.

6. Morrissy RT, Haynes DW: Acute hematogenous osteomyelitis: A model with trauma as an etiology. *J Pediatr Orthop* 1989;9:447-456.

7. Whalen JL, Fitzgerald RH Jr, Morrissy RT: A histological study of acute hematogenous osteomyelitis: Following physeal injuries in rabbits. *J Bone Joint Surg Am* 1988;70:1383-1392.

8. Modic MT, Pflanze W, Feiglin DH, Belhobek G: Magnetic resonance imaging of musculoskeletal infections. *Radiol Clin North Am* 1986;24:247-258.

9. Tang JS, Gold RH, Bassett LW, Seeger LL: Musculoskeletal infection of the extremities: Evaluation with MR imaging. *Radiology* 1988;166:205-209.

10. Unger E, Moldofsky P, Gatenby R, Hartz W, Broder G: Diagnosis of osteomyelitis by MR imaging. *AJR Am J Roentgenol* 1988;150:605-610.

11. Merkel KD, Fitzgerald RH Jr, Brown ML: Scintigraphic evaluation in musculoskeletal sepsis. *Orthop Clin North Am* 1984;15:401-416.

12. Ash JM, Gilday DL: The futility of bone scanning in neonatal osteomyelitis: Concise communication. *J Nucl Med* 1980;21:417-420.

13. Herndon WA, Alexieva BT, Schwindt ML, Scott KN, Shaffer WO: Nuclear imaging for musculoskeletal infections in children. *J Pediatr Orthop* 1985;5:343-347.

14. Bressler EL, Conway JJ, Weiss SC: Neonatal osteomyelitis examined by bone scintigraphy. *Radiology* 1984;152:685-688.

15. Canale ST, Harkness RM, Thomas PA, Massie JD: Does aspiration of bones and joints affect results of later bone scanning? *J Pediatr Orthop* 1985;5:23-26.

16. Howie DW, Savage JP, Wilson TG, Paterson D: The technetium phosphate bone scan in the diagnosis of osteomyelitis in childhood. *J Bone Joint Surg Am* 1983;65:431-437.

17. Deysine M, Rafkin H, Russell R, Teicher I, Aufses AH Jr: The detection of acute experimental osteomyelitis with 67Ga citrate scannings. *Surg Gynecol Obstet* 1975;141:40-42.

18. Ganel A, Horoszowski H, Zaltzman S, Farine I: Sequential use of 99mTc-MDP and 67GA imaging in bone infection. *Orthop Rev* 1981;10:73-77.

19. Merkel KD, Brown ML, Dewanjee MK, Fitzgerald RH Jr: Comparison of indium-labeled-leukocyte imaging with sequential technetium-gallium scanning in the diagnosis of low-grade musculoskeletal sepsis: A prospective study. *J Bone Joint Surg Am* 1985;67:465-476.

20. Kuhn JP, Berger PE: Computed tomographic diagnosis of osteomyelitis. *Radiology* 1979;130:503-506.

21. Hald JK, Sudmann E: Acute hematogenous osteomyelitis: Early diagnosis with computed tomography. *Acta Radiol Diagn (Stockh)* 1982;23:55-58.

22. Mollan RA, Piggot J: Acute osteomyelitis in children. *J Bone Joint Surg Br* 1977;59:2-7.

23. Winters JL, Cahen I: Acute hematogenous osteomyelitis: A review of sixty-six cases. *Am J Orthop* 1960;42:691-704.

24. Edwards MS, Baker CJ, Wagner ML, Taber LH, Barrett FF: An etiologic shift in infantile osteomyelitis: The emergence of the group B streptococcus. *J Pediatr* 1978;93:578-583.

25. Freedman RM, Ingram DL, Gross I, Ehrenkranz RA, Warshaw JB, Baltimore RS: A half century of neonatal sepsis at Yale: 1928 to 1978. *Am J Dis Child* 1981;135:140-144.

26. Fox L, Sprunt K: Neonatal osteomyelitis. *Pediatrics* 1978;62:535-542.

27. Ogden JA, Lister G: The pathology of neonatal osteomyelitis. *Pediatrics* 1975;55:474-478.

28. Green WT, Shannon JG: Osteomyelitis of infants: A disease different from osteomyelitis of older children. *Arch Surg* 1936;32:462-493.

29. Lim MO, Gresham EL, Franken EA Jr, Leake RD: Osteomyelitis as a complication of umbilical artery catheterization. *Am J Dis Child* 1977;131:142-144.

30. Mok PJ, Reilly BJ, Ash JM: Osteomyelitis in the neonate: Clinical aspects and the role of radiography and scintigraphy in diagnosis and management. *Radiology* 1982;145:677-682.

31. Overturf GD, Balfour G: Osteomyelitis and sepsis: Severe complications of fetal monitoring. *Pediatrics* 1975;55:244-247.

32. Lilien LD, Harris VJ, Ramamurthy RS, Pildes RS: Neonatal osteomyelitis of the calcaneus: Complication of heel puncture. *J Pediatr* 1976;88:478-480.

33. Kandel SN, Mankin HJ: Pyogenic abscess of the long bones in children. *Clin Orthop* 1973;96:108-117.

34. King DM, Mayo KM: Subacute haematogenous osteomyelitis. *J Bone Joint Surg Br* 1969;51:458-463.

35. Beretta-Piccoli BC, Sauvain MJ, Gal I, et al: Synovitis, acne, pustulosis, hyperostosis, osteitis (SAPHO) syndrome in childhood: A report of ten cases and review of the literature. *Eur J Pediatr* 2000;159:594-601.

36. Duffy CM, Lam PY, Ditchfield M, Allen R, Graham HK: Chronic recurrent multifocal osteomyelitis: Review of orthopaedic complications at maturity. *J Pediatr Orthop* 2002;22:501-505.

37. Huber AM, Lam PY, Duffy CM, et al: Chronic recurrent multifocal osteomyelitis: Clinical outcomes after more than five years of follow-up. *J Pediatr* 2002;141:198-203.

38. Kramer SJ, Post J, Sussman M: Acute hematogenous osteomyelitis of the epiphysis. *J Pediatr Orthop* 1986;6:493-495.

39. Tong CW, Griffith JF, Lam TP, Cheng JC: The conservative management of acute pyogenic iliopsoas abscess in children. *J Bone Joint Surg Br* 1998;80:83-85.

40. Hendrix RW, Lin PJ, Kane WJ: Simplified aspiration or injection technique for the sacro-iliac joint. *J Bone Joint Surg Am* 1982;64:1249-1252.

41. Reilly JP, Gross RH, Emans JB, Yngve DA: Disorders of the sacro-iliac joint in children. *J Bone Joint Surg Am* 1988;70:31-40.

42. Antoniou D, Conner AN: Osteomyelitis of the calcaneus and talus. *J Bone Joint Surg Am* 1974;56:338-345.

43. Feigin RD, McAlister WH, Joaquin VH, Middelkamp JN: Osteomyelitis of the calcaneus: Report of eight cases. *Am J Dis Child* 1970;119:61-65.

44. Skevis XA: Primary subacute osteomyelitis of the talus. *J Bone Joint Surg Br* 1984;66:101-103.

45. Robb JE: Primary acute haematogenous osteomyelitis of an isolated metatarsal in children. *Acta Orthop Scand* 1984;55:334-338.

46. Cabanela ME, Sim FH, Beabout JW, Dahlin DC: Osteomyelitis appearing as neoplasms: A diagnostic problem. *Arch Surg* 1974;109:68-72.

47. Lindenbaum S, Alexander H: Infections simulating bone tumors: A review of subacute osteomyelitis. *Clin Orthop* 1984;184:193-203.

48. Gillespie R: Septic arthritis of childhood. *Clin Orthop* 1973;96:152-159.

49. Dingle JT: The role of lysosomal enzymes in skeletal tissues. *J Bone Joint Surg Br* 1973;55:87-95.

50. Mitchell GP: Management of acquired dislocation of the hip in septic arthritis. *Orthop Clin North Am* 1980;11:51-64.

51. Morrey BF, Bianco AJ, Rhodes KH: Suppurative arthritis of the hip in children. *J Bone Joint Surg Am* 1976;58:388-392.

52. Obletz BE: Acute suppurative arthritis of the hip in the neonatal period. *Am J Orthop* 1960;42:23-30.

53. Paterson D: Septic arthritis of the hip joint. *Orthop Clin North Am* 1978;9:135-142.

54. Griffin PP, Green WT Sr: Hip joint infections in infants and children. *Orthop Clin North Am* 1978;9:123-134.

55. Morrissy RT: Bone and joint sepsis, in Morrissy RT, Weinstein SL (eds): *Lovell and Winter's Pediatric Orthopaedics*, ed 5. Philadelphia,

PA, Lippincott Williams & Wilkins, 2001, pp 459-505.

56. Unkila-Kallio L, Kallio MJ, Peltola H: The usefulness of C-reactive protein levels in the identification of concurrent septic arthritis in children who have acute hematogenous osteomyelitis: A comparison with the usefulness of the erythrocyte sedimentation rate and the white blood-cell count. *J Bone Joint Surg Am* 1994;76:848-853.

57. Kocher MS, Zurakowski D, Kasser JR: Differentiating between septic arthritis and transient synovitis of the hip in children: An evidence-based clinical prediction algorithm. *J Bone Joint Surg Am* 1999;81:1662-1670.

58. Jaramillo D, Treves ST, Kasser JR, Harper M, Sundel R, Laor T: Osteomyelitis and septic arthritis in children: Appropriate use of imaging to guide treatment. *AJR Am J Roentgenol* 1995;165:399-403.

59. Kim SJ, Choi NH, Ko SH, Linton JA, Park HW: Arthroscopic treatment of septic arthritis of the hip. *Clin Orthop* 2003;407:211-214.

60. Maraqa NF, Gomez MM, Rathore MH: Outpatient parenteral antimicrobial therapy in osteoarticular infections in children. *J Pediatr Orthop* 2002;22:506-510.

61. Kim HK, Alman B, Cole WG: A shortened course of parenteral antibiotic therapy in the management of acute septic arthritis of the hip. *J Pediatr Orthop* 2000;20:44-47.

62. Howard AW, Viskontas D, Sabbagh C: Reduction in osteomyelitis and septic arthritis related to Haemophilus influenzae type B vaccination. *J Pediatr Orthop* 1999;19:705-709.

63. Lundy DW, Kehl DK: Increasing prevalence of Kingella kingae in osteoarticular infections in young children. *J Pediatr Orthop* 1998;18:262-267.

64. Birgisson H, Steingrimsson O, Gudnason T: Kingella kingae infections in paediatric patients: 5 cases of septic arthritis, osteomyelitis and bacteraemia. *Scand J Infect Dis* 1997;29:495-498.

65. Folland DS, Burke RE, Hinman AR, Schaffner W: Gonorrhea in preadolescent children: An inquiry into source of infection and mode of transmission. *Pediatrics* 1977;60:153-156.

66. Rose CD, Fawcett PT, Eppes SC, Klein JD, Gibney K, Doughty RA: Pediatric Lyme arthri-

tis: Clinical spectrum and outcome. *J Pediatr Orthop* 1994;14:238-241.

67. McLaughlin TP, Zemel L, Fisher RL, Gossling HR: Chronic arthritis of the knee in Lyme disease: Review of the literature and report of two cases treated by synovectomy. *J Bone Joint Surg Am* 1986;68:1057-1061.

68. Weissman SL: Transplantation of the trochanteric epiphysis into the acetabulum after septic arthritis of the hip: Report of a case. *J Bone Joint Surg Am* 1967;49:1647-1651.

69. Choi IH, Pizzutillo PD, Bowen JR, Dragann R, Malhis T: Sequelae and reconstruction after septic arthritis of the hip in infants. *J Bone Joint Surg Am* 1990;72:1150-1165.

70. Harmon PH: Surgical treatment of the residual deformity from suppurative arthritis of the hip occurring in young children. *J Bone Joint Surg Am* 1942;24:576-585.

71. Campagnaro JG, Donzelli O, Urso R, Valdiserri L: Treatment of the sequelae of septic osteoarthritis of the hip during pediatric age. *Chir Organi Mov* 1992;77:223-245.

72. Weber EJ: Plantar puncture wounds: a survey to determine the incidence of infection. *J Accid Emerg Med* 1996;13:274-277.

73. Schwab RA, Powers RD: Conservative therapy of plantar puncture wounds. *J Emerg Med* 1995;13:291-295.

74. Green NE, Bruno J III: Pseudomonas infections of the foot after puncture wounds. *South Med J* 1980;73:146-149.

75. Fitzgerald RH Jr, Cowan JD: Puncture wounds of the foot. *Orthop Clin North Am* 1975;6:965-972.

76. Fustes-Morales A, Gutierrez-Castrellon P: Duran-Mckinster C, Orozco-Covarrubias L, Tamayo-Sanchez L, Ruiz-Maldonado R: Necrotizing fasciitis: A report of 39 pediatric cases. *Arch Dermatol* 2002;138:893-899.

77. Childers BJ, Potyondy LD, Nachreiner R, et al: Necrotizing fasciitis: A fourteen-year retrospective study of 163 consecutive patients. *Am Surg* 2002;68:109-116.

78. Yen ZS, Wang HP, Ma HM, Chen SC, Chen WJ: Ultrasonographic screening of clinically-suspected necrotizing fasciitis. *Acad Emerg Med* 2002;9:1448-1451.

79. Stamenkovic I, Lew PD: Early recognition of potentially fatal necrotizing faciitis: The use of frozen-section biopsy. *N Engl J Med* 1984;310:1689-1693.

80. Ring D, Johnston CE II, Wenger DR: Pyogenic infectious spondylitis in children: The convergence of discitis and vertebral osteomyelitis. *J Pediatr Orthop* 1995;15:652-660.

81. Scoles PV, Quinn TP: Intervertebral discitis in children and adolescents. *Clin Orthop* 1982;162:31-36.

82. Nolla-Sole JM, Mateo-Soria L, Rozadilla-Sacarell A, Mora-Salvador J, Valverde-Garcia J, Roig-Escofet D: Role of technetium-99m diphosphonate and gallium-67 citrate bone scanning in the early diagnosis of infectious spondylodiscitis: A comparative study. *Ann Rheum Dis* 1992;51:665-667.

83. Song KS, Ogden JA, Ganey T, Guidera KJ: Contiguous discitis and osteomyelitis in children. *J Pediatr Orthop* 1997;17:470-477.

84. Jebson PJ: Infections of the fingertip: Paronychias and felons. *Hand Clin* 1998;14:547-555.

85. Abrams RA, Botte MJ: Hand infections: Treatment recommendations for specific types. *J Am Acad Orthop Surg* 1996;4:219-230.

86. Kanavel AB: *Infections of the Hand: A Guide to the Surgical Treatment of Acute and Chronic Suppurative Processes in the Fingers, Hand, and Forearm*, ed 7. Philadelphia, PA, Lea and Febiger, 1939.

87. Behr JT, Daluga DJ, Light TR, Lewis NS: Herpetic infections in the fingers of infants: Report of five cases. *J Bone Joint Surg Am* 1987;69:137-139.

88. Walker LG, Simmons BP, Lovallo JL: Pediatric herpetic hand infections. *J Hand Surg [Am]* 1990;15:176-180.

89. Faciszewski T, Coleman DA: Human bite wounds. *Hand Clin* 1989;5:561-569.

90. Rayan GM, Putnam JL, Cahill SL, Flournoy DJ: Eikenella corrodens in human mouth flora. *J Hand Surg [Am]* 1988;13:953-956.

91. Snyder CC: Animal bite infections of the hand. *Hand Clin* 1998;14:691-711.

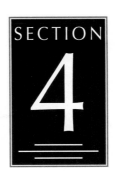

SECTION 4

Spinal Deformities in Children

Spinal Deformities in Children

The etiology, diagnosis, and treatment of spinal deformities in children has been extensively researched in the last 10 years. A lot of time and energy have been spent identifying the etiology of adolescent idiopathic scoliosis (AIS), and exciting research and early results into the genetic basis for this condition are ongoing. A better understanding of what constitutes AIS, how it is classified, and what advances have been made in treatment has distinct advantages compared with more traditional techniques and improved radiographic outcomes for these patients. Kyphosis, which is the primary sagittal plane deformity seen in children, often is challenging to treat because of the varied indications and options for treatment; there also is a significant neurologic risk associated with surgical treatment. Spondylolisthesis is one of the most controversial conditions treated in the pediatric population, with a variety of available surgical approaches and techniques. The main challenges in the treatment of high-grade spondylolisthesis are achieving fusion and correcting kyphosis without creating neurologic injury.

The articles in this section address each of these key topics. The expert authors provide excellent reviews of each topic, supplying state-of-the-art knowledge about the etiology, diagnosis, and treatment options. Each author succinctly summarizes information from the literature and provides specific personal insights on the subject. Specific surgical treatments are outlined for AIS, including video-assisted thoracoscopic surgery, kyphosis, and spondylolisthesis. The authors' vast experience managing these conditions provides key points to successful treatment. The articles in this collection are useful for residents, fellows, and attending surgeons alike to better understand, diagnose, and treat these conditions effectively.

The first article by Parent and associates reviews the etiology, anatomy, natural history, and bracing of AIS. The discussion on etiology covers genetic, hormonal, tissue abnormalities, neuromuscular, and spinal growth and biomechanical theories. Significant research on the genetic basis for AIS recently has been conducted using techniques such as genomic screening and statistical linkage analysis. The early results have identified multiple genes on a variety of chromosomes, and continued research into further gene identification is ongoing.

The authors expertly review the spinal anatomy and nicely outline the three-dimensional deformity characteristic of AIS. They focus on the subtle sagittal plane parameters that define AIS; understanding these parameter is important for us as we evaluate these patients. The pedicle anatomy and some of authors' work in this area also are reviewed, given the recent popularity of thoracic pedicle screws. Issues surrounding spinal growth and the risk factors for progression are outlined, which provides the reader with an excellent guide to treatment based on curve progression risk. Finally, current strategies for orthotic management and its results are summarized. This article is outstanding because it addresses a wide variety of important topics on AIS and supplies us with current literature-based knowledge and the authors' personal insights about AIS, the combination of which provides an excellent foundation to best understand this condition.

In the second article, Lawrence Lenke describes his surgical classification for AIS, developed as an improvement on the classic King-Moe system that was published in 1983. The Lenke classification provides a two-dimensional analysis of spinal deformity based on posteroanterior and lateral radiographs and defines three parameters with which to evaluate the deformity. The goal of his system is to provide a treatment-based classification to best define curves that require surgical treatment. The classification system is composed of three components: (1) curve type; (2) a thoracic modifier that defines the amount of thoracic kyphosis; and (3) a lumbar modifier based on the position of the lumbar apical vertebra relative to the center sacral vertical line. The article includes an excellent illustration of this comprehensive classification system, which makes it easy to understand. Dr. Lenke then specifically describes each curve type and defines the best surgical treatment for each type. General information regarding appropriate fusion levels is provided as well. He also points out that this classification system should be used in conjunction with results of the physical examination for optimal treatment.

In the next article, the use of video-assisted thoracoscopic surgery in the treatment of AIS is expertly discussed by Peter Newton, one of the pioneers of this technique. He provides a comprehensive literature review and also describes his experience using this technique in the treatment of spinal deformity. Indications and contraindications are thoroughly discussed. Importantly, the specifics of the surgical technique are outlined, with specific pearls provided by Dr. Newton from both his experience and that of others.

Two techniques are described in this article: anterior thoracoscopic release for severe deformity and/or prevention of the crankshaft phenomenon and thoracoscopic instrumentation and fusion. Useful illustrations of the diskectomy and instrumentation are provided. Preoperative and postoperative radiographs of a patient with AIS who undergoes thoracoscopic instrumentation show excellent curve correction.

In the last section of the article, outcomes of thoracoscopic surgery are discussed, which puts the technical challenge of thoracoscopy into perspective and provides a succinct list of the advantages and disadvantages of the technique.

The next three articles describe kyphosis and its treatment. In the first article, Peter Pizzutillo reviews kyphosis, defining the distinction between postural and Scheuermann's kyphosis. He supplies a very detailed review of the diagnosis and nicely summarizes the indications for nonsurgical treatment, including the use of orthoses and cast treatment. In this age of increased use of surgical treatment for most conditions, including kyphosis, the perspective that non-surgical treatment is a viable option is invaluable for orthopaedic surgeons treating patients with Scheuermann's kyphosis.

Thomas Lowe reviews the surgical treatment of thoracic and thoracolumbar kyphosis, distinguishing between large radius (principally Scheuermann's kyphosis) and short radius kyphosis. The indications for surgery as well as the various types of surgical treatment are clearly described. Dr. Lowe is an expert on kyphosis with many publications; he draws from his own research to describe the indications for anterior fusion. His pearls regarding fusion levels and anchor points are to be carefully read as they demonstrate his significant knowledge in this area. His discussion on the complex subject of short radius kyphosis clearly describes both the conditions treated and the variety of techniques that can be used. Dr. Lowe also describes congenital kyphosis and cautions the treating surgeon to be mindful of the neurologic danger associated with this condition. A number of illustrative cases that describe successful surgical treatment are included as well.

The final article concerning kyphosis is written by Lawrence Lenke, who describes the prevention and treatment of surgical complications associated with this condition. He provides a logical strategy to identify the cause of failure of the initial treatment. He then defines each of these causes specifically and describes ways in which to avoid and treat them.

The most feared complication is neurologic injury, an issue that each surgeon is concerned about during treatment of kyphosis. The increased rate of associated neurologic injury can be attributed to two factors: (1) tension applied to the anterior portion of the spinal cord and (2) limited anterior spinal cord blood supply. Thus, the spinal cord must be assessed intraoperatively with spinal cord monitoring to help prevent these complications or to identify when they may be occurring.

The article concludes with an algorithm that details how to treat these complex conditions, with Dr. Lenke drawing on his vast experience in the treatment of spinal deformities. The use of a variety of osteotomies is nicely outlined, specifically the Smith-Peterson osteotomy, the pedicle subtraction osteotomy, and an anterior-posterior osteotomy. Add-itional modalities such as intraoperative halo traction also are described. A case example shows the power of the combined use of segmental instrumentation and multiple oste-otomies to restore sagittal plane balance.

The final article addresses what may be one of the most controversial subjects in spinal deformity—high-grade spondylolisthesis. Lenke and Bridwell review the radiographic evaluation of this condition, concentrating on the kyphosis angle, which is most important to address when treating these patients. The clinical evaluation is reviewed, with special emphasis placed on the preoperative neurologic examination.

A variety of treatment options are available but are associated with high complication rates, specifically pseudarthrosis and neurologic injury. Treatment options and the authors' preferred technique are also described. Treatment options include in situ fusion, posterior instrumentation and fusion, circumferential fusion with reduction and L5 vertebrectomy for spondyloptosis. The authors prefer circumferential fusion with reduction of the kyphosis. Their instrumentation construct includes distal fixation with sacral screws supplemented with iliac screws. They strongly suggest decompression of the L5 nerve root past the transverse processes and careful monitoring of the L5 nerve root, which they state is best performed with direct nerve root stimulation.

This article is an outstanding discussion of a very controversial subject, and the authors provide excellent insight that should be carefully considered when these patients are treated.

This collection of articles provides outstanding information for all orthopaedic surgeons who treat these challenging conditions. Study of the etiology of AIS continues and is always changing as groups throughout the United States and the world are investigating the genetic basis of this multifactorial condition. Nonsurgical treatment of AIS continues as well, very similar to what the authors describe, and newer techniques of "internal bracing" are being investigated. Thoracoscopic instrumentation and fusion has declined over the last few years, most likely due to the long surgical time and the increased use of thoracic pedicle screw fixation, which has become widespread throughout the spine community with overall excellent correction.

The treatment of kyphosis has become safer as we better understand spinal cord monitoring and with increased use of posterior-only instrumentation with closing wedge-type osteotomies. As the number of revision surgeries continues to increase, the use of segmental fixation and complex osteotomies will improve results. High-grade spondylolisthesis continues to be a challenging problem because many surgical techniques are available, and the number of cases is somewhat limited compared with more common AIS-type surgeries.

The articles in this section are written by some of the world's experts in spinal deformity. They provide an outstanding reference for evaluating and treating patients with AIS, kyphosis, and spondylolisthesis. The same authors continue to research the topics they have discussed, and the future of diagnosis and treatment of spinal deformity is bright. Future directions include improved early diagnosis with prevention of progressive deformity, greater tools to predict deformity progression, nonfusion techniques to correct deformity without immobilizing or fusing the spine, and advancements in minimally invasive surgery for spinal deformity.

Daniel J. Sucato, MD, MS
Texas Scottish Rite Hospital for
 Children
Dallas, Texas

Adolescent Idiopathic Scoliosis: Etiology, Anatomy, Natural History, and Bracing

Stefan Parent, MD, PhD
Peter O. Newton, MD
Dennis R. Wenger, MD

Abstract

Adolescent idiopathic scoliosis is a three-dimensional deformity of the spine. Despite active efforts by different research teams, the etiology of scoliosis remains unclear. Treatment of scoliosis requires a solid understanding of the natural history of the disorder as well as sound clinical judgment. The evaluation, monitoring, and institution of conservative treatment such as bracing can present a challenge to the orthopaedic surgeon. Clinical monitoring is the only intervention necessary in most patients. A detailed review of the patient's history as well as a careful physical examination can help establish the diagnosis and the risk for progression. Skeletal maturity, gender, growth velocity, curve location, and magnitude are factors that can help assess the likelihood of progression. Bracing is the only nonsurgical measure proven to have any effect on halting the progression of scoliosis. Other forms of conservative treatment have not been shown to significantly modify the natural history of idiopathic scoliosis. Bracing results are directly related to compliance with brace treatment; therefore, optimal results cannot be achieved without the patient's cooperation and family support.

The etiology of idiopathic scoliosis remains unknown, but recent developments in the fields of genetics and molecular biology may ultimately provide insights into the etiology and pathophysiology of scoliosis. Several etiologic theories exist and include genetic factors, hormonal factors, growth abnormalities, biomechanical and neuromuscular theories, as well as different tissue disorders of bone, muscle, and fibrous tissue.

Etiology
Genetic Factors

Several studies suggest there is a genetic component in the development of idiopathic scoliosis. Population studies have shown an increased incidence in families of patients with idiopathic scoliosis compared with the general population.[1-7] In one study, daughters of women with idiopathic scoliosis had a 27% prevalence of scoliotic curves greater than 15°.[8] Another study on familial prevalence showed an 11% prevalence for first-degree relatives, and a 2.4% and 1.4% prevalence for second- and third-degree relatives, respectively.[2] A meta-analysis of 68 sets of twins with scoliotic curves (37 sets of monozygotic and 31 sets of dizygotic twins) showed a prevalence of scoliosis in 73% of monozygous twins compared with 36% in dizygous twins.[9] Curve severity has also been evaluated,

and monozygotic twins had greater correlation than in dizygotic twins.

Despite the accumulating evidence for a genetic etiology, the exact inheritance pattern, genes, and gene product causing scoliosis remain unknown. The most likely inheritance pattern is multifactorial.[2] Genomic screening and statistical linkage analysis are research methods used to help identify the genetic features of scoliosis.[10]

Hormonal Factors

An observation that pinealectomized chickens develop scoliosis has led to the hypothesis that melatonin (secreted by the pineal gland) deficiency may lead to scoliosis.[11,12] Levels of melatonin were then evaluated in a group of 30 patients with idiopathic scoliosis. Patients showing curve progression of more than 10° in 1 year showed a decrease of 35% of nighttime melatonin secretion compared with the patients without progression and normal controls.[13] However, in another study, Bagnall and associates[14] could not demonstrate a statistically significant difference in melatonin secretion in a group of patients with idiopathic scoliosis.

Rapid progression of scoliotic curves has been reported in patients taking growth hormone, but scoliosis is a problem in less than 1% of patients taking growth hormone.[15] Growth hormone seems to be related to melatonin activity because it has a diurnal secretion pattern, but unlike melatonin, the concentrations of growth hormone are higher during the daytime. The pineal gland could be responsible for growth control by melatonin's modulation on growth hormone activity.[14] Injection of growth hormone in pinealectomized chickens also seems to produce greater scoliotic curves.[14] An attractive theory relating to melatonin is that a deficiency in the receptor, not the ligand, is responsible for curve development. If changes in the receptor for melatonin render the hormone inactive, this could explain the variations in melatonin levels observed in different studies. Melatonin receptors have been identified in different tissues including bones and muscle. However, the exact relationship between melatonin and scoliosis development, if one exists, remains to be elucidated.

Tissue Abnormalities

The observed associations between scoliosis and disorders such as Marfan syndrome and osteogenesis imperfecta have led to research efforts evaluating the role of connective tissue in the pathogenesis of scoliosis. Collagen fibers and elastin fibers are important components of the spine that provide stability and support. A histomorphometric study of intervertebral disks has shown changes associated with the distribution of collagen fibers in patients with scoliosis, but these changes were not constant.[16]

Several investigators have proposed that scoliosis could be secondary to a functional deficit of muscular components.[17-21] Several studies have demonstrated structural changes in muscle fibers, with asymmetric changes found on the concavity and convexity of scoliotic curves.[22-25] However, these convexity/concavity modifications could easily be secondary changes associated with the alterations in muscle length or loading that follow scoliosis development.

Similarities between platelet contractile elements and skeletal muscle fibers have led researchers to study the cellular structure of thrombocytes. Because platelets are not located primarily in the spine, the changes observed in their contractile elements could represent a primary systemic process as opposed to secondary changes caused by scoliosis.[7] Elevated levels of intracellular calcium and phosphorus have been observed in patients with scoliosis.[25] Other investigators have identified abnormal calmodulin levels in patients with scoliosis.[26,27] These observations support the hypothesis of a general cellular membrane anomaly (possibly present in both platelets and muscle fibers) as a cause for idiopathic scoliosis, but this theory remains to be proven.

Neuromuscular Theories

Neuromuscular theories are based on the observations that patients with neuromuscular disease often develop scoliosis. The hypothesis is that a subclinical dysfunction of the central nervous system could result in scoliosis. Syringomyelia is associated with an increase in scoliosis incidence, possibly secondary to direct pressure on the sensory or motor tracts of the spinal cord.[28,29] Irritation of the brain stem may result from Chiari malformation or enlargement of the fourth ventricle and result in scoliosis. Cerebral asymmetry[30] and postural equilibrium dysfunction[31] have been observed in patients with scoliosis. These changes in equilibrium have been shown to be proportional to curve severity but returned to normal at maturity.[32,33] Abnormalities in the vestibulo-ocular system have also been identified in patients with scoliosis.[34,35]

Spinal Growth/Biomechanical Theories

Mechanical influences on spinal growth are thought to play an important role in curve progression because scoliosis occurs mainly during the rapid growth period of adolescence. The biomechani-

cal theories can be divided between the causative (etiologic) theories and the secondary, self-sustaining curve progression model occurring after an initial event. Several authors have proposed an etiologic theory for the development of scoliosis based on the modification of the sagittal profile.[36-42] According to this model, patients with idiopathic scoliosis develop progressive hypokyphosis, followed by lordosis of the thoracic spine, causing the spine to "buckle" under the physiologic load applied on the spine. Smith and associates[43] later described a transverse plane deformity and a bone drift phenomenon toward the concavity of the curve. More recently, Porter[44] proposed that the length of the spinal canal was shorter than the anterior length of the vertebral body, thus creating an effect similar to a posterior tether causing spinal "buckling" and finally the typical three-dimensional deformity of idiopathic scoliosis. However, the cause for this theorized "mismatch" of anterior and posterior spinal column growth has not been determined. It may relate to differences in the rates of endochondral and intramembranous growth of the vertebral elements.[27]

Once the scoliotic deformity has been established, most agree that some component of curve progression is regulated by the Hueter-Volkmann principle,[45,46] which states that growth is retarded by increased compression and accelerated when compressive loads are reduced. Stokes and associates[47,48] have proposed a mechanical modulation theory of vertebral growth based on the Hueter-Volkmann principle, and they believe that once asymmetric loading occurs, a "vicious circle" ensues, with progressive vertebral wedging promoting further asymmetric loading and further vertebral deformity. Perdriolle and associates[49] have proposed that a small thoracic curve could create asymmetric loading causing curve progression once the curve reaches a certain level.

Spinal Anatomy

The vertebral column constitutes the central structure of the human body. Along with the thoracic cage, it serves as a scaffold attaching the upper and lower extremities while supporting the head. It surrounds and protects the spinal cord and transfers the weight of the trunk to the lower extremities through the pelvis. Because of the erect posture adopted by humans during evolution, the vertebral column is composed of physiologic curvatures allowing prolonged standing. Cervical lordosis, thoracic kyphosis, and lumbar lordosis constitute the normal sagittal contour. In the frontal plane, the vertebral column is normally straight.

Idiopathic scoliosis is a three-dimensional deformity affecting the orientation and position of the spinal elements in space (Figure 1). The regional and global changes are characterized by a deviation in the frontal plane, a modification of the sagittal profile, as well as alterations in the shape of the rib cage. The most characteristic feature of scoliosis is the coronal plane curvature of the spine, the most common being a right-sided convex deviation of the thoracic spine. Although originally thought to be associated with kyphosis, in most instances the apical region of thoracic scoliosis is in fact hypokyphotic. The "apparent kyphosis" results from the convex side rib prominence that results from axial rotation of the vertebra in the transverse plane. Maximal at the apex, vertebral rotation alters the shape and orientation of the ribs, creating the rib prominence that makes the trunk appear kyphotic.

A morphometric analysis of anatomic specimens with scoliosis has demonstrated deformation of the vertebrae. This altered shape consists of progressive vertebral wedging with the transitional vertebra demonstrating minimal or no wedging and maximum wedging located at the apex of a typical scoliotic curve. In addition, pedicle width was modified significantly on the concave side of the sco-

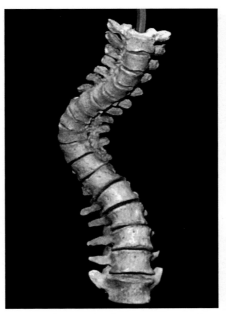

Figure 1 Photograph of an anatomic specimen with right thoracic scoliosis, demonstrating a marked change in shape of the spinal column (anterior view).

liotic curve with progressive thinning of the pedicle toward the apex of the curve.[50,51] Because of the scoliosis, the spinal cord tends to lie closer to this smaller concave apical pedicle[52] (Figure 2).

Prevalence and Natural History of Idiopathic Scoliosis

The prevalence of idiopathic scoliosis varies greatly based on the minimal curvature selected as the lower limit for diagnosis. The reported prevalence for scoliotic curves greater than 10° ranges from 0.5% to 3%.[53-58] For curves greater than 30°, the prevalence decreases to 1.5 to 3 per 1,000.[58,59] Thus, small to moderate curves are common and severe curves that require treatment are rare. Idiopathic scoliosis is most common during adolescence. The ratio of boys to girls affected is equal for minor curves, yet dominated by girls as the curve magnitude increases, reaching a ratio of 1:8 for those requiring treatment.[60]

Risk factors for scoliosis progression

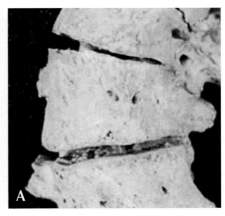

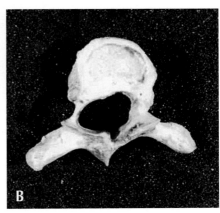

Figure 2 A, Anterior view photograph of an anatomic specimen demonstrating the vertebral wedging that results from long-standing scoliotic deformity. The Hueter-Volkmann principles result in alterations in growth, resulting in these shape changes. **B,** Superior view photograph of an anatomic specimen with scoliotic deformity, demonstrating asymmetry of the pedicles.[51]

that have been identified include gender, remaining skeletal growth, curve location, and curve magnitude, with scoliosis progression being the most rapid during peak skeletal growth. Peak growth velocity of adolescence averages 6 to 8 cm of overall height gain per year. Bone age and menarcheal status help determine the growth spurt in females, with the onset of menses generally following the most rapid stage of skeletal growth by approximately 12 months. When the Risser sign is grade 1 or less, the risk for progression is increased to 60% to 70%. However, if

Table 1
Risk of Scoliosis Progression and Relation to Curve Magnitude and Patient Skeletal Maturity

	Curves That Progressed (%)	
	5° to 19° Curves	20° to 29° Curves
Risser sign		
Grade 0 or 1	22	68
Grade 2, 3, or 4	2	23

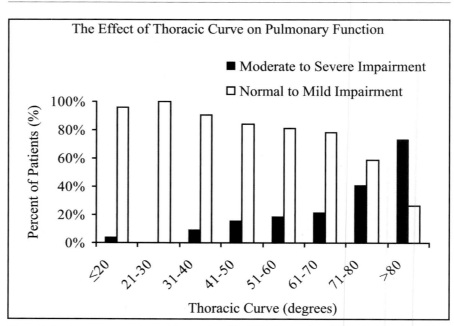

Figure 3 Graphic representation of the relationship between predicted forced vital capacity (% predicted) and thoracic Cobb angle.

the Risser sign is grade 3, the risk is reduced to less than 10%.[61,62] Unfortunately, many of the readily identified markers of maturity (for example, menarcheal status and Risser sign) are variable and appear just after the adolescent growth spurt. Therefore, it is impossible to tell whether a patient who is premenarcheal and has a Risser sign of grade 0 is approaching, in the midst of, or past the most rapid growth stage and thus at risk for scoliosis progression. Closure of the triradiate cartilage of the acetabulum has been identified as a radiographic sign, which more closely approximates the time of peak growth velocity.[63]

Curve pattern has also been identified as an important variable for predicting the probability of progression. Curves with an apex above T12 are more likely to progress than isolated lumbar curves.[61] Curve magnitude at the initial diagnosis appears to be a factor predicting progression.[62,64] Larger curves are more likely to continue to increase in magnitude with growth (Table 1).

Pulmonary function becomes limited as thoracic scoliosis becomes more severe (> 60° to 70°).[65,66] Forced vital capacity and forced expiratory volume in 1 second decrease linearly, with an approximate 20% reduction in predicted values with 100° curves.[66] The associated deformity of the chest cavity causes restrictive lung disease. Thoracic lordosis also decreases lung volume and increases the deleterious effects of scoliosis on pulmonary function[67] (Figure 3).

Estimates regarding the frequency of back pain and associated disability in adults with scoliosis vary, but most studies have shown slightly higher rates of back pain compared with control groups.[66-69] Although the risk of curve progression is highest during the rapid phases of growth, not all curves stabilize after growth. In long-term studies, many patients experience progression after skeletal maturity.[70,71] Curves less than 30° tend not to progress, with the most marked progression occurring in curves that are between 50° and 75° at the completion of growth (progression continuing at a rate of nearly 1° per year). Lumbar curves are more likely to progress if they are greater than 30° at skeletal maturity. This risk of progression in adults after skeletal maturity has led to many of the treatment recommendations regarding surgical management of scoliosis.

Nonsurgical Treatment and Bracing
The treatment approach for any condition should be based on both long-term

and short-term outcomes. Treatment decisions often are made with incomplete data, particularly with regard to the longer-term results. The three general options for treatment are observation, use of an orthotic device, or some form of surgical stabilization (Figure 4). Although other forms of treatment have been proposed (such as electrical muscle stimulation, exercise, postural training, spinal manipulation, and nutritional supplementation), it seems that only bracing and surgical fusion have scientific evidence of affecting the outcome compared with observation alone. Even the efficacy of brace treatment, which has been extensively evaluated, remains in question.

Early Detection/School Screening Programs
The objective of school screening for scoliosis is to detect scoliosis early enough to allow brace treatment instead of a later time when surgical correction is the only option. To be effective, screening programs must have early treatment

methods available for the specific disorder, and the condition must be frequent enough to justify the cost of screening. Although screening programs for scoliosis are widespread in North America, some authors have suggested that school screening is not justified based on variable sensitivity and specificity of the screening examination and the efficacy of bracing.[72-74]

School screening is routinely performed in children in the fifth and sixth grades (age 10 to 12 years). The Adams forward-bend test and the scoliometer are used in combination to evaluate the maximal angle of trunk rotation[75] (Figure 5). It has been shown that an angle of trunk rotation greater than 7° detects nearly all curves over 30°, but also refers a large number of patients (2 to 3 per 100 children screened)[74,75] for radiographs in children only presenting with spinal asymmetry (Cobb angle < 10°) or mild scoliosis (Cobb angle < 25°) not needing treatment. Despite the high number of referrals and the high costs associated with school screening, these programs have increased the awareness of scoliosis among primary care physician and the general population.

Observational Monitoring
Most patients with adolescent idiopathic scoliosis only require observational monitoring, which may create anxiety in the patient and family who are concerned about living with scoliosis. However, the natural history of most minor curves is benign. Patients with growth remaining are at risk for progression, and thus those skeletally immature patients with curves between 11° and 25° warrant periodic evaluation. Radiographs (standing PA view) are recommended every 4 to 12 months depending on the rate of growth at the time. During peak adolescent growth (6 to 10 cm per year), monitoring every 4 to 6 months may be appropriate, especially if the scoliosis is approaching a magnitude to consider brace treatment.

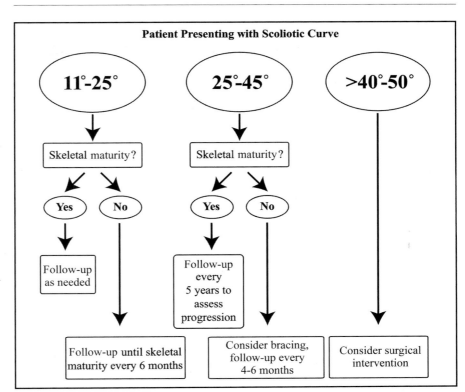

Figure 4 Treatment algorithm for adolescent idiopathic scoliosis based on curve magnitude and skeletal maturity at presentation.

Once skeletal maturity is reached, the rate of scoliosis progression, when it occurs, is much slower (approximately 1° per year) than during adolescent growth. As such, the requirements for monitoring are much less. Curves less than 25° in adults are at low risk for progression and do not require routine follow-up. Above this 25° limit, follow-up every 5 to 10 years will allow detection of a slow progression should it occur.

Brace Treatment
The use of a thoracolumbosacral orthosis is the only nonsurgical method of controlling scoliosis progression that has had any evidence of success. Current recommendations are to use a scoliosis brace to prevent progression of moderate curves only during growth. The exact upper and lower limits of curve magnitude that are appropriate for brace usage are debatable; however, the Scoliosis Research Society

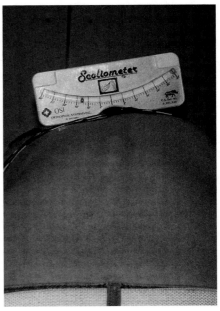

Figure 5 Photograph of a patient during Adams forward bending test, with scoliometer demonstrating right thoracic prominence and angle of trunk rotation.

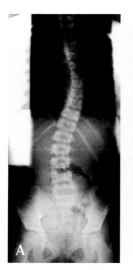
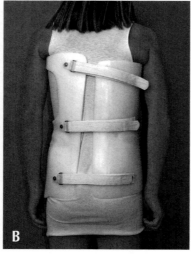
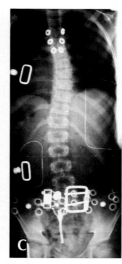

Figure 6 A, PA radiograph of patient before bracing with a Boston brace. **B,** Photograph of a patient wearing a Boston brace. **C,** PA radiograph of patient in a Boston brace shows good correction of the main thoracic curve.

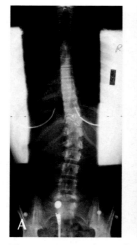
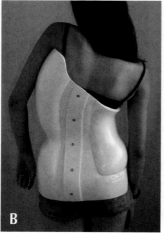
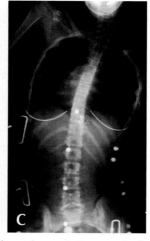

Figure 7 A, PA radiograph of patient before bracing with a Charleston brace. **B,** Photograph of a patient in Charleston nighttime bending brace. **C,** PA radiograph of patient in a Charleston brace shows good correction of the main lumbar curve.

has stated the following guidelines: a curve that has documented progression to greater than 25° or a patient presenting with a curve initially greater than 30° should be treated with bracing if the patients is still growing (Risser grade 0, 1, or 2). It is clear that brace efficacy is impacted by curve size, and those curves greater than 45° to 50° will likely benefit little from bracing.

The goal of brace treatment is to limit further curve progression, ideally keeping the scoliosis from reaching surgical indications. Although curve severity is reduced after appropriate brace fitting, this correction primarily occurs only when the brace is worn. In most patients, lasting correction of the deformity does not remain when use of the brace is discontinued. Thus, if a patient presents with a clinical deformity and scoliosis that suggests a need for surgical treatment, the same situation is likely to remain even if a brace is worn during the period of remaining growth. Currently, methods for nonsurgical reversal of a scoliotic curvature do not exist. This is often a difficult and frustrating circumstance for the patient and family because the best outcome of brace treatment is only prevention of further progression.

Brace correction is thought to occur by constant molding of the trunk and spine during growth. Full-time bracing was therefore originally suggested and remains the method of choice at several centers.[76,77] However, full-time brace wear is difficult. As such, brace-wearing schedules have been modified, reducing the time in the brace to 15 to 16 hours per day.[78,79] A dose-dependent relationship between the time per day in the brace and success in preventing curve progression was found in a meta-analysis of the literature[80] and suggests that the more time the patient spends in the brace, the less likely the curve is to progress.

Although brace treatment was deemed successful for many years, only recently have controlled treatment trials been completed.[81,82] The Scoliosis Research Society sponsored a study that compared the results of observation, bracing, and electrical stimulation in 286 patients in a prospective controlled trial.[81] Curve progression at the end of treatment was limited to less than 5° in 74% of patients treated with a brace compared with 34% in the group without treatment and 33% in the group that received electrical stimulation. Although the methodology of this study was criticized,[55] many centers continue to advise brace treatment in adolescent idiopathic scoliosis patients presenting with substantial growth remaining.

The effect of brace design on outcome is difficult to compare because most studies do not use the same inclusion criteria, and indications for brace use depends on the type and localization of the curve. In two recent studies, the underarm brace design worn full time was found to be more effective both at preventing progression and preventing further surgery than the Charleston nighttime brace design.[82,83] However, for single lumbar and thoracolumbar curves, the results of using the Charleston nighttime brace equaled those of the Boston brace.[82] (Figures 6 and 7)

The decision to include bracing in the treatment algorithm is debatable; however, if bracing is to have any chance of success, a coordinated effort must be made among the treating physician, the patient, and family as well as an orthotist with a strong interest in scoliosis treatment. Careful fitting and continued adjustment of the brace optimize curve correction while intermittent radiographs (every 4 to 6 months) are used to monitor for progression. Optimal curve correction cannot be achieved without the patient's cooperation in conforming to the brace-wearing schedule.

Summary

The cause of scoliosis remains a subject of active research. Many etiologic theories exist with different levels of evidence to support them. Adolescent idiopathic scoliosis carries a strong genetic component. Both the parents and the patient with scoliosis should be advised about the increased risk to siblings and offspring of developing scoliosis.

Treatment of scoliosis requires a solid understanding of the natural history of the disorder as well as sound clinical judgment. Adolescent idiopathic scoliosis treatment is based on curve magnitude at presentation, skeletal maturity, risk factors for progression, and clinical deformity (Figure 4). Clinical monitoring is the only intervention necessary in most patients. Brace treatment remains the standard of care in several countries for curves between 25° and 45° when significant growth remains. However, the sci-

entific basis for brace use in scoliosis is limited. Surgical treatment is advocated in skeletally immature patients when the curve reaches 40° to 50°. The small margin between bracing and surgical indications represents a challenge to the treating physician, the patient, and the family.

References

1. De George FV, Fisher RL: Idiopathic scoliosis: genetic and environmental aspects. *J Med Genet* 1967;4:251-257.

2. Risenborough EJ, Wynne-Davies R: A genetic survey of idiopathic scoliosis in Boston, Massachusetts. *J Bone Joint Surg Am* 1973;55:974-982.

3. Robin GC, Cohen T: Familial scoliosis: A clinical report. *J Bone Joint Surg Br* 1975;57:146-148.

4. Wynne-Davies R: Familial (idiopathic) scoliosis: A family survey. *J Bone Joint Surg Br* 1968;50:24-30.

5. Wynne-Davies R: Genetic aspects of idiopathic scoliosis. *Dev Med Child Neurol* 1973;15:809-811.

6. Hadley MN: Spine update: Genetics of familial idiopathic scoliosis. *Spine* 2000;25:2416-2418.

7. Miller NH: Cause and natural history of adolescent idiopathic scoliosis. *Orthop Clin North Am* 1999;30:343-352.

8. Harrington PR: The etiology of idiopathic scoliosis. *Clin Orthop* 1977;126:17-25.

9. Kesling KL, Reinker KA: Scoliosis in twins: A meta-analysis of the literature and report of six cases. *Spine* 1997;22:2009-2014.

10. Justice CM, Miller NH, Marosy B, Zhang J, Wilson AF: Familial idiopathic scoliosis: Evidence of an X-linked susceptibility locus. *Spine* 2003;28:589-594.

11. Machida M, Dubousset J, Imamura Y, Iwaya T, Yamada T, Kimura J: An experimental study in chickens for the pathogenesis of idiopathic scoliosis. *Spine* 1993;18:1609-1615.

12. Machida M, Dubousset J, Imamura Y, Iwaya T, Yamada T, Kimura J: Role of melatonin deficiency in the development of scoliosis in pinealectomised chickens. *J Bone Joint Surg Br* 1995;77:134-138.

13. Machida M, Dubousset J, Imamura Y, Miyashita Y, Yamada T, Kimura J: Melatonin: A possible role in pathogenesis of adolescent idiopathic scoliosis. *Spine* 1996;21:1147-1152.

14. Bagnall KM, Raso VJ, Hill DL, et al: Melatonin levels in idiopathic scoliosis: Diurnal and nocturnal serum melatonin levels in girls with adolescent idiopathic scoliosis. *Spine* 1996;21:1974-1978.

15. Allen DB: Safety of human growth hormone therapy: Current topics. *J Pediatr* 1996;128:S8-13.

16. Roberts S, Menage J, Eisenstein SM: The cartilage end-plate and intervertebral disc in scolio-sis: Calcification and other sequelae. *J Orthop Res* 1993;11:747-757.

17. Fidler MW, Jowett RL: Muscle imbalance in the aetiology of scoliosis. *J Bone Joint Surg Br* 1976;58:200-201.

18. Langenskiold A, Michelsson J: Experimental progressive scoliosis in the rabbit. *J Bone Joint Surg Br* 1961;43:116.

19. Spencer GS, Zorab PA: Spinal muscle in scoliosis: Comparison of normal and scoliotic rabbits. *J Neurol Sci* 1976;30:405-410.

20. Spencer GS, Eccles MJ: Spinal muscle in scoliosis: Part 2. The proportion and size of type 1 and type 2 skeletal muscle fibres measured using a computer-controlled microscope. *J Neurol Sci* 1976;30:143-154.

21. Spencer GS, Zorab PA: Spinal muscle in scoliosis: Part 1. Histology and histochemistry. *J Neurol Sci* 1976;30:137-142.

22. Bylund P, Jansson E, Dahlberg E, Eriksson E: Muscle fiber types in thoracic erector spinae muscles: Fiber types in idiopathic and other forms of scoliosis. *Clin Orthop* 1987;214:222-228.

23. Yarom R, Robin GC, Gorodetsky R: X-ray fluorescence analysis of muscles in scoliosis. *Spine* 1978;3:142-145.

24. Yarom R, Robin GC: Studies on spinal and peripheral muscles from patients with scoliosis. *Spine* 1979;4:12-21.

25. Yarom R, Blatt J, Gorodetsky R, Robin GC: Microanalysis and x-ray fluorescence spectrometry of platelets in diseases with elevated muscle calcium. *Eur J Clin Invest* 1980;10:143-147.

26. Cheung WY: Calmodulin. *Sci Am* 1982;246:62-70.

27. Kindsfater K, Lowe T, Lawellin D, Weinstein D, Akmakjian J: Levels of platelet calmodulin for the prediction of progression and severity of adolescent idiopathic scoliosis. *J Bone Joint Surg Am* 1994;76:1186-1192.

28. Zadeh HG, Sakka SA, Powell MP, Mehta MH: Absent superficial abdominal reflexes in children with scoliosis: An early indicator of syringomyelia. *J Bone Joint Surg Br* 1995;77:762-767.

29. Samuelsson L, Lindell D: Scoliosis as the first sign of a cystic spinal cord lesion. *Eur Spine J* 1995;4:284-290.

30. Goldberg CJ, Dowling FE, Fogarty EE, Moore DP: Adolescent idiopathic scoliosis and cerebral asymmetry: An examination of a nonspinal perceptual system. *Spine* 1995;20:1685-1691.

31. Yamada K, Yamamoto H, Nakagawa Y, Tezuka A, Tamura T, Kawata S: Etiology of idiopathic scoliosis. *Clin Orthop* 1984;184:50-57.

32. Sahlstrand T, Lidstrom J: Equilibrium factors as predictors of the prognosis in adolescent idiopathic scoliosis. *Clin Orthop* 1980;152:232-236.

33. Lidstrom J, Friberg S, Lindstrom L, Sahlstrand T: Postural control in siblings to scoliosis patients and scoliosis patients. *Spine* 1988;13:1070-1074.

34. Sahlstrand T, Petruson B: A study of labyrinthine function in patients with adoles-

cent idiopathic scoliosis: I. An electro-nystag-mographic study. *Acta Orthop Scand* 1979;50: 759-769.

35. Sahlstrand T, Petruson B, Ortengren R: Vestibulospinal reflex activity in patients with adolescent idiopathic scoliosis: Postural effects during caloric labyrinthine stimulation recorded by stabilometry. *Acta Orthop Scand* 1979;50:275-281.

36. Somerville EW: Rotational lordosis: The development of the single curve. *J Bone Joint Surg Br* 1952;34:421-427.

37. Deacon P, Berkin CR, Dickson RA: Combined idiopathic kyphosis and scoliosis: An analysis of the lateral spinal curvatures associated with Scheuermann's disease. *J Bone Joint Surg Br* 1985;67:189-192.

38. Dickson RA: The etiology and pathogenesis of idiopathic scoliosis. *Acta Orthop Belg* 1992;58(suppl 1):21-25.

39. Roaf R: The basic anatomy of scoliosis. *J Bone Joint Surg Br* 1966;48:786-792.

40. Cruickshank JL, Koike M, Dickson RA: Curve patterns in idiopathic scoliosis: A clinical and radiographic study. *J Bone Joint Surg Br* 1989;71:259-263.

41. Murray DW, Bulstrode CJ: The development of adolescent idiopathic scoliosis. *Eur Spine J* 1996;5:251-257.

42. Willner S, Johnson B: Thoracic kyphosis and lumbar lordosis during the growth period in children. *Acta Paediatr Scand* 1983;72:873-878.

43. Smith RM, Pool RD, Butt WP, Dickson RA: The transverse plane deformity of structural scoliosis. *Spine* 1991;16:1126-1129.

44. Porter RW: Idiopathic scoliosis: The relation between the vertebral canal and the vertebral bodies. *Spine* 2000;25:1360-1366.

45. Hueter C: Anatomische Studien an den Extramitaetengelenken Neugeborener en Erwachsener. *Virkows Archiv Path Anat Physiol* 1862;25:572-599.

46. Volkmann R: Verletzungen end Krankenheiten des Bewegungsorgane, in von Pitha B (ed): *Handbuch der allgemeine und speciellen Chirurgie Bd II Teil II.* Stuttgart, Germany, Ferdinand Enke, 1882.

47. Stokes IA, Aronsson DD, Spence H, Iatridis JC: Mechanical modulation of intervertebral disc thickness in growing rat tails. *J Spinal Disord* 1998;11:261-265.

48. Stokes IA, Spence H, Aronsson DD, Kilmer N: Mechanical modulation of vertebral body growth: Implications for scoliosis progression. *Spine* 1996;21:1162-1167.

49. Perdriolle R, Becchetti S, Vidal J, Lopez P: Mechanical process and growth cartilages: Essential factors in the progression of scoliosis. *Spine* 1993;18:343-349.

50. Parent S, Labelle H, Skalli W, Latimer B, De Guise J: Morphometric analysis of anatomic scoliotic specimens. *Spine* 2002;27:2305-2311.

51. Parent S, Labelle H, Skalli W, De Guise J: Thoracic pedicle morphometry in vertebrae from scoliotic spines. *Spine* 2004;29:239-248.

52. Liljenqvist UR, Allkemper T, Hackenberg L, Link TM, Steinbeck J, Halm HF: Analysis of vertebral morphology in idiopathic scoliosis with use of magnetic resonance imaging and multiplanar reconstruction. *J Bone Joint Surg Am* 2002;84:359-368.

53. Kane WJ, Moe JH: A scoliosis-prevalence survey in Minnesota. *Clin Orthop* 1970;69: 216-218.

54. Stirling AJ, Howel D, Millner PA, Sadiq S, Sharples D, Dickson RA: Late-onset idiopathic scoliosis in children six to fourteen years old: A cross-sectional prevalence study. *J Bone Joint Surg Am* 1996;78:1330-1336.

55. Dickson RA, Weinstein SL: Bracing (and screening): Yes or no? *J Bone Joint Surg Br* 1999;81:193-198.

56. Rogala EJ, Drummond DS, Gurr J: Scoliosis: Incidence and natural history. A prospective epidemiological study. *J Bone Joint Surg Am* 1978;60:173-176.

57. Morais T, Bernier M, Turcotte F: Age- and sex-specific prevalence of scoliosis and the value of school screening programs. *Am J Public Health* 1985;75:1377-1380.

58. Montgomery F, Willner S: The natural history of idiopathic scoliosis: Incidence of treatment in 15 cohorts of children born between 1963 and 1977. *Spine* 1997;22:772-774.

59. Kane WJ: Scoliosis prevalence: A call for a statement of terms. *Clin Orthop* 1977;126: 43-46.

60. Bunnell WP: The natural history of idiopathic scoliosis before skeletal maturity. *Spine* 1986;11:773-776.

61. Peterson LE, Nachemson AL: Prediction of progression of the curve in girls who have adolescent idiopathic scoliosis of moderate severity: Logistic regression analysis based on data from The Brace Study of the Scoliosis Research Society. *J Bone Joint Surg Am* 1995;77:823-827.

62. Lonstein JE, Carlson JM: The prediction of curve progression in untreated idiopathic scoliosis during growth. *J Bone Joint Surg Am* 1984;66:1061-1071.

63. Sanders JO, Little DG, Richards BS: Prediction of the crankshaft phenomenon by peak height velocity. *Spine* 1997;22:1352-1356.

64. Karol LA, Johnston CE, Browne RH, Madison M: Progression of the curve in boys who have idiopathic scoliosis. *J Bone Joint Surg Am* 1993;75:1804-1810.

65. Pehrsson K, Bake B, Larsson S, Nachemson A: Lung function in adult idiopathic scoliosis: A 20 year follow up. *Thorax* 1991;46:474-478.

66. Weinstein SL, Zavala DC, Ponseti IV: Idiopathic scoliosis: Long-term follow-up and prognosis in untreated patients. *J Bone Joint Surg Am* 1981;63:702-712.

67. Winter RB, Lovell WW, Moe JH: Excessive thoracic lordosis and loss of pulmonary function in patients with idiopathic scoliosis. *J Bone Joint Surg Am* 1975;57:972-977.

68. Mayo NE, Goldberg MS, Poitras B, Scott S, Hanley J: The Ste-Justine Adolescent Idiopathic Scoliosis Cohort Study: Part III. Back pain. *Spine* 1994;19:1573-1581.

69. Dickson JH, Erwin WD, Rossi D: Harrington instrumentation and arthrodesis for idiopathic scoliosis: A twenty-one-year follow-up. *J Bone Joint Surg Am* 1990;72:678-683.

70. Weinstein SL: Idiopathic scoliosis: Natural history. *Spine* 1986;11:780-783.

71. Weinstein SL, Ponseti IV: Curve progression in idiopathic scoliosis. *J Bone Joint Surg Am* 1983;65:447-455.

72. Pruijs JE: van der MR, Hageman MA, Keessen W, van Wieringen JC. The benefits of school screening for scoliosis in the central part of The Netherlands. *Eur Spine J* 1996;5:374-379.

73. Goldberg CJ, Dowling FE, Fogarty EE, Moore DP: School scoliosis screening and the United States Preventive Services Task Force: An examination of long-term results. *Spine* 1995;20:1368-1374.

74. Grossman TW, Mazur JM, Cummings RJ: An evaluation of the Adams forward bend test and the scoliometer in a scoliosis school screening setting. *J Pediatr Orthop* 1995;15:535-538.

75. Bunnell WP: Outcome of spinal screening. *Spine* 1993;18:1572-1580.

76. Price CT, Scott DS, Reed FE Jr, Riddick MF: Nighttime bracing for adolescent idiopathic scoliosis with the Charleston bending brace: Preliminary report. *Spine* 1990;15:1294-1299.

77. Blount WP, Schmidt A: The Milwaukee brace in the treatment of scoliosis. *J Bone Joint Surg Am* 1957;39:693.

78. Allington NJ, Bowen JR: Adolescent idiopathic scoliosis: treatment with the Wilmington brace: A comparison of full-time and part-time use. *J Bone Joint Surg Am* 1996;78:1056-1062.

79. Green NE: Part-time bracing of adolescent idiopathic scoliosis. *J Bone Joint Surg Am* 1986;68:738-742.

80. Rowe DE, Bernstein SM, Riddick MF, Adler F, Emans JB, Gardner-Bonneau D: A meta-analysis of the efficacy of non-operative treatments for idiopathic scoliosis. *J Bone Joint Surg Am* 1997;79:664-674.

81. Nachemson AL, Peterson LE: Effectiveness of treatment with a brace in girls who have adolescent idiopathic scoliosis: A prospective, controlled study based on data from the Brace Study of the Scoliosis Research Society. *J Bone Joint Surg Am* 1995;77:815-822.

82. Howard A, Wright JG, Hedden D: A comparative study of TLSO, Charleston, and Milwaukee braces for idiopathic scoliosis. *Spine* 1998;23:2404-2411.

83. Katz DE, Richards BS, Browne RH, Herring JA: A comparison between the Boston brace and the Charleston bending brace in adolescent idiopathic scoliosis. *Spine* 1997;22:1302-1312.

Lenke Classification System of Adolescent Idiopathic Scoliosis: Treatment Recommendations

Lawrence G. Lenke, MD

Abstract

The Lenke and associates classification system of adolescent idiopathic scoliosis (AIS) was developed to provide a comprehensive and reliable means to categorize all surgical AIS curves. This classification system requires analysis of the upright coronal and sagittal radiographs along with the supine side bending radiographic views. The triad classification system consists of a curve type (1-6), a lumbar spine modifier (A, B, C), and a sagittal thoracic modifier (-, N, +). All three regions of the radiographic coronal and sagittal planes, the proximal thoracic, main thoracic, and thoracolumbar/lumbar are designated as either the major curve (largest Cobb measurement) or minor curves with the minor curves separated into structural and nonstructural types. The recommendations are that the major and structural minor curves are included in the instrumentation and fusion and the nonstructural minor curves are excluded. Overall, the classification system is treatment directed; however, there are other aspects of the radiographic and clinical deformity that may suggest deviation from the recommendations of the classification system. The ultimate goal of this classification system is to allow organization of similar curve patterns to provide comparisons of various treatment methods to provide optimal treatment for each AIS surgical patient.

Although the King-Moe system has been the gold standard for classification of adolescent idiopathic scoliosis (AIS) since its publication in 1983,[1] several authors have found that the system has several shortcomings when used to evaluate the surgical treatment of various types of scoliosis curves with modern segmental spinal instrumentation.[2,3] Thus, a new classification system was developed that requires use of the upright coronal and sagittal radiographs, along with the supine side bending views for complete curve classification.

The development of this new triad, modular classification system for the surgical treatment of AIS was based on six goals:[4] the classification system would be comprehensive for all curve types; two-dimensional, with increased emphasis placed on the sagittal plane; treatment-based to recommend surgery on the major and structural minor regions of the spine but not on the nonstructural minor regions; able to recommend selective fusions of the spine when appropriate; able to have specific objective criteria to help separate curve types which would then optimize both interobserver and intraobserver reliability; and easily understood and usable for surgeons and their trainees on a routine basis.

Using the Lenke Classification System

The classification system begins with the evaluation of the upright coronal, sagittal, and right and left side bending radiographs. On the upright coronal radiograph, the three spinal column regions that may develop surgical curves are evaluated: the proximal thoracic (PT), main thoracic (MT), and thoracolumbar/lumbar (TL/L) regions. The major curve is the curve with the largest Cobb measurement, and that will always be included in the fusion of surgical AIS. The minor curves are the two other regions, and one of the main decisions in scoliosis surgery is whether or not to include these minor curves in the fusion along with the major curve. To help in this decision, minor curve structural criteria were established to help guide the surgeon and also create a classification scheme template. In the coronal plane, inflexibility on side bending radiographs where the residual minor curve is greater than or equal to 25° in each of the three regions will render that region a structural minor curve. In addition, hyperkyphosis greater than or equal to 20° in the PT region (T2-T5) or TL junction (T10-L2) renders the associated region of the spine a structural minor curve as well. Thus, a schematic can be created for six different curve types that are defined in this new system based on

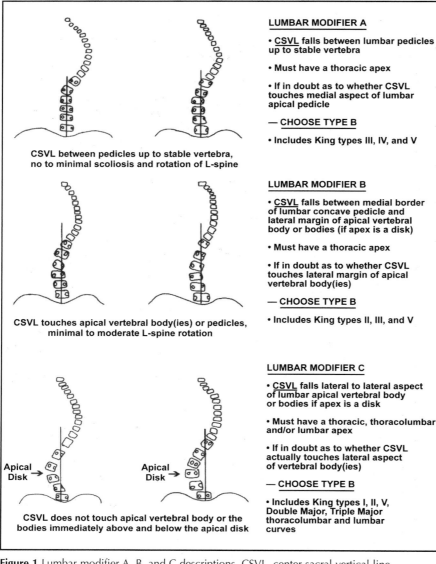

LUMBAR MODIFIER A

• <u>CSVL</u> falls between lumbar pedicles up to stable vertebra

• Must have a thoracic apex

• If in doubt as to whether CSVL touches medial aspect of lumbar apical pedicle

— **CHOOSE TYPE B**

• Includes King types III, IV, and V

LUMBAR MODIFIER B

• <u>CSVL</u> falls between medial border of lumbar concave pedicle and lateral margin of apical vertebral body or bodies (if apex is a disk)

• Must have a thoracic apex

• If in doubt as to whether CSVL touches lateral margin of apical vertebral body(ies)

— **CHOOSE TYPE B**

• Includes King types II, III, and V

LUMBAR MODIFIER C

• <u>CSVL</u> falls lateral to lateral aspect of lumbar apical vertebral body or bodies if apex is a disk

• Must have a thoracic, thoracolumbar and/or lumbar apex

• If in doubt as to whether CSVL actually touches lateral aspect of vertebral body(ies)

— **CHOOSE TYPE B**

• Includes King types I, II, V, Double Major, Triple Major thoracolumbar and lumbar curves

Figure 1 Lumbar modifier A, B, and C descriptions. CSVL, center sacral vertical line. (Reproduced with permission from Lenke LG, Betz RR, Harms J, et al: Adolescent idiopathic scoliosis: A new classification to determine the extent of spinal arthrodesis. *J Bone Joint Surg Am* 2001;83:1171).

whether each of the regions, the PT, MT, or TL/L, is a structural curve (major or minor) or a minor nonstructural curve. The six curve types are type 1, main thoracic (MT); type 2, double thoracic (DT); type 3, double major (DM); type 4, triple major (TM); type 5, thoracolumbar/lumbar (TL/L); and type 6, thoracolumbar/lumbar—main thoracic (TL/L-MT).

Next, two modifiers are added to the curve type—a lumbar spine modifier and

a sagittal thoracic modifier. The lumbar spine modifier is based on the position of the center sacral vertical line to the apex of the lumbar curve preoperatively[5] (Figure 1). For lumbar modifier A, the center sacral vertical line falls between the pedicles of the lumbar spine up to the stable vertebra. For lumbar modifier B, the center sacral vertical line touches the apex of the lumbar curve (pedicles). For lumbar modifier C, the apex (pedicles) of

the lumbar curve falls completely off the center sacral vertical line, thus documenting complete deviation of the apex of the lumbar curve off the midline. Finally, a sagittal thoracic modifier is added based on the T5-T12 sagittal Cobb measurement. When the T5-T12 Cobb measurement is less than +10°, a "-" modifier signifying thoracic hypokyphosis or lordosis is assigned. When the T5-T12 Cobb measurement is between +10° and +40°, a normal or "N" sagittal thoracic modifier is assigned. When the T5-T12 Cobb measurement is more than +40° a "+" or hyperkyphotic sagittal modifier is assigned.

Thus, this triad classification system of AIS combines the three components of curve type (1-6), lumbar spine modifier (A, B, C), plus the sagittal thoracic modifier (-, N, or +) to create the full classification system (eg, 1BN). There are 42 different curve classifications possible with this system. Thus it is very important to use the modularity of this system to help determine the appropriate classification. One must determine the curve type, then add the lumbar spine and sagittal thoracic modifiers to the curve type rather than trying to memorize all 42 different configurations. On premeasured radiographs, this classification system has been evaluated by the developers of the system, as well as an independent group of Scoliosis Research Society surgeons, and also an independent group of surgeons from a different country.[2,6] These studies have all found this system to be more reliable than the King-Moe system in its interobserver and intraobserver reliability.

Specific Treatment Recommendations

One of the general guidelines from this classification system is that the major structural curve as well as the structural minor curves should be fused, but not the nonstructural minor curves. In addition, for type 1, MT curves, the MT region should be fused exclusively either posteriorly or anteriorly. For type 2, DT curves, both the PT and MT regions should be fused posteriorly. For type 3, DM curves, both the MT and TL/L regions should be fused posteriorly. For type 4, TM major curves, all three regions, the PT, MT, and TL/L should be fused posteriorly. For type 5, TL/L curves, the TL/L region should be fused either anteriorly or posteriorly. Finally, for type 6, TL/L—MT curves, the MT and TL/L regions should be fused posteriorly. Obviously, there are certain circumstances where a circumferential approach will be considered for either the MT or TL/L regions for very large curve magnitudes, increased stiffness on side bending, increased kyphosis, or skeletal immaturity with those patients at risk for crankshaft phenomenon. The general rules of fusing the major and structural minor curves will still need to be followed as described.

Type 1: MT Curves

In type 1, MT curves, the general rule is to fuse the MT region only either via a posterior or anterior route.[7] These curve patterns can either have a lumbar modifier A, B, or C, with the 1C pattern representing a true selective fusion of the MT region. The sagittal modifier can be -, N, or +, which may affect whether the curve is approached posteriorly or anteriorly.[7]

Type 1, MT curves are primarily treated posteriorly. The posterior approach for these curves is universal, with all type 1 curves being amenable to posterior instrumentation and fusion.[8] Recently, pedicle screw anchors have been used as the spinal implants of choice for AIS surgeries.[9] In addition to the strong corrective forces applied by these posterior screw constructs, the ability to truly derotate the apical vertebrae is being achieved with multilevel segmental pedicle screw constructs through direct apical vertebral derotation maneuvers[10] (Figure 2).

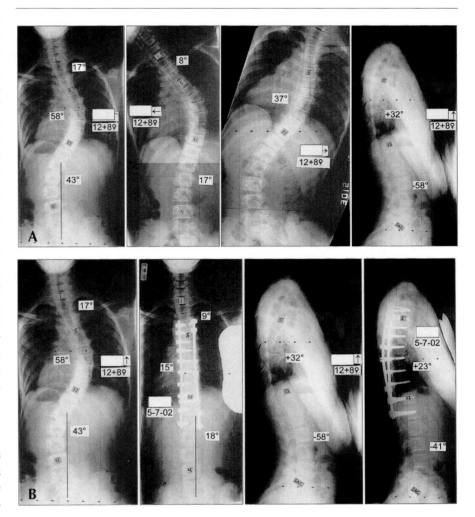

Figure 2 Radiographs of a 12-year-old girl with a 17° PT, 58° MT, 43° lumbar AIS curve. **A,** The left side bender shows the PT curve decreases to 8°, and the lumbar curve to 17°. The right side bender shows the MT curve decreases to 37°. T5-T12 kyphosis is +32°, thus the sagittal modifier is "N." The center sacral vertical line falls just off the apical lumbar pedicles, thus the lumbar modifier is a C. The PT and lumbar curves are nonstructural, and the Lenke curve classification is 1CN. **B,** The patient underwent a segmental pedicle screw instrumentation and fusion from T4 to L1 for correction of the MT curve to 15° and excellent overall coronal and sagittal balance.

However, an anterior approach could be considered for a type 1 curve in those patients who have a lordotic sagittal thoracic alignment with a minus sagittal modifier; those with a true C lumbar modifier position where selective anterior thoracic fusion may optimize spontaneous lumbar curve positioning; those patients who are skeletally immature and are at risk for crankshaft phenomenon with posterior-only fusion without the use of apical pedicle screws (which may prevent crankshaft phenomenon by the posterior route); when one to three distal fusion levels can be saved with an anterior approach by stopping at the thoracic lower end vertebra; and for those patients who can be treated with an endoscopic anterior approach to minimize morbidity during the surgical instrumentation and fusion. An anterior approach for main thoracic curves can be performed with an open, mini-open, or pure endoscopic approach, and pulmonary function should be evaluated because of the anticipated postoperative decline[11,12,] similar to that seen with a posterior thoracoplasty.[13] The instrumentation choices include a single screw/single rod, single screw/dual rod, or dual screw/dual rod construct. An anterior release and fusion combined with a posterior instrumentation and fusion of a type 1 main thoracic curve can also be done. Indications for this would be for those MT curves with very large curve magnitudes (> 90°-100° upright, with increased stiffness on side bending with a > 60°-70° residual Cobb measurement), severe lordosis or hyperkyphosis in the sagittal plane, and in those patients who are very skeletally immature and thus at high risk for crankshaft phenomenon. Currently, this circumferential approach is being used less frequently because of the powerful corrective and holding forces of multilevel segmental pedicle screw constructs, which are commonly used on these patients.

Type 2: DT Curves

Type 2, DT curve patterns require posterior instrumentation and fusion of the PT and MT regions.[14] Occasionally, a preliminary anterior release and fusion will be required for a very large and/or stiff main thoracic curve, similar to the criteria listed for type 1 MT curves. Most commonly, posterior instrumentation and fusion will extend from T2, or occasionally T3, down to the most proximal lumbar vertebra intersected by the center sacral vertical line, whether the lumbar spine modifier is A, B, or C.[15] It is very important to optimize clinical and radiographic shoulder alignment when treating the type 2, DT curve patterns, for it is not uncommon that the left shoulder will be elevated with maximal correction of the right MT curve.[16] This is especially true when the left shoulder is clinically elevated preoperatively, or even when the shoulders are level preoperatively.[17] The

PT region must be corrected with posterior convex compression forces and concave distraction forces on the appropriate sides of the curve. Usually the convex compression force is applied first to reverse kyphosis in that region.

Type 3: DM Curves

The type 3, DM curve pattern requires posterior instrumentation and fusion of the MT and TL/L regions. The most common DM curve pattern will have a lumbar C modifier position with the lumbar curve completely deviated from the midline. Varying degrees of thoracolumbar kyphosis can be seen in the junction between the thoracic and lumbar curves, and a significant amount of thoracolumbar kyphosis, 20° or more between T10 and L2, will automatically designate both curves as structural when surgically planning to treat one of them as the major curve. These DM curve patterns usually require posterior instrumentation and fusion down to either L3 or L4[9,15] (Figure 3). Occasionally a 3C curve can undergo a selective thoracic fusion if the spine can be maintained in good balance and there is a lack of junctional kyphosis between the two curves preoperatively.[18,19] In this circumstance, it is extremely important to evaluate the clinical examination of the patient very carefully to make sure that the thoracic region is still the more prominent clinical part of the deformity and will allow a successful selective thoracic fusion procedure to be performed. Also, occasionally a circumferential approach will be required for either the thoracic or lumbar portions of a double major curve pattern in those curves that are very large in curve magnitude, and/or have marked sagittal plane malalignment as described above.

Type 4: TM Curves

Type 4, TM curves are somewhat rare curve patterns that require all three structural regions of the spine (PT, MT, and TL/L) to be instrumented and fused pos-

teriorly. Commonly, these are 4C patterns with complete apical deviation off of the midline of the lumbar curve. Fusion levels normally need to extend from T2 or T3 proximal to L3 or L4 distal. Occasionally, a preliminary anterior release and fusion of the MT or TL/L regions may be required when one of those regions is disproportionately much larger and stiffer than the other region.

Type 5: TL/L Curves

In this curve pattern, the major curve is in the TL/L region, and the minor PT and MT curves above are nonstructural. Thus, the isolated TL/L curve can be treated anteriorly or posteriorly. Traditionally, most of these curves have been treated anteriorly either using single or dual rod anterior instrumentation systems.[20,21,22] In this manner, these curves are fused from the upper end vertebra to the lower end vertebra. Usually this will be one level shorter distally than what posterior instrumentation would require. It is important to maintain adequate sagittal alignment during these anterior procedures with the use of structural interbody grafts or cages, appropriate rod contouring, and/or the use of dual rod instrumentation constructs to maintain sagittal alignment over time during healing.[21] With the use of transpedicular screw fixation, these curve patterns can also be treated posteriorly, occasionally to the lower end vertebra of the TL/L curve, or one level caudal to that.

Type 6: TL/L-MT Curves

The type 6 curve pattern has the major curve in the TL/L region, with the MT region being the structural minor curve above. These curves will require posterior instrumentation and fusion of both the MT and TL/L regions. Normally the instrumentation and fusion will extend down to L3 or L4. Occasionally, an isolated selective TL/L fusion may be performed, leaving the MT region unfused when specific clinical and radiograph criteria are met that will allow the selective TL/L fusion.

Curve Prevalence

A multicenter study was performed to evaluate 606 surgical AIS cases to determine the prevalence of various curve types, lumbar and sagittal modifiers, and overall curve classification.[23] With respect to the curve types, type 1 MT curves were found in 51% of all cases; type 2 DT in 20%; type 3 DM in 11%; type 4 TM in 3%; type 5 TL/L in 12%; type 6 TL/L-MT curves, in 3%. For the lumbar spine modifiers, the lumbar modifier A position was found in 41%, lumbar spine modifier B in 37% , and lumbar spine modifier C in 32%. Finally, with respect to sagittal thoracic spine modifier, the "-" or hypokyphotic modifier was found in 14%, the "N" or normal sagittal thoracic modifier was found in 75%, and the "+" or hyperkyphotic sagittal thoracic modifier was found in 11%. Although there are 42 different configurations of all curve classifications, the top five most commonly seen curves accounted for almost 60% of all curves treated surgically. The most common classifications include: 1AN (19%), 1BN (11%), 2AN (10%), 5CN (10%), and 1CN (8%).

To help judge whether the classification system truly makes treatment recommendations, a retrospective review of 606 surgical curves (treated before the classification system was developed) was performed to investigate whether the treatment recommendations by this new system were actually used.[23] In this manner, it was investigated whether the instrumentation and fusion included the major and structural minor curves, and excluded the nonstructural minor curves during surgical treatment. The study found that for approximately 90% of cases, the treatment guidelines were followed as recommended by the classification system. Looking at individual curve types, the results ranged from a low of 75% to a high of 95% as far as following

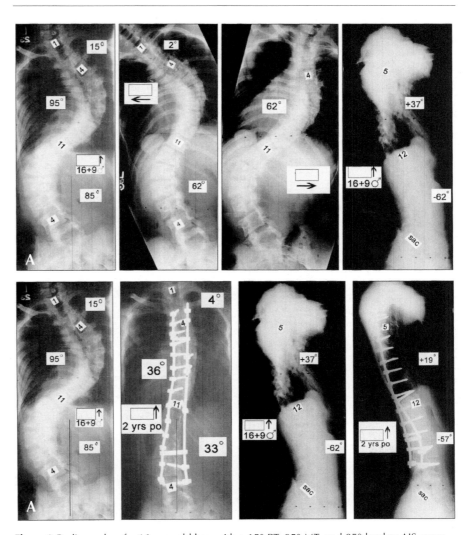

Figure 3 Radiographs of a 16-year-old boy with a 15° PT, 95° MT, and 85° lumbar AIS curve pattern. **A,** On left side bending, the PT curve decreases to 2° and the lumbar curve decreases to only 62°. On right side bending, the major MT curve decreases to 62°. T5-T12 sagittal kyphosis is +37°, thus the sagittal modifier is an "N." The center sacral vertical line falls far medial off the laterally displaced lumbar apex, thus denoting a C lumbar modifier position. The Lenke curve classification is 3CN. **B,** The patient underwent a posterior segmental pedicle screw instrumentation and fusion from T3 to L4 with excellent coronal and sagittal alignment at 2 years after initial surgery.

the treatment guidelines. Obviously, no radiographic classification system will ever be 100% predictive of treatment. Other important issues such as the clinical examination, the level of skeletal maturity of the patient, surgeon bias, and the overall radiographic structural criteria ratios between the MT and TL/L regions will often provide significant input to the surgical treatments rendered.[24]

Summary

The Lenke classification system of AIS is a comprehensive, two-dimensional, and reliable system. It is not completely treatment directed because of variations that will occur in the radiographic and clinical examination of the patient that will suggest deviation from the recommendations of the system. The ultimate goal of this classification system is to allow organization of similar patterns of surgical curves to allow comparison of various treatment methods. This will then provide surgeons with the information needed to select the optimal treatment of each particular curve pattern when discussing treatment options with AIS surgical patients and their families.

References

1. King HA, Moe J, Bradford DS, Winter RB: The selection of fusion levels in thoracic idiopathic scoliosis. *J Bone Joint Surg Am* 1983;65:1302-1313.

2. Lenke LG, Betz RR, Bridwell KH, et al: Intraobserver and interobserver reliability of the classification of thoracic adolescent idiopathic scoliosis. *J Bone Joint Surg Am* 1998;80:1097-1106.

3. Cummings RJ, Loveless EA, Campbell J, Samelson S, Mazur JM: Interobserver reliability and intraobserver reproducibility of the system of King et al for the classification of adolescent idiopathic scoliosis. *J Bone Joint Surg Am* 1998;80:1107-1111.

4. Lenke LG, Betz RR, Harms J, et al: Adolescent idiopathic scoliosis: A new classification to determine extent of spinal arthrodesis. *J Bone Joint Surg Am* 2001;83:1169-1181.

5. Lenke LG, Betz RR, Bridwell KH, Harms J, Clements DH, Love TG: Spontaneous lumbar curve coronal correction after selective anterior or posterior thoracic fusion in adolescent idiopathic scoliosis. *Spine* 1999;24:1663-1671.

6. Ogon M, Giesinger K, Behensky H, et al: Interobserver and intraobserver reliability of Lenke's new scoliosis classification system. *Spine* 2002;27:858-862.

7. Betz RR, Harms J, Clements DH III, et al: Comparison of anterior and posterior instrumentation for correction of adolescent thoracic idiopathic scoliosis. *Spine* 1999;24:225-239.

8. Lenke LG, Bridwell KH, Blanke K, Baldus C, Weston J: Radiographic results of arthrodesis with Cotrel-Dubousset instrumentation for the treatment of adolescent idiopathic scoliosis: A five to ten-year follow-up study. *J Bone Joint Surg Am* 1998;80:807-814.

9. Hamill CL, Lenke LG, Bridwell KH, Chapman MP, Blanke K, Baldus C: The use of pedicle screws to improve correction in the lumbar spine of patients with idiopathic scoliosis: Is it warranted? *Spine* 1996;21:1241-1249.

10. Rinella AS, Kim JA, Lenke LG: Posterior spinal instrumentation techniques for spinal deformity, in Bradford DS (ed): *Masters Series in Orthopaedic Surgery.* Philadelphia, PA, Lippincott Williams and Wilkins, 2004, pp 231-246.

11. Vedantam R, Lenke LG, Bridwell KH, Haas J, Linville DA: A prospective evaluation of pulmonary function in patients with adolescent idiopathic scoliotics relative to the surgical approach used for spinal arthrodesis. *Spine* 2000;25:82-90.

12. Graham EJ, Lenke LG, Lowe TG, et al: Prospective pulmonary function evaluation following open thoracotomy for anterior spinal fusion in adolescent idiopathic scoliosis. *Spine* 2000;25:2319-2325.

13. Lenke LG, Bridwell KH, Blanke K, Baldus C: Analysis of pulmonary function and chest cage dimension changes after thoracoplasty in idiopathic scoliosis. *Spine* 1995;20:1343-1350.

14. Lenke LG, Bridwell KH, O'Brien MF, Baldus C, Blanke K: Recognition and treatment of the proximal thoracic curve in adolescent idiopathic scoliosis treated with Cotrel-Dubousset instrumentation. *Spine* 1994;19:1589-1597.

15. Lenke LG, Bridwell KH, Baldus C, Blanke K, Schoenecker PL: Ability of Cotrel-Dubousset instrumentation to preserve distal lumbar motion segments in adolescent idiopathic scoliosis. *J Spinal Disord* 1993;6:339-350.

16. Kuklo T, Lenke LG, Won DS, et al: Spontaneous proximal thoracic curve correction following isolated fusion of the main thoracic curve in adolescent idiopathic scoliosis. *Spine* 2001;26:1966-1975.

17. Kuklo TR, Lenke LG, Graham EJ, et al: Correlation of radiographic, clinical, and patient assessment of shoulder balance following fusion versus nonfusion of the proximal thoracic curve in adolescent idiopathic scoliosis. *Spine* 2002;27:2013-2020.

18. Lenke LG, Bridwell KH, Baldus C, Blanke K: Preventing decompensation in King Type II curves treated with Cotrel-Dubousset instrumentation: Strict guidelines for selective thoracic fusion. *Spine* 1992;17(suppl 8):S274-S281.

19. Edwards CC II, Lenke LG, Peelle M, Sides B, Rinella AS, Bridwell KH: Time dependent response of the unfused lumbar curve after selective thoracic fusion: A 2-16 year radiographic and clinical follow-up. *Spine* 2004;29:536-546.

20. Lenke LG, Rhee J: Adolescent scoliosis: Anterior surgical techniques for adolescent idiopathic scoliosis. *Curr Opin Orthop* 2001;12:199-205.

21. Sweet FA, Lenke LG, Bridwell KH, Blanke KM: Maintaining lumbar lordosis with anterior single solid-rod instrumentation in thoracolumbar and lumbar adolescent idiopathic scoliosis. *Spine* 1999;24:1655-1662.

22. Sweet F, Lenke LG, Bridwell KH, Blanke KM, Whorton J: Prospective radiographic and clinical outcomes and complications of single solid rod instrumented anterior spinal fusion in adolescent idiopathic scoliosis. *Spine* 2001;26:1956-1965.

23. Lenke LG, Betz RR, Clements D, et al: Curve prevalence of a new classification of operative adolescent idiopathic scoliosis: Does classification correlate with treatment? *Spine* 2002;27:604-611.

24. Lenke LG, Betz RR, Haher T, et al: Multisurgeon assessment of surgical decision-making in adolescent idiopathic scoliosis: Curve classification, operative approach, and fusion levels. *Spine* 2001;26:2347-2353.

The Use of Video-Assisted Thoracoscopic Surgery in the Treatment of Adolescent Idiopathic Scoliosis

Peter O. Newton, MD

Abstract

The video-assisted thoracoscopic approach has become a useful adjunct in the treatment of scoliosis. This minimally invasive anterior approach allows access to the thoracic spine, providing a means of achieving disk excision and anterior body fusion. The advantage of this technique is the limited chest wall dissection required to reach the anterior thoracic spine. More recently, techniques have been developed to allow anterior instrumentation for an entirely endoscopic method of performing scoliosis correction. This approach is appropriate for curves less than 70° when only the thoracic curve is structural. The outcomes of this approach are promising and suggest reduced morbidity compared with open anterior approaches.

The video-assisted thoracoscopic approach has been used for a variety of diagnoses in the chest cavity,[1-3] and more recently, it has been used for spinal deformity treatment.[4-6] The thoracoscopic approach is a minimally invasive method of accessing the anterior spine through the chest cavity. It has its appeal in the limited chest wall dissection required to reach the anterior spine. In the surgical treatment of scoliosis, the anterior approach to the thoracic spine is commonly indicated. Anterior thoracic scoliosis procedures are often well suited for the thoracoscopic approach because the chest cavity is typically spacious and it is relatively easy to manipulate the endoscope and instruments within.

The thoracoscopic approach uses three to five small incisions through which instruments can be placed to visualize and perform anterior spinal surgery.

Visualization using the latest video technology can be quite spectacular; however, loss of this visualization (because of poor camera position, bleeding, and lung tissue) can make it impossible to safely perform surgery. Thoracoscopic anterior spinal release and fusion for the treatment of scoliosis continues to gain acceptance and popularity within the orthopaedic community. In addition, thoracoscopic anterior instrumentation techniques, which now allow for an entirely endoscopic correction of scoliosis, have been developed and may be appropriate for select patients.

Thoracoscopic Anterior Release and Fusion

The indications for anterior release and fusion in patients with scoliosis generally relate to the treatment of large or rigid curves,[6,7] which require increased flexi-

bility to obtain maximal correction during posterior instrumentation and fusion. The upper limits of curve magnitude as well as flexibility may be debated. However, it is clear that removal of the disk anteriorly increases curve flexibility,[8-11] providing both greater coronal and sagittal plane correction with posterior implant systems. The degree to which flexibility can be increased is dependent on the completeness of removal of both the anulus fibrosus and internal disk material. In the most severe cases of scoliosis, resection of the rib head and/or costovertebral joint may be required to optimize mobility. An additional indication for anterior disk excision and fusion is in the prevention of crankshaft growth, which has been reported to occur following an isolated posterior instrumentation and fusion procedure in skeletally immature patients.[12] In general, patients being treated posteriorly before their peak growth are at risk for crankshaft development.[13] The triradiate cartilage closure may be a reasonable marker to determine which patients such an anterior procedure would benefit. Thus, patients being treated posteriorly with open triradiate cartilage who are Risser 0 are considered for an anterior release and fusion with the primary goal of limiting later anterior growth.[14,15] An additional indication for anterior release and fusion may exist in those patients at greater risk for pseudarthrosis. Examples include patients with the diagnosis of neurofibromatosis, Marfan syndrome, or prior irradiation. Anterior fusion generally provides a large cancellous bony surface for fusion once the disk has been adequately removed, increasing the likelihood of solid arthrodesis. The thoracoscopic approach is applicable for release and fusion between the T4-T12 vertebral levels and may be extended both proximally to T2 and distally to L1 as additional experience is gained.[16] As with any open procedure, the goal is to obtain complete release with thorough disk excision to allow grafting and ultimately solid interbody arthrodesis.

Contraindications to the Thoracoscopic Approach

The thoracoscopic approach requires an adequate working space within the chest cavity to manipulate both the endoscope and working instruments. This generally requires selective ventilation of the lungs, with collapse of the lung in the chest cavity to be operated. As such, the pulmonary status of the patient must allow single lung ventilation. In addition, any past medical history that would suggest intrathoracic pleural adhesions should be considered a relative contraindication. Pleural adhesions between the lung and chest wall limit the ability of the lung to adequately collapse. If minor, these adhesions can be divided, although a nearly complete pleural symphysis between the chest and lung can make this an extremely challenging proposition. This scenario is most often encountered in patients with a prior thoracotomy or significant pulmonary infection. In addition, the requirement for an adequate working space dictates that curves in which the spine has become closely approximated to the rib cage may also be relatively contraindicated. A working distance of 2 to 3 cm should be considered the minimum when reviewing the preoperative radio-

graphs. Achieving single lung ventilation in young children as well as having an adequate space to work within the chest is a challenge. Children who weigh less than 30 kg have been safely treated with this method;[17] however, the relative benefit of the minimally invasive approach seems to be reduced in very small patients.

If visualization is inadequate at any point during the endoscopic procedure, conversion to an open approach must be considered. It is certainly unwise to proceed with an operation when visualization is compromised. Visualization is most often limited by excessive bleeding or inconsistent lung deflation.

Surgical Technique for Thoracoscopic Disk Excision

Thoracoscopic removal of multiple thoracic disks for the purpose of increasing flexibility of the spine, as mentioned, requires single lung ventilation. The patient is placed in the lateral decubitus position with plans to approach the chest via the convex side of the curve. In the typical right thoracic scoliosis pattern, the right lung is deflated with either a double lumen endotracheal tube or a mainstem bronchial blocker on the right side. There are occasions in which the prone position may be used rather than the lateral decubitus position. In the prone position it is possible to reach the spine endoscopically without complete deflation of the lung. With the lungs hypoventilated, a posterior working space is created that, when combined with a retractor, allows access to the spine. This situation has been found to be less satisfactory than the lateral approach, which allows for more anterior portals and greater access to the concave side of the spine.

In either position, typically three to four portals are used for both visualization and working instruments. Skin incisions (1.5 cm in length) are used to place rigid tubular ports between the ribs along the anterior axillary line. A 10-mm endo-

scope, both with straight-ahead and angled optics, is used for visualization. A 45° angulation of the endoscope provides the best opportunity to see deep within the disk space during disk removal and is recommended over the 30° angulated endoscope. Care should be taken in placing the portals, particularly when placing them distally to avoid penetration below the diaphragm. Upon entering the chest cavity with the endoscope, a fan retractor is often required to provide initial additional displacement and protection of the lung. After establishing the levels of release by counting from the proximal ribs, a longitudinal opening of the pleura is performed using an ultrasonic dissecting device. Segmental vessels may be isolated and preserved or more commonly coagulated with the ultrasonic device. This provides excellent hemostasis and allows circumferential exposure of the spine. The azygos vein, esophagus, and aorta are reflected anteriorly off the spine, and a space between the anterior longitudinal ligament and these structures is maintained by packing sponges within the interval (Figure 1).

Following exposure of the spine, disk excision is initiated after incising the anulus of the disk with an ultrasonic scalpel. Diskectomy is performed using a combination of rongeurs and curets, first removing the most anterior and concave aspects of the anulus. Clear identification of the direction and path of diskectomy is required to avoid removing excessive bone, which will result in additional bleeding and difficulties in visualization. Additional disk material is then removed centrally and on the convex lateral side of the spine. Disk mobility can be confirmed with the use of an end plate shaver. By carefully peeling the end plate cartilage off the vertebral body, in most pediatric patients the disk can be excised with very little bleeding from the vertebral body itself (Figure 2). In patients with osteopenia or when the disk excision inadvertently involves portions of

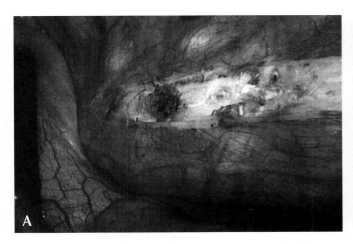

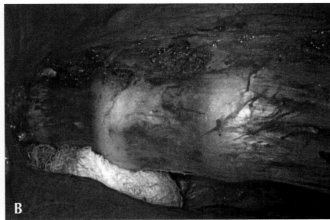

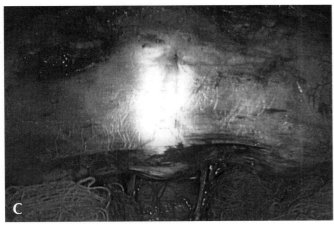

Figure 1 A, Endoscopic view of the midthoracic spine demonstrating a longitudinal incision of the pleura just anterior to the rib heads. The segmental vessels have been divided using the ultrasonic device. **B,** After stripping the pleura from the anterior aspect of the spine, a sponge has been packed in this interval, protecting the azygos vein, aorta, and esophagus. **C,** A close-up view of the concave side of the spine demonstrates that the segmental vessels have been pushed off of the concave lateral aspect of the spine. The view is directly anterior with the margins of the anterior longitudinal ligament easily seen.

the vertebral body, bleeding can make visualization more problematic. The deep aspects of the disk should only be taken under direct visualization, maintaining the integrity of the posterior longitudinal ligament to protect the neural elements. Bone grafting of the disk space can be performed with either autograft or allograft bone, based on the surgeon's preference and requirements of the individual patient. The endoscope and working instruments are moved within the various portals to gain access to each disk space with the rongeur or other working instrument directed inline with the disk space. Following diskectomy and grafting, it is recommended that the pleura be closed with a running suture using the Endo-Stitch (US Surgical, Norwalk, CT) device. The running closure reapproxi-

mates the pleura, minimizing intrathoracic scar and chest tube drainage, while maintaining the graft within the intervertebral spaces.

Results Following Thoracoscopic Release and Fusion

The thoracoscopic method of removing disk and performing anterior interbody fusion is comparable to that of open approaches.[4] There is, however, a substantial learning curve associated with this procedure.[16] The procedure typically requires the skills of both an endoscopic surgeon as well as a spinal surgeon. As with any endoscopic approach, the limitation in direct visualization can be challenging but generally mastered. There have been several studies published in the literature that demonstrate comparable

degrees of disk excision in both clinical series and animal models.[8-11] The safety of the thoracoscopic approach has been evaluated in clinical series with relatively few perioperative complications and rates similar to those for open procedures.[16] The potential complications include excessive bleeding, injury to the lung parenchyma, spinal cord injury, chylothorax, nonunion, and postoperative pulmonary complications typical for anterior thoracic surgery. The surgical time for many of these procedures has been longer than in the open series; however, with experience surgical time has been consistently reduced. In one study, the length of the procedure is comparable to that of an open thoracotomy, with a surgical time of 2 to 2.5 hours.[17] In most series, patients with neuromuscular con-

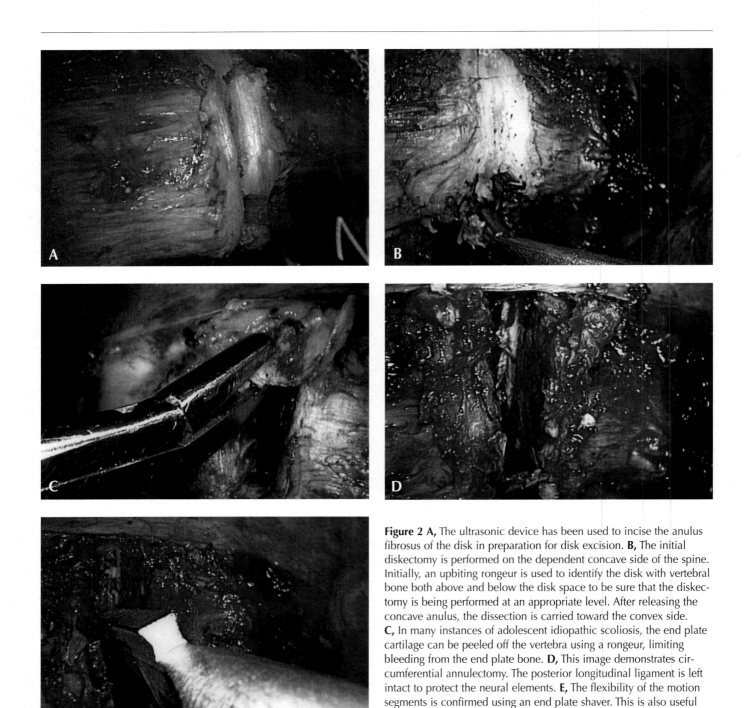

Figure 2 A, The ultrasonic device has been used to incise the anulus fibrosus of the disk in preparation for disk excision. **B,** The initial diskectomy is performed on the dependent concave side of the spine. Initially, an upbiting rongeur is used to identify the disk with vertebral bone both above and below the disk space to be sure that the diskectomy is being performed at an appropriate level. After releasing the concave anulus, the dissection is carried toward the convex side. **C,** In many instances of adolescent idiopathic scoliosis, the end plate cartilage can be peeled off the vertebra using a rongeur, limiting bleeding from the end plate bone. **D,** This image demonstrates circumferential annulectomy. The posterior longitudinal ligament is left intact to protect the neural elements. **E,** The flexibility of the motion segments is confirmed using an end plate shaver. This is also useful for scoring the end plate before placing bone graft to encourage union.

ditions provide the greatest challenges because of curve magnitude, small patient size, preoperative pulmonary compromise, and osteopenia associated with increased blood loss. However, in patients with idiopathic scoliosis, many of these issues are less problematic and outcomes have been similar to open series but without the chest wall dissection required of an open thoracotomy. Anterior fusion rates have been measured and assessed critically, demonstrating that in most of the disk spaces treated with either autograft or allograft some degree of fusion exists.[18] Clinical failures associated with a thoracoscopic anterior release/fusion followed by posterior instrumentation and fusion have been exceedingly rare.

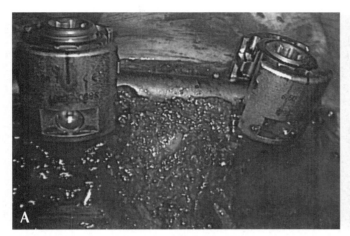

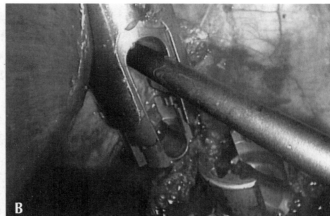

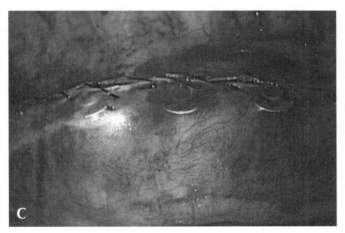

Figure 3 A, This photograph demonstrates the rod having been placed in the proximal two screws of a scoliosis construct. The disk space has been fully packed with autogenous iliac crest bone, which has been placed through a bone mill. Prior to tightening the screw on the left, interbody compression will be performed. **B,** Distally, the rod requires cantilevering to engage the lower screws. An approximating device is used to achieve this aspect of the correction. **C,** This photograph demonstrates the closure of the pleura following multilevel scoliosis instrumentation performed endoscopically.

Indications for Thoracoscopic Anterior Scoliosis Correction

Anterior scoliosis correction has been popularized over the past 10 years with the use of single-rod thoracic constructs placed generally through a thoracotomy approach.[19] These techniques have been adapted for thoracoscopic placement as well. Single structural thoracic scoliosis is generally amenable to a selective fusion of the thoracic curve.[20-22] This may be accomplished by either anterior or posterior methods. The anterior approach has the advantage of typically fewer levels of instrumentation. However, the open anterior approach has had the disadvantages of the morbidity associated with an extensive thoracotomy. As such, the thoracoscopic minimally invasive approach has been developed to limit the morbidi-

ty associated with this approach. The specific curve patterns that are appropriate for such instrumentation include the Lenke 1A, 1B, and 1C curve patterns in which there is reduced or normal kyphosis (see chapter 51). The anterior approach tends to be kyphogenic, and the use of this approach in patients with increased thoracic kyphosis should be avoided. In addition, the approach is believed to be contraindicated in obese patients, who will overstress a single rod anterior construct. The upper limit in weight is roughly 60 to 70 kg. In addition, the approach is contraindicated in very small patients in whom the vertebral bodies have limited ability to maintain the purchase of a vertebral body screw. Curves less than 70° with greater than 50% flexibility are amenable to the thora-

coscopic approach. Larger curves have been instrumented; however, the challenges associated with such curves seem to favor a posterior approach.

Surgical Technique for Anterior Thoracoscopic Scoliosis Correction

The patient is positioned and prepared for surgery just as for a thoracoscopic release and rigidly stabilized in the direct lateral position. The image intensifier is critical for identifying the orientation of each vertebra in the coronal plane within the levels to be instrumented. In this way, the trajectory of each screw can be anticipated before making skin incisions for screw placement. Generally, three portals are required along the posterior axillary line for screw insertion. This is supple-

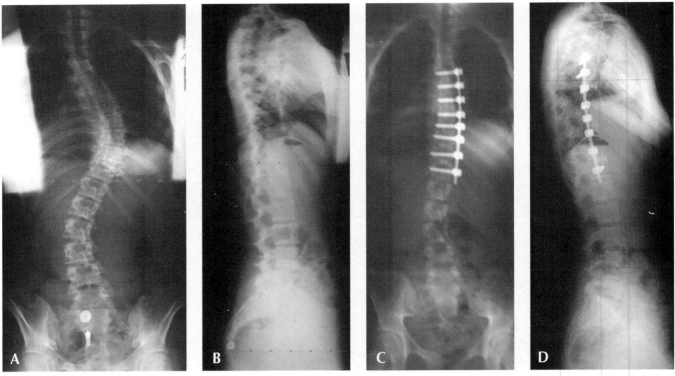

Figure 4 Preoperative standing PA **(A)** and lateral **(B)** radiographs demonstrate the typical right thoracic adolescent idiopathic scoliosis, which is appropriate for thoracoscopic anterior instrumentation. Postoperative PA **(C)** and lateral **(D)** radiographs demonstrate the correction achieved with a thoracoscopic instrumentation system. This was accomplished using five portals. The iliac crest was harvested for graft material, and the patient wore a brace for 3 months postoperatively.

mented by two anterior axillary line portals, which are used during disk excision and for placement of the endoscope. The levels to be instrumented generally include those of the measured Cobb angle. The procedure is initiated by thoracoscopic exposure of the spine and disk excision as described previously. The disk spaces are packed with an oxidized cellulose hemostat to reduce bleeding from the vertebral end plates. Next, screw insertion is initiated proximally. A 15-mm Thoracoport (US Surgical) is placed between the ribs through the proximal skin incision. The starting point for the screw is in the mid to superior aspect of the vertebral body just anterior to the rib head articulation with the vertebral body. An awl is used to initiate the hole, followed by a tap. The screw path is tapped through the far cortex, and using a ball-tipped calibrated probe the exact length of the screw is determined. Typically, 6.5-mm diameter screws are used. Moving the portal one rib space distally, the adjacent screw is placed in similar fashion, with care being taken to appropriately align each screw to make later rod insertion as straightforward as possible. Each of the screws should be placed with bicortical purchase; however, excessive screw penetration should be avoided, given the location of the aorta on the left side of the vertebral bodies. Following screw placement, each of the disk spaces should be grafted with autogenous bone, from either the iliac crest or rib. At more distal levels, the interspace may require structural support, in which case an interbody device or cortical allograft is used. Deformity correction is accomplished by cantilevering a rod into position, beginning by engaging the proximal screws first. Segmental compression is performed at each of the levels with an endoscopic compressing device. This combination of rod cantilevering facilitated with an approximating device and segmental vertebral body compression provide coronal plane correction of the scoliosis, sagittal restoration of kyphosis, and axial plane derotation of the spine. Following rod insertion, the pleura may be closed with a running suture (Figure 3).

Outcomes of Thoracoscopic Anterior Scoliosis Correction

The thoracoscopic method of anterior scoliosis correction remains relatively new, but follow-up data are limited. In 1998, Picetti and associates[23] first reported on the clinical use of a thoracoscopic anterior scoliosis system. The worldwide experience since then has been increasing.[24,25] In the author's initial experience, curve correction has averaged 60%, with operating time averaging 5.5 hours.[24] The number of vertebra instrumented in such constructs has ranged from six to nine levels, with the uppermost instrumented vertebra being T4 and the distal most level being L1. The author continues to brace thoracoscopically instrumented patients for 3 months postoperatively; with this protocol, one instance of rod failure has occurred in the first 30 idiopathic cases performed (follow-up of 2 years or longer). Comparative studies of anterior and posterior approaches have suggested similar degrees of deformity correction when curve patterns were matched.[24] Complication rates, however, have been greater in nearly all surgeons' initial experience with the technique. This approach remains technically demanding and requires thorough disk excision and grafting to obtain early solid union (Figure 4).

The functional benefits associated with the thoracoscopic approach have begun to be quantified. Shoulder girdle strength and range of motion return to normal within 3 to 6 months following surgery. This is a more rapid return than noted in open anterior procedures. In addition, the reduction in pulmonary function following thoracoscopic instrumentation is less than that associated with open anterior instrumentation (Figure 5). All of these data suggest that there are benefits to the thoracoscopic approach that may be realized once the surgeon is able to master the technique.

Summary

The role of thoracoscopy in the treatment of pediatric spinal deformity is evolving, and surgeon experience with the technique continues to grow. Early reports of this approach suggested its safety and efficacy. Refinements in the technique and instrumentation used for

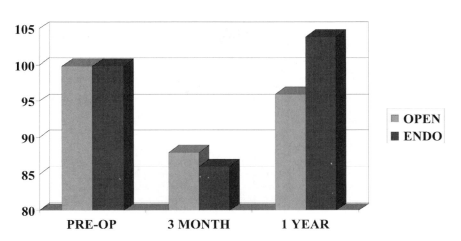

Figure 5 This graph represents the reduction in pulmonary function, as a percentage of preoperative value (y-axis), associated with open and thoracoscopic (endoscopic) anterior scoliosis correction. At 1 year, the thoracoscopic group has returned to greater than baseline forced vital capacity, whereas the open anterior instrumentation patients have not completely recovered to baseline. The difference in the return of function between these two groups is statistically significant. Pre-op = preoperative; endo = endoscopic.

this surgery will also continue to evolve. There is room for cautious optimism with regard to the continued development of this field. The approach requires the careful selection of patients and a surgeon with the appropriate temperament and judgment to negotiate the challenges of the early learning curve. It is likely that continued advances with this technique will reduce the learning curve and allow this technique to have greater indications in the future.

References

1. Dickman CA, Karahalios DG: Thoracoscopic spinal surgery. *Clin Neurosurg* 1996;43:392-422.

2. Mack MJ, Regan JJ, Bobechko WP, et al: Application of thoracoscopy for diseases of the spine. *Ann Thorac Surg* 1993;56:736-738.

3. Dickman CA, Rosenthal D, Karahalios DG, et al: Thoracic vertebrectomy and reconstruction using a microsurgical thoracoscopic approach. *Neurosurgery* 1996;38:279-293.

4. Newton PO, Wenger DR, Mubarak SJ, et al: Anterior release and fusion in pediatric spinal deformity: A comparison of early outcome and cost of thoracoscopic and open thoracotomy approaches. *Spine* 1997;22:1398-1406.

5. Crawford AH, Wall EJ, Wolf R: Video-assisted thoracoscopy. *Orthop Clin North Am* 1999;30:367-385.

6. Waisman M, Saute M: Thoracoscopic spine release before posterior instrumentation in scoliosis. *Clin Orthop* 1997:130-136.

7. Kokoska ER, Gabriel KR, Silen ML: Minimally invasive anterior spinal exposure and release in children with scoliosis. *J Soc Laparoendosc Surg* 1998;2:255-258.

8. Wall EJ, Bylski-Austrow DI, Shelton FS, et al: Endoscopic discectomy increases thoracic spine flexibility as effectively as open discectomy: A mechanical study in a porcine model. *Spine* 1998;23:9-15.

9. Newton PO, Cardelia JM, Farnsworth CL, et al: A biomechanical comparison of open and thoracoscopic anterior spinal release in a goat model. *Spine* 1998;23:530-535.

10. Huntington CF, Murrell WD, Betz RR, et al: Comparison of thoracoscopic and open thoracic discectomy in a live ovine model for anterior spinal fusion. *Spine* 1998;23:1699-1702.

11. Connolly PJ, Ordway NR, Sacks T, et al: Video-assisted thoracic diskectomy and anterior release: A biomechanical analysis of an endoscopic technique. *Orthopedics* 1999;22:923-926.

12. Dubousset J, Herring JA, Shufflebarger H: The crankshaft phenomenon. *J Pediatr Orthop* 1989;9:541-550.

13. Sanders JO, Little DG, Richards BS: Prediction of the crankshaft phenomenon by peak height velocity. *Spine* 1997;22:1352-1356.

14. Gonzalez Barrios I, Fuentes Caparros S, Avila Jurado MM: Anterior thoracoscopic epiphysiodesis in the treatment of a crankshaft phenomenon. *Eur Spine J* 1995;4:343-346.

15. Lapinksy AS, Richards BS: Preventing the crankshaft phenomenon by combining anterior fusion with posterior instrumentation. Does it work? *Spine* 1995;20:1392-1398.

16. Newton PO, Shea KG, Granlund KF: Defining the pediatric spinal thoracoscopy learning curve: sixty-five consecutive cases. *Spine* 2000;25:1028-1035.

17. Early SD, Newton PO, White KK, et al: The feasibility of anterior thoracoscopic spine surgery in children under 30 kilograms. *Spine* 2002;27:2368-2373.

18. Newton PO, Faro F, Gaynor TP, et al: Anterior fusion after thoracoscopic disc excision: Analysis of 112 consecutive deformity cases. *71st Annual Meeting Proceedings*. Rosemont, IL, American Academy of Orthopaedic Surgeons, 2004, p 541.

19. Betz RR, Harms J, Clements DH, et al: Comparison of anterior and posterior instrumentation for correction of adolescent thoracic idiopathic scoliosis. *Spine* 1999;24:225-239.

20. Newton PO, Faro FD, Lenke LG, et al: Factors involved in the decision to perform a selective versus nonselective fusion of Lenke 1B and 1C (King-Moe II) curves in adolescent idiopathic scoliosis. *Spine* 2003;28:S217-S223.

21. Lenke LG, Betz RR, Clements D, et al: Curve prevalence of a new classification of operative adolescent idiopathic scoliosis: does classification correlate with treatment? *Spine* 2002;27:604-611.

22. Lenke LG, Betz RR, Bridwell KH, et al: Spontaneous lumbar curve coronal correction after selective anterior or posterior thoracic fusion in adolescent idiopathic scoliosis. *Spine* 1999;24:1663-1671.

23. Picetti G III, Blackman RG, O'Neal K, et al: Anterior endoscopic correction and fusion of scoliosis. *Orthopedics* 1998;21:1285-1287.

24. Newton PO, Marks M, Faro F, et al: Use of video-assisted thoracoscopic surgery to reduce perioperative morbidity in scoliosis surgery. *Spine* 2003;28:S249-S254.

25. Sucato DJ: Thoracoscopic anterior instrumentation and fusion for idiopathic scoliosis. *J Am Acad Orthop Surg* 2003;11:221-227.

Nonsurgical Treatment of Kyphosis

Peter D. Pizzutillo, MD

Abstract

An increase in thoracic kyphosis in children and adolescents is usually the result of postural kyphosis or Scheuermann's kyphosis. Although no structural deformity of the spine is observed in postural kyphosis, wedging of vertebral bodies and disk space narrowing are noted radiographically in patients with Scheuermann's kyphosis. Effective interventions for adolescents with postural kyphosis include exercises to relieve lower extremity contractures and strengthen abdominal musculature coupled with practiced normal posture in stance and in sitting. Skeletally immature patients with Scheuermann's kyphosis benefit from a similar exercise program but also require the use of a spinal orthosis. Bracing of the spine in patients with Scheuermann's kyphosis results in permanent correction of vertebral deformity, unlike bracing in patients with idiopathic scoliosis. The evaluation of children and adolescents with increased thoracic kyphosis is an important aspect of the decision process used to determine appropriate interventions.

The term kyphosis is derived from the Greek work kyphos, meaning humpbacked, and refers to the posterior rounding of the spine when viewed from the side. Conversely, lordosis refers to the anterior curving of the spine in the sagittal plane. In the past 2 decades, there have been extensive efforts to better understand and define the sagittal alignment of the human spine.[1-5] Although this work may have been initiated to improve surgical techniques for correction of spinal deformity, the observations have had broader applications for understanding the normal human spine and its development at various stages of growth and development. The normal mature pattern of sagittal alignment of the spine is established by 6 years of age. The average cervical lordosis, measured from C2 to C7, is 15°; thoracic kyphosis, measured from T5 to T12 ranges between 20° and 40°; and lumbar lordosis, measured from L1 to L5, ranges between 20° and 55°.

A host of clinical problems may result in increased or decreased kyphosis. Although congenital, neuromuscular, infectious, iatrogenic, and neoplastic etiologies exist, the most common causes of increased kyphosis are postural kyphosis and Scheuermann's kyphosis. Decreased kyphosis or flattening of the thoracic spine is observed in patients with bone dysplasia, myopathy, myelodysplasia, idiopathic scoliosis, congenital scoliosis, and as a secondary deformity in association with severe spondylolisthesis and lumbar Scheuermann's disease. Decreased kyphosis may create significant cosmetic concerns because of the flat appearance of the back; of even greater importance is the development of restrictive pulmonary disorder that has implications for impaired health and decreased longevity.

Postural Kyphosis

Increased kyphosis in the preadolescent and adolescent patient often causes parental anxiety because of the child's development of back pain or the possibility of permanent spinal deformity. Patients with postural kyphosis are readily identified because of their ability to voluntarily correct their deformity. They are asymptomatic, unconcerned about the appearance of their back, and may be tall for their peer group. Early breast development is also a common reason for adolescent girls to stand with a round-back posture. The older adolescent female, with ponderous breasts and increased thoracic kyphosis, may experience significant upper back pain that will require intervention. Strengthening exercises for the upper back and abdominal muscles, the use of a supportive figure-of-8 brace, or breast reduction may be indicated for relief of pain.

Physical examination of the erect patient shows forward posturing of the shoulders, gentle posterior rounding of the thoracic spine, increased lumbar lordosis, and mild protuberance of the abdomen. The increased thoracic kyphosis and lumbar lordosis are flexible. No focal areas of back deformity, tenderness, or spasm are found. Physical examination also reveals contracture of the pectoral and hamstring muscle groups and weakness of the abdominal muscles.

Radiographic evaluation of the spine is not necessary in postural kyphosis unless there is concern that structural changes may be present. The AP radiograph taken with the patient in an erect position is normal. Standing lateral radiographs of the thoracic and lumbar spine may show increased dorsal kyphosis, but no vertebral body wedging, end plate irregularity, disk space narrowing, or Schmorl's nodes will be observed. In clinical practice, there is great variation in the quality of standing lateral radiographs of the spine. Radiologic techniques may result in overexposure or underexposure with resultant difficulty in seeing clear anatomic landmarks for measurement of curve magnitude. The interobserver error in measurement of lateral radiographs of the spine is 11°.[6] In addition, unorthodox positioning of the upper extremities as well as the tendency to lean forward or backward will alter the true spinal curve measurements. The current positioning technique requires the patient to stand erect with hips and knees in extension and with the arms resting comfortably at shoulder height on a crossbar positioned directly in front of the patient. Positioning for more reliable and reproducible evaluation

of lateral radiographs of the spine is currently under investigation.

The motivated patient is able to correct the postural kyphosis by practicing more normal posture and by performing exercises to stretch contracted pectoral and hamstring muscles and strengthen abdominal muscles. The use of figure-of-8 straps or spinal orthoses is not indicated in this patient population. An exercise program, which eliminates contracture and weakness, will facilitate the patient's efforts to stand in a more normal posture. There is no evidence that persistence of postural kyphosis will result in the development of fixed spinal deformity or an increased risk for back pain.

Scheuermann's Kyphosis

Scheuermann's kyphosis refers to the condition characterized by increased posterior rounding of the thoracic spine in association with structural deformity of the vertebral elements. Multiple theories on the etiology of Scheuermann's kyphosis have suggested osteonecrosis of the vertebral ring apophyses, intrinsic weakness of the cartilaginous end plate, osteochondrosis, transient osteoporosis, malabsorption, infection, and endocrine disorders as contributing factors; none have been established as the primary cause. Histologic evaluations of vertebrae from patients with Scheuermann's kyphosis have not confirmed the presence of osteoporosis or osteonecrosis; however, altered endochondral ossification in the vertebral end plates and growth cartilage has been found, which results in abnormal longitudinal growth of the end plate.[7] These biologic alterations may then be worsened by mechanical factors that increase compressive forces on the anterior portion of the vertebral body. Although familial incidence of

this condition has been recognized, recent studies suggest that Scheuermann's kyphosis is inherited by a major gene allele model in which all male carriers of the mutant gene and one half of the female carriers will manifest the kyphosis.[8] The study group showed a higher frequency of scoliosis with 0.08 per 1,000 compared with 0.02 per 1,000 for the general population.

Scheuermann's kyphosis occurs more often in males and typically develops between 10 and 14 years of age. Preadolescent and adolescent patients seek evaluation for increased rounding of the thoracic spine and infrequently report back pain. When pain is present, it is usually localized at the interscapular area. Parental concerns primarily involve cosmetic deformity, progressive spinal deformity, and the possible development of back pain in the asymptomatic patient.

The natural history of patients with Scheuermann's kyphosis has been reported by several investigators. Progression of deformity has been documented by Travaglini and Conte[9] who noted increased structural spinal changes in 40 of 50 untreated patients who had been followed for 25 years. Pain developed more frequently in those patients with thoracolumbar kyphosis; however, no significant functional problems were noted. Lowe[10] reported that, with deformity less than 75°, no long-term disability or significant pain problems should be expected. Murray and associates'[11] review indicated that low back pain occurs in patients with Scheuermann's kyphosis but patients do not experience a major effect on life activities. No correlations were found for pain that interfered with activities of daily living, numbness of lower extremities, use of medication for back pain, level of recreational activity, fatigue, self-esteem, social limitations, occupation, sick leave usage, psychologic disorders, or cardiopulmonary insufficiency when comparing patients with Scheuermann's kyphosis with a control group. Spondylolisthesis was not observed in their study population.

Physical examination of the standing patient shows findings similar to those seen in postural kyphosis except for the inability to voluntarily correct the deformity. Young patients, who are referred for evaluation after school screening for scoliosis, may show a mild thoracic scoliosis but may also exhibit a previously undetected increase in thoracic kyphosis. In the erect position, increased thoracic kyphosis with sloping shoulders and forward posturing of the head and neck and increased lumbar lordosis will be seen. The Adam's forward flexion test is used to critically observe the patient from behind to detect truncal asymmetry associated with scoliosis. Although forward flexion of the back is typically restricted in these patients, examination from the side is important because increases in thoracic kyphosis will be exaggerated and easier to identify (Figure 1). Patients with Scheuermann's kyphosis will show abrupt posterior angulation of a segment of the thoracic spine compared with the harmonious curvature of the normal flexed spine. A frequently observed pattern of deformity in forward flexion is that of a sharply angulated, short segment kyphosis of the midthoracic spine with flattening of the upper thoracic spine and loss of reversal of the lumbar spine. A less common pattern of deformity is the sharply angulated kyphosis that is centered at the low thoracic or thoracolumbar junction and is associated with marked hypokyphosis of the

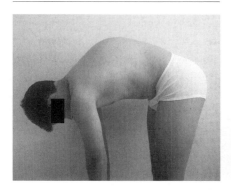

Figure 1 In forward flexion, dorsal kyphosis is accentuated and more easily detected.

upper thoracic spine. The latter pattern is usually evident on observation of the erect patient and results in greater cosmetic deformity.

The patient with Scheuermann's kyphosis is not able to voluntarily correct the sagittal deformity of the spine. When the patient is examined prone or supine, it is difficult to passively correct the increased kyphosis by direct pressure, whereas the increased lumbar lordosis may be reversible. Increased lordosis of the cervical spine is cosmetically objectionable and may become fixed. Contracture of the pectoral and hamstring muscle groups is common, as is weakness of the abdominal and upper paraspinal muscle groups. Neurologic evaluation is normal.

Standing AP radiographs of the spine will show scoliosis of the thoracic or thoracolumbar spine. Scoliosis associated with Scheuermann's kyphosis is characterized by a thoracic curve that is not progressive and rarely exceeds a 25° Cobb angle. This radiographic view also provides an estimate of skeletal maturity by inspection of the Risser sign.

A standing lateral radiograph of the spine will show thoracic kyphosis greater than 40° with anterior wedg-

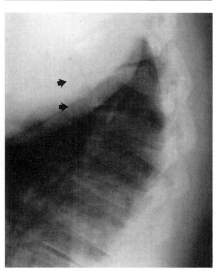

Figure 2 A lateral radiograph shows wedging of vertebrae with end plate irregularities and Schmorl's nodes (*arrows*).

ing of three or more vertebral bodies, end plate irregularities, disk space narrowing, and Schmorl's nodes (Figure 2). There is also a concomitant increase in cervical lordosis and lumbar lordosis. Attention to the increased lordosis of the cervical spine associated with Scheuermann's kyphosis has not been emphasized in medical literature. Loder[2] studied the sagittal profile of the cervical and lumbar spine in children with Scheuermann's kyphosis to determine whether significant correlations existed. He found that the flexible cervical and lumbar areas are linked by a rigid intermediate thoracic segment. As the residual sagittal difference (for example, thoracic kyphosis/lumbar lordosis) became more kyphotic, the cervical lordosis became more lordotic. Significant fixed deformity of the cervical spine may be an important limiting factor in the surgical correction of the thoracic kyphosis.

When the initial clinical and radiographic evaluation is consistent with a diagnosis of Scheuermann's kyphosis in a skeletally immature patient, brace treatment may be considered. The use of a cross-table stress lateral radiographic view of the spine, which passively extends the kyphos, provides helpful information to determine the appropriateness of bracing for a given patient. The stress radiograph is obtained by placing the patient supine with a bolster positioned at or below the apex of the kyphosis. The patient should be resting comfortably with hips and knees flexed to control the lumbar spine. The weight of the freely hanging head and upper back provide the force needed to passively extend the thoracic spine. After a 5-minute period, a cross-table lateral radiograph is obtained in the stress position. It is important to measure the stress lateral radiograph at the same vertebral landmarks as the previously obtained standing lateral radiograph.

If the kyphosis is flexible and reduces to less than 40° on the stress radiograph, brace treatment may be initiated. If the kyphosis remains more than 40°, there is a decreased likelihood of success with the use of bracing. In the patient with rigid kyphosis that exceeds 50°, surgical intervention may be more appropriate.

In an immature patient with rigid kyphosis that does not reduce to less than 40° on the stress lateral radiograph, serial casting may result in reduction of kyphosis to normal parameters that would then allow application of a brace. An underarm cast is applied with the patient supine on a Risser table with hips and knees in flexed position to reduce the lumbar lordosis; the cast is molded well over the pectorals anteriorly. By using a muslin strap that is positioned under the apex of the kyphosis, a posterior mold is created to provide strong anterior forces directed at passive correction of the kyphosis. The

patient will require cast changes every 2 weeks until the thoracic kyphosis is reduced to less than 40°. At that time, the patient may be transitioned from cast to brace treatment.

Brace treatment for patients with Scheuermann's kyphosis includes a regular program of physical therapy to complement the effects of bracing. Stretching of pectoral muscles, lumbosacral fascia, and hamstring muscles is uniformly indicated. Supine hyperextension maneuvers over a bolster or exercise ball aid in stretching the thoracic spine and are helpful in achieving passive correction. Strengthening of thoracic paraspinal muscles and abdominal muscles is important for maintenance of good postural alignment.

Orthotic treatment of Scheuermann's kyphosis is indicated in the skeletally immature patient with progressive kyphosis, unacceptable cosmesis, or kyphosis greater than 60° that is flexible. The goals of orthotic treatment include the prevention of increasing deformity, the reduction of compressive forces on the anterior aspect of the vertebral bodies to foster restoration of vertebral height, the reduction of hyperlordosis of the lumbar spine, and the restoration of normal sagittal alignment of the spine. Orthotic treatment of patients with idiopathic scoliosis can prevent curve progression but does not offer the likelihood of curve correction. Orthotic treatment of patients with Scheuermann's kyphosis not only prevents curve progression but may result in significant curve correction.

The Milwaukee brace is the most commonly used brace for the treatment of Scheuermann's disease. It is indicated when the apex of the kyphosis is at or above T8 and for the overweight patient or the female patient with large breasts. The pelvic

girdle serves as the base for the superstructure and decreases the lumbar lordosis. Posterior pads are positioned at or just below the apex of the kyphosis but should not be placed above the apex where they would apply forces that block correction or increase deformity. The Milwaukee brace neck ring and occipital pads are rarely used.

The underarm orthosis or thoracolumbosacral orthosis (TLSO) is indicated in the trim patient when the apex of the kyphosis is at or below T9. The anterior upper portion of the TLSO is molded tightly to the sternal area or is augmented with shoulder outrigger extensions. As the patient's kyphosis becomes more flexible, the shoulder outriggers may be adjusted or anterior chest pads may be added to the TLSO to obtain more correction in the brace. The upper border of the posterior aspect of the TLSO is trimmed at the level of the apex of the kyphosis and the lower portion of the TLSO is molded to decrease lumbar lordosis (Figure 3).

Treatment protocols for brace treatment of Scheuermann's kyphosis are similar for all of the spinal orthoses and all include a concomitant exercise regimen. Wear time varies from 16 to 22 hours per day. Earlier treatment programs recommended continued bracing until vertebral ring apophyses were fused; more recent studies suggest that weaning from brace usage may proceed rapidly when Risser 4 capping of the iliac crest is observed.[12]

Sachs and associates[12] reported on 120 patients with an established diagnosis of Scheuermann's kyphosis who were treated with the Milwaukee brace and reevaluated at least 5 years after completion of treatment. Ten patients showed no change in kyphosis when final radiographic studies were compared with initial studies. Seventy-six patients had improvement in the kyphosis and 24 patients had more kyphosis than found in their initial studies. Ten patients did not fully comply with the recommended brace treatment and were included in the failure group of 44 patients; ie, 37% of the 120 in the study sample group. One third of patients with initial kyphosis of 75° or greater subsequently underwent surgical treatment. The authors noted a 41% correction of the prebrace kyphosis with 69% maintenance of correction when evaluated 5 years after completion of brace wear.

Gutowski and Renshaw[13] reported the results of 41 patients with Scheuermann's kyphosis who were treated with either a Milwaukee or Boston brace. The authors noted significant difficulty in determining actual hours of brace usage and documented a progressive degradation in curve improvement with 30% correction recorded at evaluation 2 years after completion of brace wear.

Ponte and associates[14,15] reported the results of using antigravity and localizer-type casts in 1,043 patients with Scheuermann's kyphosis. Patients with mean initial curves of 57° were treated in casts from 8 to 16 months with 40% improvement. Subsequent treatment included night wear of a Milwaukee brace and physical therapy until maturity. At 3-year follow-up, an average 62% mean wedge improvement was observed, thus suggesting that prolonged use of the Milwaukee brace lessens the loss of correction.

The nonsurgical treatment of Scheuermann's kyphosis is effective if brace treatment is pursued in the skeletally immature patient with flexible kyphosis less than 74° (Figure 4). The best results have been

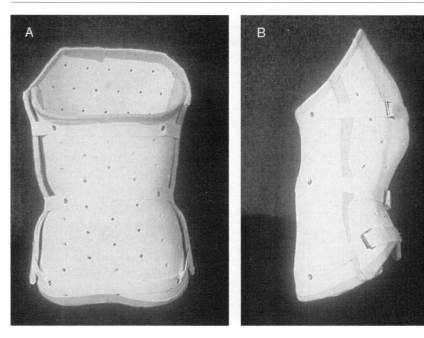

Figure 3 A and **B,** A clamshell TLSO molded to decrease lumbar lordosis and to decrease dorsal kyphosis.

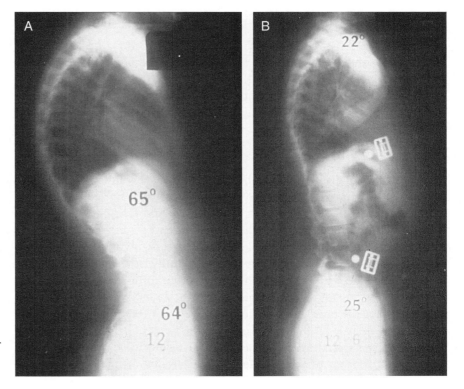

Figure 4 A, A standing lateral radiograph of the spine shows 65° of thoracic kyphosis. **B,** A standing lateral radiograph of the spine in a TLSO show reduction of dorsal kyphosis and lumbar lordosis.

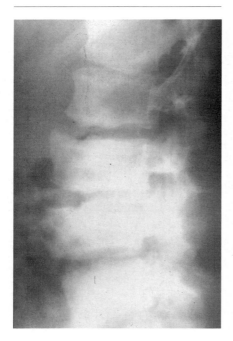

Figure 5 Lateral radiograph of the thoracolumbar spine shows anterosuperior segmental defects of the vertebral body with significant enlargement of involved vertebral bodies.

achieved with full-time use of the Milwaukee brace program. With more rigid kyphosis (more than 75°) surgical intervention becomes more appropriate.

Lumbar Scheuermann's Disease

Adolescent patients with lumbar Scheuermann's disease typically have insidious onset of severe low back pain that is unrelated to activity.[16] Progressive increase in severity of pain precludes involvement in athletic activities and may even interfere with activities of daily living. Radiation of pain to the buttocks or lower extremities, night pain that awakens the patient, and episodes of sphincter dysfunction are not present in this population. These patients are in good health and have no prior experience of similar back pain. In general, although significant deformity

may be obvious on physical examination, neither the patients nor their family members will initially report cosmetic concerns.

Physical examination reveals significant flattening of the lumbar lordosis with a thoracolumbar kyphosis. In more advanced stages of this disorder, the patient may exhibit kyphosis of the lumbar spine and compensatory thoracic lordosis. Although true muscle spasm is not usually present, the rigidity of the flat lumbar region may suggest spasm. Spinal movement is painful and markedly limited in flexion, extension, and rotation. No scoliosis is noted, and the neurologic evaluation is normal. No tenderness is noted with palpation of the sacroiliac joints or the sciatic notch. Severe contracture of the hamstrings is present with no evidence of knee flexion contractures.

Standing AP radiographs of the spine usually will not show scoliosis. If a mild curvature is noted, there is usually no rotational change. Standing lateral radiographs of the spine show marked distortions from normal sagittal alignment. The lumbar spine is minimally lordotic to kyphotic with a concomitant kyphotic deformity at the thoracolumbar junction. Scalloped, lucent defects are noted at the anterosuperior corner of involved vertebral bodies (Figure 5). Schmorl's nodes are not typical but end plate irregularities may be seen. The involved vertebrae are significantly larger in the AP dimension when compared with more normal vertebral bodies.

Orthotic treatment is indicated for the relief of pain and to halt progressive deformity of the spine. The TLSO used for patients with lumbar Scheuermann's disease is molded or padded in a manner to encourage more normal lumbar lordosis compared with the TLSO used in pa-

tients with Scheuermann's kyphosis. In the author's experience, low back pain quickly subsides with brace treatment. The patient is instructed to wear the brace between 16 and 22 hours per day for a period of 18 months in conjunction with an exercise program of abdominal strengthening and hamstring stretching exercises.

Brace treatment quickly relieves pain and stimulates bone formation in the lucent defects of the anterosuperior corner of vertebral bodies but has been ineffective in improving the sagittal alignment of the spine.

Lumbar Scheuermann's disease is not hereditary but is believed to be caused by anterior herniation of disk material under the anterior longitudinal ligament.[17] Longitudinal studies of patients with lumbar Scheuermann's kyphosis are not available but concern exists for future disk degeneration in this population.

Summary

Increased roundback deformity of the upper back or kyphosis may be postural or structural in nature. Patients with postural kyphosis will respond to an exercise program, whereas those with Scheuermann's kyphosis will demonstrate improved spinal alignment and relief of pain after a combined program of exercises and bracing.

References

1. Bernhardt M: Spinal anatomy: Normal sagittal plane alignment, in Bridwell KH, DeWald RL (eds): *The Textbook of Spinal Surgery*, ed 2. Philadelphia, PA, Lippincott-Raven, 1997, pp 185-191.

2. Loder RT: The sagittal profile of the cervical and lumbosacral spine in Scheuermann thoracic kyphosis. *J Spinal Disord* 2001;14:226-231.

3. Propst-Poctor L, Bleck EE: Radiographic determination of lordosis and kyphosis in normal and scoliotic children. *J Pediatr Orthop* 1983;3:344-346.

4. Stagnara P, De Mauroy JC, Dran G, et al: Reciprocal angulation of vertebral bodies in the sagittal plane: Approach to references for the evaluation of kyphosis and lordosis. *Spine* 1982;7:335-342.

5. Voutsinas SA, MacEwen GD: Sagittal profiles of the spine. *Clin Orthop* 1986;210:235-242.

6. Stotts AK, Smith JT, Santora SD, Roach JW, D'Astous JL: Measurement of spinal kyphosis: Implications for the management of Scheuermann's kyphosis. *Spine* 2002;27:2143-2146.

7. Ippolito E, Ponseti IV: Juvenile kyphosis: Histologic and histochemical studies. *J Bone Joint Surg Am* 1981;63:175-182.

8. Axenovich TI, Zaidman AM, Zorkoltseva IV, Kalashnikova EV, Borodin PM: Segregation analysis of Scheuermann disease in ninety families from Siberia. *Am J Med Genet* 2001;100:275-279.

9. Travaglini F, Conte M: Untreated kyphosis: 25 years later, in *Kyphosis*. Bologna, Italy, Italian Scoliosis Research Group, 1984, pp 21-27.

10. Lowe TG: Scheuermann's disease. *Orthop Clin North Am* 1999;30:475-487.

11. Murray PM, Weinstein SL, Spratt KF: The natural history and long-term follow-up of Scheuermann kyphosis. *J Bone Joint Surg Am* 1993;75:236-248.

12. Sachs B, Bradford DS, Winter R, Lonstein J, Moe J, Willson S: Scheuermann kyphosis: Follow-up of Milwaukee brace treatment. *J Bone Joint Surg Am* 1987;69:50-57.

13. Gutowski WT, Renshaw TS: Orthotic results in adolescent kyphosis. *Spine* 1988;13:485-489.

14. Ponte A, Gebbia F, Eliseo F: Nonoperative treatment of adolescent hyperkyphosis. *Annual Meeting Proceedings*. Milwaukee, WI, Scoliosis Research Society, 1984.

15. Ponte A, Vero B: Siccardi Gl, et al: Ipercifosi Dell' adolescenza: Il trattamento incruento. *Prog Pat Vert* 1988;12:85.

16. Edgren W, Vaino S: Osteochondrosis juvenilis lumbalis. *Acta Chir Scand Suppl* 1957;227:1.

17. Blumenthal SL, Roach J, Herring JA: Lumbar Scheuermann's: A clinical series and classification. *Spine* 1987;12:929-932.

Kyphosis of the Thoracic and Thoracolumbar Spine in the Pediatric Patient: Surgical Treatment

Thomas G. Lowe, MD

Abstract

Kyphosis of the thoracic or thoracolumbar spine is a common deformity in pediatric and adolescent populations. When it progresses to the point at which nonsurgical treatment is no longer an option, surgery is indicated. Surgical options available for the treatment of different types of pediatric kyphosis of the thoracic and thoracolumbar spine include posterior instrumentation and fusion, posterior instrumentation and fusion combined with anterior fusion, and anterior instrumentation and fusion.

Two basic patterns of kyphosis are found in pediatric patients: nonfixed and fixed. Nonfixed kyphosis, the most common pattern, is a rounded, flexible deformity commonly associated with postural kyphosis and Scheuermann's disease. Nonfixed kyphosis is rarely associated with neurologic compromise. Progression of the deformity and/or significant pain in adults may occur when kyphosis is greater than 80° in the thoracic spine or greater than 50° in the thoracolumbar spine. Kyphosis of lesser degree rarely results in progressive deformity or significant pain.

Fixed kyphosis is an angular, rigid deformity that is often associated with congenital kyphosis, neurofibromatosis, postlaminectomy kyphosis, and infectious diseases of the spine. This curve pattern has a high incidence of neurologic compromise if a high degree of deformity develops and is untreated.[1,2] Progression of fixed kyphosis into adulthood is an unpredictable but frequent sequelae.

Differences in pediatric kyphotic deformities are based on the location of the apex of the deformity. Kyphosis, which occurs in the thoracic spine, is inherently stable because of the rib cage, and pulmonary complications are rare unless kyphosis exceeds 100°.[3-5] Pediatric patients who seek surgical treatment for thoracic kyphosis usually do so because of pain, progression of the deformity, or poor cosmesis.[3,4] Thoracolumbar kyphosis has a much higher incidence of progression because of the lack of support provided by surrounding musculature. When the deformity exceeds 50° to 55°, sagittal imbalance and pain are common, and the deformity is readily apparent.

Clinical Evaluation

Preoperative clinical evaluation should include a history of the onset and progression of the deformity, degree of severity, and location of associated pain. The flexibility, severity, and location of the deformity and any associated coronal deformity should be carefully assessed. When any cutaneous lesions, foot deformities, or muscle contractures are present, a complete neurologic examination should be done to determine the etiology of the deformity and the urgency of treatment.

Diagnostic Studies

Routine preoperative radiographic studies should include standing PA and lateral 36-inch radiographs as well as a supine hyperextension bolster lateral at the level of the apex of the deformity. A preoperative MRI should be obtained for patients with atypical or rapidly progressive kyphosis, any neurologic signs and symptoms, or congenital kyphosis or neurofibromatosis. A three-dimensional CT with coronal and sagittal reconstruction should be obtained for patients with

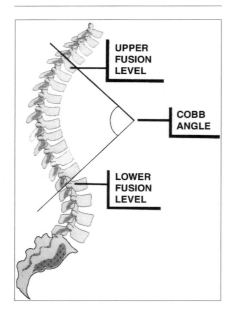

Figure 1 The degree of kyphosis is determined by measuring the intersecting lines of the most tilted vertebrae above and below the apex of the deformity. Levels of fusion should include the upper Cobb vertebra and the first lordotic vertebra and the first lordotic vertebra below the lower Cobb vertebra. (Reproduced with permission from Lowe TG: Scheuermann's disease, in Bridwell K, DeWald R (eds): *The Textbook of Spinal Surgery.* Philadelphia, PA, Lippincott-Raven, 1997, pp 1173-1198.)

congenital deformities for preoperative planning.

Large Radius Kyphosis
Surgical Indications and Options
Surgical indications for large radius, flexible kyphosis include thoracic kyphosis greater than 80° or thoracolumbar kyphosis greater than 50° and progression of the deformity despite brace treatment, thoracic back pain interfering with activities of daily living, or cosmetic deformity that the surgeon, patient, and patient's family believe to be significant.[4] Unusual indications include pulmonary or neurologic compromise, both of which would be un-

usual in kyphosis less than 100°.

Surgical options for large radius kyphosis include posterior instrumentation and fusion alone, posterior instrumentation and fusion combined with anterior fusion, and occasionally anterior instrumentation and fusion alone.

Posterior Instrumentation and Fusion Posterior instrumentation and fusion is useful in the skeletally immature individual with a flexible deformity. Because of remaining anterior vertebral body growth, continued anterior growth will frequently occur, creating a stable anterior column for load sharing. Posterior instrumentation and fusion should also be considered for skeletally mature individuals in whom the deformity corrects to less than 50° on the hyperextension bolster lateral radiograph. Levels of posterior instrumentation, shown in Figure 1, should include the upper and lower Cobb levels and the first lordotic level distally to minimize the risk of junctional kyphosis.[6] If there is a significant associated thoracolumbar coronal deformity, a lower level of instrumentation may be required.

The basic posterior instrumentation construct should include a minimum of eight anchors above and below the apex of the kyphosis. Pedicle screws below the apex provide better fixation than hooks. Above the apex, either two double-level, pedicle-transverse process claws with hooks (Figure 2) or five or six pedicle screws on each side (Figure 3) provide the best fixation. Smooth 5.5- to 6.0-mm rods are first contoured to the anticipated corrected kyphosis based on the hyperextension lateral radiograph. The rods are then inserted into the hooks or screws above the apex of the kyphosis and cantilevered into the distal implants below the apex; compression is applied to-

ward the apex of the kyphosis. Transverse connectors are applied to the proximal and distal ends of the construct. Iliac and local bone graft are packed into each of the facetectomy sites and along the transverse processes. For additional correction, two to three periapical Smith-Petersen osteotomies are often helpful.

Posterior Instrumentation and Fusion Combined With Anterior Fusion
Posterior instrumentation and fusion combined with anterior fusion is recommended for adolescent patients with less flexible kyphotic deformities (> 50° on the hyperextension lateral radiograph).[3,4,7] Combined procedures are normally done at the same sitting. An anterior release and fusion is usually done first to achieve increased flexibility of the deformity. Levels for anterior release and fusion should include all "fixed" levels above and below the apex of the kyphosis based on the hyperextension lateral radiographs (usually six to eight segments) and distally across the thoracolumbar junction to the distal level of the planned posterior instrumented fusion. This would generally include the distal Cobb level and the first lordotic level. Single-lung ventilation is mandatory to achieve adequate exposure whether a thorascopic or open approach is selected. For an open procedure, a standard right-sided thoracotomy or thoracoabdominal approach is usually used, depending on whether exposure below L1 is needed. During the exposure, segmental vessels can easily be preserved and retracted with vessel loops while the diskectomies are being performed.[4] Morcellized rib graft alone is normally used above T10, whereas structural cages or grafts should be added from T10 distally where the disk spaces are larger to provide load sharing. After the insertion of a chest tube and wound closure, the patient

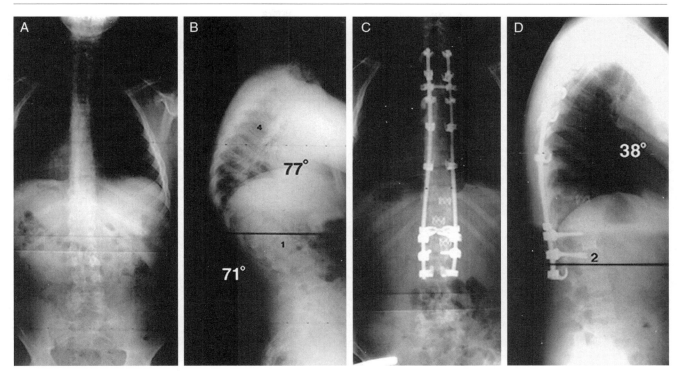

Figure 2 A and **B,** Preoperative radiographs of a 16-year-old patient with a progressive low thoracic 77° kyphosis caused by Scheuermann's disease. **C** and **D,** Postoperative radiographs at 2-year follow-up. Double two-level pediculotransverse process claws with hooks for fixation above the apex and an additional pedicle hook just below the apex of the deformity were used. Pedicle screws and infralaminar hooks were used distally.

is positioned for the posterior procedure.

Anterior Instrumentation and Fusion In pediatric patients with flexible kyphosis, the deformity can be corrected with anterior instrumentation and fusion[4] (Figure 4). This technique allows for saving several fusion levels proximally and distally. In addition to complete diskectomy, structural grafts or cages must be inserted at each level for arthrodesis and instrumentation. Next, bicortical vertebral body screws are inserted transversely at each level, followed by insertion of a single 6.5- to 7.0-mm rod that is contoured to the corrected sagittal profile of the kyphotic deformity.

Surgical Outcomes

Surgical outcomes for correction of this type of kyphosis in the pediatric population have been very good, with long-term correction returning the spinal curvature to within normal range and maintaining good sagittal and coronal balance. In general, clinical outcomes have been good, with patients reporting significant improvements in back pain and cosmesis.[4,6,8,9]

Short Radius Kyphosis
Surgical Indications and Options

Several special considerations must be taken into account in the treatment of short radius, rigid kyphosis in pediatric patients. Kyphosis created by congenital spine deformity is related to developmental vertebral anomalies that impair longitudinal growth anteriorly or anterolaterally. These curves have been classified as caused by anterior failure of vertebral body formation (type I), anterior failure of vertebral body segmentation (type II), and a combination of failure of formation and segmentation (type III).[1,2,10] All three types may cause potentially serious deformities; even type I congenital spinal deformity can lead to cord compression and paraplegia. As a result, brace treatment is ineffective, and surgery is frequently necessary. No single surgical procedure is effective for all types and magnitudes of congenital spinal deformity. The method of treatment depends on the age of the patient, size of the deformity, type of anomaly, and presence or absence of spinal cord compression. Before surgical treatment is undertaken, possible cardiopulmonary, urinary, and neurologic anomalies must be assessed because such anomalies may affect the timing and approach to treatment.

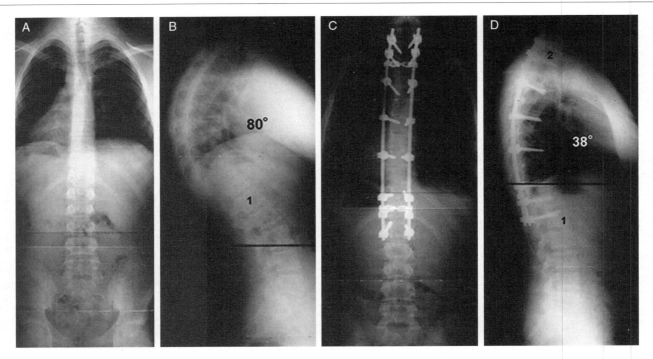

Figure 3 A and **B,** Preoperative radiographs of a 17-year-old boy with a painful 80° thoracic kyphosis caused by Scheuermann's disease. **C** and **D,** Postoperative radiographs following a combined anterior-posterior spinal fusion using a pedicle screw construct extending from T2 to L1. Note that pedicle screws are used distally and proximally in two levels and then every other level in between.

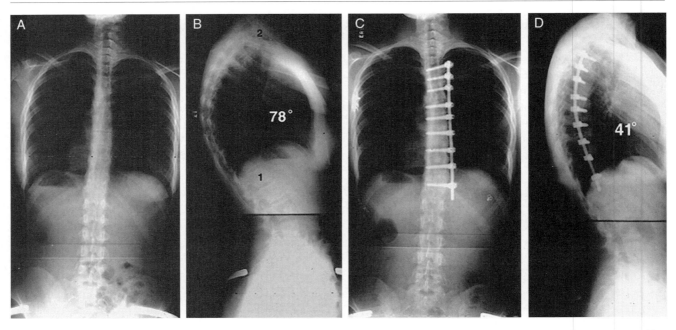

Figure 4 A and **B,** Preoperative radiographs of a 16-year-old girl with a progressive flexible 78° kyphotic deformity caused by Scheuermann's disease. Postoperative PA (**C**) and lateral (**D**) radiographs 2 years after an anterior instrumented fusion. Structural interbody support was placed at each instrumented level, followed by a single anterior rod and vertebral screws. One level was saved distally by this technique.

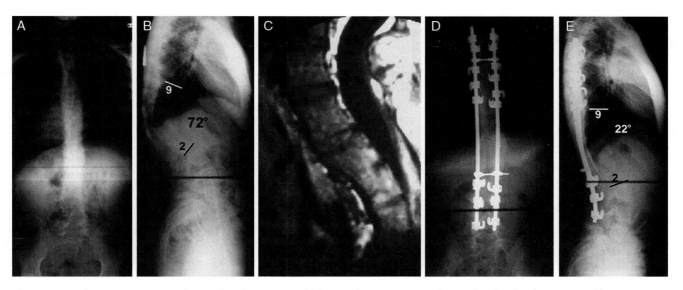

Figure 5 A and **B,** Preoperative radiographs of a 15-year-old boy with a progressive thoracolumbar kyphosis caused by a congenital anterior bar. Congenital kyphosis extends from T9 to L2. Preoperative kyphosis was 72°. **C,** MRI of the thoracolumbar spine shows the anterior bar with formation of a portion of the disks posteriorly. **D** and **E,** Postoperative radiographs 4 years after three osteotomies of the bar and posterior instrumentation and fusion. Postoperative kyphosis was 22°.

Posterior In Situ Fusion With or Without Instrumentation In pediatric patients with a congenital spinal deformity that meets treatment criteria, a posterior in situ fusion with or without instrumentation is usually all that is necessary to treat both type I and II deformities.[1,10] A posterior epiphysiodesis is created that allows for continued anterior growth through the remaining anterior growth plates and some degree of correction. Posterior instrumentation may decrease the incidence of pseudarthrosis and provide some additional correction.

Combined Anterior and Posterior Fusion With Instrumentation In pediatric patients with a congenital spinal deformity greater than 60° to 70° and for whom correction of the deformity is appropriate, a combined anterior and posterior fusion with instrumentation is indicated.[1,10] For type I deformities, the anterior procedure should consist of a release of ligamentous structures and any remaining disk followed by grafting with morcellized autogenous graft and strut grafting to fill in large gaps. For type II deformities, the anterior procedure should consist of one or more osteotomies of the unsegmented bar followed by packing of the defects with morcellized autograft. After the anterior procedure is completed, a posterior instrumented fusion of the entire deformity is performed.

Combined Anterior and Posterior Instrumented Fusion In pediatric patients with a congenital spinal deformity ranging from 60° to 80°, a combined anterior and posterior instrumented fusion of the entire deformity is usually the treatment of choice.[1] Excessive correction should be avoided because of the high risk of neurologic complications. In type I deformities, the anterior procedure consists of an anterior soft-tissue release and diskectomy followed by strut grafting. In type II deformities, single or multiple osteotomies of the anterior bar followed by grafting of the defects should be done to facilitate correction (Figure 5).

Combined Anterior-Posterior In Situ Fusion With Strut Grafting or Spine Shortening In pediatric patients with a congenital spinal deformity greater than 80°, either a combined anterior-posterior in situ fusion with strut grafting or a spine shortening procedure can limit the risk of neurologic complications (Figure 6). If a spine shortening procedure is selected, a single-stage posterior vertebrectomy is the best option for treating type I deformities. Following the hemivertebrectomy, a posterior fusion with instrumentation should be done to maximize correction of the spine. For type II deformities, a pedicle subtraction osteotomy offers the best solution.[11] Before the osteotomy, pedicle screws should be inserted above and below the proposed osteotomy site. After completion of one side of the osteotomy, temporary fixation should always be inserted to avoid displacement and possible spinal cord injury once the opposite side of the osteotomy is completed. After controlled correction of the osteotomy, bilateral pedicle screw fixation is obtained. Although excellent

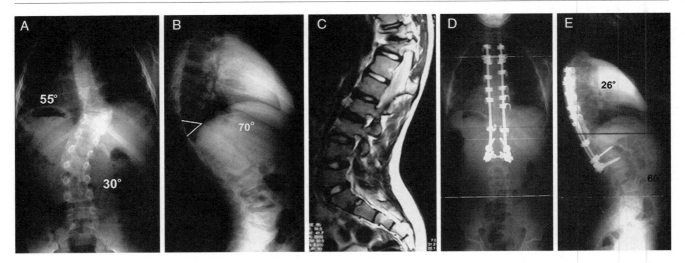

Figure 6 **A** and **B,** Preoperative radiographs of an 11-year-old boy with a progressive thoracic kyphoscoliosis (55°) caused by a posterolateral hemivertebra. Lumbar scoliosis was 30°. Thoracic kyphosis was 70°. **C,** MRI of the hemivertebra reveals no spinal cord impingement. **D** and **E,** Postoperative radiographs 2 years after excision of the hemivertebra and correction of the thoracic hyperkyphosis, which were done through a posterior approach. Thoracic kyphosis was 26°.

correction can be obtained with either of these procedures, they require the expertise of experienced surgeons to avoid neurologic complications.

Other Surgical Options When there is major spinal cord compression, either formal anterior cord decompression or a spine shortening procedure combined with correction of the kyphosis should be done along with a posterior fusion with instrumentation (Figure 7). Mild spinal cord compression without motor loss can usually be treated effectively with a standard combined anterior-posterior instrumented fusion. This procedure achieves only a modest amount of correction of the kypho-

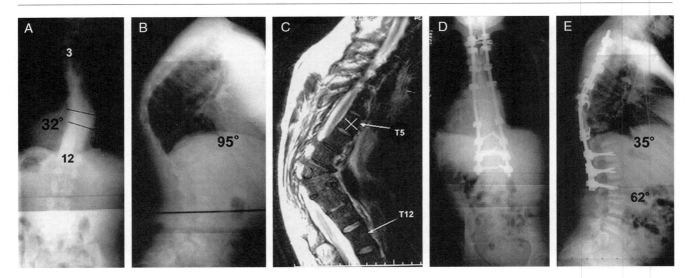

Figure 7 **A** and **B,** Radiographs of a 17-year-old boy with a progressive thoracic kyphosis caused by two hemivertebrae (T8-T9) and the subsequent acute onset of paraparesis. The patient was also undergoing routine renal dialysis because of chronic renal failure. Scoliosis extends from T3 to T12 and measures 32°. Thoracic kyphosis is 95° and lumbar lordosis is 62°. **C,** Sagittal MRI of the spine shows severe stenosis at the apex of the deformity. **D** and **E,** Postoperative radiographs 2 years after complete excision of T8 and partial excision of T9, which was done through a posterior approach. A long construct was required because of osteopenia related to dialysis. 35° is the corrected thoracic kyphosis.

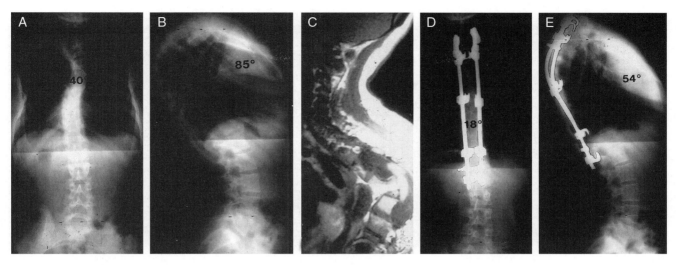

Figure 8 **A** and **B,** Preoperative radiographs of a 12-year-old girl with a fixed 85° thoracic kyphosis and an associated 40° thoracic scoliosis caused by neurofibromatosis. She reported mild weakness in both lower extremities, hyperreflexia, and bilateral ankle clonus. Thoracic scoliosis is 40°. Thoracic kyphosis is 85°. **C,** MRI shows the sharp angular deformity as well as compression of the spinal cord. **D** and **E,** Postoperative radiographs 3 years after a combined anterior cord decompression and strut grafting followed by posterior instrumentation and fusion. The patient's myelopathic findings resolved postoperatively.

sis, but it is often enough to resolve the paresis.

The role of skeletal traction for fixed deformities remains controversial because of an increased risk of neurologic complications.[1] It may, however, be useful in the treatment of flexible, high-magnitude deformities. A pretraction MRI and frequent, careful neuromonitoring are essential.

Patients with dystrophic kyphoscoliosis caused by neurofibromatosis usually require a combined anterior-posterior fusion.[12-14] These patients have an increased risk of spinal cord compression if a high-magnitude deformity develops. These deformities are usually fixed and difficult to correct. The surgical goal in kyphosis associated with neurofibromatosis is to achieve permanent stabilization of the spine and avoid neurologic injury. Surgical treatment should consist of a combined anterior-posterior in situ fusion. When a high-magnitude residual deformity is present, either a vascularized rib pedicle graft and/or fibular strut grafts should be consid-

ered[15] (Figure 8). Dystrophic thinning of posterior elements and dural ectasia make posterior instrumentation more difficult, resulting in a high rate of pseudarthrosis. Any loss of correction or implant failure warrants reexploration and reinforcement of the fusion mass.[12,14,16]

With aggressive surgical treatment of malignant spinal tumors with laminectomy, chemotherapy, and radiation, many children survive and develop postlaminectomy kyphosis.[17-19] The treatment of postlaminectomy kyphosis poses some special problems. Obviously, prevention of the deformity is the best treatment. In pediatric patients, the younger the patient and the higher the level of the laminectomy, the greater the likelihood of postlaminectomy kyphosis to occur.[17,18] A posterolateral fusion should always accompany a multilevel decompression, especially if facetectomies are a required part of the decompression. Bracing after decompression is ineffective in preventing or treating the deformity.

A combined anterior-posterior fu-

sion of the entire deformity is required because of the poor posterior fusion bed related to missing posterior elements.[17,19] Although posterior instrumentation is often difficult because of missing posterior elements and osteopenia, pedicle screws can usually be used and provide excellent fixation when combined with double-rod systems; postoperative bracing is usually not needed (Figure 9).

Summary

The treatment of large radius kyphosis in pediatric patients is primarily nonsurgical. Surgery should be reserved for patients with kyphosis of 80° or more and painful or progressive deformities. Congenital kyphosis requires early diagnosis and treatment using posterior fusion to prevent worsening of the deformity. Short radius, fixed deformities that have progressed significantly before initial evaluation require combined anterior-posterior fusion. Patients who have developed neurologic complications require a formal anterior decompression and strut grafting as well as an in-

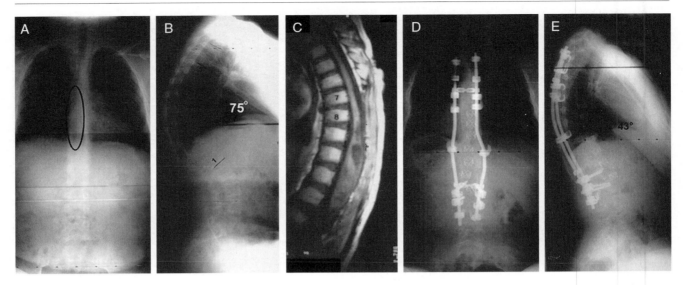

Figure 9 A and **B,** Radiographs of a 12-year-old boy 1 year after he underwent a multilevel laminectomy; a progressive thoracic kyphosis developed within a few months of the surgery. The black line in **A** identifies the extent of the multilevel laminectomy. **B,** thoracic kyphosis that developed after the laminectomy was 75°; the levels of kyphosis are identified by the lines and spaces. **C,** MRI demonstrates the presence of a spinal cord tumor (astrocytoma). **D** and **E,** Postoperative radiographs following a combined anterior-posterior fusion. Note that anterior cages were used for structural support for the length of the laminectomy defect.

strumented posterior fusion. Patients with kyphosis caused by neurofibromatosis or postlaminectomy always require combined anterior-posterior fusion because of a high risk of pseudarthrosis.

References

1. Lonstein JE: Congenital spine deformities: Scoliosis, kyphosis, and lordosis. *Orthop Clin North Am* 1999;30:387-405.

2. McMaster MJ, Singh H: Natural history of congenital kyphosis and kyphoscoliosis: A study of one hundred and twelve patients. *J Bone Joint Surg Am* 1999;81:1367-1383.

3. Lowe TG: Scheuermann disease. *J Bone Joint Surg Am* 1990;72:940-945.

4. Lowe TG: Scheuermann's disease. *Orthop Clin North Am* 1999;30:475-487.

5. Murray PM, Weinstein SL, Spratt KF: The natural history and long-term follow-up of Scheuermann kyphosis. *J Bone Joint Surg Am* 1993;75:236-248.

6. Lowe TG, Kasten MD: An analysis of sagittal curves and balance after Cotrel-Dubousset instrumentation for kyphosis secondary to Scheuermann's disease: A review of 32 patients. *Spine* 1994;19:1680-1685.

7. Bradford DS, Ahmed KB, Moe JH, Winter RB, Lonstein JE: The surgical management of patients with Scheuermann's disease: A review of twenty-four cases managed by combined anterior and posterior spine fusion. *J Bone Joint Surg Am* 1980;62:705-712.

8. Bradford DS, Moe JH, Montalvo FJ, Winter RB: Scheuermann's kyphosis: Results of surgical treatment by posterior spine arthrodesis in twenty-two patients. *J Bone Joint Surg Am* 1975;57:439-448.

9. Bradford DS, Ahmed KB, Moe JH, Winter RB, Lonstein JE: The surgical management of patients with Scheuermann's disease: A review of twenty-four cases managed by combined anterior and posterior spine fusion. *J Bone Joint Surg Am* 1980;62:705-712.

10. McMaster MJ, Singh H: The surgical management of congenital kyphosis and kyphoscoliosis. *Spine* 2001;26:2146-2155.

11. Thiranont N, Netrawichien P: Transpedicular decancellation closed wedge vertebral osteotomy for treatment of fixed flexion deformity of spine in ankylosing spondylitis. *Spine* 1993;18:2517-2522.

12. Crawford AH: Neurofibromatosis, in Weinstein SL (ed): *The Pediatric Spine: Principles and Practice*, ed 2. Philadelphia, PA, Lippincott Williams & Wilkins, 2001, pp 471-490.

13. Fienman NL: Pediatric neurofibromatosis: Review. *Compr Ther* 1981;7:66-72.

14. Kim HW, Weinstein SL: Spine update: The management of scoliosis in neurofibromatosis. *Spine* 1997;22:2770-2776.

15. Bradford DS, Daher YH: Vascularised rib grafts for stabilisation of kyphosis. *J Bone Joint Surg Br* 1986;68:357-361.

16. Hsu LC, Lee PC, Leong JC: Dystrophic spinal deformities in neurofibromatosis: Treatment by anterior and posterior fusion. *J Bone Joint Surg Br* 1984;66:495-499.

17. Lonstein JE: Post-laminectomy kyphosis. *Clin Orthop* 1977;128:93-100.

18. Munechica Y: Influence of laminectomy on the stability of the spine. *J Jpn Orthop Assoc* 1973;47:111-126.

19. Peterson HA: Spinal deformity secondary to tumor, irradiation and laminectomy, in Bradford DS, Hensinger RN (eds): *The Pediatric Spine*. New York, NY, Thieme, 1985, pp 273-285.

Kyphosis of the Thoracic and Thoracolumbar Spine in the Pediatric Patient: Prevention and Treatment of Surgical Complications

Lawrence G. Lenke, MD

Abstract

The successful outcome of surgical treatment of pediatric kyphosis depends on careful preoperative identification of the etiology of the problem as well as identification of any associated medical conditions or syndromes that may render surgical reconstruction more challenging. Many perioperative surgical factors can lead to an unsuccessful surgical outcome, including inadequate preoperative patient or kyphosis assessment; inappropriate selection of proximal and/or distal instrumentation and fusion levels; inadequate spinal fixation applied at the ends of the posterior construct where tension forces are greatest; inadequate performance of a meticulous posterior spinal fusion; absence and/or an inadequate performance of an anterior spinal fusion when required either before or after the posterior procedure; overcorrection of the kyphotic deformity based on the ability of the spine above and below to compensate for the correction; a higher risk of neurologic complications with correction of kyphotic deformities; and inadequate postoperative support with an orthosis. Revision surgery for failed pediatric kyphosis surgeries requires careful reexamination of all these factors to correct any shortcomings. In addition, adjunctive procedures such as spinal osteotomies, perioperative traction, and/or anterior fusion techniques may be required to optimize spinal alignment, balance, and ultimate successful fusion. When following these guidelines, pediatric spinal kyphosis disorders can be successfully treated and complications avoided.

It is generally more difficult and dangerous to surgically treat kyphosis pathology than scoliosis pathology.[1] Because the management of complications related to the surgical treatment of pediatric kyphosis can be particularly challenging, it is important to stress preventive measures to avoid complications in the first place.

When postoperative problems arise, however, the reasons why the kyphosis reconstruction failed must be identified and a treatment plan developed to correct and overcome the complications.

This chapter discusses the etiology of failed pediatric kyphosis reconstructive surgery along with specific treatment plans to surgically manage these difficult complications. Preventive measures are also discussed that can help avoid the complications of failed surgery.

Etiology

Before treating complications arising from failed pediatric kyphosis surgery, it is extremely important to accurately determine what caused the initial reconstruction to fail.[2,3] Various causes include but are not limited to the following: inadequate preoperative patient or deformity assessment; fusion done at inappropriate proximal and/or distal levels; the application of inadequate fixation, especially at the ends of the posterior construct; inadequate abundant posterior spinal fusion; inadequate anterior spinal fusion; overcorrection of kyphosis as determined by the ability of the spine above and below to compensate for the correction; neurologic complications; and any combination of the above. The type of kyphosis and the particular patient characteristics must also be determined. For example, the surgical treatment of kyphosis will fail for

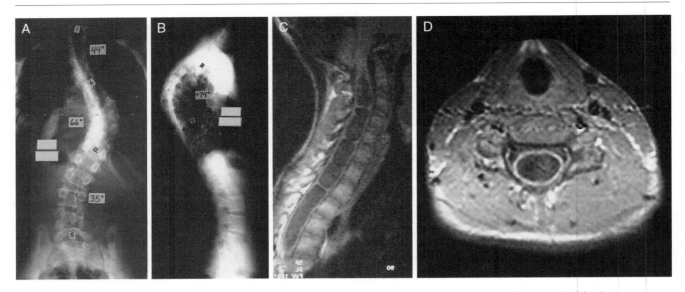

Figure 1 **A** and **B**, Radiographs of a 15-year-old boy with a 44° proximal thoracic and 66° main thoracic double-thoracic curve pattern. Although the coronal plane is idiopathic in presentation, the sagittal plane demonstrates 74° of kyphosis in the mid-thoracic region. Because of the presence of thoracic hyperkyphosis, which is atypical for adolescent idiopathic scoliosis, the patient underwent total spine MRI examination. **C** and **D**, Total spine MRI shows a large cervical-thoracic syrinx extending from C2 down to T10 as well as an Arnold-Chiari malformation. This condition required neurosurgical intervention before anterior and posterior spinal fusion.

different reasons in a 3-year-old patient who weighs 30 lb and has a congenital dislocation of the proximal thoracic spine and an adult patient who weighs 275 lb and has a Scheuermann's kyphosis. In addition to identifying the type of kyphosis being treated (for example, congenital, Scheuermann's, postlaminectomy, posttraumatic, or myelokyphosis), it must also be determined whether sagittal plane malalignment is associated with any coronal plane malalignment (scoliosis). Although rare, an otherwise idiopathic scoliosis apparent on a coronal plane radiograph can be associated with a thoracic hyperkyphosis malalignment.[4] Therefore, a preoperative total spine MRI should be obtained to exclude any associated spinal canal anomalies (Figure 1). Because medical problems such as heart disease, lung disease, and connective tissue disorders can complicate the surgical treatment of pediatric kyphosis, a thor-

ough medical history must be obtained and a careful physical examination performed when revision surgery is being planned.

Problems with the surgical treatment of pediatric kyphosis most often arise as the result of inappropriate selection of proximal and/or distal fusion levels, which often occurs in combination with inadequate fixation.[3,5] Much has been written regarding the selection of appropriate proximal and distal fusion levels in the treatment of coronal plane abnormalities such as scoliosis; however, much less has been written regarding the selection of appropriate proximal and distal fusion levels in the treatment of kyphosis. One published method recommends including the first lordotic disk in the upper to midlumbar spine as the distal fusion level.[5] This will usually be a safe distal fusion level in the majority of patients. However, in some patients, a neutral disk above the first lordotic

disk is present, and the vertebra between these disks can occasionally be the distal fusion level. The concept of the "stable" vertebra on the sagittal radiographs can be used to denote the safe distal fusion level and draw the posterior sacral vertical line, a vertical line drawn from the posterior edge of the S1 body, proximally until it intersects (or bisects) one of the lumbar vertebra (Figure 2). Similarly, the center sacral vertical line is drawn on the coronal plane radiograph to determine the "stable" vertebra in the coronal plane. As is true in the coronal plane, occasionally the vertebra immediately above the true "stable" vertebra can be the distal fusion level in the sagittal plane. As long as the posterior sacral vertical line intersects some part of this more proximal vertebra, this vertebra is a safe distal fusion level, particularly when the disk above it is lordotic or neutral. If the disk above it is in any degree of kyphosis, the safe fusion level normally will have to be extended one level more distal.

For choosing the proximal level of instrumentation and fusion, symmetry is normally defined above the apex of a deformity to make symmetric moment arms both above and below the apex. For example, if a kyphosis has an apex of T10, and the posterior sacral vertical line selected L3 as the stable vertebra (five levels below the apex T10), then T4 would be selected as the proximal starting point, which is five levels above the apex. Occasionally, one more proximal level can be added for additional fixation, if required.

With posterior fixation, the strength and security of the fixation increases as sublaminar wires, various supralaminar and infralaminar hooks, and then pedicle screws are used for fixation.[6-11] The three-column support of multisegmented pedicle screw constructs provides extremely secure purchase and construct stability for primary and revision kyphosis reconstructions. The number of pedicle screw implants required to optimally stabilize a kyphosis reconstruction, especially in a revision reconstruction, is unknown. But because of the difficulty in healing of kyphosis surgeries as a result of the tension-band forces of posteriorly applied implants, more fixation points are used.[7,12] This is particularly appropriate in a revision reconstruction for which previous posterior implants have failed to secure a strong posterior fusion mass for long-term stability. Also, failed hook purchase in the low thoracic and upper- and midlumbar spine can be revised with appropriate distal screw fixation (Figure 3).

Another distinct advantage of using transpedicular fixation for proximal and distal kyphosis implants is the lack of any iatrogenic ligamen-

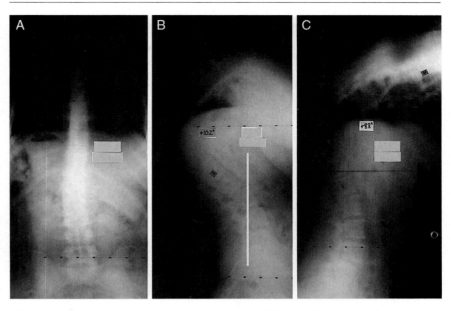

Figure 2 A through **C**, Radiographs of a 17-year-old boy with a large Scheuermann's kyphosis. The posterior sacral vertical line as drawn from the back edge of the sacrum most closely bisects the L3 vertebral body, which is known as the "stable" sagittal vertebra. This was the lowest instrumented vertebra for anterior and posterior spinal reconstruction.

tous injury when the implants are properly placed. Generally, with any type of sublaminar wire or hook fixation, implants placed supra-adjacent to the proximal fusion level and infra-adjacent to the inferior instrumented level will disrupt ligamentous tissue. To avoid junctional problems, it is important to maintain the posterior ligamentous tension band. If radical posterior tension-band disruption occurs, as it can when the bilateral supralaminar hooks used as proximal implants are placed following complete removal of the interspinous ligaments and ligamentum flavum at the supra-adjacent level, then proximal junctional kyphosis will ensue (Figure 4). Regardless of the type of implant used, injury to the supra-adjacent and infra-adjacent soft tissue and ligamentous structures must also be avoided when performing any type of primary or revision reconstruction for kyphosis.

Overcorrection of the kyphotic

deformity can also cause surgery to fail.[5] If overcorrection occurs, a problem is usually evident more proximally at the cervicothoracic junction than distally at the lumbosacral junction. Thus, for severe kyphotic deformities, such as those associated with Scheuermann's disease, it is advisable to plan for correction of approximately 50%. Attempting to correct these deformities to within the 25° to 30° range may result in overcorrection for those patients with deformities within the 80° to 100° range. Regardless of the amount of correction, a thorough posterior fusion with autogenous bone graft is mandatory to create a thick posterior fusion mass that will prevent loss of correction, which can occur over time as a result of constant posterior tension forces. Additionally, posterior implants should be left in place long term, even when a solid posterior fusion mass is present. A fusion mass with a resid-

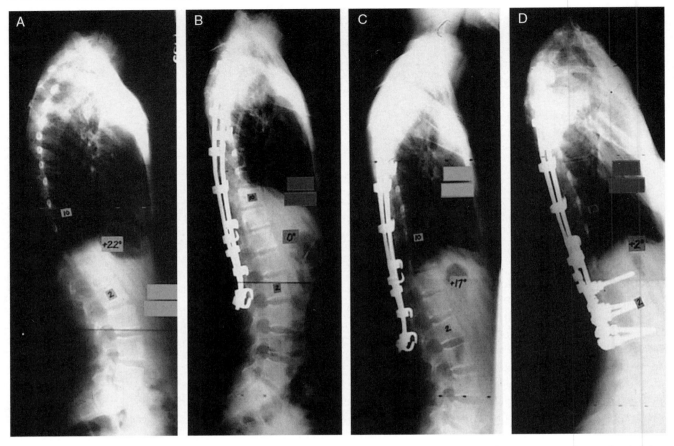

Figure 3 A, Preoperative radiograph of a female patient with adolescent idiopathic scoliosis and a 22° T10-L2 thoracolumbar kyphosis. **B**, The patient underwent posterior instrumentation and fusion down to L2 with a segmental hook construct. **C**, Four weeks postoperatively, the patient reported increased pain and a palpable mass in the lower part of her incision. A lateral radiograph demonstrated hook pull-off distally. **D**, The patient had a revision posterior instrumentation with extension to L3 with transpedicular screws with good sagittal realignment.

ual large kyphosis can still bend and/ or break over time, in which case revision surgery involving an anterior fusion mass (intradiskal and/or strut) will be required to prevent further bending (Figure 5).

Some of the more common complications associated with pediatric kyphosis surgery are neurologic. It is well known that the primary and revision surgical treatment of conditions such as congenital kyphosis have an extremely high rate of neurologic complications. Two factors account for this high rate: tension applied to the anterior portion of the spinal cord[13,14] and limitation of the anterior spinal cord blood supply[15-17] resulting from straightening of the kyphosis. Although it is difficult to distinguish these two etiologies clinically, spinal cord monitoring during pediatric kyphosis surgery can help identify problems occurring as a result of concomitant hypotension. With combined somatosensory-evoked potential and neurogenic motor-evoked potential monitoring, hypotension-induced spinal cord monitoring signal losses can be abruptly reversed by the delivery of hypertensive agents. This intervention occasionally requires administering a dopamine drip intraoperatively and immediately postoperatively to maintain blood pressures at a level that will maintain adequate spinal cord blood flow.

Because it is so important to maximize spinal cord blood flow during kyphosis reconstruction, harvesting of segmental vessels anteriorly should be avoided. The placement of instrumentation anteriorly should also be avoided because it often requires segmental vessel ligation. Inducing hypotension during the posterior correction of kyphosis is not recommended. A mean arterial blood pressure of 70 to 80 mm Hg can maintain optimal spinal cord perfusion. Because dim-

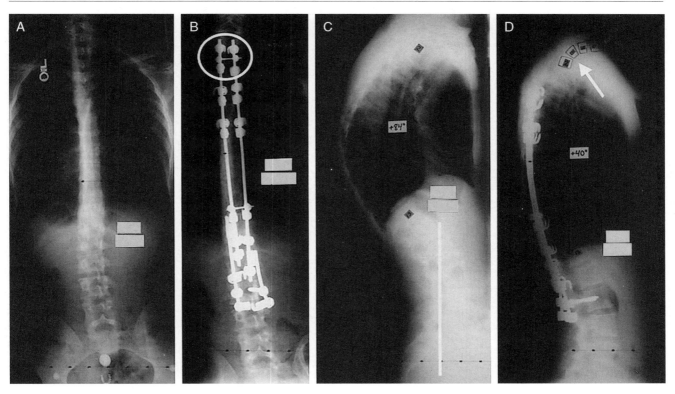

Figure 4 A, Preoperative radiograph of a male patient with a Scheuermann's kyphosis. **B**, The patient underwent anterior and posterior spinal fusion with posterior instrumentation from T2 to L3. His proximal construct consisted of bilateral pedicle-supralaminar claw hooks. **C**, These bilateral supralaminar hooks are detrimental for cervical thoracic junctional stability because of the iatrogenic ligamentous disruption required to place the hooks. **D**, The patient subsequently developed a cervicothoracic junctional kyphosis.

inution of spinal cord data with hypotension is more often seen initially with neurogenic motor-evoked potential than somatosensory-evoked potential monitoring, multimodality spinal cord monitoring should be used when surgically treating patients with kyphosis.[15,18-21] The intraoperative wake-up test can definitively confirm appropriate lower extremity neurologic function; however, results of this test provide data for only one moment in time, and waiting for results may delay the correction of a hypotension-induced neurologic dysfunction. In addition, the problem may not be appropriately identified if correction of deformity has not yet been performed.

The etiology of failed pediatric kyphosis surgery may be multifacto-rial, with several of the previously discussed factors resulting in an unsuccessful reconstruction that requires revision. Thus, before revision takes place, all previous surgical procedures must be carefully reviewed and the factors that contributed to the ultimate failure definitively identified (Figures 6 through 8). Only then can corrective surgery be planned that will ultimately result in a solid spinal fusion and a well-balanced spine.

Surgical Treatment

The basic options available for pediatric patients in whom previous kyphosis surgery has failed include revision posterior spinal fusion with instrumentation; anterior spinal fu-sion either as a primary or revision procedure; spinal osteotomies to improve segmental, regional, and global spinal kyphotic malalignment; and potentially adjunctive procedures, such as halo traction, to assist in overall realignment.

If the previous fusion and existing instrumentation needs to be extended proximally and/or distally, the entire spinal region can be exposed to confirm that adequate fusion exists in those regions as well. Although an existing rod can be added to extend the patient's proximal and/or distal fusion and instrumentation in simple reconstructions, in complex reconstructions (ie, in patients who have undergone multiple previous surgeries), the entire "fusion" mass

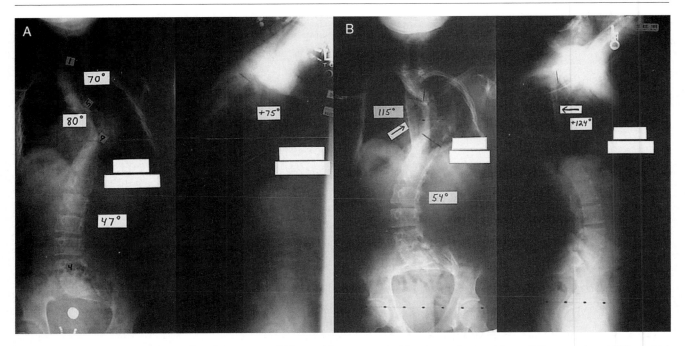

Figure 5 A, Preoperative radiographs of a 17-year-old boy with a congenital kyphoscoliosis with an 80° coronal and 75° sagittal plane deformity and a solid posterior fusion. A progressive deformity occurred as a result of chronic bending of the fusion mass caused by severe residual kyphosis. **B**, Radiographs of the same patient at 5-year follow-up. The patient underwent an anterior allograft fibular structural fusion from a concave thoracotomy approach. This vertically placed fibular graft supports the spine from bending, providing an "I" beam type of support for the 115° coronal and 124° sagittal plane deformity.

should be explored to make sure that it is solid rather than simply noting pseudarthrotic areas that will require revision posteriorly and/or anteriorly. Previous fixation points, such as hooks or screws, can be reused, although it is recommended that old implants be exchanged for new implants to ensure that the connection between the longitudinal member and the implants is as strong and secure as possible. If the previous wire or hook fixation was inadequate, then placing pedicle screws is usually possible in these regions, even with altered anatomy. Fluoroscopy or image-guided techniques (eg, computerized stealth systems) can be helpful, if required. In these situations, more rather than less fixation will be indicated to fully immobilize the spine and provide the best chance of obtaining a solid fusion.

Posterior osteotomies may help realign the kyphotic spine into a more neutral or even lordotic position. Osteotomies may also improve segmental and regional lordosis and sagittal balance. Three types of osteotomies can be used: the Smith-Petersen osteotomy (SPO), the pedicle subtraction osteotomy (PSO), and the anterior-posterior osteotomy (APO).

The SPO is a posterior column osteotomy that opens the anterior column (disk), hinges on the middle column, and closes the posterior column the amount that is removed posteriorly. This is done in a V-shaped fashion in the infralaminar spaces posteriorly between the spinous processes and lamina. Five to 10 mm of posterior element bone and ligament is usually removed to allow posterior closure, which is best accomplished with multisegmented

screw fixation. If the anterior column is fused, SPO may not work. Additionally, once done, the anterior defects created by closing the posterior column must be examined and may require secondary intradiskal grafting to optimize the fusion rate. SPO can be very helpful in the treatment of thoracic and thoracolumbar pathologies in which a modest amount of correction can be obtained over multiple segments to nicely contour the spine into a better alignment.

The PSO is a more extensive three-column osteotomy that resects the posterior column, the pedicles (middle column), and the lateral portion of the vertebral body, while hinging on the anterior aspect of the body. Approximately 30° to 40° of kyphosis correction can often be obtained at one level. The PSO is quite

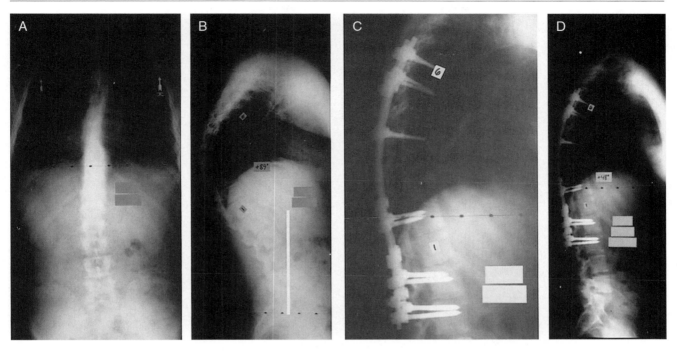

Figure 6 Preoperative PA (**A**) and lateral (**B**) radiographs of an 18-year-old man with a presumed Scheuermann's kyphosis. **C** and **D**, The patient underwent anterior and posterior spinal fusion. A diagnosis of connective tissue disorder was made later. His posterior instrumentation initially ended at L1, which was far proximal to his stable vertebra at L3. He experienced early screw pull-out and 1 week postoperatively underwent surgery for extension down to L3. However, because of the connective tissue disorder in his neutral thoracolumbar alignment, his deformity below the instrumentation progressed with a rounded kyphosis extending to L5.

stable because, when done correctly, a bone-on-bone position of all three columns of the spine is produced once the posterior column is closed. It is preferable to perform this osteotomy in the midlumbar and upper-lumbar spine (below the spinal cord) because of the amount of dural retraction and tension created when this osteotomy is closed. A PSO in the midlumbar spine can be combined with multiple SPOs in the thoracolumbar junction and thoracic spine for marked deformity correction of stiff global kyphotic deformities (Figure 6).

The APO is rarely used because it is only indicated to treat fixed kyphosis in the thoracic spine and thoracolumbar junction for which the PSO may not be as appropriate. For example, an APO is potentially indi-cated to correct congenital kyphosis over multiple segments in the thoracic spine. Regardless of the posterior approach used, secure segmental instrumentation and the abundant application of autogenous bone graft from either the iliac crest or ribs (as in a thoracoplasty procedure) are mandatory for the long-term success of primary and/or revision posterior kyphosis surgery.

Appropriate anterior spinal fusion can also help achieve long-term fusion in patients undergoing posterior kyphosis surgery. If the anterior spine has not been approached during the initial operation, then performing anterior spinal fusion either before or after the posterior procedure may be indicated, especially over any pseudarthrotic area where the posterior fusion bed may not be adequate for obtaining a secure fusion. In the thoracic spine, this usually entails the application of morcellized autogenous bone after a thorough diskectomy. However, in the lower thoracic and throughout the lumbar and lumbosacral spine, intradiskal structural support should be provided using allograft bone or vertical mesh cages that help support the loads applied to the anterior and middle columns through the disk spaces. Applying strut graft as an "I" beam support is indicated for large severe kyphoses in which intradiskal grafting alone may not provide enough support to prevent postoperative fusion mass bending or breakage because of the large kyphotic angulation and long moment arm involved in the spinal malalignment. Applying allograft or autograft fibula

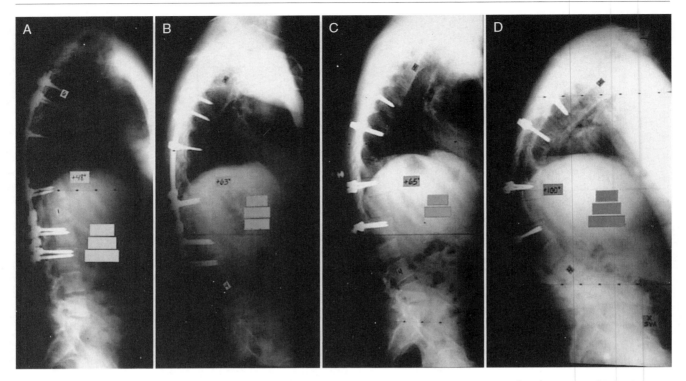

Figure 7 Same patient as shown in Figure 6. **A** and **B,** When exploring the patient's posterior wound, a deep wound infection was noted with multiple organisms cultured out. Thus, the rods were removed, several critical screws kept and he was placed on long-term intravenous antibiotics. **C** and **D,** Although the patient's wound infection healed, he developed a stiff progressive global thoracic and lumbar kyphosis all the way to his sacrum measuring 100°.

is the preferred method of treatment of these types of deformities in pediatric patients with vertebral bodies large enough to accept these grafts. Rarely, a vascularized rib or autogenous fibula graft will be required for high-risk patients undergoing revision kyphosis surgery.[22-24]

Perioperative or intraoperative halo traction can be used to help realign the kyphotic spine. When used perioperatively, halo traction can gradually and safely stretch the spinal column and cord, with the patient awake and able to respond to any type of excessive stretching to the neural axis. Although halo traction has been used selectively to treat very severe deformities, it can be especially helpful in patients who have undergone surgical revision because previous anterior surgery and vessel harvest or

ligation or anterior or posterior scar formation with previous laminectomies can put them at increased risk for neurologic complications. Additionally, the halo device can be used to optimize intraoperative positioning for deformity correction. Preoperative halo traction can be used for patients with kyphosis greater than 100°, especially those who will undergo revision and those who are smaller or in ill health to maximize their respiratory status perioperatively. In addition, patients with a concomitant scoliosis deformity greater than 90° to 100° would also be candidates for simultaneous coronal and sagittal plane correction. Thus far, no major complications resulting from the use of perioperative halo gravity traction have been reported, and traction has not been stopped be-

cause of any type of cranial nerve or upper or lower extremity neurologic complication (A Rinella, MD, LG Lenke, MD, St Louis, MO, unpublished data, 2003).

Summary

Although prevention is often the best way to avoid the need for revision surgery, surgical treatment of pediatric kyphosis is a significant undertaking. Thorough preoperative evaluation is required to identify not only the nature of the deformity but also the patient's overall health and any existing conditions/syndromes. Selection of the best approach (posterior alone or circumferential), appropriate fusion levels, placement of secure segmental spinal instrumentation, the judicious use of both anterior (if needed) and posterior spi-

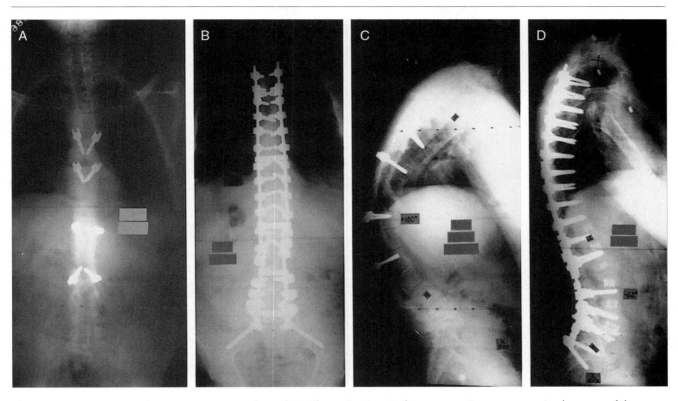

Figure 8 Same patient as shown in Figure 6. **A** through **D,** The patient's spinal reconstruction was extensive because of the complicated nature of his pathology. He underwent a first-stage posterior instrumentation and fusion with bilateral transpedicular screws at every level from T3 to the sacrum except L3, where a PSO was done. Pseudarthrosis was noted at every level of his previous fusion attempt. Thus, multilevel SPOs were done to contour his lower thoracic and thoracolumbar junction and to achieve a more appropriate amount of sagittal alignment. An anterior spinal fusion was subsequently done from T10 to the sacrum using structural cages, autogenous, and allograft bone. Postoperative radiographs show excellent sagittal realignment with normal sagittal contours throughout.

nal fusion techniques with autogenous bone are necessary for success. Revision for failed surgery requires careful reexamination of all of these factors and compensation for any shortcomings. In addition, adjunctive procedures such as spinal osteotomies, perioperative traction, and anterior fusion techniques may be required to optimize spinal alignment, balance, and ultimately successful fusion. When following these guidelines, kyphosis in pediatric patients can be successfully treated and complications avoided.

References

1. Bridwell KH, Lenke LG, Baldus C, Blanke K: Major intraoperative neurologic deficits in pediatric and adult spinal deformity patients: Incidence and etiology at one institution. *Spine* 1998;23:324-331.

2. Johnston CE II, Schoenecker PL: Letter: Cervical kyphosis in patients who have Larsen syndrome. *J Bone Joint Surg Am* 1997;79:1590-1591.

3. Wiggins GC, Rauzzino MJ, Bartkowski HM, Nockels RP, Shaffrey CI: Management of complex pediatric and adolescent spinal deformity. *J Neurosurg* 2001;95(suppl 1):17-24.

4. Betz RR, Harms J, Clements DH III, et al: Comparison of anterior and posterior instrumentation for correction of adolescent thoracic idiopathic scoliosis. *Spine* 1999;24:225-239.

5. Wenger DR, Frick SL: Scheuermann kyphosis. *Spine* 1999;24:2630-2639.

6. Abumi K, Shono Y, Taneichi H, Ito M, Kaneda K: Correction of cervical kyphosis using pedicle screw fixation systems. *Spine* 1999;24:2389-2396.

7. Belmont PJ Jr, Polly DW Jr, Cunningham BW, Klemme WR: The effects of hook pattern and kyphotic angulation on mechanical strength and apical rod strain in a long-segment posterior construct using a synthetic model. *Spine* 2001;26:627-635.

8. Brown CA, Lenke LG, Bridwell KH, Greideman WM, Hasan SA, Blanke K: Complications of pediatric thoracolumbar and lumbar pedicle screws. *Spine* 1998;23:1566-1571.

9. Lenke LG, Padberg AM, Russo MH, Bridwell KH, Gelb DE: Triggered electromyographic threshold for accuracy of pedicle screw placement: An animal model and clinical correlation. *Spine* 1995;20:1585-1591.

10. Lewis SJ, Lenke LG, Raynor B, Long J, Bridwell KH, Padberg A: Triggered

electromyographic threshold for accuracy of thoracic pedicle screw placement in a porcine model. *Spine* 2001;26:2485-2490.

11. Papagelopoulos PJ, Klassen RA, Peterson HA, Dekutoski MB: Surgical treatment of Scheuermann's disease with segmental compression instrumentation. *Clin Orthop* 2001;386:139-149.

12. Oda I, Cunningham BW, Buckley RA, et al: Does spinal kyphotic deformity influence the biomechanical characteristics of the adjacent motion segments? An in vivo animal model. *Spine* 1999;24:2139-2146.

13. Birnbaum K, Siebert CH, Hinkelmann J, Prescher A, Niethard FU: Correction of kyphotic deformity before and after transection of the anterior longitudinal ligament: A cadaver study. *Arch Orthop Trauma Surg* 2001;121:142-147.

14. Bridwell KH, Kuklo TR, Lewis SJ, Sweet FA, Lenke LG, Baldus C: String test measurement to assess the effect of spinal deformity correction on spinal canal length. *Spine* 2001;26:2013-2019.

15. Kai Y, Owen JH, Lenke LG, Bridwell KH, Oakley DM, Sugioka Y: Use of sciatic neurogenic motor evoked potentials versus spinal potentials to predict early-onset neurologic deficits when intervention is still possible during overdistraction. *Spine* 1993;18:1134-1139.

16. Pelosi L, Jardine A, Webb JK: Neurological complications of anterior spinal surgery for kyphosis with normal somatosensory evoked potentials (SEPs). *J Neurol Neurosurg Psychiatry* 1999;66:662-664.

17. Tribus CB: Transient paraparesis: A complication of the surgical management of Scheuermann's kyphosis secondary to thoracic stenosis. *Spine* 2001;26: 1086-1089.

18. Komanetsky RM, Padberg AM, Lenke LG, et al: Neurogenic motor evoked potentials: A prospective comparison of stimulation methods in spinal deformity surgery. *J Spinal Disord* 1998;11:21-28.

19. Padberg AM, Russo MH, Lenke LG, Bridwell KH, Komanetsky RM: Validity and reliability of spinal cord monitoring in neuromuscular spinal deformity surgery. *J Spinal Disord* 1996;9:150-158.

20. Wilson-Holden TJ, Padberg AM, Parkinson JD, Bridwell KH, Lenke LG, Bassett GS: A prospective comparison of neurogenic mixed evoked potential stimulation methods: Utility of epidural elicitation during posterior spinal surgery. *Spine* 2000;25:2364-2371.

21. Wilson-Holden TJ, Padberg AM, Lenke LG, Larson BJ, Bridwell KH, Bassett GS: Efficacy of intraoperative monitoring for pediatric patients with spinal cord pathology undergoing spinal deformity surgery. *Spine* 1999;24:1685-1692.

22. Govender S, Kumar KP, Med PC: Long-term follow-up assessment of vascularized rib pedicle graft for tuberculosis kyphosis. *J Pediatr Orthop* 2001;21:281-284.

23. Harwant S: Factors influencing the outcome of arthrodesis for congenital kyphosis and kyphoscoliosis. *Med J Malaysia* 2001;56:18-24.

24. Zeller RD, Dubousset J: Progressive rotational dislocation in kyphoscoliotic deformities: Presentation and treatment. *Spine* 2000;25:1092-1097.

Evaluation and Surgical Treatment of High-Grade Isthmic Dysplastic Spondylolisthesis

Lawrence G. Lenke, MD
Keith H. Bridwell, MD

Abstract

In children and young adults who seek medical treatment for high-grade isthmic dysplastic spondylolisthesis, common clinical symptoms are referable to the lumbosacral spine and/or the lower extremities. Pain in the lumbosacral spine may be secondary to altered lumbosacral alignment and biomechanics. It also may be caused by malalignment of the entire spinal-pelvic axis as a result of anterior sagittal imbalance. Lower extremity radiculopathies involving the L5 nerve root(s) may be present, and in severe forms of spondylolisthesis crisis, marked entrapment of the cauda equina at L5-S1 may occur.

High-grade isthmic dysplastic spondylolisthesis are treated surgically and should include appropriate central and foraminal decompressions at the L5-S1 level, followed by lumbosacral fusion. Partial reduction aiming at improving the slip angle (lumbosacral kyphosis) is more beneficial and provides less risk to the L5 nerve roots than complete reduction of the translational component of the slip. Solid anterior and posterior spinal fusion at L5-S1 appears to provide the best long-term results.

Spondylolisthesis, or the forward slippage of one particular segment of the spine onto the next lower segment, comes in many forms and levels of severity. When discussing the higher-grade forms (Meyerding translation grade III, IV, and V),[1] the traditional classification of Wiltse and Winter[2] does not always fully represent the pathoanatomy involved.

One or more of the authors or the departments with which they are affiliated have received something of value from a commercial or other party related directly or indirectly to the subject of this chapter.

Patients with high-grade spondylolisthesis, especially those in the pediatric age range, invariably have a dysplastic component to their lumbosacral bony anatomy.[3-5] They also may or may not have actual defects of the pars interarticularis. The pars area may be stretched or elongated, with cracks developing later. The L5-S1 facet joints are almost universally dysplastic, as well as the posterior arch at L5 and, often, the proximal sacrum. Spina bifida occulta is a common finding.[4]

Marchetti and Bartolozzi[6] developed a classification system for spondylolisthesis that places the dysplastic form in a completely separate category. They fur-

ther subdivided this category into low and high dysplastic forms that occur either with or without an intact pars interarticularis. Patients with high-grade dysplastic spondylolisthesis invariably have a high slip angle or high degree of lumbosacral kyphosis, which further alters the lumbosacral alignment and makes achievement of surgical success more challenging.

Radiographic Evaluation

The two most important radiographic parameters are the Meyerding grading of L5 translation on the sacrum and the slip angle.[1-3] Meyerding[1] divided the position of L5 on the sacrum into quarters (I through IV) with the high grade slips present in grades III, IV, and V. Grade V is unique in that it represents the position of L5 completely below the top of the sacrum, which is termed spondyloptosis. The slip angle, or measurement of lumbosacral kyphosis, is measured as perpendicular from the back edge of the sacrum to the angle subtended by a line drawn along the inferior or superior edge of the L5 vertebral end plate (Fig. 1). The normal slip angle in a patient without spondylolisthesis should be a lordotic value because the L5-S1 disk is normally in 20° to 25° of lordosis. However, with a high-grade spondylolisthesis, this number

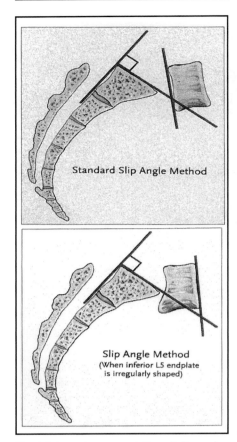

Fig. 1 Schematic representation of slip angle or kyphotic malalignment of the lumbosacral junction present in high-grade isthmic dysplastic spondylolisthesis.

is neutral or, more commonly, kyphotic. The degree of kyphosis may become quite large, representing a severe form of segmental kyphosis present at L5-S1.[4]

The standard radiographic series for evaluation of patients with a presumed or known high-grade isthmic spondylolisthesis includes a spot lateral view of the lumbosacral region that provides an optimal profile of the translational and angular measurements of L5-S1. In addition, a Ferguson coronal view should be obtained; this view is taken in an attempt to place the angle of the x-ray beam parallel with the L5-S1 disk. The profile of the L5 pedicles, transverse processes, and the sacral ala should be seen easily, and the surgeon should be able to note whether

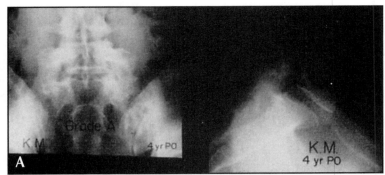

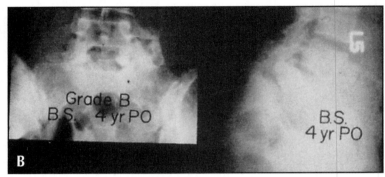

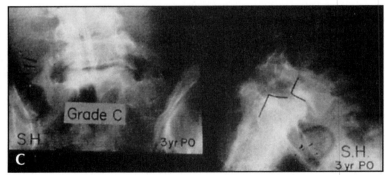

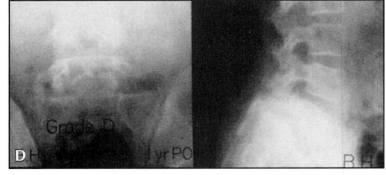

Fig. 2 The Ferguson coronal view provides a means of categorically analyzing the posterolateral fusion mass after fusion for spondylolisthesis. Fusions can be categorized into grade A, bilaterally, definitely solid (**A**); grade B, unilaterally solid with questionable fusion on the contralateral side (**B**); grade C, questionable solid fusion masses bilaterally (**C**); and grade D, definite pseudarthrosis bilaterally with possible graft resorption (**D**).

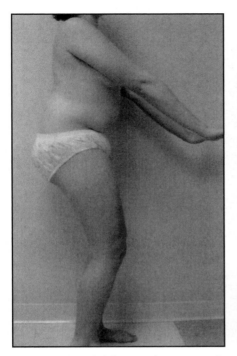

Fig. 3 The clinical deformity of a patient with high-grade isthmic dysplastic spondylolisthesis. Note the forward posture, prominent buttocks, and knee flexion present in this patient.

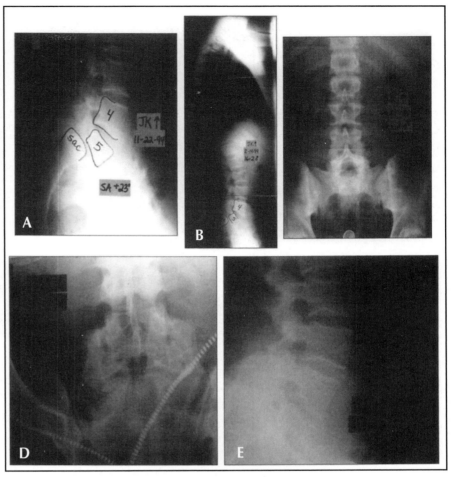

Fig. 4 A through **C,** Radiographs of a 16-year-old boy with a grade III isthmic dysplastic spondylolisthesis. Overall sagittal balance is good and L5 transverse processes are quite large. **D** and **E,** Radiographs show posterolateral fusion in situ at L4 to the sacrum with postoperative cast immobilization. At 5 years after surgery, grade A fusion bilaterally is solid with a stable slip. The patient has no clinical symptoms.

spina bifida occulta is present in the L5 segment and sacrum. The Ferguson view also has been reported to be a helpful way to determine the presence or absence of a solid lumbosacral fusion following surgical intervention[7,8] (Fig. 2).

To check the patient's overall coronal and sagittal balance, long cassette upright frontal and lateral radiographs should be obtained. The C7 plumb line should be evaluated with reference to the anterior and/or posterior edge of the sacrum. The degree of thoracolumbar and lumbar lordosis above the lumbosacral kyphotic segment should be noted because this lordosis is a common compensatory response. Any degree of associated scoliosis above the lumbosacral region should also be noted on the frontal view. This scoliosis may be secondary to a slippage that is somewhat angled in the frontal plane, or it may be an actual idiopathic scoliosis that may be associated with the spondy-

lolisthesis. In addition, patients with high-grade spondylolisthesis and nerve root tension may develop a sciatic scoliosis as a result of pressure on the lumbosacral cauda equina and/or nerve roots. A hyperextension view of the lumbosacral region with that area positioned over a bolster also will show any mobility in either the translational or sagittal rotational deformity. This mobility also can be noted on formal flexion-extension lateral radiographs taken with the patient in the supine position and showing the lumbosacral region.

A lumbosacral MRI study should be obtained on all patients being prepared for surgery in order to further define the lumbosacral alignment with the patient in a supine position. The health of disk spaces above L5 should be noted, especially that of L4-5.[8] This level often begins to degenerate in the second and third decades of life because of its proximity to the altered L5-S1 malalignment, which results in retrolisthetic forces on the L4-L5 segment. The MRI study also details the neuroanatomy quite well. Of the two most common findings, one will

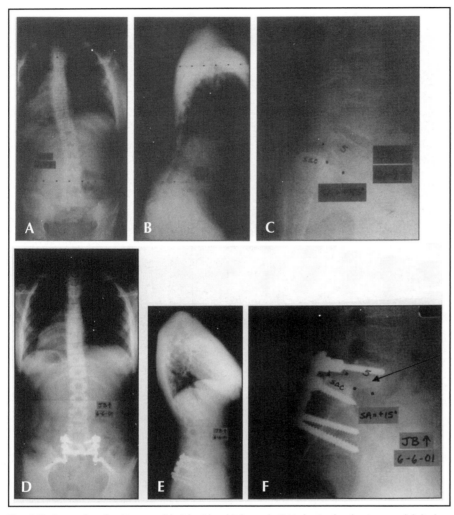

the facet dysplasia and possible central stenosis, especially when the arch at L5 remains intact and is being dragged forward into the canal.

Clinical Evaluation

In most patients who come to a spinal specialist with a high-grade spondylolisthesis,[5,10,11] low lumbosacral pain often is present but usually is not severe. This pain seems to correlate somewhat with the degree of postural malalignment that may be present from the overall spinal deformity. Specific areas of leg pain, numbness, and any bowel or bladder symptomatology, especially in those patients who have high-grade spondylolisthesis with central canal stenosis that can impinge on the cauda equina, should be noted.[5,10-13] It is fairly common for patients to have an L5 radiculopathy with posterior lateral thigh, anterior calf, and foot pain and/or numbness. Unilateral pain is more common than bilateral pain in our experience. The pain usually prevents athletic activity and is often the reason for initial evaluation.

Clinical examination focuses on the overall clinical deformity, postural alignment, spinal mobility, and neurologic examination. Patients with a high-grade spondylolisthesis often have a fairly marked clinical deformity involving a foreshortened trunk, a protruding abdomen, and a lower rib cage[4] (Fig. 3). They often flex their hips and knees in an attempt to counterbalance the forward position of the entire trunk on the pelvis. Patients have flattened buttocks and, occasionally, a scoliosis deformity caused by their altered spinal malalignment and tight spinal canal. Spinal mobility is usually restricted, and patients have marked limited flexion as well as severely limited extension of the spine. Patients invariably have tight hamstrings, which is a neurologic sign to their lower extremities. This is caused by tension on the L5 nerve roots by the slippage.[8] The straight-leg raising test is usually positive in these patients,

Fig. 5 Radiographs of a 12-year-old girl with a high-grade IV isthmic dysplastic spondylolisthesis. The patient has a small amount of sciatic scoliosis on the coronal view (**A** and **B**). Her sacrum is quite vertical on the sagittal radiograph (**C**), and she is positioned with her trunk anterior to her pelvis, demonstrating anterior sagittal imbalance. The patient underwent posterior decompression, partial reduction, sacral dome osteotomy, and posterolateral fusion with instrumentation from L5 to the sacrum. One week later, she underwent an anterior fibular dowel graft placement from L5 to the sacrum. Radiographs in **D** through **F** demonstrate the improved position of L5 on the sacrum and excellent alignment in her overall coronal (**D**) and sagittal (**E**) radiographs (**F**). The arrow points to the anterior edge of the fibular graft.

be central stenosis present at L5-S1, which usually is caused by a pincer effect from the posterior elements of L5, with an intact pars interarticularis being dragged forward into the spinal canal, thus narrowing it centrally. In addition, it is quite common to have L5 foraminal stenosis with high-grade dysplastic spondylolisthesis at L5-S1, which opti-

mally is evaluated by parasagittal MRI slices that can detail the foramina nicely.[9] This area is not evaluated very well on CT myelography because the nerve root sleeve does not extend into the foramen; thus, the myelographic dye is not present in that region. For those patients obtaining a CT myelogram, the axial view of the lumbosacral junction often displays

although the examiner must be sure that the trunk is not extended when a sitting straight-leg raise is performed. Gait often is altered, with hip and knee flexion posture continuing during forward gait.

A lower extremity neurologic examination should evaluate the motor, sensory, and reflex functions. The most common motor level involved will be L5, with weakness to the extensor hallucis longus as well as possibly to the anterior tibialis (ankle extensors) unilaterally and/or bilaterally. Dynamic assessment includes asking the patient to stand on tiptoe and back on the heels as well as ambulation. Sensory function is tested with a light touch over the L4, L5, and S1 dermatomes. In addition, patients with very high-grade spondylolisthesis, who are at risk for a cauda equina syndrome, should have sacral sensory testing as well as a rectal examination both preoperatively and postoperatively when sacral nerve root function is of concern. Lower extremity reflex function should not be altered in this condition, except for diminished ankle jerks. It is extremely important to get a good sense of motor function in the L5 distribution because this is the nerve root at highest risk for postoperative weakness and diminished function.[9]

Treatment Options

The treatment of high-grade isthmic dysplastic spondylolisthesis in the pediatric and young adult population is with surgery.[4,14-17] Even in those rare patients who are relatively asymptomatic with a grade III or more slip along with a fair degree of dysplasia to their lumbosacral region, surgical treatment is recommended. Many options for posterior treatment are available, including posterior in situ fusion with or without a decompression;[7,8,16,17] adding instrumentation to an in situ fusion;[8] posterior decompression, partial reduction, instrumentation, and fusion;[8,15,17] posterior decompression, complete reduction, instrumentation, and posterior fusion;[14,15,18,19] and for those

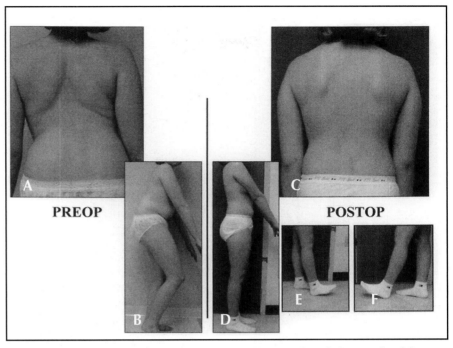

Fig. 6 Preoperative (**A** and **B**) and postoperative (**C** through **F**) clinical photographs of the patient whose radiographs are shown in Figure 5. Note the postoperative improvement in the coronal and sagittal alignment and also the excellent foot dorsiflexion function bilaterally.

patients with a true spondyloptosis, an L5 spondylolectomy with L4-sacrum fusion as popularized by Gaines[20,21] Additional posterior treatment options that can address the anterior spine include a posterior lumbar interbody fusion or a transforaminal interbody fusion using either nonstructural or structural bone graft or metallic cages. In addition, for higher-grade spondylolisthesis with a kyphotic slip angle, a posterior fibular dowel graft can be placed from posterior on the sacrum into the body of L5, through the L5-S1 disk as popularized by Smith and Bohlman.[22]

Various options for anterior treatment include anterior anulus and disk release in preparation for a posterior reduction. The technique of performing an anterior spinal fusion following a posterior reduction with either an intradiskal graft or structural cage is popular. However, the use of anterior instrumentation in the form of threaded screws compress-

ing the bone graft is possible. For those patients with only a partial posterior reduction, sparing the L5 segment through the disk space into S1 with a fibular dowel graft is also an option for solidifying the anterior column.[23,24]

So how does a surgeon decide the approach for a specific patient with a high-grade isthmic dysplastic spondylolisthesis? The first step is to determine exactly how much reduction should be obtained. The risk of surgery, especially neurologic risk to the L5 root with subsequent dorsiflexion weakness or complete foot drop, is highest in those patients who undergo a more aggressive reduction procedure.[9,15] However, the pseudarthrosis risks are higher for patients who are left in a biomechanically unstable position with marked residual forward translation and, especially, angulation in the sagittal plane with a kyphotic slip angle[7,8] One attractive option appears to be a partial reduction aimed at improve-

50%. Risk factors for pseudarthrosis with these in situ fusions included female gender with excessive L5-S1 mobility, a dysplastic lumbosacral region and small lumbar transverse processes, a markedly kyphotic slip angle, and signs of sacral root stretch and overall global anterior sagittal imbalance. In one group of in situ fusion patients, the size of the transverse processes in cm² was a statistically significant predictor of successful in situ fusion.[8] Patients with transverse process surface areas that averaged 3.59 cm² had successful fusions, whereas those with a surface area of only 1.59 cm² had pseudarthroses. A patient having only L5-S1 fusion had a higher pseudarthrosis risk than those patients having fusions from L4 to the sacrum. It is important to critically assess the fusion using a good quality Ferguson coronal view of the lumbosacral region[7] (Fig. 2).

The Authors' Preferred Treatment

Our current approach to patients with high-grade isthmic dysplastic spondylolisthesis with a kyphotic slip angle, with or without trunk imbalance, and signs of L5 and/or sacral nerve root impingement includes a wide decompression, posterior instrumentation with partial reduction, sacroplasty if required, and posteralateral fusion of L4 or L5 to the sacrum.[8] An anterior fusion by the posterior route is always planned; when adequate access cannot be obtained to the L5-S1 disk posteriorly, it is done by a formal anterior route on a different day.[23] Patients are positioned flexed at the hips and knees prior to the decompression. A Gill laminectomy and bilateral L5 and S1 nerve root decompressions are performed. It is extremely important to decompress the L5 nerve roots widely past the tips of the L5 transverse processes. Pedicle screws are placed at L5 and S1, and we also recommend an additional point of sacral pelvic fixation that includes bilateral distal iliac wing screws.[25] After placing mild distraction on the

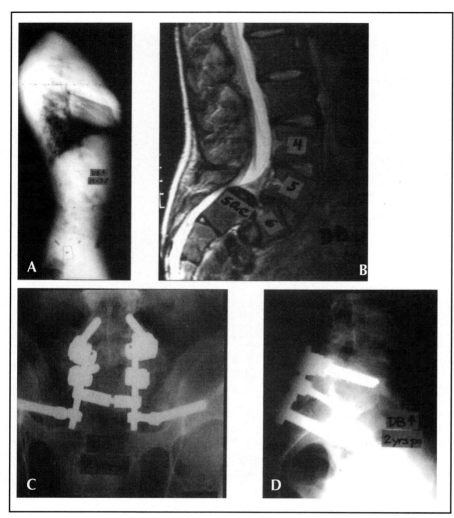

Fig. 7 A and **B,** Imaging studies of a teenager with a severe spondyloptosis of L6 on the sacrum. **C** and **D,** The patient underwent a L6 spondylolectomy and anterior and posterior spinal fusion with instrumentation placing L5 onto the sacrum. Radiographs at 2 years after surgery demonstrate a solid fusion between L5 and the sacrum, with near normal alignment.

ment of the slip angle, which will improve the biomechanics of the slipped segment while limiting the neurologic risk to the L5 nerve root. Postural reduction using a cast postoperatively is also an option for children, although its use seems to be declining with the advent of more versatile spinal instrumentation systems that can accommodate smaller children.[8] Each surgeon needs to form a risk/benefit ratio for each patient based on many factors, including patient presentation, the exact type of pathology, the

tolerance of the parents and the patient to accepting the risks associated with a partial reduction, and the subsequent risks of pseudarthrosis if less aggressive treatment is planned. In addition, the experience of the surgeon in these various techniques is also important in deciding the best approach.

In situ fusions with postoperative cast immobilizations were initially performed on patients with high-grade isthmic dysplastic spondylolisthesis[7] (Fig. 4); however, the pseudarthrosis rate approached

L5-S1 segment, a sacroplasty may be performed to shorten the sacrum and decrease the stretch of the L5 nerve roots. Next, the patient is placed with the hips and knees in an extension that will secondarily flex the pelvis to meet the L5 segment. Rods are contoured, placed into the distal fixation (S1 and iliac screws), and flexed to meet the L5 segment. An attempt is made to gain access to the L5-S1 disk to place morcellized graft and/or structural cages if the reduction is such that the disk is accessible through the posterior route. The instrumentation is then locked in place. Intraoperative AP and lateral radiographs are carefully reviewed, and the patient undergoes a formal wake-up test to assess bilateral foot and ankle movement. Iliac crest bone graft already harvested proximal to the iliac screws is then placed over the decorticated transverse processes and sacral ala bilaterally (Figs. 5 and 6).

If formal anterior spinal fusion has not been performed, the patient usually will be brought back 5 to 7 days postoperatively for the procedure. Depending on the degree of reduction obtained, a formal diskectomy with structural grafts or metallic cages is used with the anterior iliac crest graft for the fusion. If the slip angle and translation correction have not been enough to allow access to the L5-S1 disk, then an allograft fibular graft is reamed over a Kirschner wire that is placed from the midportion of the L5 body through the L5-S1 disk and into the proximal sacrum.[23,24] The patient is placed in a single pantaloon brace and may begin ambulation soon after surgery depending on the security of fixation obtained.

Careful monitoring of the L5 nerve roots during these surgeries is of paramount importance. We have found that somatosensory-evoked potential monitoring, which is a mixed nerve assessment, often does not provide the best information regarding L5 nerve root function. In addition, spontaneous electromyograms have not been very helpful

in evaluating excessive L5 nerve root stretch or dysfunction noted postoperatively by toe/ankle dorsiflexion weakness. Thus, we have been using direct nerve stimulation as an attempt to carefully monitor the L5 nerve root before decompression, after decompression, and after reduction. We have found this to be the best way to keep a close eye on L5 nerve root function along with an intraoperative postinstrumentation and postreduction wake-up test to optimize foot and ankle dorsiflexion function postoperatively.

The results of these procedures at our institution have been reported by Molinari and associates,[8] who studied 60 patients with high-grade isthmic dysplastic spondylolisthesis treated by two attending spinal surgeons. Three groups were evaluated: posterior spinal fusion in situ (n = 15); posterior spinal fusion with instrumentation and postural reduction (n = 19); and posterior spinal fusion with instrumentation, partial reduction, and formal anterior spinal fusion (n = 26). The fusion rates in these three groups were 55%, 71%, and 98%, respectively. The patients with a solid fusion had the best clinical outcomes with respect to function, pain relief, and overall satisfaction with the procedure. All seven patients with pseudarthrosis following in situ fusion were revised with instrumented posterior spinal fusion and have undergone solid fusion. Three patients in the partial reduction group had temporary L5 neurapraxia. One patient had posterior migration of bilateral intrasacral rods with loss of reduction, and we have abandoned that technique for sacral pelvic fixation. Another patient had pseudarthrosis following circumferential fusion and required a revision fusion.

For those patients with a true spondyloptosis with the last vertebral segment sitting well below the top of the sacrum, the two best options appear to be in situ fusion with fibular dowel grafts placed either from posterior to anterior or vice versa[22] and a spondylolectomy or Gaines

procedure.[20,21] In this challenging procedure, the lowest vertebral segment is resected and the supra-adjacent segment is placed back onto the sacrum and held with posterior instrumentation and fusion (Fig. 7). This procedure should be done only by those surgeons who are experienced in the surgical treatement of patients with high-grade isthmic dysplastic spondylolisthesis.

Summary

Surgical treatment of patients with high-grade isthmic dysplastic spondylolisthesis is still somewhat controversial. Our surgical approach includes wide nerve root decompression, partial reduction with improvement of the slip angle, posterior instrumentation, and posterior as well as anterior fusion. This approach has proven to provide the best fusion rates and clinical outcomes with acceptable complication rates. Using sound surgical techniques and principles, a high degree of clinical success can be achieved in this patient population.

References

1. Meyerding HW: Spondylolisthesis. *Surg Gynecol Obstet* 1932;54:371-377.

2. Wiltse LL, Winter RB: Terminology and measurement of spondylolisthesis. *J Bone Joint Surg Am* 1983;65:768-772.

3. Boxall D, Bradford DS, Winter RB, Moe JH: Management of severe spondylolisthesis in children and adolescents. *J Bone Joint Surg Am* 1979;61:479-495.

4. DeWald RL, Faut MM, Taddonio RF, Neuwirth MG: Severe lumbosacral spondylolisthesis in adolescents and children: Reduction and staged circumferential fusion. *J Bone Joint Surg Am* 1981;63:619-626.

5. Muschik M, Zippel H, Perka C: Surgical management of severe spondylolisthesis in children and adolescents: Anterior fusion in situ versus anterior spondylodesis with posterior transpedicular instrumentation and reduction. *Spine* 1997;22:2036-2043.

6. Marchetti PG, Bartolozzi P: Classification of spondylolisthesis as a guideline for treatment, in Bridwell KH, DeWald RL, Hammerberg KW, et al (eds): *The Textbook of Spinal Surgery*, ed 2. Philadelphia, PA, Lippincott-Raven, 1997, vol 2, pp 1211-1254.

7. Lenke LG, Bridwell KH, Bullis D, Betz RR, Baldus C, Schoenecker PL: Results of in-situ

fusion for isthmic spondylolisthesis. *J Spinal Disord* 1992;5:433-442.

8. Molinari RW, Bridwell KH, Lenke LG, Ungacta FF, Riew KD: Complications in the surgical treatment of pediatric high-grade, isthmic dysplastic spondylolisthesis: A comparison of three surgical approaches. *Spine* 1999;24:1701-1711.

9. Petraco DM, Spivak JM, Cappadona JG, Kummer FJ, Neuwirth MG: An anatomic evaluation of L5 nerve stretch in spondylolisthesis reduction. *Spine* 1996;21:1133-1139.

10. Freeman BL III, Donati NL: Spinal arthrodesis for severe spondylolisthesis in children and adolescents: A long-term follow-up study. *J Bone Joint Surg Am* 1989;71:594-598.

11. Harris IE, Weinstein SL: Long-term follow-up of patients with grade-III and IV spondylolisthesis: Treatment with and without posterior fusion. *J Bone Joint Surg Am* 1987;69:960-969.

12. Maurice HD, Morley TR: Cauda equina lesions following fusion in situ and decompressive laminectomy for severe spondylolisthesis: Four case reports. *Spine* 1989;14:214-216.

13. Schoenecker PL, Cole HO, Herring JA, Capelli AM, Bradford DS: Cauda equina syndrome after in situ arthrodesis for severe spondylolisthesis at the lumbosacral junction. *J Bone Joint Surg Am* 1990;72:369-377.

14. Dick WT, Schnebel B: Severe spondylolisthesis: Reduction and internal fixation. *Clin Orthop* 1988;232:70-79.

15. Hu SS, Bradford DS, Transfeldt EE, Cohen M: Reduction of high-grade spondylolisthesis using Edwards instrumentation. *Spine* 1996;21:367-371.

16. Johnson JR, Kirwan EO: The long-term results of fusion in situ for severe spondylolisthesis. *J Bone Joint Surg Br* 1983;65:43-46.

17. Poussa M, Schlenzka D, Seitsalo S, Ylikoski M, Hurri H, Osterman K: Surgical treatment of severe isthmic spondylolisthesis in adolescents: Reduction or fusion in situ. *Spine* 1993;18:894-901.

18. Ani N, Keppler L, Biscup RS, Steffee AD: Reduction of high-grade slips (grades III-V) with VSP instrumentation: Report of a series of 41 cases. *Spine* 1991;16(suppl 6):S302-S310.

19. Boos N, Marchesi D, Zuber K, Aebi M: Treatment of severe spondylolisthesis by reduction and pedicular fixation: A 4-6 year follow-up study. *Spine* 1993;18:1655-1661.

20. Gaines RW, Nichols WK: Treatment of spondyloptosis by two stage L5 vertebrectomy and reduction of L4 onto S1. *Spine* 1985;10:680-686.

21. Lehmer SM, Steffee AD, Gaines RW Jr: Treatment of L5-S1 spondyloptosis by staged L5 resection with reduction and fusion of L4 onto S1 (Gaines procedure). *Spine* 1994;19:1916-1925.

22. Smith MD, Bohlman HH: Spondylolisthesis treated by a single stage operation combining decompression with in situ posterolateral and anterior fusion: An analysis of eleven patients who had long-term follow-up. *J Bone Joint Surg Am* 1990;72:415-421.

23. Hanson DS, Bridwell KH, Rhee JM, Lenke LG: Dowel fibular strut grafts for high-grade dysplastic isthmic spondylolisthesis. *Spine* 2002;27:1982-1988.

24. Smith JA, Deviren V, Berven S, Kleinstueck F, Bradford DS: Clinical outcome of trans-sacral interbody fusion after partial reduction for high-grade L5-S1 spondylolisthesis. *Spine* 2001;26:2227-2234.

25. McCord DH, Cunningham BW, Shono Y, Myers JJ, McAfee PC: Biomechanical analysis of lumbosacral fixation. *Spine* 1992;17(suppl 8):S235-S243.

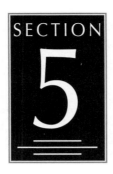
Problems of the Cervical Spine

Problems of the Cervical Spine

The articles in this section address the evaluation of children who have cervical spine problems. The injured child is difficult to evaluate. Because of the potential for serious consequences, cervical spine injuries in all children must be evaluated promptly and expeditiously. These three articles describe current methods available to evaluate cervical spine problems in children and offer excellent background for anyone who treats children, particularly those on the front line such as the emergency department.

Assessment of the immature spine poses several problems. Vertebral ossification is incomplete because a high percentage of the spine is still cartilaginous, which often confuses the examiner. No comparison views are available, and each child's ossification pattern is unique. There are few developmental markers, such as in the elbow. In addition, children may not cooperate with the examination or are unable to communicate. Children who can communicate often cannot be specific about their complaints. With many cervical spine injuries, the mechanism of injury is not clear, or the injury is associated with a violent force, such as that which occurs in a motor vehicle accident or a collision between a pedestrian and a vehicle. In these situations, patients typically have many associated injuries as well.

Children are very elastic, and their joints are hypermobile. This hyperelasticity is not limited to the extremities, but it also is characteristic in the axial skeleton, particularly in the cervical spine motion segments, which can give the false impression of instability. Growth in children is disproportionate. As we know, children do not begin as small adults and then just gradually grow larger. Rather, the various segments grow at different rates. Initially, the skull is much larger than the trunk, and simply placing a child in a supine position can lead to significant flexion of the cervical spine. These excellent articles help the reader to analyze each problem and put the various elements in perspective.

Peter Pizzutillo's article on cervical spine injury focuses on the clinical assessment of the injured child, highlighting associated problems that suggest cervical injury such as skull trauma, mandibular injuries, and posturing of the child's head and neck. He provides an excellent discussion about hypermobility that can be associated with normal growth but may be misinterpreted as an injury, such as pseudosubluxation of C2-C3. He describes various mechanisms of injury, including compression from vertical loads leading to the Jefferson fracture and hyperextension that can result in the hangman's fracture. Odontoid fractures in the young child are the result of flexion and shear, similar to an epiphyseal injury. Although these fractures are the most commonly recognized cervical fractures in children, the diagnosis may be confusing to the inexperienced.

John Dormans article describes the developmental anatomy of the atlas and axis and its relationship with the occiput, emphasizing how the unique features of the immature spine influence injury pattern. This article also offers an excellent discussion of a perplexing problem that occurs in the young child—spinal cord injury without observable radiograph abnormality (SIWORA). In children, the elasticity of the vertebral spine exceeds that of the spinal cord, which can result in significant spinal cord injuries that may not be detected on routine radiographs. He notes that the axis of normal flexion and extension in the cervical spine changes with the age of the child, eventually descending to the adult level of C5-C6, as the ratio of the head to the thorax approaches that of the adult. This changing motion pattern greatly influences the level of injury in the cervical spine.

This article also provides an excellent discussion of the radiographic evaluation after acute injury. Dr. Dormans offers step-by-step recommendations on how to evaluate the upper cervical spine, and he describes its relationship with the skull. The role of special tests, such as CT, dynamic views, and three-dimensional reconstructions is described, as is the role of MRI evaluation in the acute period.

In the third article in this section, Martin Herman reviews torticollis in infants and children. Torticollis is a common complaint that demands evaluation. He reminds us that torticollis is head rotation and tilt, not just head tilt, which is an important point because true torticollis suggests problems in the upper cervical spine. The article includes an excellent discussion of the etiology and treatment of congenital muscular torticollis, which is the most common cause of torticollis in the first year of life.

The article also describes the complete and rather extensive range of problems that cause torticollis, including infection, neurologic problems, gastrointestinal problems, trauma, and tumors. Anyone who examines children must have more than a passing familiarity with these problems. Although these problems are uncommon, once identified, diagnosis and treatment should proceed promptly.

We now have technology available to extensively evaluate cervical spine problems in children. CT scanners are faster and becoming more readily available in the emergency department. MRI allows evaluation of the spinal cord and its relationship to the spinal canal. This collection of articles provides excellent algorithms for evaluation and management of these very complex cervical problems. Implementation of these guidelines will significantly reduce the potential for further deformity and neurologic injury.

Robert N. Hensinger, MD
Professor
Department of Orthopaedic Surgery
University of Michigan Health
  System
Ann Arbor, Michigan

Injury of the Cervical Spine in Young Children

Peter D. Pizzutillo, MD

Abstract

The evaluation of injury of the cervical spine in children is complicated by biomechanics of the pediatric cervical spine that differ from those in the adult, by incomplete maturation and ossification of the vertebral segments, and by difficulties the physician may have in communicating with the child. Because the upper cervical region, from occiput to C2, is most susceptible to injury in children, it is important to have an understanding of mechanisms of injury, diagnostic imaging modalities, and therapeutic interventions. A clear understanding of adult and pediatric cervical spine differences will facilitate early diagnosis and appropriate treatment of cervical spine injuries in young children.

Although spine injury in the child is rare, a high index of suspicion of injury must be maintained when evaluating the traumatized child to avoid delay in diagnosis and potential injury to the spinal cord. Important differences exist in evaluating the young child compared with the adult. Extracting a reliable history of injury in the absence of a mature witness may be impossible. Communication is stifled when the patient is a nonverbal toddler or when the child is panicked and unable to respond to questions about the injury. Loss of consciousness in the child imposes the same limitations in evaluation as in the unconscious adult.

In addition to problems in communication, the anatomy of the skull and cervical spine in the young child is sufficiently different than that of the adult to influence the patterns of cervical spine injury that are observed in the immature population. Children younger than 8 years exhibit a higher ratio of skull diameter to chest diameter. The importance of this increased ratio resides in the observation that in children with suspected neck injury who are secured in the supine position to a flat spinal board, the cervical spine will be passively positioned in flexion because of the large occipital area.[1] This flexed position may jeopardize the integrity of the cervical cord if the patient has a neck injury that has produced instability in flexion. To place the cervical spine in a more neutral position, specialized pediatric spinal boards are available that incorporate a cutout for the occiput. If a specialized transport spinal board is not available, a towel roll should be placed under the shoulders to allow the head to drop into mild extension and effectively position the neck in neutral.

The young child's relatively large head is also a factor that focuses the fulcrum of flexion and extension of the cervical spine at the C2-3 or C3-4 levels as opposed to the more caudal fulcrum at C5-6 in the child older than 8 years and thus exposes the upper cervical spine in this group to greater loads.[2] This observation is consistent with the clinical observation of increased frequency of injury of the upper cervical spine in children younger than 8 years when compared with older children. Rotatory subluxation of C1-C2 is rarely the result of trauma in the young child and is usually secondary to inflammation of the posterior pharynx.

Incomplete ossification of the cervical spine with an increased cartilage-to-bone ratio and the intrinsic flexibility of the immature spine make radiographic interpretation more difficult in children younger than 8 years. It is important to appreciate these differences and avoid applying established parameters of radiographic stability from the adult population to the immature spine.

Assessment of the Injured Child

Every attempt should be made to obtain a history of injury from a reliable witness. A comprehensive initial examination of the entire musculoskeletal and neurologic systems is mandatory and must be clearly documented for meaningful comparison with later observations.

The presence of scalp or skull injury, submental injury, local tenderness of the cervical spinous processes or surrounding muscles, unwillingness to actively flex or rotate the neck, or cradling of the head (by grasping the skull with both hands to prevent passive motion of the neck) are factors that strongly suggest cervical spine injury.[3] The thoracic and lumbar spine and all limbs should be diligently examined to rule out coexistent injury. Documentation of the initial neurologic examination is essential as a standard to permit recognition of progressive deterioration in neurologic status.

A lateral radiograph of the skull and cervical spine with the child lying restrained in a supine position will serve as a baseline evaluation before more specialized studies are undertaken. When physical examination of the neck, neurologic evaluation, and radiographic studies are normal, gentle active motion of the neck in flexion and rotation may be permitted. When active motion can be accomplished without guarding, limitation of motion, or pain, the cervical spine may be cleared and no other imaging studies are indicated.

Radiographic evaluation of the immature cervical spine is complicated by increased flexibility and incomplete ossification in comparison with the mature spine. Increased flexibility of the cervical spine is the result of incomplete ossification of vertebral elements, laxity of joint capsules and interspinous ligaments, undeveloped posterior uncinate joints, horizontal orientation of the facet joints, and immature development of the muscles of the neck.

The ossification centers of subaxial cervical vertebral bodies fuse with their neural arches at the neurocentral synchondrosis by age 6 years, and the posterior vertebral arches fuse by age 4 years. In children younger than 6 years, the radiographic appearance of unfused neurocentral synchondroses, which lie anterior to the pedicles of the subaxial cervical spine, may be misinterpreted as fractures.

Ossification of the atlas and axis differs from that of the remaining cervical vertebrae. At birth, a primary center of ossification is radiographically present in each of the lateral masses of the atlas. The ossification of the anterior arch of the atlas may not appear radiographically until 12 months of age and may initially be seen as a single center or as multiple centers. The posterior neural arches of the atlas will usually fuse together by age 7 years but may remain unfused into adulthood. The absence of ossification of the anterior arch of the atlas in children younger than 12 months complicates the evaluation of atlantoaxial instability and eliminates the ability to measure the atlantodens interval. The presence of multiple ossification centers of the anterior arch of the atlas and unfused posterior neural arches of the atlas may suggest the presence of a fracture on radiographic evaluation. Congenital failure of formation of the posterior arch of the atlas may be noted radiographically as an isolated ossicle that is distant from the remainder of the atlas, or as a flange of bone that is fused to the base of the occiput (occipitalization of the atlas). CT has allowed more specific analysis of the immature atlas and more precise determination of injury.

Five primary ossification centers contribute to the formation of the axis. Two parallel ossification centers fuse by age 3 months to form the dens. The summit ossification center is a secondary center that appears by age 6 years and fuses with the remainder of the dens by age 12 years. The remaining primary centers of ossification occur at the two neural arches and at the body of the axis. The junction of the dens with the body of the axis is the basilar synchondrosis. Fusion of the basilar synchondrosis is noted between 6 and 11 years of age with rare persistence of vestiges of the synchondrosis in the mature spine. In the young child, the radiographic presence of the basilar synchondrosis or failure of the summit ossification center to fuse with the remainder of the dens (ossiculum terminale) may be confused with fractures of the dens (Figure 1). The basilar synchondrosis is situated at a more caudal level within the body of the axis than fractures of the base of the dens. Fractures through the basilar synchondrosis do occur and usually result in anterior or posterior tilting of the odontoid process and an increase in the width of the retropharyngeal space at the base of the axis.[4-7]

When increased width of the retropharyngeal space is noted on lateral radiographs of the cervical spine, it should be carefully evaluated. Although an increase in width of the retropharyngeal space beyond established limits may indicate occult injury of the cervical spine, it is also present in association with forced expiration, such as crying, or with breath holding. In the absence of forced expiration, a width of up to 3.5 mm at the anterior base of the vertebral body of the axis or up to 7.5 mm at the anterior base of the vertebral body of C6 is normal in children.

Ossification of vertebral bodies of the subaxial cervical spine is more advanced at the dorsal aspect of the body and progresses anteriorly with full maturation at age 24 years. In the young child, incomplete ossification of vertebral bodies creates the radiographic appearance of anterior wedging of vertebral bodies. Although the immature cervical vertebral bodies will appear to be rectangular in shape by age 7 years, before that time wedging of vertebral bodies may be confused with anterior compression fractures.

Pseudosubluxation is the apparent presence of intersegmental instability that is noted on neutral lateral radiographs of the immature cervical spine. Relative forward displacement of a cervical vertebra in relation to the next inferior vertebral body with the appearance of flattening of the cervical axis or mild kyphosis at the level of concern may suggest that the cervical spine is unstable. Pseudosubluxation is most commonly noted at the C2-3 level but may also occur at C3-4. Forty percent of children younger than 8 years and 16% of those between 8 and 16 years of age will experience pseudosubluxation.[8] Persistence of pseudosubluxation into adulthood is rare. Lateral radiographs of the cervical spine in patients with pseudosubluxation will reveal that the retropharyngeal space is not widened and the posterior spinolaminar line of C2 is positioned behind Swischuk's line, which is drawn from the posterior spinolaminar line of C1 to the posterior spinolaminar line of C3[9] (Figure 2). If the posterior spinolaminar line of C2 is positioned anterior to Swischuk's line, true instability must be considered.

Experimental studies[10] have shown that elongation of the spinal column to a distance of 2 inches can

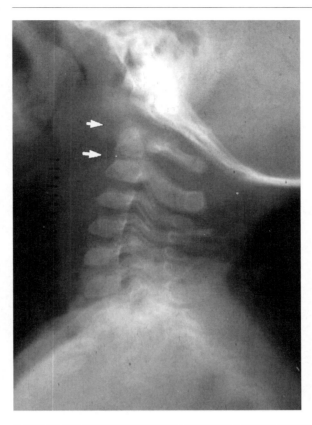

Figure 1 Incomplete ossification of the cervical spine demonstrates persistence of the basilar synchondrosis, apparent anterior wedging of the vertebral bodies, and apparent absence of the anterior arch of the atlas. The top arrow points to the unossified anterior arch of the atlas, and the bottom arrow points to the basilar synchondrosis.

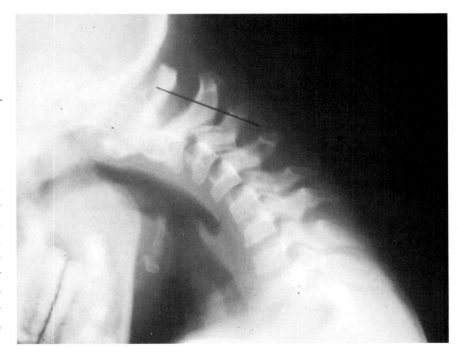

Figure 2 Swischuk's line is anterior to the posterior spinolaminar line of C2 and indicates the presence of pseudosubluxation.

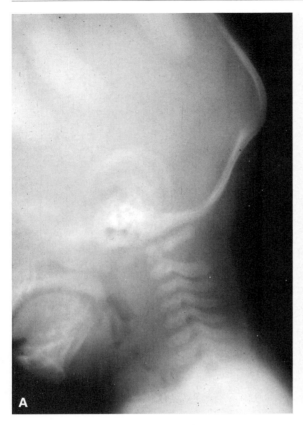
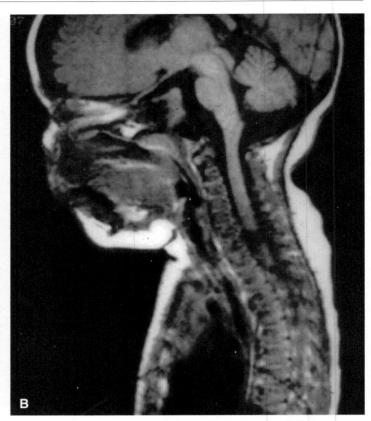

Figure 3 **A,** Lateral radiograph of the cervical spine reveals no evidence of vertebral column injury despite significant neurologic deficits (SCIWORA). **B,** MRI reveals disruption of the spinal cord in the absence of injury of the spinal column in a patient with SCIWORA.

be accomplished without disruption of the bone-cartilage-ligament complex; however, the spinal cord can only be stretched 0.25 inches before injury occurs. This occurrence may explain the mechanism of injury in patients with spinal cord injury without radiographic abnormality (SCIWORA), which has been more frequently reported in children than in adults. Prior to the advent of MRI, young patients with SCIWORA would have significant neurologic deficits and no radiographic evidence of spinal column disruption (Figure 3, *A*). MRI evaluation of the spinal cord in this patient population has subsequently documented the presence of spinal cord edema, hemorrhage within the spinal cord, disrup-

tion of the spinal cord, (Figure 3, *B*) vertebral body injury, and disk injury.[11,12] Autopsies have revealed spinal cord injury as the result of infarction, spinal cord traction, spinal cord impingement by ligamentum flavum or herniated disk, and injury at the vertebral end plate. Complete spinal cord lesions have been documented in most patients with SCIWORA; however, a significant number of patients will have incomplete spinal cord injuries and must be protected to prevent progressive deterioration in neurologic status.

Occipitoatlantal Instability

The occipitoatlantal junction does not have the benefit of osseous confines of many joints, such as the hip

joint, that impose a degree of stability. The junction is stabilized by soft tissues, including the tectorial membrane and the apical and alar ligaments. Attention to injuries at this level has been stimulated by Bucholz and Burkhead[13] in a review of fatalities as the result of severe injury caused by a vehicular accident. Although most patients with severe injury to the occipitoatlantal junction caused by a vehicular accident will die as a result of their neural injury, survivors may have a spectrum of motor deficits that vary from mild limb weakness to quadriplegia. Cranial nerve palsy is frequently noted and is the result of stretching of the nerves during displacement of the skull on the cervical axis. The most

commonly involved are the third and sixth cranial nerves.

A nontraumatic form of occipitoatlantal instability is uncommon and has been most frequently observed in patients with Down syndrome as an incidental finding on screening flexion and extension lateral radiographs of the cervical spine. The patient with Down syndrome and hypermobility at the occipitoatlantal junction is typically asymptomatic and neurologically intact but is restricted from high-risk activities that involve the cervical spine. A small group of patients who have no chromosomal abnormalities have been reported to have nontraumatic occipitoatlantal instability.[14] These individuals had no associated history of trauma and presented with the insidious onset of vertebrobasilar signs such as headache, nausea, vomiting, vertigo, and a sense of ill being. Lateral flexion and extension radiographs of the cervical spine revealed translation of the occiput on the cervical axis. Symptoms were believed to be the result of traction on the vertebral arteries as they course through the foramen of the atlas into the foramen magnum. No neurologic deficits were noted on examination.

True lateral radiographs of the cervical spine are mandatory for accurate analysis. Use of cineradiography (to position the head and neck in neutral) or CT may be necessary to define specific anatomic markers for measurement of instability. Wiesel and Rothman[15] conducted a radiographic study of the measurement of motion from the basion to the odontoid tip and found that 1 mm of motion is the limit of normal motion in the adult. These results have not been reported in children.

Power's ratio is defined as the distance from the opisthion to the anterior arch of the atlas over the distance from the basion to the posterior arch of the atlas. These landmarks may be difficult to identify on lateral radiographs of the cervical spine but are more reliably identifiable on CT sagittal reconstructions of the cervical spine. Power's ratio is 1.0 in the normal, stable cervical spine; if the ratio is 0.8 or less, it is diagnostic of instability at the occipitoatlantal junction.[16]

The patient with occipitoatlantal instability must be immobilized and protected. Although treatment options have included external immobilization, no longitudinal studies are available to support external immobilization as a reliable method of stabilizing this junction. Because the occipitoatlantal junction is stabilized primarily by ligaments and because continued or recurrent instability at this level is life threatening, surgical fusion of occiput to C1 or C2 is recommended as the primary treatment in eliminating instability and protecting the vital neural tissues. Once stability has been obtained, patients may return to most activities, excluding those that create significant risk for the cervical spine, such as football, ice hockey, rugby, and wrestling.

Jefferson Fracture

Jefferson fracture of the atlas is rare in children and is caused by axial loading of the cervical spine. Scalp lacerations and skull fractures are commonly associated with the occurrence of Jefferson fractures. Patients may have nonspecific neck pain and headache and are usually neurologically intact.[17] Physical examination may reveal guarding and limitation of neck motion, muscle spasm, and local tenderness with palpation of the base of the skull and upper cervical spine. Radiographic evaluation should include the skull

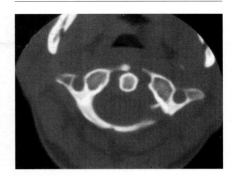

Figure 4 CT clearly documents fractures in the ring of the atlas and aids in differentiating fractures from incomplete ossification.

and the cervical spine. Nondisplaced or minimally displaced fractures of the ring of the atlas are frequently undetected with three-dimensional CT reconstructions of the cervical axis but are clearly demonstrated by standard CT (Figure 4). In the adult, an open-mouth AP radiograph that demonstrates combined overhang of 7 mm of the lateral masses of C1 over the lateral masses of C2 is diagnostic of disruption of the transverse atlantal ligament. This finding is not reliable in the immature spine because incomplete ossification of the lateral masses of C2 creates the impression of substantial overhang of the lateral masses of C1. CT provides detailed information regarding the ring of C1 and aids in differentiating immature development of elements of the ring from injury.

In the young patient with Jefferson fracture of the atlas with no evidence of disruption of the transverse atlantal ligament, external immobilization with a cervical collar is sufficient. When disruption of the transverse atlantal ligament occurs, more stringent immobilization in a halo vest or Minerva cast is indicated to prevent progressive displacement of the fracture and to promote healing.

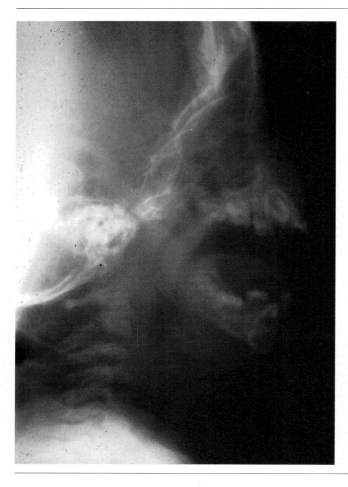

Figure 5 Radiograph of the cervical spine with a lucent defect noted at the posterior element of the axis (Hangman's fracture).

tebral levels.[18] MRI is indicated in patients with neurologic deficits to evaluate the status of the spinal cord and the integrity of the C2-3 disk.[19]

Treatment of patients with Hangman's fracture involves immobilization with a halo vest or Minerva cast when minimal displacement exists at the fracture site. When displacement of the fracture results in spinal cord compression, reduction may be obtained through the use of halter traction that will gently extend the neck. Traction is applied with minimal weight and is primarily positional in nature. Frequent radiographic evaluation of the spinal alignment is indicated. Once acceptable reduction is achieved, the patient's alignment can be maintained through external immobilization with a halo vest or Minerva cast.[20] Surgical intervention is rarely indicated.

Odontoid Fractures

Odontoid fractures are common in children and are the result of birth trauma, falls, and motor vehicle crashes.[21] Patients may have nonspecific neck pain, acute torticollis, apprehension with range of motion of the neck, or neck cradling. Physical examination reveals local tenderness at the upper cervical spine, spasm of neck muscles, limited motion of the neck, or fixed torticollis. The neurologic evaluation is usually normal. Torticollis is discussed in more detail in chapter 65.

Open-mouth AP radiographs of the upper cervical spine are difficult to obtain in the uncooperative child. Lateral radiographs of the cervical spine will show the presence of the basilar synchondrosis in the young child and complicate the evaluation of the upper cervical spine. CT will more precisely evaluate the upper cervical spine as well as the adjacent C2-3

Surgical intervention is rarely indicated.

Hangman's Fracture

Hangman's fracture, involving the posterior elements of the axis, may occur in the young child when significant injury imposes extension and distraction forces on the cervical axis or with indirect or minimal trauma that result in compressive forces generated by a relatively large head on the pedicles of the axis.[3] The presence of facial, skull, or submental injury emphasizes the need for special attention in the evaluation of the upper cervical spine. The child may guard the neck or cradle the head and have limited motion of the neck and neurologic deficits. Physical examination reveals spasm of the neck muscles, limited motion of the neck, and local tenderness with palpation of the spinous processes of the upper cervical spine. The results of neurologic evaluation range from normal status to hemiparesis.

A lateral radiograph of the cervical spine in a protected position may reveal injury (Figure 5). If no injury is noted on the screening lateral radiograph, active lateral flexion and extension radiographs of the cervical spine will show the presence of fractures at the base of the pedicles of the axis. When adequate radiographic evaluation of the cervical spine is not obtained, CT scan evaluation may be used to document the presence of fracture as well as the degree of displacement and the presence of concomitant injury at other cervical ver-

disk and the subaxial cervical spine. In the patient with neurologic deficits, MRI is indicated to evaluate the spinal cord and the status of the disk.

Treatment of the young patient with an odontoid fracture requires stabilization of the spine with gentle positional traction. Aggressive traction that may distract a disrupted spinal column and cause injury to an unprotected spinal cord should be avoided. After 1 to 2 weeks in traction, early bone healing provides sufficient clinical stability of the cervical spine to allow transition to a halo vest or Minerva cast immobilization. Healing of odontoid fractures in children is the rule with external immobilization (Figure 6). As opposed to odontoid fractures in the adult, the need for surgical intervention is rare in a child.[22]

Summary

The evaluation and treatment of infrequent injuries of the immature cervical spine require an understanding of the differences that exist in the anatomy and imaging of the growing patient and a high index of suspicion for injury that will allow early diagnosis and protection of vital neural structures. A detailed history, physical examination, neurologic evaluation, and appropriate imaging studies will result in a specific diagnosis that directs effective therapeutic interventions.

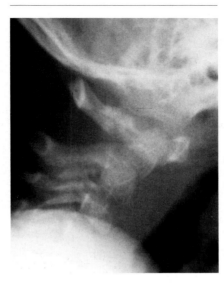

Figure 6 Lateral radiograph reveals a healing fracture of the base of the odontoid with anterior tilting of the dens.

References

1. Price AE: Unique aspects of pediatric spine injuries, in Ervico TJ, Bauer RO, Waugh T (eds): *Spinal Trauma*. Philadelphia, PA, JB Lippincott, 1991, pp 581-625.

2. Ruge JR, Sinson GP, McLane DG, et al: Pediatric spinal injury: The very young. *J Neurosurg* 1988;68:25-30.

3. Pizzutillo PD, Rocha EF, D'Astous J, et al: Bilateral fracture of the pedicle of the second cervical vertebra in the young child. *J Bone Joint Surg Am* 1986;68:892-896.

4. Allen B, Ferguson RL: Cervical spinal trauma in children, in Bradford DS, Hensinger RN (eds): *The Pediatric Spine*. New York, NY, Thieme, 1985, pp 89-104.

5. Bohn D, Armstrong D, Becker L, et al: Cervical spine injuries in children. *J Trauma* 1990;30:463-469.

6. Ogden JA: Spine, in Wickland E (ed): *Skeletal Injury in the Child*, ed 2. Philadelphia, PA, WB Saunders, 1990, pp 571-625.

7. Magerl F, Brunner C, Zoch K, et al: Fractures and dislocations of the vertebral column, in Weber BG, Brunker C, Freuler F (eds): *Treatment of Fractures in Children and Adolescents*. Berlin, Germany, Springer-Verlag, 1980, pp 226-243.

8. Cattell HS, Filtzer DL: Pseudosubluxation and other normal variations in the cervical spine in children. *J Bone Joint Surg Am* 1965;47:1295-1309.

9. Swischuk LE: Anterior displacement of C2 in children: Physiologic or pathologic? *Radiology* 1977;122:759-763.

10. Leventhal HR: Birth injuries of the spinal cord. *J Pediatr* 1960;56:447-453.

11. Pang D, Wilberger J: Spinal cord injury without radiographic abnormalities in children. *J Neurosurg* 1982;57:114-129.

12. Aufdermaur M: Spinal injuries in juveniles: Necropsy findings in 12 cases. *J Bone Joint Surg Br* 1974;56:513-519.

13. Bucholz RW, Burkhead WZ: The pathological anatomy of fatal atlanto-occipital dislocation. *J Bone Joint Surg Am* 1979;61:248-250.

14. Georgopoulos G, Pizzutillo PD, Lee MS: Occipito-atlantal instability in children. *J Bone Joint Surg Am* 1987;69:429-436.

15. Wiesel S, Rothman RH: Occiptoatlantal hypermobility. *Spine* 1979;4:187-191.

16. Powers B, Miller MD, Kramer RS, Martinez S, Gehweiler JA Jr: Traumatic anterior atlanto-occipital dislocation. *Neurosurgery* 1979;4:12-17.

17. Marlin AE, Gayle RW, Lee JF: Jefferson fractures in children. *J Neurosurg* 1983;58:277-279.

18. Keenan HT, Hollingshead MC, Chung CJ, Ziglar MK: Using CT of the cervical spine for early evaluation of pediatric patients with head trauma. *AJR Am J Roentgenol* 2001;177:1405-1409.

19. Rocha EF, Pizzutillo PD, D'Astous J, Kling TF, McCarthy RE: Bilateral pedicle fracture of the second cervical vertebra in the young child. *J Bone Joint Surg Am* 1986;58:892-896.

20. Frank JB, Lim CK, Flynn JM, et al: The efficacy of magnetic resonance imaging in pediatric cervical spine clearance. *Spine* 2002;27:1176-1179.

21. Brown RL, Brunn MA, Garcia VF: Cervical spine injuries in children: A review of 103 patients treated consecutively at a level 1 pediatric trauma center. *J Pediatr Surg* 2001;36:1107-1114.

22. Givens TG, Polley KA, Smith GF, et al: Pediatric cervical spine injury: A three year experience. *J Trauma* 1996;41:310-314.

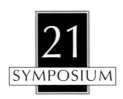

Evaluation of Children With Suspected Cervical Spine Injury

John P. Dormans, MD

Cervical spine injuries in infants and children are usually associated with motor vehicle accidents, falls, diving accidents, sports injuries, gunshot injuries, and, occasionally, child abuse. They range broadly, from minor soft-tissue injuries to severe fracture-dislocations with spinal cord injury or sudden death. Although rare, the injuries are worthy of special attention because of particular aspects relating to the pediatric cervical spine, including unique features of developmental anatomy, injury patterns, treatment, and prognosis. Appropriate algorithms for evaluation and management are essential for the care of these injured children. Deformity, instability, posttraumatic stenosis, and neurologic sequelae may be prevented with early recognition and appropriate management of those at risk.

Developmental Anatomy of the Cervical Spine

In order to adequately understand the differences in injury patterns unique to the pediatric cervical spine, it is essential to understand the anatomic and developmental features that are unique to infants and children.

The notochord is formed by week 2 of fetal development and is in close proximity to the paraxial mesoderm (mesenchymal tissue running parallel to the notochord), which becomes segmented into four cranial and eight cervical somites at weeks 2 and 3.[1,2] The somites each differentiate into cranial and caudal halves, which then reunite with the caudal and cranial halves, respectively, of the adjacent somite, forming each provertebra.[1,2] The notochord eventually constitutes the apical and alar ligaments as well as the nucleus pulposus of each intervertebral disk.[1,2] During weeks 5 and 6, chondrification takes place in each half of the vertebral body and neural arch.[1,2] Finally, ossification takes place in each body and lateral mass.[1-3]

The Atlas

The atlas develops from three ossification centers: the two primary ossification centers of the lateral masses, which are ossified at birth, and one secondary ossification center for the body, which ossifies at approximately 1 year of age (Fig. 1).[4,5] The posterior arches fuse by the age of 3 or 4 years; the neurocentral synchondroses between the lateral masses and the body fuse at approximately 7 years of age.[6]

The Axis

The axis is derived from five primary ossification centers, including two lateral masses (or neural arches), an odontoid process (which comprises two condensed longitudinally oriented halves at birth), and a body or centrum (Fig. 1). There are also two secondary centers: the ossiculum terminale at the tip of the odontoid process and the inferior ring apophysis.[6] The two halves of the odontoid process are generally fused or condensed at birth but may persist as two centers known as a dens bicornis.[6] The odontoid process is separated from the body by a dentocentral, or basilar, synchondrosis, which lies well caudad to the level of the superior articular facets, giving the ossification centers the overall appearance of a "cork in a bottle" on an open-mouth radiograph of the axis, with the odontoid process being the "cork" and the lateral masses and the body together forming the "bottle" (Fig. 1).[4,6] The dentocentral synchondrosis of the axis remains open in most children until the age of 3 years, is present in 50% by the age of 4 to 5 years, and is absent in most by the age of 6 years.[2,4,6] The tip of the odontoid process is not ossified at birth but appears around the age of 3

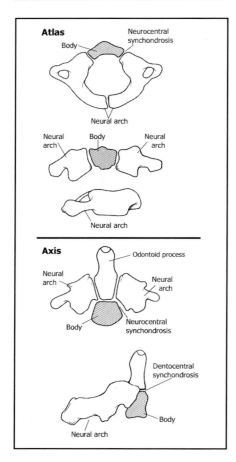

Fig. 1 Ossification centers of the atlas and axis during development. (Reproduced with permission from Copley LA, Dormans JP: Cervical spine disorders in infants and children. *J Am Acad Orthop Surg* 1998;6:205.)

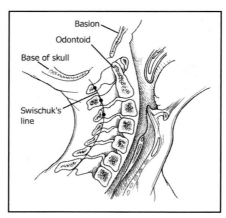

Fig. 2 The spinolaminar line (Swischuk's line) used to determine the presence of pseudo-subluxation of the second cervical vertebra on the third. (Reproduced with permission from Copley LA, Dormans JP: Cervical spine disorders in infants and children. *J Am Acad Orthop Surg* 1998;6:207.)

years and fuses to the odontoid process by the age of 12 years.[6] Occasionally, it remains as a separate ossiculum terminale persistens.[6]

The Lower Cervical Spine
The vertebrae of the lower cervical spine are each composed of three primary ossification centers: one for the body and one each for the two neural arches. The ring apophyses (the two secondary ossification centers) eventually ossify during late childhood and fuse in the early 20s. The neural arches fuse posteriorly by the age of 2 or 3 years, and

the neurocentral synchondroses fuse between the ages of 3 and 6 years. The vertebral bodies are wedge-shaped until age 7 years, when they begin to "square off."

Unique Features of the Immature Cervical Spine
There are several physiologic differences between the cervical spine in children and that in adults. For instance, children who are younger than 8 years old have increased neck motion, which is due to the relative laxity of the ligaments, relative muscle weakness, and incomplete ossification of the cartilaginous elements of the pediatric cervical spine as well as to other factors such as the horizontal orientation of the shallow facet joints.[4,7-10] As mentioned earlier, incomplete ossification in the cervical spine in children accounts for differences in measurements of certain relationships, including the basion-odontoid interval and the atlanto-odontoid interval (4 mm is considered the upper limit of the normal range for children). Furthermore, in chil-

dren, the vertebral bodies are more wedge-shaped than are those in adults. The cervical spine approaches adult size and shape by the age of 8 years as the vertebral bodies gradually lose their oval or wedge shape and become more rectangular.[11] The facet orientation changes to become more vertical, the uncinate processes increase in vertical height, and the ligaments and facet capsules increase in tensile strength.[10]

These factors help to explain the occurrence of spinal cord injury without radiographic abnormality (SCIWORA), which is seen in infants and young children and has been reported in a substantial percentage of young children with spinal cord injury.[4,7,12,13] SCIWORA is due to stretching of the vertebral column beyond the tolerance of the spinal cord or to spontaneous reduction of a dislocation or apophyseal separation. Biomechanical testing has shown that the immature cervical spine stretches as much as 2 in (5 cm) prior to failure. The spinal cord can tolerate stretching of only about 0.25 in (0.64 cm).[14]

When a SCIWORA occurs, careful neurologic evaluation is indicated to document the level and type of injury, to determine whether the cord injury is complete or incomplete, and to assess for the presence of spinal shock. MRI may be useful to identify the nature of the injury. In children with associated head trauma, monitoring of somatosensory evoked potentials has also been useful.[13] Multilevel spinal injuries also occur more frequently in children. In one study of 105 patients (mostly children and young adults) with cervical spine injuries, 24% of the injuries involved more than one level.[15] The use of steroid protocols soon after injury may be helpful in children with a spinal cord injury.[16]

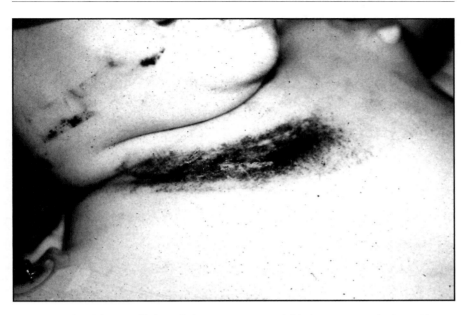

Fig. 3 Example of the so-called seat belt sign in a young child after a motor vehicle accident.

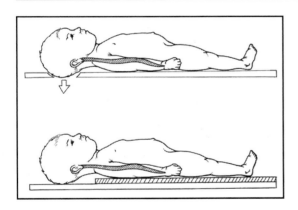

Fig. 4 Diagrams of young children on modified spine boards with either an occipital recess (top figure) or a mattress pad (bottom figure) to raise the chest.

Spinal cord injuries occur at different levels in children than in adults. In a study of 227 consecutively treated children with a traumatic fracture of the cervical spine, 87% of those who were younger than 8 years old had an injury of the third cervical vertebra or higher and had an increased risk of dying from the injury.[17] Conversely, children who were older than 8 years old had an injury pattern similar to that of adults (predominantly caudad to the fourth cervical vertebra), and none died.[17] Physiologic motion of the cervical

vertebrae in children is greater than that in adults, and a normal pediatric cervical spine may appear to have a subluxation. When a subluxation is not present, the movement is termed a pseudosubluxation; this condition does not require treatment. Pseudosubluxation of the second cervical vertebra on the third or of the third cervical vertebra on the fourth is common in children.[4,8,9,18,19] In one study, pseudosubluxation of the second cervical vertebra on the third was seen in 19% of children who were 1 to 7 years old; pseudo-

subluxation of the third cervical vertebra on the fourth was seen less frequently.[19] Another study showed that pseudosubluxation occurs in 40% of children younger than age 8 years.[9] Up to 4 mm of AP step-off of the second cervical vertebra on the third in flexion may be seen in children with a normal cervical spine.[9] The differentiation of this phenomenon from true injury can be facilitated by the use of Swischuk's line,[4,19] which is drawn along the posterior arch (the spinolaminar line) from the first cervical vertebra to the third (Fig. 2). The line should pass within 1.5 mm of the posterior arch of the second cervical vertebra.[19] When a fracture is present, the line is disrupted. Furthermore, pseudosubluxation reduces with extension, whereas acute traumatic subluxation generally does not reduce with extension, usually because of pain and muscle spasm.

Additionally, localized kyphosis in the midcervical spine (that is, the absence of cervical lordosis) can be a normal finding on lateral radiographs of children, occurring in up to 14% of children who are younger than 16 years old;[8] this finding in the adult cervical spine strongly indicates an abnormality. In children, localized kyphosis in the midcervical spine that occurs normally disappears with extension, whereas kyphosis resulting from an injury does not.

Apparent overriding of the anterior arch of the atlas on the odontoid process may also be seen, in extension, in very young children; it occurs in 20% of those between the ages of 1 and 7 years.[8] Children who are younger than 7 years old may have displacement of as much as two thirds of the arch above the odontoid process. (This finding is due to the fact that the body of the atlas is not ossified at birth, and the tip of the

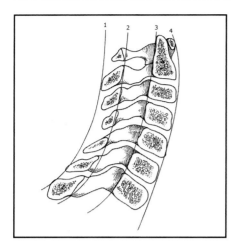

Fig. 5 Normal relationships in the lateral aspect of the cervical spine. 1 = spinous processes, 2 = spinolaminar line, 3 = posterior vertebral body line, and 4 = anterior vertebral body line. (Reproduced with permission from Copley LA, Dormans JP: Cervical spine disorders in infants and children. *J Am Acad Orthop Surg* 1998;6:207.)

odontoid process is cartilaginous.) In addition, anterior angulation of the odontoid process is seen in as many as 4% of children.[9] The presence or persistence of the basilar odontoid synchondrosis of the axis may result in the false impression of fracture of the base of the odontoid process at this level.[6] The synchondrosis is normally seen in 50% of all children up to the age of 11 years and can mimic an odontoid fracture. The synchondrosis appears sclerotic, unlike an acute fracture, and is located well caudad to the base of the odontoid process, where most fractures occur in adults.[7]

Initial Evaluation

Traumatic injury of the spinal column is uncommon in children. In most series of cervical spine injuries in adults and children, only 2% to 3% of all spinal injuries involve children.[4] In a study performed at a large, busy children's hospital, the incidence of injuries of the cervical spine averaged only 1.3 per year during a 15-year time period.[20] In another large series of 631 cervical spine injuries, only 12 (1.9%) occurred in children who were younger than 15 years old.[21] The common causes of injury include motor vehicle accidents, diving and other sports accidents, falls from a height, gunshot wounds, and child abuse.[4,22] Most spinal injuries in children who are younger than 8 years old involve the third cervical vertebra or higher, and most deaths from cervical spine injury occur in this age group.

When a child has a suspected injury of the cervical spine, the cervical spine should be immobilized in an adequate manner to prevent motion that could cause spinal cord or other additional injury. At my institution, the indications for immobilization after trauma include loss of consciousness (a Glasgow Coma Scale score of <13 points), altered mental status, a mechanism of injury that could be consistent with spinal injury (including, but not limited to, a motor vehicle–pedestrian or motor vehicle–cyclist accident, a fall from a considerable height, and a motor vehicle accident in which the patient was an unrestrained passenger), neck pain or guarding of the neck, or associated head or facial trauma. A physical finding such as a seat belt sign may also be indicative of cervical spine injury (Fig. 3).

Proper immobilization of the cervical spine on a spine board must allow for the disproportionately large size of the infant's or child's head with respect to the body. This may be accomplished either by using a spine board with an occipital recess or, more commonly, by placing a mattress or blankets beneath the shoulders and trunk of the child[23] (Fig. 4).

When an infant or child has a known or suspected cervical spine injury, the cervical spine should initially be immobilized with a rigid cervical orthosis, specifically designed and appropriate for infants or children, and there should be sandbags on each side of the head to prevent motion.[7] Movement should be minimized, and the child should be moved only as necessary. The back is inspected in a log-roll fashion with gentle in-line cervical traction until all screening AP and lateral radiographs of the spine as well as an open-mouth radiograph of the odontoid process (if appropriate) have been reviewed. The cervical spine remains immobilized until either initial radiographs are made and evaluated and injury is ruled out or definitive treatment is rendered.

Neurologic signs and symptoms, including the inability to move the extremities or a history of numbness, tingling, or weakness, are sought and may indicate a cervical spine injury. Examination of the spine begins with inspection and palpation for abnormalities, including sites of tenderness, deformity, ecchymosis, head tilt, contusion, and abrasion. A high index of suspicion for occult cervical spine injury should be maintained when patients have sustained multiple trauma.

The range of motion should be evaluated only when the child is conscious and cooperative and an unstable injury is not suspected. If the child has no neck pain or cervical spine tenderness and has a full, painless range of motion of the neck and spine, then the cervical collar may be removed and the child can be taken off the spine board. If the patient has tenderness or limitation of motion despite normal findings on a high-quality radiographic trauma series of the cervical spine, lateral radiographs with voluntary flexion and extension of the spine can be made to rule out injury or instability that was not detected on the initial radiographs. These studies should be performed only if the child is alert, oriented, and of an appropriate age to cooperate with the study. If the findings are negative and tenderness persists, a soft collar can be used for comfort, and other studies, such as MRI, can be considered. Ideally, the patient should not leave the emergency department unless the physician in charge has either ruled out injury of the cervical spine or made a diagnosis of a specific injury.

Radiographic Evaluation

The Trauma Series

Initial radiographs include high-quality cross-table lateral and AP radiographs and an open-mouth radiograph of the odontoid process. It is mandatory that the cervicothoracic junction (the disk space between the seventh cervical and first thoracic vertebrae) be visualized radiographically in every patient with adequate lateral plain radiographs (sometimes requiring careful downward traction on the arms to lower the shoulders), a so-called swimmer's view radiograph, or a CT scan with fine cuts through this portion of the spine.

Because of the variability in radiographic findings in children, care must be taken in reviewing these studies and in correlating this information with the history and physical findings in the child. Serial physical examinations may be useful when attempting to determine if a radiographic finding represents true abnormality or a normal variant for that child. Rapid resolution of symptoms with restoration of a voluntary range of motion suggests a normal variation, whereas persistence of tenderness, limitation of motion,

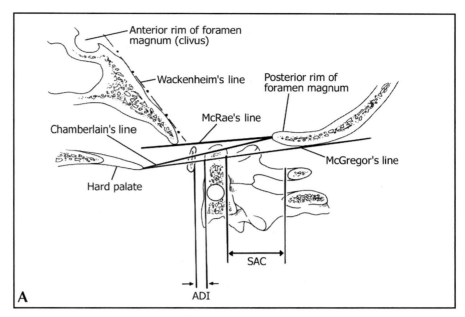
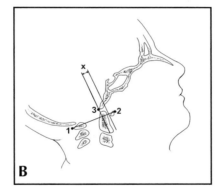
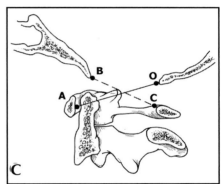

Fig. 6 Lateral craniometry. A, The lines commonly used to determine basilar impression and the measurements for determining atlantoaxial instability. ADI = atlanto-odontoid interval; SAC = space available for the cord. B, Method of measuring atlanto-occipital instability according to Wiesel and Rothman.[26] The atlantal line joins points 1 and 2. A line perpendicular to the atlantal line is made at the posterior margin of the anterior arch of the atlas. The distance (x) from the basion (3) to the perpendicular line should not vary by more than 1 mm in flexion and extension. C, The ratio of Powers and associates is determined by drawing a line from the basion (B) to the posterior arch of the atlas (C) and a second line from the opisthion (O) to the anterior arch of the atlas (A). The length of line BC is divided by the length of line OA. A ratio of greater than 1.0 is diagnostic of anterior occipitoatlantal dislocation. (Reproduced with permission from Copley LA, Dormans JP: Cervical spine disorders in infants and children. J Am Acad Orthop Surg 1998;6:206.)

paraspinal muscle spasm, or torticollis suggests the need for additional investigation.

Evaluation of the lateral radiograph begins with an assessment of the four lines corresponding to the

anterior vertebral bodies, the posterior vertebral bodies, the inside of the lamina (the spinolaminar line), and the tips of the spinous processes from the first to the seventh cervical vertebra[24] (Fig. 5). All four of these lines

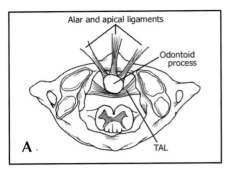

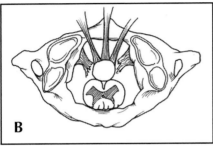

Fig. 7 Atlantoaxial joint viewed from above, demonstrating **(A)** normal relationships of the alar and apical ligaments and the transverse atlantal ligament (TAL) and **(B)** the checkrein effect of the alar ligaments, which prevents cord compression after rupture of the transverse atlantal ligament. (Reproduced with permission from Copley LA, Dormans JP: Cervical spine disorders in infants and children. *J Am Acad Orthop Surg* 1998;6:207.)

should follow a smooth, even contour. There should be a parallelism of the articular facets and a balance of the interspinous distances and the posterior aspect of the disk spaces.[18] The retropharyngeal space should be less than 7 mm, and the retrotracheal space should be less than 14 mm in children; however, these may be difficult to interpret in a normal, crying child.[25] Subtle findings suggestive of an injury at these levels include a widened disk space (apophyseal separation), avulsion fracture of the vertebral end plates, fractures of the spinous processes, and an increased distance between two spinous processes.

Another area of particular interest is the relationship of the first cervical vertebra, the second cervical vertebra, and the spinal cord as described by the atlanto-odontoid interval and the space available for the cord[26] (Fig. 6). The atlanto-odontoid interval should be less than 4 mm in children who are younger than 8 years old (some consider 5 mm to be acceptable[4]), whereas the value should be 3 mm or less in older children and adults.[27] In a child with atlantoaxial instability associated with a traumatic rupture or avulsion of the transverse ligament, the atlanto-odontoid interval may be substantially increased (Fig. 7).

The space available for the spinal cord is roughly defined by the "rule of thirds" proposed by Steel.[27] At the level of the odontoid process, one third of the space is occupied by the spinal cord, one third is occupied by the odontoid process, and one third is so-called free space.

At this level, the transverse ligament serves as the first line of defense, maintaining the atlanto-odontoid interval at 4 mm or less. The alar, or check, ligaments form the second line of defense. When the atlanto-odontoid interval exceeds 10 to 12 mm, then all ligaments have failed and the space available for the spinal cord is negligible, resulting in cord compression (Fig. 6).[27,28] MRI or CT scans can also be used to evaluate for instability and resultant compression in this area.[29] These findings should be correlated with the history and the findings of the physical examination to determine the clinical relevance of the instability for each child.

As shown in Figure 6, several other lines (McGregor's, McRae's, Chamberlain's, and Wackenheim's lines; the line used in the ratio of Powers and associates; and the lines described by Wiesel and Rothman[8,30-32]) have been described to help to evaluate the upper cervical spine as seen on lateral static radiographs. McGregor's line is one of the best for detecting basilar impression because the osseous landmarks are usually clearly seen at all ages.[8] The line is drawn from the superior surface of the posterior edge of the hard palate to the most caudad point of the occiput. If the tip of the odontoid process lies more than 4.5 mm above McGregor's line, the finding is consistent with basilar impression.[8] McRae's line defines the opening of the foramen magnum. The odontoid process projects above this line in patients with basilar invagination.[8] The lines of Wiesel and Rothman[26] are used to measure AP translation at the atlanto-occipital joint, which should be no more than 1 mm[31] (Fig. 6, *B*). The ratio of Powers and associates[32] is used to evaluate atlanto-occipital dislocation (Fig. 6, *C*). Values of 1.0 or more are abnormal, and values of less than 1.0 are normal.[32] If there is suspicion of abnormalities, a more detailed evaluation with MRI or CT may be indicated.[7,29]

Wholey and associates noted that the middle half of the odontoid process lies directly beneath the basion (the anterior lip of the foramen magnum) at an average distance of 5 mm on the lateral radiograph.[4,25] This distance may be increased up to 1 cm in children younger than age 8 years because of incomplete ossification.[25] More recently, the occipitovertebral relationship has been evaluated by measurement of the basion axial interval,[33] which is the distance between the basion and the posterior axial line (the rostral extension of the posterior cortex of the body of the axis). It has been observed that this interval should not exceed 12 mm in children who are younger than 13 years old.[33] The

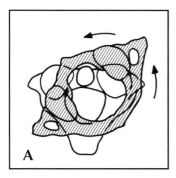 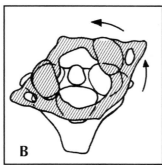 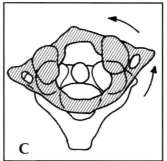 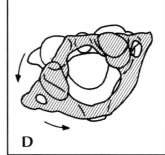

Fig. 8 Drawings of the Fielding and Hawkins classification of atlantoaxial rotatory displacement, showing the four types of rotatory fixation:[35] type I—rotatory fixation with no anterior displacement and the odontoid acting as the pivot (**A**), type II—rotatory fixation with anterior displacement of 3 to 5 mm and with one lateral articular process acting as the pivot (**B**), type III—rotatory fixation with anterior displacement of greater than 5 mm (**C**), and type IV—rotatory fixation with posterior displacement (**D**).

basion-odontoid interval has been found to be less reliable in young children.

At the base of the odontoid process, an optical phenomenon that can be mistaken for a fracture can occasionally be produced on plain radiographs. Mach bands are dark and light lines that appear at the borders of structures with different radiodensities and commonly occur at the base of the odontoid process where it joins the body of the axis and where the lateral masses join the odontoid.[34] CT may be useful to demonstrate definitively the presence or absence of a fracture in patients with persistent tenderness following trauma.

Special Studies

Special studies may supplement plain radiographs of the cervical spine in children. Oblique radiographs are useful in showing detail of the facet joints and pedicles. Lateral radiographs made under careful supervision, with the cervical spine in flexion and extension as mentioned previously, are used to evaluate for instability but may be inappropriate for very young or obtunded infants and children with head injury. False-negative findings may also occur

when the child has pain, is guarding the neck, or is frightened. Flexion and extension radiographs of the cervical spine should never be made when the patient is unconscious.

Tomography is very helpful for the evaluation of trauma of the upper cervical spine. However, these studies are associated with an increased amount of radiation compared with CT scans and MRI. At many hospitals, CT scanning with three-dimensional (3-D) reconstruction has replaced tomography.

CT scans allow better definition of bone injury, but fractures in the same plane as the plane of the imaging (such as fractures of the odontoid process with transverse images) may be missed without 3-D reconstruction or reformatted sagittal or coronal images. A CT scan with 3-D reconstruction should be used when plain radiographs are not definitive.[29] CT scans do not visualize ligaments and soft tissue well. Dynamic CT scans with neutral cuts and rotation cuts to the left and right are used to evaluate atlantoaxial rotatory displacement.[35] CT scans with 3-D reconstructions and reformatted sagittal and coronal images are also helpful at times to examine children with congenital anomalies of the cervical spine.

Myelography and CT myelography are used less commonly but may be indicated occasionally to demonstrate the presence of dural bands or compression in cases of stenosis or basilar impression.

MRI (either static, or dynamic in flexion and extension) is an excellent technique for examination of the brainstem and spinal cord, soft tissues (disks, ligaments, and so on), and bone of the cervical spine and for detection of hemorrhage associated with injury. MRI is very helpful in evaluating a comatose or unconscious child who cannot safely undergo dynamic radiography. When appropriate, an MRI study of the cervical spine can be easily added to an MRI study of the head. Sedation usually is required. MRI is also useful in the evaluation of a child with SCIWORA.[12]

Cervical Spine Injury

Clearance Protocols

Once a cervical collar or other immobilization device is in place (that is, applied either before or after the child arrives at the hospital), formal clearance (that is, a determination that the cervical spine is free of injury) to remove the collar is required. Clinical examination can be used if the patient is awake and alert, has no signs or symptoms of neck injury, and does not have a mechanism of injury consistent with a spine injury (as described previously).

If, after adequate plain radiographs have been made, an unconscious child with a suspected cervical spine injury is to undergo MRI or CT scanning for evaluation of a head or abdominal injury, one can consider performing those studies to evaluate the cervical spine as well.

For unconscious, uncooperative, or very young patients, MRI may be used to reveal soft-tissue and osseous injury of the cervical spine and its supporting structures that are not visible on plain radiographs. These studies may be the best way to rule out cervical spine injury and allow the removal of the cervical collar from unconscious individuals, thereby preventing the skin breakdown that can occur from prolonged use of such a collar.

The value of clearance protocols to rule out pediatric cervical spine injuries is still debated. Suspected cervical spine injuries are more difficult to rule out in young children not only for the reasons already mentioned, but also because the children are often unable to describe pain and are often uncooperative. Plain radiographs alone may not demonstrate occult injuries (for example, synchondrosis injury) and do not visualize the soft tissues (that is, the ligaments and disks) well. The cephalad and caudad ends of the cervical spine are also often difficult to evaluate, especially in children.

The role of MRI in identifying spinal injuries is well established; however, its role in evaluating children with suspected spinal injuries is less clear. MRI is the study of choice

for the evaluation of the spinal cord and is the most sensitive for the evaluation of soft tissue, ligaments, disks, and growth cartilage.

A retrospective study[36] performed at my institution between 1993 and 1997 identified 237 children with an ICD-9 (International Classification of Diseases, Ninth Revision) coding for neck injury. Ninety-three of these children had a cervical spine injury, and 79 had MRI studies that revealed injuries not seen on plain radiographs. Fifteen (19%) of the 79 patients had negative findings on radiographs and positive findings on MRI. Seven of them had ligamentous injuries, mostly at the first and second cervical levels. Seven others had other soft-tissue (muscle) injury only. One had a fracture (of the first cervical lateral mass) not seen on plain radiographs. MRI also made it possible to rule out injuries suspected on plain radiographs. Seven children had radiographs with suspicious findings (two had questionable subluxation of the second on the third cervical vertebra, one had an anomaly of the first cervical vertebra, three had a suspected fracture of the odontoid process, and one had a suspected fracture of the fourth cervical vertebra) that were later discounted with MRI as indications of injury. MRI also made it possible to rule out injuries suspected on CT. Three children who had a suspected odontoid fracture on CT scans had negative findings on MRI. Of those with evidence of ligamentous injuries on MRI, six were successfully treated with immobilization only and one died of associated injuries. MRI was also helpful in definitively ruling out cervical spine injury in intubated, obtunded, or uncooperative children. Twenty-five intubated or uncooperative children had MRI of the cervical spine. Three of them were found to

have serious injuries. The remaining 22 children had negative findings, their collars were removed, and they had no problems later.

MRI is a very sensitive method for evaluating children with suspected cervical spine injuries. It is useful when plain radiographs or CT scans are equivocal. MRI is the treatment of choice for ruling out injury of the cervical spine in obtunded, intubated, or uncooperative children. The sequence protocol for MRI currently includes sagittal T1-weighted images, conventional sagittal T2-weighted images, axial T1-weighted and T2-weighted images, and coronal T2-weighted images (if there is suspicion of unilateral injury). Determining which of the more subtle findings on MRI constitute instability requires further study.

Atlantoaxial Rotatory Subluxation

Trauma is a common cause of atlantoaxial rotatory subluxation. Other causes include infection, postoperative inflammation, and other inflammatory conditions, such as rheumatologic conditions. Children with atlantoaxial rotatory subluxation present with pain and torticollis and are best evaluated with plain radiographs and a dynamic rotation CT scan. Atlantoaxial rotatory subluxation represents a spectrum of abnormalities ranging from mild displacement to severe fixed displacement (atlantoaxial rotatory fixation). The Fielding and Hawkins classification is used to describe the abnormal relationship between the first and second cervical vertebrae in this disorder and to guide management (Fig. 8).[35]

Immobilization

There are several commercially available rigid cervical orthoses specifically designed for infants or children with a known or suspected cervical spine injury. Sandbags can also be used on each side of the head in combination with the spine board to prevent motion. Once the child arrives in the hospital and a diagnosis is made, traction can be used if appropriate. Traction can be applied with Gardner-Wells tongs or a halo ring. The advantage of a Minerva brace or cast is that no skeletal pins are needed, but the disadvantage is that contact dermatitis can develop under the brace or cast, especially the chin portion, and can contribute to temporomandibular joint pain and difficulties with eating.

A halo ring and vest has been used for immobilization of the cervical spine in children for some time. The advantages include ease of application, better immobilization and positioning, earlier mobilization of the patient than is possible when traction is used, fewer skin complications than occur with other orthoses, ease of access to wounds of the neck or scalp, and freedom of mandibular motion for eating and talking.

The technique for applying the halo ring and vest in children differs from that in adults as children have thinner skulls. A CT scan made prior to halo application may be helpful in the placement of pin sites so that cranial sutures in infants and other thin areas of the skull in young children can be avoided.

Eight to 12 pins are used with low insertional torques (1 to 5 in-lb) in children, whereas the standard construct in adults consists of four pins with an insertional torque of 6 to 8 in-lb. Complication rates for children treated with pediatric halo constructs (including multiple-pin constructs) are similar to those reported in adult series, with infection at anterior pin sites being the most common complication seen in children.[37]

Summary

The evaluation of a child with a suspected cervical spine injury differs substantially from that of an adult. Knowledge of the developmental anatomy and injury patterns is necessary to evaluate and manage these children effectively. Improved imaging techniques are facilitating the radiographic evaluation of such patients, and the understanding of trauma patterns and how these patterns influence the stability of the cervical spine is increasing. With the growing awareness of the pathoanatomy and natural history of these injuries, it will be possible to manage the issues related to the cervical spine in children more effectively.

References

1. Keynes RJ, Stern CD: Segmentation and neural development in vertebrates. *Trends Neurosci* 1985;8:220-223.

2. Tachdjian MO (ed): *Pediatric Orthopedics*, ed 2. Philadelphia, PA, WB Saunders, 1990, vol 1 & 3, pp 112-128, 2230-2238.

3. Bailey DK: The normal cervical spine in infants and children. *Radiology* 1952;59:712-719.

4. Sullivan JA: Fractures of the spine in children, in Green NE, Swiontkowski MF (eds): *Skeletal Trauma in Children*. Philadelphia, PA, WB Saunders, 1994, pp 283-306.

5. Ogden JA: Radiology of postnatal skeletal development: XI. The first cervical vertebra. *Skeletal Radiol* 1984;12:12-20.

6. Ogden JA: Radiology of postnatal skeletal development: XII. The second cervical vertebra. *Skeletal Radiol* 1984;12:169-177.

7. Flynn JM, Dormans JP: Spine trauma in children. *Semin Spine Surg* 1998;10:7-16.

8. Loder RT: The cervical spine, in Morrissy RT, Weinstein SL (eds): *Lovell and Winter's Pediatric Orthopaedics*, ed 4. Philadelphia, PA, Lippincott-Raven, 1996, vol 2, pp 739-779.

9. Cattell HS, Filtzer DL:Pseudo-subluxation and other normal variations in the cervical spine in children: A study of one hundred and sixty children. *J Bone Joint Surg Am* 1965;47:1295-1309.

10. Penning L: Normal movements of the cervical spine. *AJR Am J Roentgenol* 1978;130:317-326.

11. Swischuk LE, Swischuk PN, John SD: Wedging of C-3 in infants and children: Usually a normal finding and not a fracture. *Radiology* 1993;188:523-526.

12. Grabb PA, Pang D: Magnetic resonance imaging in the evaluation of spinal cord injury without radio-graphic abnormality in children. *Neurosurgery* 1994;35:406-414.

13. Pang D, Pollack IF: Spinal cord injury without radiographic abnormality in children: The SCIWORA syndrome. *J Trauma* 1989;29:654-664.

14. Leventhal HR: Birth injuries of the spinal cord. *J Pediatr* 1960;56:447-453.

15. Hadden WA, Gillespie WJ: Multiple level injuries of the cervical spine. *Injury* 1985;16:628-633.

16. Bracken MB, Shepard MJ, Collins WF Jr, et al: A randomized, controlled trial of methylprednisolone or naloxone in the treatment of acute spinal-cord injury: Results of the Second National Acute Spinal Cord Injury Study. *N Engl J Med* 1990;322:1405-1411.

17. Nitecki S, Moir CR: Predictive factors of the outcome of traumatic cervical spine fracture in children. *J Pediatr Surg* 1994;29:1409-1411.

18. Pennecot GF, Gouraud D, Hardy JR, Pouliquen JC: Roentgenographical study of the stability of the cervical spine in children. *J Pediatr Orthop* 1984;4:346-352.

19. Swischuk LE: Anterior displacement of C2 in children: Physiologic or pathologic. *Radiology* 1977;122:759-763.

20. Jones ET, Loder RT, Hensinger RN: Fractures of the spine, in Rockwood CA Jr, Wilkins KE, Beaty JH, Green DP (eds): *Fractures in Children*, ed 4. Philadelphia, PA, Lippincott Williams & Wilkins, 1996, pp 1023-1105.

21. Henrys P, Lyne ED, Lifton C, Salciccioli G: Clinical review of cervical spine injuries in children. *Clin Orthop* 1977;129:172-176.

22. Garfin SR, Shackford SR, Marshall LF, Drummond JC: Care of the multiply injured patient with cervical spine injury. *Clin Orthop* 1989;239:19-29.

23. Herzenberg JE, Hensinger RN, Dedrick DK, Phillips WA: Emergency transport and positioning of young children who have an injury of the cervical spine: The standard backboard may be hazardous. *J Bone Joint Surg Am* 1989;71:15-22.

24. Williams C, Bernstein TW, Jelenko C: Essentiality of the lateral cervical spine radiograph. *Ann Emerg Med* 1981;10:198-204.

25. Wholey MH, Bruwer AJ, Baker HL Jr: Lateral roentgenogram of the neck: With comments on the atlanto-odontoid-basion relationship. *Radiology* 1958;71:350-356.

26. Wiesel SW, Rothman RH: Occipitoatlantal hypermobility. *Spine* 1979;4:187-191.

27. Steel HH: Abstract: Anatomical and mechanical considerations of the atlanto-axial articulations. *J Bone Joint Surg Am* 1968;50:1481-1482.

28. Fielding JW, Cochran GV, Lawsing JF, Hohl M: Tears of the transverse ligament of the atlas: A clinical and biomechanical study. *J Bone Joint Surg Am* 1974;56:1683-1691.

29. McAfee PC, Bohlman HH, Han JS, Salvagno RT: Comparison of nuclear magnetic resonance imaging and computed tomography in the diagnosis of upper cervical spinal cord compression. *Spine* 1986;11:295-304.

30. Copley LA, Dormans JP: Cervical spine disorders in infants and children. *J Am Acad Orthop Surg* 1998;6:204-214.

31. Gabriel KR, Mason DE, Carango P: Occipito-atlantal translation in Down's syndrome. *Spine* 1990;15:997-1002.

32. Powers B, Miller MD, Kramer RS, Martinez S, Gehweiler JA: Traumatic anterior atlanto-occipital dislocation. *Neurosurgery* 1979;4:12-17.

33. Harris JH, Carson GC, Wagner LK: Radiologic diagnosis of traumatic occipitovertebral dissociation: 1. Normal occipitovertebral relationships on lateral radiographs of supine subjects. *AJR Am J Roentgenol* 1994;162:881-886.

34. Daffner RH: Pseudofracture of the dens: Mach bands. *AJR Am J Roentgenol* 1977;128:607-612.

35. Fielding JW, Hawkins RJ: Atlanto-axial rotatory fixation: Fixed rotatory subluxation of the atlanto-axial joint. *J Bone Joint Surg Am* 1977;59:37-44.

36. Closkey R, Flynn J, Dormans J, Mahboubi S: Abstract: The role of MRI in the assessment of pediatric cervical spine injuries. *Annual Meeting Proceedings of the Pediatric Orthopaedic Society of North America*. Rosemont, IL, Pediatric Orthopaedic Society of North America, 1999, p 70.

37. Dormans JP, Criscitiello AA, Drummond DS, Davidson RS: Complications in children managed with immobilization in a halo vest. *J Bone Joint Surg Am* 1995;77:1370-1373.

22

Torticollis in Infants and Children: Common and Unusual Causes

Martin J. Herman, MD

Abstract

Torticollis is a clinical symptom and sign characterized by a lateral head tilt and chin rotation toward the side opposite to the tilt. Many conditions cause torticollis. The differential diagnosis is different for infants than for children and adolescents. Congenital muscular torticollis associated with a contracture of the sternocleidomastoid muscle is the most common etiology of torticollis in infants. The condition of most infants with congenital muscular torticollis improves with a regimen of manual cervical stretching. Congenital anomalies of the occipital condyles and upper cervical spine must be ruled out before performing a release of the sternocleidomastoid muscle in a child who fails to improve with physical therapy. Unusual nonmuscular causes of torticollis in the infant also must be considered and include ocular torticollis caused by eye muscle weakness, Sandifer's syndrome resulting from gastroesophageal reflux, neural axis abnormalities, and benign paroxysmal torticollis. Torticollis in the older child is most frequently a manifestation of atlantoaxial rotatory displacement resulting from trauma or oropharyngeal inflammation (Grisel's syndrome). Retropharyngeal abscesses and pyogenic cervical spondylitis are unusual infectious causes of torticollis. Intermittent torticollis associated with headaches, vomiting, or neurologic symptoms may be caused by tumors of the posterior fossa. Benign and malignant neoplasms of the upper cervical spine are rare causes of torticollis in children. Torticollis resulting from cervical dystonia is also rare in children but may be seen in older adolescents.

Torticollis describes a lateral head tilt with rotation of the chin toward the side opposite to the tilt. This position is often called the cock-robin position. Torticollis is a clinical symptom and sign, not a diagnosis. For the clinician, identifying the etiology of torticollis and treating the underlying pathology can be challenging. Torticollis in an infant has a different list of potential etiologies

than torticollis in the older child or adolescent. Congenital muscular torticollis (CMT), caused by a contracture of the sternocleidomastoid (SCM) muscle, is the most common etiology of torticollis in infants. Children with torticollis are diagnosed most commonly with inflammatory conditions of the ear, nose, and throat (such as Grisel's syndrome) and traumatic atlantoaxial

rotatory displacement (AARD). These conditions frequently occur and are well known to most clinicians who care for children; therefore, diagnosis is relatively easy in most patients. Other less common etiologies, including upper cervical congenital anomalies, ocular pathology, gastroesophageal reflux, and neoplasia of the spinal column and neural axis demand a high index of suspicion by the physician to appropriately diagnose. Delay in establishing the correct etiology of torticollis is not uncommon, and may worsen the outcome for some children. This chapter will provide a framework for the clinical evaluation of torticollis to facilitate efficient and prompt diagnosis of the many potential etiologies of this condition. Common and unusual causes of torticollis will be discussed and treatment recommendations for each diagnosis will be presented.

Torticollis in the Infant
Congenital Muscular Torticollis
CMT, caused by contracture or shortening of the SCM muscle, is the most common etiology of torticollis in infants. Two different etiologies of CMT have been proposed. Because CMT can occur in associa-

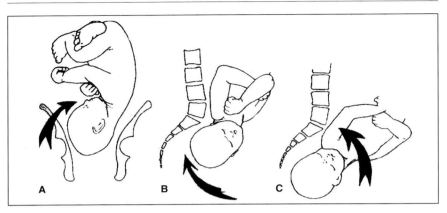

Figure 1 With normal progression of the fetus through the birth canal, the head and neck undergo flexion (**A**),lateral bending (**B**), and rotation (**C**). Difficult labor may cause a fixed and prolonged positioning of the head within the canal leading to increased pressure and a compartment syndrome of the SCM muscle. The resultant muscle fibrosis is a possible etiology of CMT. (Reproduced with permission from Davids J, Wenger D, Mubarak S: Congenital muscular torticollis: Sequela of intrauterine or perinatal compartment syndrome. *J Pediatr Orthop* 1993;13:141-147.)

tion with oligohydramnios, multiple births, developmental dysplasia of the hip, and metatarsus adductus, one theory is that restricted fetal motion coupled with head and neck malpositioning in utero results in contracture and fibrosis of the SCM muscle. A second theory is that CMT is the end-product of a compartment syndrome of the SCM that occurs toward the end of intrauterine life.[1] As the fetus descends the birth canal with the progression of labor, the head forward flexes, laterally bends, and rotates (Figure 1). With prolonged labor, the fetus' head and neck may be severely malpositioned for several hours, elevating the pressure of the SCM compartment. Muscle ischemia and fibrosis result, akin to injury seen in the muscle compartments of the tibia that have sustained a compartment syndrome.[1] The resulting SCM muscle contracture manifests as CMT in the neonate.

Treatment for the infant with CMT is typically sought by the parents when the infant is 3 weeks to 3 months of age because of a noted head tilt, and/or facial or skull asym-

metry. On examination, a defined mass or fullness of the SCM muscle on one side is noted. Lateral bending of the head away from the tight SCM muscle and rotation toward the same side of the tight SCM muscle are the most consistent clinical findings (Figure 2). The occiput often is flattened on the side opposite to the contracted SCM muscle because the infant's head will preferentially roll toward the unaffected SCM muscle when supine. Ortolani and Barlow tests of the hip may be abnormal; approximately 8% of children with CMT will have associated developmental dysplasia of the hip. Internal tibial torsion and metatarsus adductus also may be seen in association with torticollis.[2]

If examination findings and history are consistent with CMT, plain radiographs of the cervical spine and a diagnostic evaluation of the hips is recommended. Ultrasound of the hip is used for infants younger than 3 or 4 months of age, and a plain AP radiograph of the pelvis is used in older infants. Cervical imaging may identify congenital vertebral anoma-

lies. Hip studies are necessary to rule out developmental dysplasia of the hip. MRI and CT of the brain and cervical spine are not necessary unless the clinical examination is not fully consistent with CMT. Ultrasound evaluation of an affected SCM muscle is helpful to assess a palpable mass within the SCM if a cervical cyst or a mass other than that caused by focal scarring from the SCM muscle is suspected. Imaging characteristics of the contracted SCM muscle can be used to define the degree of fibrosis, which may be helpful in predicting the outcome of nonsurgical treatment.[3] A child with more significant fibrosis is less likely to respond favorably to a program of manual stretching.

Treatment of CMT is predominantly nonsurgical. A supervised regimen of passive cervical stretching and active exercises that emphasize rotation and lateral bending is successful in improving range of motion and diminishing head tilting in more than 90% of infants by 1 year of age.[4] Head and neck orthotic devices and helmets, although potentially useful for children with severe restrictions of neck motion or severe head deformity, are not routinely prescribed. Most children, after regaining cervical range of motion, show spontaneous remodeling of the skull and facial asymmetry by 3 years of age.

Surgery for CMT is indicated only for children older than 1 year of age who have not had a successful outcome after a formal stretching program lasting a minimum of 4 months. Distal unipolar release of the SCM muscle is the treatment of choice for most children with CMT who have not been successfully treated nonsurgically. The incision is placed just above the clavicle and centered over the insertion of the more prominent of the two heads of the SCM. After careful exposure and opening of the SCM muscle sheath, the insertion is released and a 1- to 2-cm segment of the distal muscle-tendon unit is resected to prevent repeat contracture. Alternatively, Z-lengthening of the SCM muscle may be performed to preserve the contour of the cervical musculature.[5] Release of the origin of the SCM muscle at the mastoid through a second incision, in addition to insertional release, is called a bipolar release. Bipolar release of the SCM muscle is indicated for more severe contractures in older children. Outcomes for surgical release by all methods are generally excellent. Improvement of cervical range of motion can be expected for most children. Significant remodeling of facial and skull asymmetry is seen in children younger than 12 years.[6] Patients older than 12 years may have improved cervical motion after SCM muscle release but are less likely to show marked improvement in facial and skull asymmetry.

Congenital Anomalies of the Cervical Spine

Prior to performing surgical release of the SCM muscle for suspected CMT, careful consideration must be given to nonmuscular etiologies of torticollis in the infant.[7] Congenital anomalies of the occiput and upper cervical spine may not be readily apparent on plain radiographs. The author recommends MRI or CT evaluation of the cervical spine before surgical release of the SCM muscle. The only manifestations of congenital anomalies of the occipital condyles, atlas, and the lower cervical spine (Klippel-Feil syndrome) may be torticollis or head tilting.[8] Renal ultrasonography, cardiac echocardiography, and auditory testing are necessary for children diagnosed with congenital anomalies of

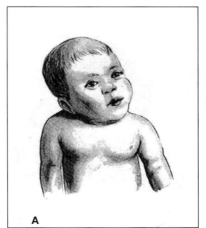
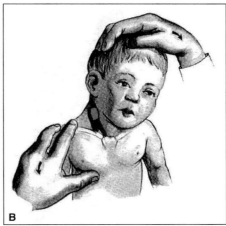
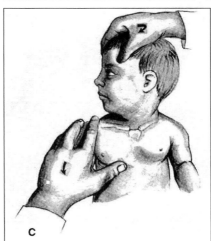

Figure 2   CMT in an infant is characterized by head tilting to one side and rotation of the chin to the opposite side—the classic "cock-robin" position (**A**). Because of contracture of the SCM muscle, lateral bending of the head toward the side opposite to the tilt occurs (**B**) and rotation of the head toward the same side of the head tilt (**C**) is restricted. A mass may be palpable within the muscle belly. (Reproduced with permission from Disorders of the neck, in Herring A (ed): *Tachjdian's Pediatric Orthopaedics,* ed. 3. Philadelphia, PA, WB Saunders, 2002, p 175.)

the cervical spine to rule out associated abnormalities. The choice of orthopaedic treatment is based on the specific patterns of occipital and vertebral malformation.

Ocular Torticollis

Eye pathology is an uncommon etiology of torticollis. Infants with ocular torticollis typically are brought for treatment at 4 to 6 months of age because of head tilting that usually occurs when the infant is awake and in a sitting position. Weakness of the superior oblique muscle or (less commonly) the lateral rectus muscle results in asymmetric eye placement in space.[9] The infant, in an attempt to reduce or eliminate the resultant disconjugate gaze pattern, tilts the head

away from the affected eye. Head tilting is not seen during sleep and passive cervical range of motion is normal. Because the ophthalmologic findings may be subtle and difficult to identify in the infant, evaluation by a pediatric ophthalmologist is necessary to confirm this uncommon diagnosis.

Sandifer's Syndrome

Sandifer's syndrome is another uncommon etiology of torticollis that results from intermittent gastroesophageal reflux. Infants with Sandifer's syndrome are poor feeders and have frequent episodes of vomiting in association with torticollis. It is hypothesized that the infant tilts the head and neck to one side, sometimes alternating from one side to the other, in an attempt to alleviate pain from esophagitis that results from the gastroesophageal reflux. Orthopaedic examination of the head and neck shows normal findings in infants with Sandifer's syndrome. Prompt referral to a pediatric gastroenterologist for medical treatment leads to resolution of torticollis as the symptoms of esophagitis abate.

Neural Axis Abnormalities

Congenital anomalies and neoplasms of the neural axis such as posterior fossa tumors are rare etiologies of torticollis in the infant. Careful clinical evaluation may detect dysfunction of the cranial nerves and asymmetry or weakness of upper extremity motion. The classic findings of SCM muscle fibrosis and restricted motion seen with CMT are not present. These diagnoses are exceedingly uncommon in infants and often are delayed because the signs and symptoms may be intermittent and subtle. Evaluation by a pediatric neurologist and MRI of the brain and cervical spine are most useful for ruling out these pathologies.

Benign Paroxysmal Torticollis of Infancy

Benign paroxysmal torticollis in the infant is characterized by intermittent episodes of head tilting or posturing that is associated with prolonged periods of crying, inconsolability, and vomiting.[10] The head position may change from one side to the other. The episodes of torticollis last hours or days. A family history of migraine headaches or benign paroxysmal torticollis may provide the only clue to help in diagnosing this rare condition. Benign paroxysmal torticollis is genetically linked to migraine headaches in adulthood. When the child is

not experiencing the paroxysm of torticollis, examination of the head and neck is normal. Neural axis anomalies and neoplasms have similar symptoms and must be ruled out by MRI. A thorough evaluation by a pediatric neurologist is necessary to confirm the diagnosis.

Torticollis in the Child

Torticollis that develops de novo in the otherwise normal, healthy child has many possible etiologies and presents a particularly challenging diagnostic dilemma. The clinical history is most useful for narrowing the differential diagnoses. Queries about an inciting event such as a fall, pain associated with the torticollis, the duration of the abnormal head tilting, and whether it is fixed or intermittently resolves provide the most important clues. Other pertinent information includes associated signs or symptoms such as fever or chills, headaches, nausea or vomiting, and neurologic dysfunction such as diminished coordination, gait abnormalities, or weakness in the extremities.

The physical examination of the child with acquired torticollis is different than the examination for the infant with CMT. A child with painful, newly acquired torticollis may have palpable spasm or tightness of the SCM muscle on the side opposite to the direction of the lateral head tilt; generalized cervical muscle spasm and tenderness also may be seen. Neck mobility is often limited and painful in all planes of motion. Findings from a neck examination may be normal in the child with intermittent torticollis. A thorough neurologic examination is mandatory for the child with torticollis. Observation of gait and coordination, cranial nerve testing, motor and sensory testing of the extremities, as-

sessment of deep tendon reflexes of the upper and lower extremities, and testing for signs of upper motor neuron dysfunction comprise a complete evaluation. Examination of the ears, nose, and throat, cardiopulmonary evaluation, and abdominal examination are indicated based on symptoms associated with the torticollis that are reported in the history.

Traumatic Atlantoaxial Rotatory Displacement and Grisel's Syndrome

Torticollis in the child is most frequently the manifestation of AARD resulting from trauma or inflammation of the oropharynx (Grisel's syndrome). Traumatic injury of the head and neck may result in rotational displacement of the atlas on the axis (Figure 3). More serious injuries of the upper cervical spine including fractures and ligamentous injuries must be ruled out using plain radiograph, CT, or MRI as indicated by the history and physical examination. For most children, the displacement spontaneously reduces with symptomatic treatment that includes application of a cervical collar and the administration of muscle relaxants and pain medication. In untreated patients with symptoms that last for more than 10 days, cervical traction may be required to effect reduction. Cervical fusion is indicated for the child who develops recurrent torticollis after treatment or develops secondary instability of the atlantoaxial vertebral segment, an uncommon but potentially devastating sequela of AARD.[11]

Upper respiratory infection, adenoiditis, and other inflammatory conditions of the oropharynx may result in AARD and torticollis; this condition is called Grisel's syndrome. The venous plexus of the posterior pharynx lies adjacent to the soft tissue of the anterior upper cervical spine. Hyperemia resulting from localized inflammation is believed to induce laxity of the capsule and ligamentous attachments of the atlantoaxial articulation that permits this rotatory displacement. Treatment of the underlying inflammatory condition results in spontaneous resolution of the associated torticollis in most patients. The algorithm for treatment of children with Grisel's syndrome whose torticollis does not resolve spontaneously is similar to that for traumatic AARD. More information about Grisel's syndrome can be found in chapter 66, "Infections and Inflammatory Conditions of the Cervical Spine."

Retropharyngeal Abscess

Retropharyngeal abscess formation is an uncommon manifestation of Grisel's syndrome. The syndrome typically occurs in a child younger than 5 years of age. Symptoms include head posturing or torticollis, painful neck flexion or extension, and a sore throat or respiratory symptoms (such as stridor or wheezing).[12] An anterior neck mass may be palpable. CT or MRI confirms the diagnosis (Figure 4). Most children respond to treatment with antibiotics. Surgical drainage of the abscess is indicated for large abscesses and for patients who do not respond to antibiotic therapy alone.

Pyogenic Cervical Spondylitis

In children, vertebral diskitis and osteomyelitis, also called pyogenic spondylitis, occur uncommonly in the cervical spine compared with the rate of occurrence in the thoracolumbar spine.[13] Pyogenic spondylitis of the cervical spine typically occurs in a child younger than 8 years of age and is characterized by symptoms of fever and neck pain.

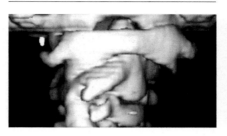

Figure 3 A three–dimensional CT scan identifies AARD in an 8-year-old girl who had neck pain and torticollis after a motor vehicle crash.

Head tilting may be seen in the child with lower cervical involvement; true torticollis occurs when the upper cervical spine is involved. The erythrocyte sedimentation rate, C-reactive protein, and white blood cell counts are usually elevated. Plain radiographs may show disk space narrowing or vertebral end plate lysis; however, radiographs often are normal early in the disease process. A bone scan is useful for children with normal radiographs whose history and physical examination raise suspicion for this condition. An increased technetium uptake in the involved disk and adjacent vertebral end plates confirms the diagnosis. MRI or CT is useful to define the extent of disk and vertebral body involvement and to detect associated paravertebral soft-tissue abscesses. Intravenous antibiotic therapy is effective in treating pyogenic spondylitis in most patients. Surgical débridement is necessary only for those children with large paravertebral abscesses and for those who do not respond to nonsurgical treatment.

Posterior Fossa Tumors

Approximately 10% of tumors of the posterior fossa initially occur with torticollis.[14] The most common neoplasms of the posterior fossa are astrocytomas, ependymomas, and

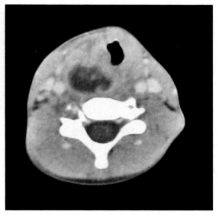

Figure 4 An axial CT scan of the neck of a 5-year-old boy with fever, neck stiffness, and respiratory stridor identifies a large retropharyngeal abscess. The abscess required urgent surgical drainage.

gliomas. The child with a tumor of the posterior fossa typically has intermittent torticollis that is associated with headaches, vomiting, or neurologic dysfunction such as clumsiness or weakness. Days or weeks may pass during which the child is asymptomatic. Pertinent examination findings include papilledema, dysfunction of cranial nerves, and focal weakness. Because the symptoms appear only intermittently and clinical findings may be subtle, a delay in the diagnosis is common. Plain radiographs are usually normal. CT and MRI of the brain are the best tests for diagnosing these neoplasms (Figure 5). Cranial tumor excision by a pediatric neurosurgeon is indicated for most children; chemotherapy and radiation may be used as adjuncts to resection depending on staging and the specific pathology of the tumor.

Nonneoplastic abnormalities of the brain stem and cervical cord, such as Arnold-Chiari malformation and syringomyelia, may occur with symptoms that are similar to those found in patients with tumors

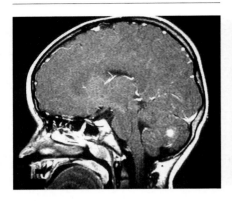

Figure 5 Sagittal MRI scan of the brain of a 7-year-old girl with intermittent headaches, vomiting, and torticollis identifies an astrocytoma of the cerebellum; she underwent successful resection.

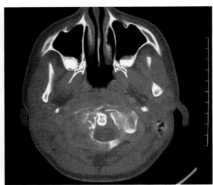

Figure 6 Axial CT scan of a 4-year-old boy with fever, malaise, severe neck pain, and torticollis shows lysis and bony destruction of C2 resulting from a lymphoma that was confirmed by a biopsy.

of the posterior fossa. Intermittent torticollis or head tilting, head and neck pain, and upper extremity weakness are symptoms associated with these rare conditions. Diagnostic imaging of the brain and cervical cord is indicated for all children with intermittent episodes of torticollis regardless of clinical findings at the time of examination. Such imaging will improve the ability of the physician to diagnosis neural axis abnormalities.

Neoplasms of the Cervical Vertebrae

Benign and malignant neoplasms of the upper cervical vertebral column are unusual causes of torticollis in the child. Osteoid osteoma, osteoblastoma, and Langerhans cell histiocytosis are the most common benign tumors of the cervical vertebrae.[15] The child with one of these neoplasms typically presents for treatment with progressively worsening neck pain, stiffness, and torticollis or head tilting. Systemic illness and neurologic symptoms and signs are not associated with benign neoplasms. Osteoid osteomas and osteoblastomas incite sclerosis in the bone

adjacent to the lesion that may be seen on plain radiographs. Bone scans show focal intense uptake at the site of the lesion. CT and MRI scans are used to confirm the diagnosis of osteoid osteoma or osteoblastoma by identifying a lytic nidus centrally within the sclerotic bone. Osteoid osteoma and osteoblastoma require excision in most patients. Langerhans cell histiocytosis characteristically is identified by plain radiographs showing flattening and collapse of the involved vertebral body (vertebra plana); this collapse also may be asymmetric. Langerhans cell histiocytosis is symptomatic for most children and is nonsurgically treated. Chemotherapy and radiation are reserved for patients with multiple sites of involvement or severe extraskeletal disease. The vertebral body affected by Langerhans cell histiocytosis reconstitutes in most patients and permanent spinal deformity and neurologic deficits are rare.

Leukemia, lymphoma (Figure 6), and primary malignancies of bone, such as Ewing's sarcoma and osteosarcoma, rarely occur in the upper cervical spine and are unusual etiologies of torticollis. The child

with a malignancy of the atlas or axis typically has torticollis, neck pain and stiffness, as well as systemic symptoms including fever, weight loss, diminished energy, and general body aches. Diagnostic imaging, laboratory studies, and tissue biopsy are used to confirm the suspicion of malignancy. Wide resection of these tumors is not always possible. Decompression of neural elements, local resection of the tumor, and spine stabilization may be necessary. Chemotherapy, with or without radiation, is used in most patients. Treatment is based on staging and the specific pathology.

Cervical Dystonia

Cervical dystonia is the most common focal dystonia in adolescents and adults.[16] It is a rare cause of torticollis in the child. This condition is characterized by episodes of painful neck stiffness and torticollis. Although some patients with cervical dystonia may report an inciting traumatic event, many patients develop abnormal head posturing and torticollis spontaneously. Psychogenic or hysterical torticollis is often difficult to distinguish clinically from cervical dystonia because imaging studies are normal for both of these conditions. Cervical dystonia is diagnosed after all other organic etiologies of torticollis have been excluded. Injection of botulinum toxin into dystonic and overactive muscle groups is the treatment of choice for patients with cervical dystonia. Surgical denervation of involved cervical muscles is a treatment option only for those who do not respond to therapy with botulinum toxin.

Summary

Torticollis is a clinical sign and symptom that has many causes. CMT results from contracture of the SCM muscle and is the most common diagnosis in infants. Congenital upper cervical anomalies, ocular torticollis and other unusual etiologies must be considered in the infant with CMT who fails to respond to physical therapy. New onset torticollis in children and adolescents is a particularly challenging diagnostic dilemma. Although atlantoaxial rotatory displacement from trauma and oropharyngeal inflammation (Grisel's syndrome) are the most common causes, careful clinical evaluation and diagnostic studies assist in narrowing the differential diagnosis. Retropharyngeal abscess, pyogenic cervical spondylitis, and tumors of the posterior fossa and spinal column are less common causes of torticollis in the child. Cervical dystonia, a condition that is rare in children, may be seen in older adolescents.

References

1. Davids J, Wenger D, Mubarak S: Congenital muscular torticollis: Sequela of intrauterine or perinatal compartment syndrome. *J Pediatr Orthop* 1993;13:141-147.

2. Walsh J, Morrissy R: Torticollis and hip dislocation. *J Pediatr Orthop* 1998;18:219-221.

3. Tang SF, Hsu KH, Wong AM, Hsu CC, Chang CH: Longitudinal follow-up study of ultrasonography in congenital muscular torticollis. *Clin Orthop* 2002;403:179-185.

4. Cheng JC, Wong MW, Tang SP, Chen TM, Shum SL, Wong EM: Clinical determinants of the outcome of manual stretching in the treatment of congenital muscular torticollis in infants: A prospective study of eight hundred and twenty-one cases. *J Bone Joint Surg Am* 2001;83:679-687.

5. Ferkel RD, Westin GW, Dawson EG, Oppenheim WL: Muscular torticollis: A modified surgical approach. *J Bone Joint Surg Am* 1983;65:894-900.

6. Ippolito E, Tudisco C, Massobrio M: Long-term results of open sternocleidomastoid tenotomy for idiopathic muscular torticollis. *J Bone Joint Surg Am* 1985;67:30-38.

7. Ballock R, Song K: The prevalence of nonmuscular causes of torticollis in children. *J Pediatr Orthop* 1996;16:500-504.

8. Dubousset J: Torticollis in children caused by congenital anomalies of the atlas. *J Bone Joint Surg Am* 1986;68:178-188.

9. Williams CR, O'Flynn E, Clarke NM, Morris RJ: Torticollis secondary to ocular pathology. *J Bone Joint Surg Br* 1996;78:620-624.

10. Giffin N, Benton S, Goadsby P: Benign paroxysmal torticollis of infancy: Four new cases and linkage to CACNA1A mutation. *Dev Med Child Neurol* 2002;44:490-493.

11. Phillips WA, Hensinger RN: The management of rotatory atlanto-axial subluxation in children. *J Bone Joint Surg Am* 1989;71:664-668.

12. Craig F, Schunk J: Retropharyngeal abscess in children: Clinical presentation, utility of imaging, and current management. *Pediatrics* 2003;111:1394-1398.

13. Song KS, Ogden JA, Ganey T, Guidera KJ: Contiguous discitis and osteomyelitis in children. *J Pediatr Orthop* 1997;17:470-477.

14. Gupta AK, Roy DR, Conlan ES, Crawford AH: Torticollis secondary to posterior fossa tumors. *J Pediatr Orthop* 1996;16:505-507.

15. Ngu BB, Khanna AJ, Pak SS, McCarthy EF, Sponseller PD: Eosinophilic granuloma of the atlas presenting as torticollis in a child. *Spine* 2004;29:E98-100.

16. Dauer WT, Burke RE, Greene P, Fahn S: Current concepts on the clinical features, aetiology and management of idiopathic of cervical dystonia. *Brain* 1998;121:547-560.

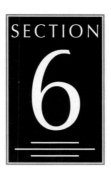

SECTION
6

Tumors

Tumors

We have made considerable advances in the treatment of malignant bone tumors in children. Thirty years ago, eight or nine of every 10 children with an osteosarcoma or Ewing tumor was likely to lose a limb or die. Today, those figures essentially are reversed. In the same 30 years, however, few advances have been made in our understanding of the etiology and treatment of benign bone tumors in children, yet they are more common, occupy a considerable amount of physician office time, may lead to significant morbidity, and be a significant cause of frustration for the child, parents, and the orthopaedist. Although benign tumors are not life threatening, they can significantly interfere with the integrity of the involved bone, often keeping budding athletes from pursuing a fav-orite sport. Benign tumors also may affect bone growth if the physis is involved, leading to foreshortened upper extremities and limb-length discrepancies in the lower extremity.

Benign tumors also are a major cause of concern for other physicians. Most radiologists, primary care physicians, emergency physicians, and unfortunately many orthopaedists are not facile with the radiographic appearance of benign bone tumors. An unsuspecting radiologist or primary care physician may interpret the radiograph of a patient with a benign tumor as possibly showing a malignancy, which can lead to many unnecessary studies such as bone scans, MRI, and CT, not to mention undue anxiety and concern for the parents. Perhaps worse is the mistaken interpretation of a malignant tumor as benign, leading to a delay in diagnosis, but this error is much less common in this age of caution and litigation. Many of these benign lesions present as pathologic fractures, which makes the differential diagnosis even more difficult because the fracture and hematoma obscure the imaging characteristics. At times it is difficult to confirm that the fracture is pathologic, and the ability to arrive at the correct underlying diagnosis often is obscured by the fracture. This results in two dilemmas: how to treat the fracture and how to treat the tumor.

Perhaps even more frustrating is the lack of readily available, adequate guidelines for evaluating whether a benign bone tumor is likely to lead to fracture and therefore in need of treatment. The literature reports that orthopaedists, even those specializing in oncology, cannot accurately predict whether a given lesion is likely to lead to fracture with various activities. For some reason, however, these lesions never seem to occur in sedentary children; rather, they always seem to affect children whose parents believe that they are destined to be Olympic or professional athletes. Hours of office time are spent educating parents about the relative advantages and risks of treatment options, including observation without any activity restriction while the lesion heals (in the hope that it will not fracture), observation with restricted sports activities (very difficult to "sell" to most parents and affected young athletes), or surgical management of some sort. Recently, as mentioned in the article by Dormans and Pill and in subsequent publications, analysis of benign bone defects with specialized CT has resulted in more precise guidelines to ascertain whether a given defect substantially reduces the ability of the affected bone to withstand axial, torsional, and bending loads. This type of biomechanical analysis can go a long way to guiding the discussion but is not yet widely available.

Dormans and Pill provide an excellent review of common benign bone defects that may lead to fracture in children. They detail the problems encountered when treating patients with fractures and nicely outline a classification and treatment algorithm for bone cysts and other benign bone tumors, particularly the difficulties with those of the proximal femur, which arguably is the most difficult site. Although treating any bone tumor can be frustrating, tumors of the proximal femur are perhaps the most challenging because they severely limit a child's mobility and are fraught with potential complications, not only associated with the lesion itself but also with the treatment, including malunion, varus neck deformities, growth arrest, and osteonecrosis of the femoral head.

One of the principal problems associated with bone cysts is that we do not understand their etiology and pathogenesis; therefore, all treatments are empiric and none uniformly successful. The authors nicely outline the suspected causes in their review. The principal goal of treatment is to stabilize the fracture and allow the defect to fill in with bone. This approach sounds simple, but none of the techniques (eg, steroid injection, autograft packing, allograft packing, or various bone graft substitutes) is predictably successful. Months or even years and multiple treatments may be required to arrive at a healed, stable lesion. The authors present a helpful classification of proximal femoral lesions that considers the location of the cyst relative to the physis and lateral cortical buttress; they also include an algorithm of fixation alternatives that will be of great assistance to the treating orthopaedist.

Any orthopaedic surgeon involved in the treatment of a child with an impending or pathologic fracture will want to read this article carefully. The authors provide excellent descriptions of the radiographic characteristics, pathology, and natural history of benign defects and how to differentiate among them. Unicameral bone cysts are radiolucent, central metaphyseal lesions that typically resolve with time. A comprehensive discussion of the current treatment options designed to speed the healing process also is presented, specifically the state of the art of corticosteroid injections, bone grafting, and newer minimally invasive techniques.

Aneurysmal bone cysts generally are not self-limiting and almost always require treatment because of pain, interference with bone integrity, and continued growth. These lesions are true neoplasms as indicated by recent findings of cytogenetic rearrangements in chromosomes 17p11-13 and/or 16q22. They also have high recurrence rates, and the article describes the techniques that maximize the likelihood of a successful curettage and the adjuvants used. At times, a resection may be appropriate, but radiation therapy should be avoided because of the potential for secondary malignancy as a result of the treatment.

Nonossifying fibromas are common lesions that are eccentrically located in the metaphysis of the bone and may lead to fracture. The treatment dilemmas associated with these lesions are similar to those with unicameral bone cysts, but because fibromas are not fluid-filled cavities, injection is not an option. Curettage, bone grafting options, and fixation techniques are nicely outlined in the article.

One issue Dormans and Pill raise is the necessity to fill tumor defects with healthy, mechanically stable bone. Traditionally, autogenous bone graft is harvested from the iliac crest. However, the morbidity associated with graft harvest often is more troubling than the morbidity of operating on the bone lesion; thus, the second article in this section by Rougraff is useful because it nicely outlines alternatives to autogenous bone graft. As noted in the article, many of these alternatives originally were developed for more common purposes such as scoliosis fusion or treatment of fracture nonunion, but they also are useful to fill benign tumor defects. An osteoinductive material is ideal for this purpose, although the osteoconductive substitutes are used much more frequently. Rougraff reviews the relative indications and appropriate use of each alternative material and cites the available evidence regarding their success rates. Some alternatives may need only injection (minimally invasive) instillation such as demineralized bone matrix gels, calcium phosphate, and hydroxyapatite preparations, whereas others such as freeze-dried allogeneic bone chips, calcium sulfate, and coralline hydroxyapatite require open techniques. Virtually all of these alternatives, except perhaps demineralized bone matrix, are osteoconductive materials, and some (eg, calcium phosphate and hydroxyapatite) do not completely resorb over time.

One point is obvious after reading this review: currently, we do not have the ideal graft material. The most promising agents are the bone morphogenetic proteins that are osteoinductive proteins. Two such proteins (rhBMP-2 and rhBMP-7) are in clinical use for anterior spine fusion and fracture nonunion, but none of the agents has been approved specifically for the treatment of benign defects. Rougraff provides an excellent review of the current data on the use of all of these bone graft substitutes.

What is apparent from these two articles is that we have much to learn about the tumors. Both sets of authors discuss the treatment options that are currently available. We attempt to treat lesions even though we understand little about their etiology and pathogenesis. With the possible exception of the recent cytogenetic finding in aneurysmal bone cysts, we truly are operating in the dark. Therefore, our treatments are destined to be unsuccessful in many cases.

More research is needed regarding the etiology of unicameral bone cysts and nonossifying fibromas so that we can more precisely direct our treatments at the cause. We need more practical methods of identifying patients who are at risk for fracture. Randomized studies of the treatment options are needed so that we have evidence-based data by which to guide patients and their families through the treatment maze that now exists. We also need to explore the use of bone morphogenetic proteins and other strategies to determine if they will yield a higher healing rate than is now available from other current techniques. Although these lesions are not malignant, they pose significant problems for our patients and we need to improve they way they are managed. These articles present state-of-the-art information in this area and are helpful to the treating orthopaedist, but it is discouraging to note that despite the passage of time, not much has changed.

Mark C. Gebhardt, MD
Frederick W. and Jane M. Ilfeld
  Professor of Orthopaedic Surgery
Harvard Medical School
Boston, Massachusetts

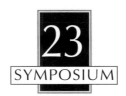

Fractures Through Bone Cysts: Unicameral Bone Cysts, Aneurysmal Bone Cysts, Fibrous Cortical Defects, and Nonossifying Fibromas

John P. Dormans, MD
Stephan G. Pill, MS, PT

Introduction

When a child presents with a fracture, orthopaedic surgeons should be aware of the possibility of pathologic fracture, especially after minimal trauma or when radiographs suggest that an underlying abnormal process is occurring in the bone.[1] A pathologic fracture is defined as a fracture that occurs through abnormal bone. The involved abnormal bone lacks the viscoelastic properties and mechanical strength of normal bone. In general, pathologic fractures can result from intrinsic processes, such as osteopenia from osteogenesis imperfecta or the replacement of normal bone with tumor, or from extrinsic processes, such as internal fixation, radiation, or a hole in bone from a biopsy, that decrease the inherent structural integrity of bone.[1]

Pathologic bone may fail with either a microfracture or complete fracture. Microfractures most commonly occur in trabecular bone, such as in the metaphysis of long bones or in a vertebral body. Isolated microfractures are typically undisplaced and heal without consequence; many go unrecognized. The energy required to produce a pathologic microfracture may be small, such as from the repeated loading of weight bearing.

Many successive microfractures can result in deformity, such as the shepherd's crook deformity of the proximal femur seen in children with fibrous dysplasia. Greater forces can often produce completely displaced fractures in pathologic bone. With these more significant fractures, the child generally has acute symptoms and more intense signs, such as pain, swelling, and an inability to bear weight (lower extremity) or reluctance to move the injured extremity (upper and lower extremity).

Several attempts have been made to predict the risk of pathologic fractures occurring in abnormal bone. In 1995, Hipp and associates[2] proposed a method to quantify the general risk of pathologic fracture. They defined the "factor of risk" as the load applied to the involved bone divided by the load required for bone failure. Other attempts have been made to determine the chance of pathologic fracture occurring in children with underlying bone conditions.[3-5] However, none of these studies were able to identify an accurate, widely used method of predicting fractures based on radiographic findings that can be applied to most clinical situations. The risk of pathologic fracture perhaps is best revealed with a careful history, physical examination, and a review of plain radiographs. New methods that apply engineering principles to information provided by CT or other advanced imaging techniques may produce better noninvasive estimates for the risk of pathologic fracture.[2]

Plain radiographs are often most helpful in determining the underlying cause of a pathologic fracture. Most tumors and tumor-like processes of bone are recognizable by their radiographic appearance. The location and radiographic features of the lesion can be helpful in making the diagnosis.[6] In many cases, biopsy is needed to determine the cause of a pathologic fracture. In these situations, the surgeon must ensure that the biopsy is taken from a representative area of the lesion. Determining the underlying diagnosis is essential for planning treatment in children with pathologic fractures.

Benign tumors can be classified according to their aggressiveness.[7] Stage 1 or latent benign lesions usually are asymptomatic, are discovered incidentally, can remain static or heal spontaneously, and are seldom associated with pathologic fracture. Stage 2 or active benign lesions comprise the majority of benign lesions; they tend to grow steadily

Table 1
Usual Treatment Priorities for Children With Pathologic Fractures Associated With Tumors and Tumor-Like Lesions

Priority for Treatment	Tumor/Tumor-Like Lesion
Fracture (lesion may heal spontaneously)	Eosinophilic granuloma* Fibrous cortical defect†
Fracture first, then lesion (if surgery is indicated and fracture is stable, may go directly to surgery)	Unicameral bone cyst Aneurysmal bone cyst Nonossifying fibroma Fibrous Dysplasia Enchondroma Chondromyxoid fibroma
Fracture and lesion (simultaneous)	Giant cell tumor Aneurysmal bone cyst (proximal femur) Angiomas of bone Malignant bone tumors, sarcoma‡
Underlying process (fracture usually heals with treatment of underlying process)	Metastatic lesions such as neuroblastoma Leukemia Selected chemosensitive or radiosensitive malignant bone tumors

*Lesion healing: months
†Lesion healing: years
‡Fracture treatment concurrent with chemotherapy and later surgery

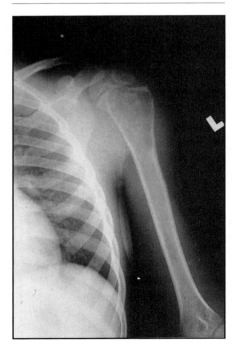

Fig. 1 AP radiograph of a UBC of the proximal humerus with microfracture.

but are limited by natural barriers and may be symptomatic. Stage 3 or aggressive benign lesions are generally symptomatic and tender, grow rapidly, are not limited by natural barriers, and may be associated with pathologic fracture. Stage 3 tumors, which often have a more aggressive natural history, include chondroblastomas, aneurysmal bone cysts (ABCs), chondromyxoid fibromas, giant cell tumors, osteoblastomas, chordomas, and adamantinomas.

This chapter reviews the evaluation and management of pathologic fractures associated with the most common underlying conditions in children: unicameral bone cysts (UBCs), ABCs, fibrous cortical defects (FCDs), and nonossifying fibromas (NOFs). The identification of an abnormal underlying condition usually alters the treatment for children with pathologic fractures. The treatment plan should include both the treatment of the fracture and management of the

condition responsible for the fracture (Table 1).

Unicameral Bone Cysts

UBCs are fluid-filled cystic lesions that are found most commonly in the metaphysis of long bones. The term unicameral suggests a single-chambered cyst. Most UBCs are indeed unicameral, but some contain septa that divide the cyst into more than one chamber, especially after treatment or previous fractures.[8] UBCs usually have a thin, fibrous, peripheral lining and contain yellow serous fluid. In order of decreasing frequency, the cysts most commonly are found in the proximal humerus, proximal femur, proximal tibia, distal tibia, distal femur, calcaneus, distal humerus, radius, fibula, ilium, ulna, and rib.[9] Approximately 70% of UBCs are found in either the proximal humerus or proximal femur. Most UBCs are diagnosed within the first two decades of life,[10-12] and the ratio of males to females is about 2:1.[13] UBCs develop from an accumulation of interstitial fluid in the bone, and some authors suggest that this is because of a defect in venous or lymphatic drainage.[11,14,15]

The usual radiographic appearance of a UBC is a centrally located, radiolucent, slightly expansile lesion in the metaphysis[16] (Fig. 1). UBCs are occasionally found in the diaphysis when the physis has migrated away from the lesion.[17] The width of the UBC rarely exceeds that of the adjacent physis. The fallen fragment sign, described by Reynolds[16] in 1969, is a fracture fragment seen on plain radiographs at the bottom of a cyst, suggesting a hollow cavity in the bone rather than a solid tumor. The diagnosis of UBC is usually straightforward, but the differential diagnosis occasionally includes ABC (Fig. 2), fibrous dysplasia with cystic component, enchondroma, and, less frequently, giant cell tumor and eosinophilic granuloma.

The natural history of UBCs is vari-

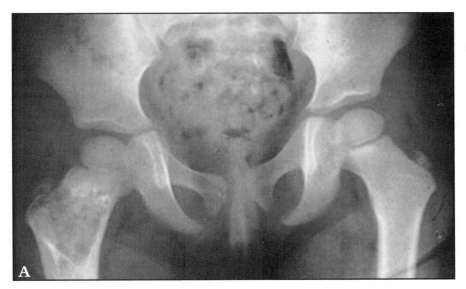

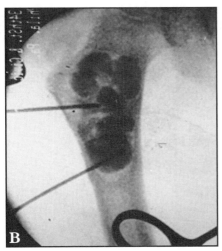

Fig. 2 Although having a similar radiographic appearance as a UBC (A), incomplete filling of the cyst after injection with radiopaque dye (ie, a cystogram) suggests an ABC (B). ABC was confirmed with open biopsy.

Pathologic fractures through UBCs heal in the typical amount of time, usually with simple immobilization. In the upper extremity, minimally displaced, stable pathologic fractures through UBCs are usually treated with simple immobilization for 4 to 6 weeks. Often a sling is adequate treatment for stable fractures of the proximal humerus. Once healing is achieved, the options for further treatment of the UBC are discussed with the patient and family.

With pathologic fractures through UBCs in the proximal femur, varus malunion is a common complication with nonsurgical treatment.[11] Other complications associated with pathologic fractures through UBCs of the femoral neck include osteonecrosis of the femoral head and growth arrest of the proximal femoral physis. Most authors recommend internal fixation when the fracture is unstable,[9,13,19,24] and some recommend preliminary traction before surgical intervention.[25]

Surgical Management

With pathologic fracture through a UBC in the proximal femur, treatment is usually more involved than is treatment for pathologic fractures in other long bones[25] (Figs. 3 and 4). For type I-A fractures, in the authors' classification system, there is enough bone in the femoral neck and lateral proximal femur (lateral buttress) to allow fixation with cannulated screws after curettage and bone grafting. A pediatric hip screw and side plate also can be used. With type I-B fractures, despite sufficient bone in the femoral neck, there is loss of lateral buttress, so a pediatric hip screw and a side plate should be considered rather than cannulated screws after biopsy, curettage, and bone grafting. Because of the lack of adequate bone beneath the physis in type II-A and II-B fractures, there are two options for treatment of these bone cysts. After curettage and bone grafting, parallel pins across the physis can be used in combination with a

able, but the cysts tend to improve gradually with time and growth. Many UBCs persist into adulthood, whereas some spontaneously resolve during puberty.[15] These cysts are described as active when they are adjacent to the physis or latent when the lesion is located farther than 0.5 cm from the physis.[15,18]

Approximately 75% of patients who have UBCs present with pathologic fractures.[19-23] Most of these fractures are microfractures or minimally displaced fractures. Although the fractures heal within 6 weeks, only about 10% of the UBCs heal, and this can lead to refracture. Neer and associates[9] observed an

additional 2.5 fractures per patient during observation periods after the initial injury. Ahn and Park[3] noted that pathologic fracture occurred when the transverse diameter of the cyst occupied 85% or more of the diameter of the affected bone. Others have reported that the likelihood of fracture is high when the width of the cyst wall is less than 0.5 mm.[5] Kaelin and MacEwen[4] further categorized the likelihood of fracture from UBCs by dividing the area of the lesion by the square of the diaphysis diameter to derive a "cyst index." They found that patients with a low cyst index were at lower risk for fracture and often did not require treatment.

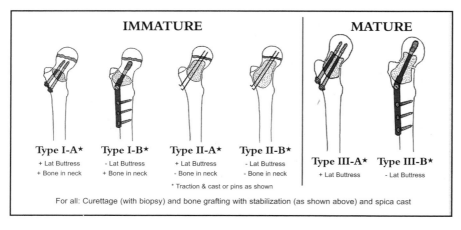

IMMATURE

Type I-A★
+ Lat Buttress
+ Bone in neck

Type I-B★
- Lat Buttress
+ Bone in neck

Type II-A★
+ Lat Buttress
- Bone in neck

Type II-B★
- Lat Buttress
- Bone in neck

* Traction & cast or pins as shown

MATURE

Type III-A★
+ Lat Buttress

Type III-B★
- Lat Buttress

For all: Curettage (with biopsy) and bone grafting with stabilization (as shown above) and spica cast

Fig. 3 The authors' classification system for the treatment of pathologic fractures of the proximal femur associated with bone cysts in children. In type I-A, a moderately sized cyst is present in the middle of the femoral neck, In type I-B, a large cyst is present at the base of the femoral neck. In types II-A and II-B, because of a large lesion present iin the femoral neck, the bone beneath the physis is insufficient to accept screws. In types III-A and III-B, the physis is closing or closed.

spica cast. As an alternative, the patient can be treated in traction until the fracture heals (with subsequent spica cast), followed by curettage and bone grafting. The lateral buttress is present in type III-A fractures, so cannulated screws (or compression screws and a side plate) can be used to stabilize the fracture after biopsy, curettage, and bone grafting. In type III-B fractures, the loss of a lateral buttress makes it necessary to use a pediatric hip screw and a side plate after curettage and bone grafting. In all types, we recommend spica cast immobilization after surgery. If fracture stabilization is relatively secure, the spica cast can be unilateral with a free ankle ("a walking hip spica cast") or unilateral hip spica cast with the hip and knee in 20° to 30° of flexion.

Many surgical techniques have been developed for treatment of the UBC itself, either before or after fracture healing. From a historic perspective, one of the earliest surgical interventions consisted of curettage and bone grafting. UBCs treated this way have a recurrence rate varying from 10% to 40%.[9,18,19,22,23,26,27] Delaying the treatment until the cyst converts from an active to a latent stage has been advocated by some, but an observation period of more than 2 years may be necessary.[19] Furthermore, some data suggest that the response to treatment may be the same for latent and active cysts.[17] After fracture (excluding the hip), many authors advocate a delay of several weeks before undertaking curettage and bone grafting, to allow the fracture to heal.[11,28]

Open curettage and bone grafting has fallen out of favor for the treatment of upper extremity and small lower extremity UBCs because of the invasive nature of the surgery and the high recurrence rate associated with this option. Curettage and bone grafting remains a popular method of treatment for larger UBCs of the proximal femur. Although some authors have advocated the use of adjuvants, such as phenol or liquid nitrogen, in combination with open curettage and bone grafting for the treatment of UBCs,[29] most prefer to avoid these materials for UBC treatment.

Corticosteroid Injection

In 1979, Scaglietti and associates[30] reported radiographic improvement in 96% of their 72 patients treated by injection of UBCs with methylprednisolone. The mechanism for cyst healing after methylprednisolone injection remains unknown. Some suggest that UBC healing occurs, at least in part, through decompression of cyst fluid pressure by multiple trephination.[10,31] This treatment option became popular because of its relatively low morbidity and an apparent effectiveness approaching that of open curettage and bone grafting. However, because incomplete healing, persistence of the UBC, and recurrence are common after the initial injection of corticosteroid,[30] other techniques for the treatment of UBCs have been developed.

A two-needle injection technique for steroid injection is most commonly used. The initial dose of methylprednisolone can vary from 40 to 200 mg.[8,21,30,32] It is important to evaluate the cyst by injecting radiopaque dye before injecting the methylprednisolone.[8,23,32] With this technique, known as a cystogram, intracystic fibrous septa can be found (92% of lesions in one series[8]); these septa may prevent complete filling of the cyst by corticosteroids and thus may result in incomplete healing. With the use of cystograms, septations can be broken up, thus allowing more even or uniform distribution of injected steroid to all areas of cyst. In most instances in which steroid injection is used, the fracture is allowed to heal before corticosteroid is injected.

Steroid injection can also be used for UBCs of the lower extremity, but if a cyst is potentially unstable and there is a risk of malunion (ie, varus of the femoral neck), a different treatment should be considered (Fig. 3).

In addition to recurrence, other complications can occur with corticosteroid treatment of UBCs. Recurrent pathologic fractures[20,23,33] and osteonecrosis of the femoral head associated with proximal femoral UBCs have been reported.[20,34] In one series, incomplete healing was a problem in 48% of 141 patients with UBCs treated by corticosteroid injec-

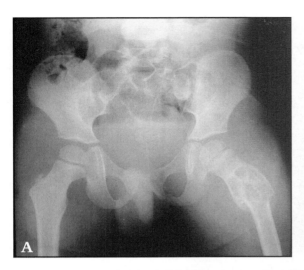
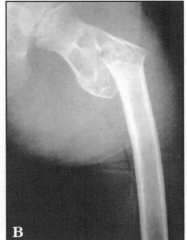
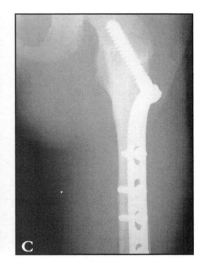
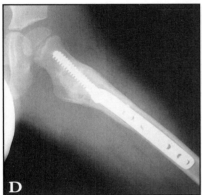
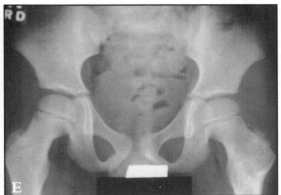

Fig. 4 AP **(A)** and lateral **(B)** radiographs showing a pathologic fracture of the proximal femur. This fracture was categorized as a type I-B fracture, the most common type. AP **(C)** and lateral **(D)** radiographs showing treatment after open biopsy, curettage with bone grafting, and open reduction and internal fixation. A walking hip spica cast was used, and follow-up radiographs showed good healing and anatomic alignment **(E)**.

tion.[34] Systemic reactions to the corticosteroid injection (eg, corticosteroid flush, increased appetite, weight gain) are rare.[23,31] Calcaneal UBCs may not respond as well to injections with methylprednisolone as those in other bones,[35,36] and several authors have recommended primary curettage and bone grafting or minimally invasive grafting techniques for these lesions.[35,36]

Decompression and Grafting

Some authors believe that relieving the pressure of the interstitial fluid in the lesions promotes the healing of the cyst. Chigira and associates[10] treated seven patients by puncturing the cyst wall with multiple Kirschner wires. The lesion recurred in two patients 4 to 5 months after the wires were extracted, and there was no clinical response in another patient who required subsequent curettage and bone grafting. Santori and associates[37] decompressed UBCs with either Ender nails or Rush pins and at short-term follow-up noted healing in all 11 patients. In a more recent study, Roposch and associates[38] reported favorable responses in all 32 patients with UBCs in their series (30 with associated pathologic fractures) who were treated with flexible intramedullary nails; 14 healed completely and 9 required a change of nails. This appears to be a useful technique for unstable fractures of long bones associated with UBCs. There is some early evidence that creating a communication between the UBC and the medullary canal of the long bone will promote healing of the cyst.

New grafting materials, such as demineralized bone matrix,[39-41] also are becoming available and are being used with minimally invasive grafting techniques. Demineralized bone matrix is composed of demineralized bone particles ranging from 100 to 500 mm in size in a glycerol base. Killian and associates[39] used demineralized bone matrix for 11 patients with UBCs and were able to obliterate cysts in 9 patients by using a single injection within 4 to 5 months. At the 2-year follow-up, no cysts appeared to be active or recurrent.

Packing of the defect with plaster of Paris pellets was described by Peltier and Jones[32] in 1978. Commercially available pellets made of radiopaque, medical-grade calcium sulfate can be placed percutaneously for UBCs. The biodegrad-

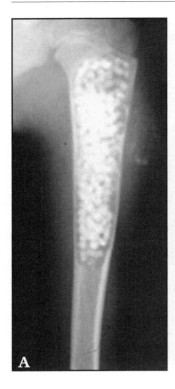
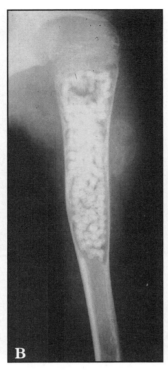
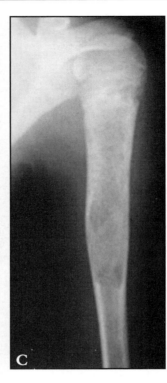

Fig. 5 A, Immediate postoperative AP radiograph showing complete packing of calcium sulfate pellets in a UBC of the proximal humerus. Follow-up AP radiographs taken at 3 weeks (**B**) and 3 months (**C**) after the surgery show good healing.

able pellets are resorbed within 30 to 60 days. This product is not intended to provide structural support during the healing process and therefore is contraindicated where such support is needed. Tricalcium phosphate also has been used as a synthetic cancellous bone to substitute for bone graft after tumor excision.[42]

Minimally Invasive Grafting: Surgical Technique Under fluoroscopic guidance, the involved bone is rotated until an area of thin cyst cortex is identified. Aspiration and a cystogram with Renografin dye (Squibb, Princeton, NJ) are done to confirm the fluid-filled nature of the cyst and to determine whether the cyst is indeed single chambered. The presence of serous fluid is indicative of UBC. If the cyst is multiloculated after fracture or a previous treatment, needles are used to break up septations. The diagnosis of UBC should be questioned if the dye does not fill a cyst cavity, and a biopsy should be considered. Calcium sulfate pellets (or other synthet-

ic materials) are then placed percutaneously under C-arm guidance. The radiopaque nature of the pellets is helpful in determining when complete packing of the UBC is accomplished (Fig. 5). To protect against recurrent fracture, the extremity is protected in a cast (sling for proximal humerus) for several weeks until structural integrity is sufficient for unprotected activities; radiographs are taken every 6 weeks to monitor healing.

Authors' Preferred Method of Treatment

Microfractures associated with UBCs in the upper extremity and lower extremity (excluding the hip) are common; more extensive fractures occur but are less common, and displacement is usually minimal. Large UBCs associated with pathologic microfractures (excluding the hip) can be treated soon after presentation. We recommend a brief period of simple immobilization for more severe fractures, if they are stable and nondis-

placed, to allow for fracture stabilization and healing. In addition to fracture healing, spontaneous cyst healing can also occur, although this is infrequent. Once the fracture has healed, the UBC can be treated when necessary and appropriate (eg, when there is high risk of refracture).

Because incomplete healing and recurrence are common after the injection of corticosteroid, and because multiple injections are necessary in most patients, percutaneous placement of new grafting materials, such as calcium sulfate, is being used more commonly at our institution.

Displaced pathologic fractures of the proximal femur can be very challenging to treat. If there is a significant loss of bone, coxa vara is likely to occur without internal fixation. Both the location of the cyst and the amount of bone loss dictate whether fixation can stabilize the fracture after grafting and what type of fixation would be most ideal. We use the classification system described in Figure 3 and

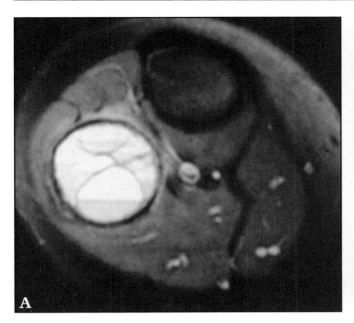 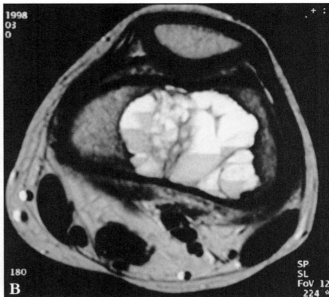

Fig 6 MRI studies showing septations and fluid-fluid levels in an ABC. **A,** ABC of the proximal fibular metaphysis. **B,** ABC of the distal femur.

use the corresponding treatment recommendations for internal fixation (Figs. 3 and 4).

Aneurysmal Bone Cysts

ABCs are central or eccentric, expansile, osteolytic lesions most commonly found in the metaphysis of long bones and in the posterior elements of the spine. ABCs involve the long bones in 75% of patients. In order of decreasing frequency, the most commonly involved long bones are the distal femur, proximal tibia, proximal humerus, and distal radius. Vertebral involvement is seen in 12% to 27% of patients;[34,43] the lumbar vertebrae are most commonly affected. There is frequent extension into the vertebral body.[44]

The lesions are not true cysts but rather a sponge-like collection of fibrous tissue, bony septa, and blood-filled spaces[43] (Fig. 2). ABCs are benign but locally aggressive. Usually at least a thin osseous shell surrounds the cyst.

Nearly 75% of ABCs are found in patients younger than 20 years, and 50% are seen in individuals between 10 and 20

years of age.[34,45] They are relatively rare, accounting for approximately 1.5% of all primary bone tumors.[45]

Radiographic findings commonly include a well-defined, radiolucent, expansile metaphyseal lesion with septations, giving rise to the so-called soap bubble or honeycomb appearance. Extension beyond the thinned cortex is uncommon. Initially, there is frank osteolysis of the margins of the bone, and with growth of the lesion, there is progressive destruction of bone. Although rare, epiphyseal involvement by the ABC through metaphyseal extension has been reported.[46,47]

Campanacci and associates[34] classified ABCs into three groups. An aggressive cyst is one with signs of reparative osteogenesis with ill-defined margins and no periosteal shell. An active cyst is one with an incomplete periosteal shell and a defined margin between the lesion and the host bone. An inactive cyst is one with a complete periosteal shell and a sclerotic margin between the cyst and the long bone.

The etiology of ABCs is not certain.

In most instances, they are primary lesions;[48] occasionally they are secondary to or associated with other lesions, such as UBCs, NOFs, fibrous dysplasia, or osteogenic sarcoma.[49] The most common presenting symptom is localized pain of less than 6 months' duration from microfracture.[34,48] A reported 11% to 35% of patients present with fractures through ABCs of the long bones,[50,51] with the humerus and femur being most commonly fractured.[51,52]

MRI is often helpful in differentiating ABCs from other lesions that can occasionally have a similar radiographic appearance, such as UBCs and cystic fibrous dysplasia. MRI of ABCs shows the septations and fluid-filled levels, which are characteristic, but not pathognomonic, for ABCs[53] (Fig. 6).

Conservative treatment with immobilization is inappropriate as the definitive treatment for pathologic fractures through ABCs. Although the pathologic fracture will heal, the ABC will usually persist and enlarge and another pathologic fracture usually will occur. Despite the potential to heal after simple biopsy,[34] this

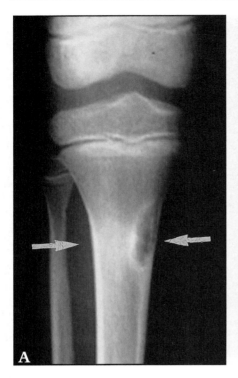
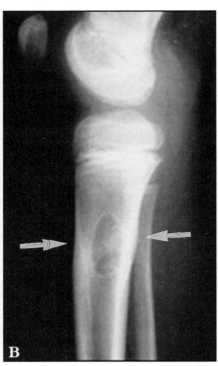

Fig 7 AP **(A)** and lateral **(B)** radiographs of an NOF with microfracture of the proximal tibia. Note the sclerotic new bone formation seen with the healing, nondisplaced pathologic fracture (*arrows*).

occurs rarely, and observation is not recommended because ABCs usually are locally aggressive. Simple curettage and bone grafting has been associated with recurrence rates as high as 20% to 30%.[34,43,46,48,54] The rate is higher in patients younger than 15 years of age.[48]

Selective arterial embolization can be used as definitive treatment or preoperatively with other procedures.[55] It is used most commonly in the spine, pelvis, and the proximal portion of the extremities when surgical exposure is more difficult and invasive and when blood loss with standard surgery can be significant. Adjuvants to curettage and bone grafting also have been described. Treatment of ABCs with cryotherapy (liquid nitrogen) in conjunction with curettage is associated with a recurrence rate of between 8% and 14%.[46,56,57] Cementation also has been described as an adjuvant treatment of ABC. Ozaki and associates[58] compared

curettage and bone grafting in 30 patients with curettage and cementation in 35 patients. At follow-up ranging from 24 to 161 months, the recurrence rate was 37% for curettage and bone grafting compared with 17% for curettage and cementation. Phenol also has been used as an adjuvant, especially for aggressive or recurrent ABCs. The use of adjuvants such as liquid nitrogen, bone cement, and phenol may be inappropriate for children with ABCs adjacent to open physes. In general, adjuvants should be used with caution.

Complete en bloc resection is reserved for active or recurrent ABCs,[44,45,51,54] and it is most feasible in the proximal fibula, distal ulna, ribs, pubic ramus, metatarsals,[34] and metacarpals.[59] Irradiation should be avoided because it has been associated with later development of sarcoma.[48] It also may damage reproductive organs and the active growth areas of long bones and cause other complications.[34]

Authors' Preferred Method of Treatment

It is important to remember that ABCs can be seen in association with or secondary to other tumors and tumor-like lesions. The first step in the effective treatment of a patient with an ABC is to confirm the diagnosis with open biopsy and frozen section. The biopsy is usually done in the same surgical setting as the definitive surgical procedure.

Because most ABCs are aggressive and grow and invade rapidly, treatment should be prompt once the diagnosis is made. Preoperative planning is important to assure adequate exposure, preparation for blood loss, internal fixation when needed, availability of grafting material, and, in selected cases, preoperative embolization.

We use a four-step approach to surgical treatment: (1) curettage, (2) exploration of the cyst wall with a cautery, (3) use of a high-speed burr, and, occasionally, (4) use of adjuvants (for example, hydrogen peroxide or phenol) for aggressive or recurrent ABCs. Achieving adequate exposure, including a large cortical window for thorough extended curettage, is essential for successful treatment. A headlamp, surgical loupes, and dental mirror can be helpful to inspect for residual tumor. Electrocautery is used to explore the walls of the cyst after curettage to identify pockets of additional tumor. The use of a high-speed burr allows systematic extended intralesional curettage. Phenol is reserved for aggressive or recurrent ABCs. Bone grafting can consist of autograft, allograft, bone substitutes, or a combination of these. For more severe or unstable fractures, internal stabilization may be needed (Fig. 3). Postoperatively, a walking hip spica cast can sometimes be used after adequate surgical stabilization of the pathologic fracture.

Fibrous Cortical Defects and Nonossifying Fibromas

FCDs are small, eccentric metaphyseal lesions ranging from 1 to 2 cm in diame-

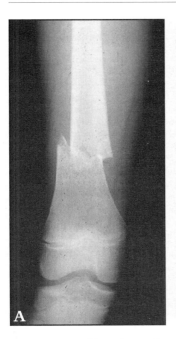 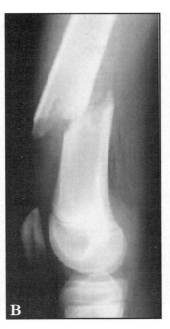 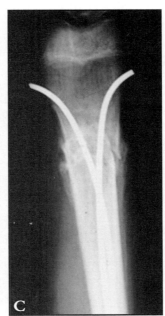 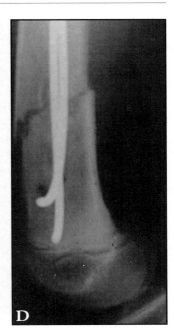

Fig. 8 AP **(A)** and lateral **(B)** radiographs of an unstable, displaced, pathologic supracondylar fracture through an NOF. Intramedullary fixation with titanium elastic nails was used to stabilize the fracture, as seen in the postoperative AP **(C)** and lateral **(D)** radiographs.

ter, most commonly seen in the distal femur, proximal tibia, and fibula. FCDs are common and are apparent on lower extremity radiographs in approximately 25% of children.[60] They usually are asymptomatic.

NOFs are larger, eccentric lesions of the metaphysis reaching lengths of 5 cm or more[61] and may occupy the entire width of the shaft in the fibula and other small bones. They follow a similar distribution of bone involvement as FCDs and present at a similar age (the first 2 decades of life). Approximately 33% of affected patients have multiple lesions.[62,63] On radiographs, the lesions are radiolucent and can be either uniloculated or multiloculated. Histologically, both lesions contain fibrous tissue, foam cells, and multinucleated giant cells. Most authors have described spontaneous regression for both lesions, with an average duration ranging from 29 months to 53 months.[61-65] As with FCDs, NOFs are typically asymptomatic unless a pathologic fracture is present.[61] Microfractures are most common (Fig.

7), and the larger the lesion, the greater the chance of fracture.

Fractures associated with these lesions exhibit excellent healing potential,[61,63,66] but the lesion usually persists after healing of the fracture. The incidence of documented refracture is low.[63,66] Fracture union takes place normally, but often multiple radiolucencies remain.[61] Arata and associates[66] noted that all pathologic fractures associated with NOF in the lower extremity occurred through lesions involving more than 50% of the transverse cortical diameter. These "large lesions" were defined as exhibiting more than 50% cortical involvement on AP and lateral radiographs and a height measurement of greater than 33 mm. Although the authors recommended careful observation of these large NOFs, they suggested that "prophylactic curettage and bone grafting be considered if there is a reasonable chance of impending fracture."[66] We recommend intramedullary fixation for displaced and unstable pathologic supracondylar fractures of the distal

femur in older children (Fig. 8).

Easley and Kneisl[67] suggested that although absolute size parameters were helpful in predicting pathologic fractures, they do not imply a requirement for prophylactic curettage and bone grafting. In their series, 13 "large" NOFs (59%) did not fracture despite exceeding the previously established size threshold. In the nine patients (41%) with pathologic fractures, healing was uneventful after closed reduction and cast immobilization, and no refractures were observed.

Authors' Preferred Method of Treatment

Most patients with NOFs can be monitored without surgical intervention because spontaneous resolution occurs in most patients. However, it may be appropriate to limit the activity of children with large NOFs. If fracture does occur, it should be remembered that most are stable, and conservative immobilization can be used until healing is noted. Whereas absolute size parameters may be useful in predicting pathologic fractures, they do not imply a requirement for prophylactic surgery. Many incidentally discovered large NOFs do not fracture and remain nonproblematic.

Surgery is indicated when the residual lesion is of sufficient size to predispose the child to further fractures or when there is doubt about the identity of the lesion. In general, patients with larger lesions (ie, a diameter greater than 50% of the width of the bone on AP and lateral radiographs) are thought to be prone to fracture and may be best managed with curettage and bone grafting. However, each patient should be approached individually, and patient and family wishes may influence the decision.

References

1. Dormans JP, Flynn JM: Pathologic fractures associated with tumors and unique conditions of the musculoskeletal system, in Bucholz RW, Heckman JD, Beaty JH, Kasser JR (eds): *Rockwood, Green, and Wilkins' Fractures*, ed 5. Philadelphia, PA, Lippincott Williams & Wilkins, 2001, pp 139-240.

2. Hipp JA, Springfield DS, Hayes WC: Predicting pathologic fracture risk in the management of metastatic bone defects. *Clin Orthop* 1995;120-135.

3. Ahn JI, Park JS: Pathological fractures secondary to unicameral bone cysts. *Int Orthop* 1994;18:20-22.

4. Kaelin AJ, MacEwen GD: Unicameral bone cysts. Natural history and the risk of fracture. *Int Orthop* 1989;13:275-282.

5. Nakamura T, Takagi K, Kitagawa T, et al: Microdensity of solitary bone cyst after steroid injection. *J Pediatr Orthop* 1988;8:566-568.

6. Copley L, Dormans JP: Benign pediatric bone tumors: Evaluation and treatment. *Pediatr Clin North Am* 1996;43:949-966.

7. Enneking W: *Musculoskeletal Tumor Surgery*. New York, NY, Churchill Livingstone, 1983, pp 741.

8. Capanna R, Albisinni U, Caroli GC, et al: Contrast examination as a prognostic factor in the treatment of solitary bone cyst by cortisone injection. *Skeletal Radiol* 1984;12:97-102.

9. Neer CS, Francis KC, Johnston AD, et al: Current concepts on the treatment of solitary unicameral bone cyst. *Clin Orthop* 1973;97:40-51.

10. Chigira M, Maehara S, Arita S, et al: The aetiology and treatment of simple bone cysts. *J Bone Joint Surg Br* 1983;65:633-637.

11. Cohen J: Unicameral bone cysts. a current synthesis of reported cases. *Orthop Clin North Am* 1977;8:715-736.

12. Gartland JJ, Cole FL: Modern concepts in the treatment of unicameral bone cysts of the proximal humerus. *Orthop Clin North Am* 1975;6:487-498.

13. Khermosh O, Weissman SL: Coxa vara, avascular necrosis and osteochondritis dissecans complicating solitary bone cysts of the proximal femur. *Clin Orthop* 1977;18:143-146.

14. Cohen J: A simple bone cyst: Studies of cyst fluid in six cases with a theory of pathogenesis. *J Bone Joint Surg Am* 1960;42:609-616.

15. Jaffe H: *Tumors and Tumorous Conditions of Bone and Joints*. Philadelphia, PA, Lea & Febiger, 1958, pp 629.

16. Reynolds J: The "fallen fragment sign" in the diagnosis of unicameral bone cysts. *Radiology* 1969;92:949-953.

17. Harrer M, Dormans J, Stanton R, et al: Diaphyseal unicameral bone cysts in children. *Orthop Trans* 1997-1998;21:1187-1188.

18. Neer C, Frands K, Marcove R, et al: Treatment of unicameral bone cyst: A follow-up study of one hundred seventy-five cases. *J Bone Joint Surg Am* 1966;48:731-745.

19. Boseker EH, Bickel WH, Dahlin DC: A clinicopathologic study of simple unicameral bone cysts. *Surg Gynecol Obstet* 1968;127:550-560.

20. Capanna R, Dal Monte A, Gitelis S, et al: The natural history of unicameral bone cyst after steroid injection. *Clin Orthop* 1982;12:204-211.

21. de Palma L, Santucci A: Treatment of bone cysts with methylprednisolone acetate: A 9 to 11 year follow-up. *Int Orthop* 1987;11:23-28.

22. Fahey JJ, O'Brien ET: Subtotal resection and grafting in selected cases of solitary unicameral bone cyst. *J Bone Joint Surg Am* 1973;55:59-68.

23. Oppenheim WL, Galleno H: Operative treatment versus steroid injection in the management of unicameral bone cysts. *J Pediatr Orthop* 1984;4:1-7.

24. Malkawi H, Shannak A, Amr S: Surgical treatment of pathological subtrochanteric fractures due to benign lesions in children and adolescents. *J Pediatr Orthop* 1984;4:63-69.

25. Weisel A, Hecht HL: Development of a unicameral bone cyst: Case report. *J Bone Joint Surg Am* 1980;62:664-666.

26. Baker DM: Benign unicameral bone cyst: A study of forty-five cases with long-term follow up. *Clin Orthop* 1970;71:140-151.

27. Spence KF, Sell KW, Brown RH: Solitary bone cyst: Treatment with freeze-dried cancellous bone allograft: A study of one hundred seventy-seven cases. *J Bone Joint Surg Am* 1969;51:87-96.

28. Robins PR, Peterson HA: Management of pathologic fractures through unicameral bone cysts. *JAMA* 1972;222:80-81.

29. Schreuder HW, Conrad EU, Bruckner JD, et al: Treatment of simple bone cysts in children with curettage and cryosurgery. *J Pediatr Orthop* 1997;17:814-820.

30. Scaglietti O, Marchetti PG, Bartolozzi P: The effects of methylprednisolone acetate in the treatment of bone cysts: Results of three years follow-up. *J Bone Joint Surg Br* 1979;61:200-204.

31. Colville MR, Aronson DD, Prcevski P, et al: The systemic and local effects of an intramedullary injection of methylprednisolone acetate in growing rabbits. *J Pediatr Orthop* 1987;7:412-414.

32. Peltier LF, Jones RH: Treatment of unicameral bone cysts by curettage and packing with plaster-of-Paris pellets. *J Bone Joint Surg Am* 1978;60:820-822.

33. Fernbach SK, Blumenthal DH, Poznanski AK, et al: Radiographic changes in unicameral bone cysts following direct injection of steroids: A report on 14 cases. *Radiology* 1981;140:689-695.

34. Campanacci M, Capanna R, Picci P: Unicameral and aneurysmal bone cysts. *Clin Orthop* 1986;127:25-36.

35. Glaser DL, Dormans JP, Stanton RP, et al: Surgical management of calcaneal unicameral bone cysts. *Clin Orthop* 1999;231-237.

36. Moreau G, Letts M: Unicameral bone cyst of the calcaneus in children. *J Pediatr Orthop* 1994;14:101-104.

37. Santori F, Ghera S, Castelli V: Treatment of solitary bone cysts with intramedullary nailing. *Orthopedics* 1988;11:873-878.

38. Roposch A, Saraph V, Linhart WE: Flexible intramedullary nailing for the treatment of unicameral bone cysts in long bones. *J Bone Joint Surg Am* 2000;82:1447-1453.

39. Killian JT, Wilkinson L, White S, et al: Treatment of unicameral bone cyst with demineralized bone matrix. *J Pediatr Orthop* 1998;18:621-624.

40. Kresler T, Kling T, Rougraff B: Unicameral bone cysts. *Curr Opin Orthop* 1994;5:75-81.

41. Rougraff B: Treatment of inactive unicameral bone cysts with injectable autogenic bone graft and autogenous bone marrow. *Orthop Trans* 1995-1996;19:788.

42. Altermatt S, Schwobel M, Pochon JP: Operative treatment of solitary bone cysts with tricalcium phosphate ceramic: A 1 to 7 year follow-up. *Eur J Pediatr Surg* 1992;2:180-182.

43. Dabska M, Buraczewski J: Aneurysmal bone cyst: Pathology, clinical course and radiologic appearances. *Cancer* 1969;23:371-389.

44. Capanna R, Albisinni U, Picci P, et al: Aneurysmal bone cyst of the spine. *J Bone Joint Surg Am* 1985;67:527-531.

45. Besse B: Aneurysmal bone cyst: Additional considerations. *Clin Orthop* 1956;7:93-102.

46. Biesecker JL, Marcove RC, Huvos AG, et al: Aneurysmal bone cysts: A clinicopathologic study of 66 cases. *Cancer* 1970;26:615-625.

47. Jaffe KA, Dunham WK: Treatment of benign lesions of the femoral head and neck. *Clin Orthop* 1990;1:134-137.

48. Tillman BP, Dahlin DC, Lipscomb PR, et al: Aneurysmal bone cyst: An analysis of ninety-five cases. *Mayo Clin Proc* 1968;43:478-495.

49. Bonakdarpour A, Levy WM, Aegerter E: Primary and secondary aneurysmal bone cyst: A radiological study of 75 cases. *Radiology* 1978;126:75-83.

50. Hooper JC: Aneurysmal bone cysts penetrating the tibial epiphysis after curettage. *Med J Aust* 1971;1:200-201.

51. Koskinen EV, Visuri TI, Holmstrom T, et al: Aneurysmal bone cyst: Evaluation of resection and of curettage in 20 cases. *Clin Orthop* 1976;1:136-146.

52. Clough JR, Price CH: Aneurysmal bone cyst: Pathogenesis and long term results of treatment. *Clin Orthop* 1973;97:52-63.

53. Sullivan RJ, Meyer JS, Dormans JP, et al: Diagnosing aneurysmal and unicameral bone cysts with magnetic resonance imaging. *Clin Orthop* 1999;79:186-190.

54. Hay MC, Paterson D, Taylor TK: Aneurysmal bone cysts of the spine. *J Bone Joint Surg Br* 1978;60:406-411.

55. De Cristofaro R, Biagini R, Boriani S, et al: Selective arterial embolization in the treatment of aneurysmal bone cyst and angioma of bone. *Skeletal Radiol* 1992;21:523-527.

56. Marcove RC, Sheth DS, Takemoto S, et al: The treatment of aneurysmal bone cyst. *Clin Orthop* 1995;157-163.

57. Schreuder HW, Veth RP, Pruszczynski M, et al: Aneurysmal bone cysts treated by curettage, cryotherapy and bone grafting. *J Bone Joint Surg Br* 1997;79:20-25.

58. Ozaki T, Hillmann A, Lindner N, et al: Cementation of primary aneurysmal bone cysts. *Clin Orthop* 1997;240-248.

59. Burkhalter WE, Schroeder FC, Eversmann WW: Aneurysmal bone cysts occurring in the metacarpals: A report of three cases. *J Hand Surg Am* 1978;3:579-584.

60. Selby S: Metaphyseal cortical defects in the tubular bones of growing children. *J Bone Joint Surg Am* 1961;43:395-400.

61. Cunningham J, Ackerman L: Metaphyseal fibrous defects. *J Bone Joint Surg Am* 1956;38:797-808.

62. Campbell C, Harkess J: Fibrous metaphyseal defect of bone. *Surg Gynecol Obstet* 1957;104:329-336.

63. Drennan DB, Maylahn DJ, Fahey JJ: Fractures through large non-ossifying fibromas. *Clin Orthop* 1974;0:82-88.

64. Hatcher C: The pathogenesis of localized fibrous lesions in the metaphyses of long bones. *Ann Surg* 1945;122:1016-1030.

65. Ritschl P, Karnel F, Hajek P: Fibrous metaphyseal defects: Determination of their origin and natural history using a radiomorphological study. *Skeletal Radiol* 1988;17:8-15.

66. Arata MA, Peterson HA, Dahlin DC: Pathological fractures through non-ossifying fibromas: Review of the Mayo Clinic experience. *J Bone Joint Surg Am* 1981;63:980-988.

67. Easley ME, Kneisl JS: Pathologic fractures through nonossifying fibromas: Is prophylactic treatment warranted? *J Pediatr Orthop* 1997;17:808-813.

Bone Graft Alternatives in the Treatment of Benign Bone Tumors

Bruce T. Rougraff, MD

Abstract

Most bone grafting procedures are done during spinal fusion and to treat patients with skeletal trauma. Very few studies have addressed the bone grafting of skeletal defects after benign bone tumor excision. Contained defects have been treated with autogenous bone grafts, fresh-frozen allografts, freeze-dried allografts, demineralized bone matrix, and ceramic materials. Additionally, bone morphogenetic proteins may provide a future treatment option for bone tumor reconstruction.

Bone grafting in the United States is most commonly used for spinal fusion and treatment of delayed unions or nonunions. It is estimated that 500,000 bone grafting procedures are performed each year.[1] Autogenous bone grafting has always been considered the gold standard for efficacy in bone grafting; however, donor site morbidity[2] and limited supply has encouraged the development of alternative bone graft materials. An ideal bone graft substitute should be osteoinductive, osteoconductive, and completely degradable by the host bone. In response to the challenge to create an ideal bone graft material and fueled by the large volume of bone grafting procedures done each year, several products have been developed over the past 50 years. These include fresh-frozen allografts, freeze-dried allografts, demineralized bone matrix, ceramic materials, and most recently, bone morphogenetic proteins (BMPs).

Although most bone grafting procedures are done during spinal fusion and to treat nonunion, malunion, or delayed union of skeletal injuries, the treatment of bone defects after benign tumor excision offers a better clinical model to study the efficacy of bone graft substitutes. In patients undergoing spinal fusion and nonunion repair, failure of the graft can be attributed to hardware failure, infection, local vascular deficiency, nutritional factors, smoking, patient compliance, and other uncontrollable issues unrelated to the quality of the graft material. Contained bone defects treated by curettage and bone grafting of a benign bone lesion give rise to fewer contaminating issues that may cause failure of the graft, but which are typically not related to the quality of the grafting material. Other than tumor recurrence and poor patient compliance with postoperative activity recommendations, most of these causes of graft failure do not commonly occur in

patients who undergo benign bone tumor grafting. Comparison studies in tumor surgery are difficult to perform, because defining outcome parameters to allow comparison among various bone graft materials in this patient population is challenging. Additionally, a single institution will rarely treat enough patients with bone tumors to identify a difference. The focus of this discussion, therefore, is on the grafting of contained bone defects after benign bone tumor excision.

After complete intralesional excision of a benign bone lesion, the treating surgeon is faced with the problem of promoting rapid bone healing and remodeling to reconstitute a competent skeleton. The void is best filled with material that has the three properties of bone healing and repair (it must be osteoinductive, osteoconductive, and completely degradable by the host bone). Osteoinduction (the ability to mediate the induction of bone formation singularly in a non-osseous location) is the process by which undifferentiated perivascular cells are stimulated to form osteoprogenitor cells. Osteoconduction (the ability of a material to act as a scaffold for new bone in a bony environment in the absence of osteoinductive factors) is the process whereby a scaffold is provided for ingrowth of immature bone. Osteoprogenitor cells are the osteoblastic cells that are capable of forming bone in the correct environment. No bone graft substitute can provide osteoprogenitor cells, but autogenous bone marrow can be added to the material. Patient considerations that can affect the choice of bone graft substitute include religious concerns and patient expectations. Patients who are Jehovah's Witnesses and some Asian patients will not accept allograft tissue. Patient concern over blood loss may keep them from choosing an autogenous bone graft, particularly if it is needed to treat a large defect. If a patient wants a rapid return to work, procurement of a large autogenous graft may not be best for that patient because the donor site can be a significant source of pain and disability. Use of bone graft substitutes in the treatment of bone tumors eliminates the potential contamination of an autogenous donor site with tumor cells.

Fresh-Frozen Allograft

Fresh frozen allografts are stored at –60°C, need cryopreservative to protect the articular cartilage, and are rarely used for the treatment of contained skeletal defects. They are commonly used for skeletal reconstruction after intercalary bone resection or for an osteoarticular reconstruction. Fresh-frozen allografts are also indicated for composite reconstructions with a complex arthroplasty for reconstruction after tumor resection or revision arthroplasty. Fresh-frozen allografts are also less commonly used in combination with a vascularized autogenous bone graft. Fresh-frozen cortical allografts retain significant structural integrity, which is considerably greater than freeze-dried cortical allograft tissue. Human immunodeficiency virus transmission has been reported with the use of fresh allograft tissue (before blood screening) but not with freeze-dried tissue. Although fresh-frozen morcellized bone allograft can be used for contained bone defects, the use of fresh-

frozen bone tissue is typically reserved for reconstruction of large skeletal defects.

Freeze-Dried Allograft

Freeze-dried (lyophilized) cancellous allograft is commonly used for grafting contained defects and for augmentation of autogenous bone graft (Figure 1). Lyophilization involves removing water from frozen tissue after which the bone may be stored in a vacuum for up to 5 years. This processed tissue has been used since 1951 and has never been associated with viral transmission.[3] Freeze-dried allograft has several advantages. It is of unlimited supply, it is readily available, it does not result in donor site morbidity, it is easy to use in the operating room, and it is osteoinductive (weak), osteoconductive, minimally immunogenic, and completely resorbed and replaced. It has several disadvantages as well. Patients who are Jehovah's Witnesses may refuse to use it, it is not a carrier for antibiotics, and it has significant structural weakness, loss of hoop and compressive strength, and requires rehydration before implantation. Spence and associates[4] reported the results of 177 unicameral bone cysts that were treated with open curettage and freeze-dried allografting. They found excellent results in the rate of healing, and the lowest recurrence rate of cysts occurred in older patients whose bone defects were completely packed with allograft. Most patients were completely healed at 1 year after surgery, but sequential radiographs were not available for exact confirmation of the time of healing. No data were recorded regarding the time to return to full activities or weight bearing. Glancy and associates[5] compared freeze-dried allograft to autograft in the treatment of 61 benign bone lesions in a retrospective review. They found no significant advantage in autograft over allograft in lesions that were less than 60 cm³ in volume. The allografts were reported to take 6 months longer to remodel radio-

graphically, but this did not result in a difference in clinical outcome. The exact time to weight bearing and return to full activities was not recorded for comparison in this study either. The authors found a greater number of tumor recurrences in the group with larger tumors and more problems in those patients who received allograft. This study was not randomized, and the authors acknowledged a study bias. The patients receiving allograft had the largest skeletal defects because not enough autogenous bone graft was available to treat large skeletal defects; therefore, allograft was used.

Demineralized Bone Matrix

Demineralized bone matrix was first reported as an osteoinductive agent in 1965 in a classic article by Urist,[6] where it was shown to have produced bone in an extraskeletal site. Demineralized bone matrix is now commercially prepared using acid extraction of mineral from freeze-dried allograft. The demineralized bone is mixed with a glycerin carrier that gives it a toothpaste-like consistency. Avoiding ethylene oxide or gamma radiation in the sterilization process protects the BMPs and enhances its osteoinductive characteristics. The advantages of demineralized bone matrix include unlimited supply; it is readily available; it is injectable through large-bore needles (11-gauge), which allows for percutaneous applications; it does not result in donor site morbidity; it is osteoinductive (weak); it is not immunogenic; and it is completely resorbed. Disadvantages include potential viral disease transfer (minimal risk); patients who are Jehovah's Witnesses may refuse to use it; it has no structural support, which may require supplemental fixation; and it is not a carrier for antibiotics. Viral transmission with demineralized bone matrix has not yet been documented despite its use in over 1.5 million patients. In addition, viral inactivation has been demonstrated by use of the decalcification tech-

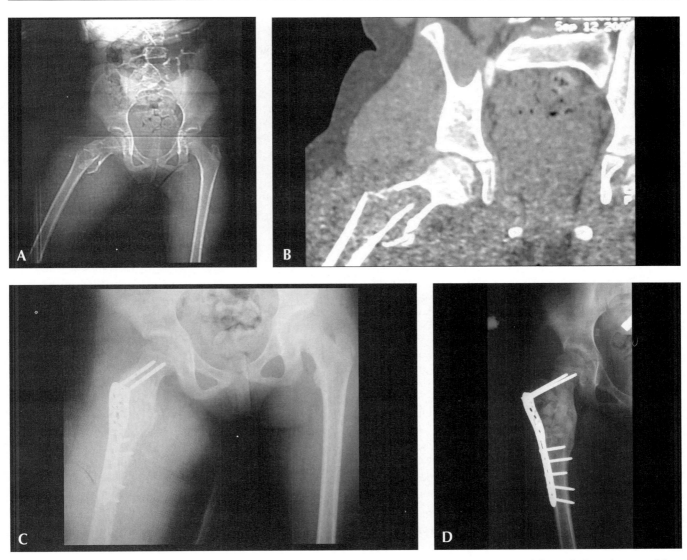

Figure 1 A, Radiograph of an 8-year-old girl who had a 6-week history of groin pain. She later fell and sustained this pathologic fracture of the right proximal femur. **B,** CT confirms the presence of a pathologic fracture through a cystic lesion. **C,** Postoperative radiograph obtained after the patient underwent open curettage, reduction, internal fixation, and grafting with freeze-dried cancellous allograft. Biopsy confirmed the presence of a unicameral bone cyst. **D,** Radiograph taken 3 months after surgery reveals a healed fracture. Patient returned to full activities without pain. Note that at this point the allograft is only partially resorbed radiographically. At 2-year follow-up, the patient has no pain and no recurrence of cyst.

nique.[7] Demineralized bone matrix (as a mixture with autogenous bone marrow) has been studied as a bone graft substitute for the treatment of unicameral bone cysts (Figure 2). Rougraff and Kling[8] reported on 23 patients with active unicameral bone cysts who were treated with percutaneous injection of demineralized bone matrix and autogenous bone mar-row. All of the patients showed good early bone formation as early as 3 months. By 1-year follow-up, excellent bone healing and remodeling occurred in 79% of patients. Five patients developed recurrent unicameral bone cysts, despite early bone healing. Of the patients treated for recurrence, a second injection was equally successful. Satisfactory osteoinduction of bone occurred using this technique, but some patients developed heterotopic ossification from extruded demineralized bone matrix into the soft tissue. The average time for pain relief after injection was 5 weeks, and the average time to return to full activities was 6 weeks. Demineralized bone matrix has also been studied in the treatment of nonunions as

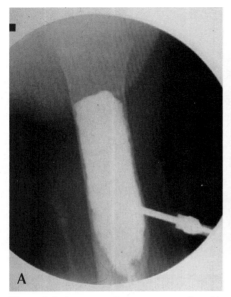
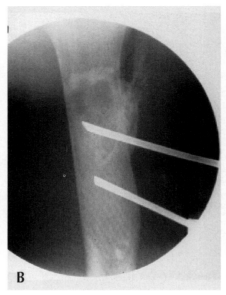
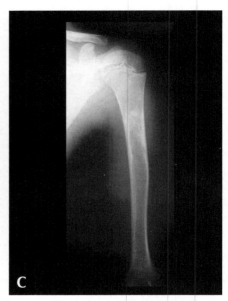

Figure 2 A, Intraoperative cystogram of an 11-year-old patient with a unicameral bone cyst of the humerus. The patient had two previous fractures and a progressively enlarging lesion. **B,** Intraoperative cystogram showing two 11-gauge needles placed into the cyst, at which time 28 cm³ of demineralized bone matrix and autogenous bone marrow were injected into the lesion percutaneously. **C,** Radiograph obtained 1 year after the injection demonstrates complete healing of the cyst; at 6-year follow-up, no further treatment was needed.

well as other clinical studies requiring grafting of skeletal defects with good results.[9-12] Because the US Food and Drug Administration (FDA) considers demineralized bone matrix to be a tissue rather than a drug or implant, as with all allograft tissue, it does not have a specific approval for use in humans.

Ceramic Materials

Ceramic materials comprise a broad category of artificial bone graft substitutes that includes tricalcium phosphate (TCP), hydroxyapatite/TCP, calcium sulfate, coralline hydroxyapatite, calcium phosphate, and injectable hydroxyapatite. Ceramic materials may be used as osteoconductive matrices for grafting contained defects with minimal osteoinductive characteristics. They can also be used successfully as autogenous graft expanders. All of these bone graft substitutes have the advantage of being in unlimited supply, they are nonimmunogenic, they are easy to package and sterilize, they are accepted by all religious groups, and they

present no risk of viral disease transmission. Mechanically, they are brittle and have very little tensile strength.

Tricalcium Phosphate

TCP is a biocompatible, random porous ceramic that is resorbed more rapidly than hydroxyapatite, with 98% resorbed by 1 year after implantation.[13] The micropore size ranges from 1 to 1,000 μm, with most being between 100 and 1,000 μm. Some of the TCP may convert to hydroxyapatite in vivo, but the rates of resorption and conversion to hydroxyapatite are inconsistent. Bucholz and associates[14] reported good results with TCP in various grafting applications, including tumor reconstruction. Nicholas and Lange[15] reported on 20 patients who were treated for benign bone lesions with curettage and grafting with granular TCP (Orthograft Large Granular, DePuy, Warsaw, IN). They reported complete healing of 12 of the 20 defects by 2-year follow-up. They concluded that graft resorption preceded trabecular bone

reconstitution radiographically. Graft resorption was seen radiographically 3 to 6 months after implantation. Of the defects that did not heal completely, they tended to be larger lesions or (in one patient) the result of a recurrence of a large aneurysmal bone cyst that destroyed the graft. Nineteen patients were released to full activities by 24 months after surgery. No adverse effects or adverse reactions to the TCP were reported in this series. It should be noted that TCP is mechanically very weak. Therefore, it is best used as an expander, a graft substitute for defects that are mechanically stable, or as a treatment modality when supplemental skeletal fixation is also used. TCP (Vitoss, Orthovita, Malvern, PA) is currently approved by the FDA for traumatic or surgically created defects of the extremities, pelvis, and spine.

Hydroxyapatite/TCP

Porous calcium phosphate and bovine-derived fibrillar collagen is marketed as a composite product to be mixed intraoperatively with autogenous bone marrow. In theory, this combines the osteoinductive and osteoconductive features of the ceramic with the osteoprogenitor cells of the marrow.[16,17] The calcium phosphate is 65% hydroxyapatite and 35% TCP. The bovine carrier is 95% type I collagen. Collagraft (Zimmer, Warsaw, IN) is a commercially available product, it has no structural strength, and to the author's knowledge, no studies assessing the use of Collagraft for the treatment of benign bone tumors have yet been published. Chapman and associates[16] and Cornell and associates[17] compared Collagraft and autogenous bone graft in the treatment of long bone fractures and reported no difference in union rate or functional outcome. Whether grafting was even necessary in most patients is not clear. It seems logical that this product is best used as an autogenous bone graft expander. Collagraft is approved by the FDA for grafting traumatic bone defects less than 30 mL.

Calcium Sulfate

Calcium sulfate (plaster of Paris) has been used for many years as a bone graft substitute with variable results.[18] In 1996, a product was released that had minimal trace elements and a uniform α-crystalline structure with the expectation of resulting in more uniform clinical outcomes. Osteoset (Wright Medical, Arlington, TN) is available as hard pellets that are biocompatible, completely resorbable, and osteoconductive (Figure 3). Kelly and associates[19] reported on 109 patients with skeletal defects resulting from trauma, benign tumor, arthroplasty failure, or fusion. Forty-six patients with benign tumors were separately studied in this report. The authors noted that 100% of the pellets were resorbed radiographically and 97% of the lesions had bone formation at 1-year follow-up. Most of the resorption occurred within the first 3 months. The healing rate of the tumor subgroup was comparable to the excellent results seen with the fracture sub-

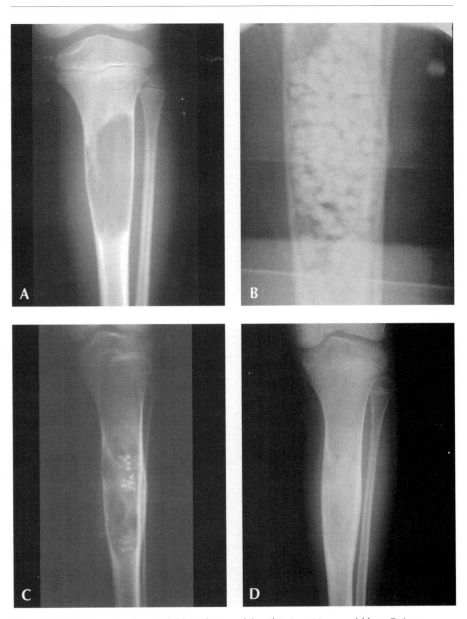

Figure 3 A, Radiograph of a painful lytic lesion of the tibia in a 10-year-old boy. **B,** Intraoperative cystogram shows the cyst was filled with calcium sulfate pellets. **C,** Radiograph obtained 3 months after surgery shows that most of the calcium sulfate has resorbed with early bone formation. **D,** Radiograph obtained 1 year after surgery shows excellent bone healing and the presence of bone remodeling.

group of patients. There was one tumor recurrence and one postoperative fracture. No data were given for the time to return to full activities. Gitelis[20] reported his results of 23 patients with benign bone tumors who received Osteoset graft with and without demineralized bone

matrix. He found no advantage of the addition of demineralized bone matrix over Osteoset alone. Ninety-four percent of the defects showed osseous repair 2 years after implantation. Osteoset is approved by the FDA for grafting all bone defects.

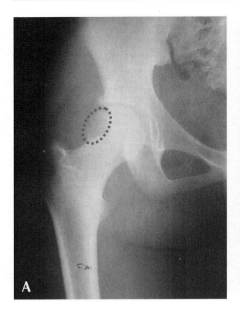
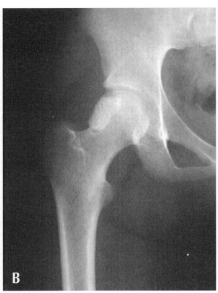
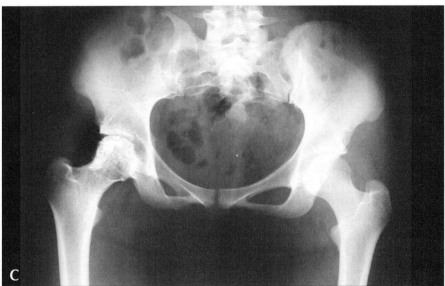

Figure 4 A, Radiograph of a painful lytic lesion (*dotted circle*) in the right femoral head of an 11-year-old girl who is a Jehovah's Witness. **B,** Radiograph obtained 4 months after curettage of the chondroblastoma and implantation of coralline hydroxyapatite shows no resorption of the implant. Weight bearing was initiated at this time. **C,** Radiograph obtained 8 years after implantation of coralline hydroxyapatite shows no tumor recurrence and very little radiographic evidence of implant resorption. The patient had normal hip function without pain.

Additionally, it has an unlimited supply, it is acceptable for use by patients who are Jehovah's Witnesses, it poses no risk of disease transfer, and it has some intrinsic strength in compression. The disadvantages include the fact that it is not completely resorbed, it requires cutting and shaping of the implant in the operating room and can be difficult to machine well, and it has brittle mechanical properties with very little tensile strength. The author's experience with this product after 8 years has shown that the coralline hydroxyapatite is still unchanged radiographically (Figure 4). Bucholz and associates[21] reported on their experience using coralline hydroxyapatite to treat patients with depressed tibial plateau fractures. They found that the coralline hydroxyapatite was equally effective as cancellous autograft at 15-month follow-up. Uchida and associates[24] reported the results of 60 patients with bone tumors that were treated with curettage and coralline hydroxyapatite. No postoperative wound healing problems, infections, or tumor recurrences were reported. Bone healing and incorporation continued to improve for the first 12 months after implantation, and no resorption of the ceramic was seen as late as 5 years postoperatively. The authors found coralline hydroxyapatite to be a useful, effective bone graft substitute for the treatment of patients with benign bone tumors. They did not report functional outcomes nor quantify the time to return to full activities. The FDA has approved coralline hydroxyapatite for use in the treatment of traumatic metaphyseal defects of long bones.

Injectable Calcium Phosphate and Injectable Hydroxyapatite

The Skeletal Repair System (SRS) (Norian, Cupertino, CA) is an injectable calcium phosphate that hardens within minutes and forms a carbonated apatite. This material has had good results in the treatment of distal radius fractures that

Coralline Hydroxyapatite

Coralline hydroxyapatite is derived from sea coral (*Porites goniopora*). The calcium phosphate of sea coral is put through a hydrothermal exchange method and converts it to hydroxyapatite with pore diameters of 200 to 500 μm, which are comparable to those of human bone.[13,21-25] Pro-Osteon (Interpore Cross International, Irvine, CA) is a coralline hydroxyapatite that is osteoinductive (very weak), osteoconductive, and nonimmunogenic.

becomes indistinguishable at 3 months from standard treatment.[26] No reports on the use of SRS to treat patients with bone tumors have yet been published in the literature. Using a similar product, Berrey and associates (unpublished data presented at the Musculoskeletal Tumor Society Meeting, Denver, CO, 1999) presented data on 22 patients with bone tumors that were treated with injectable hydroxyapatite cement (Bone Source, Howmedica/ Osteonics Inc, Allendale, NJ). They showed good preliminary results without fractures or resorption of the bone or implant. Resorption of this material is incomplete, but its role in the treatment of tumors is yet to be determined. Its best advantage over other bone graft substitutes is its mechanical strength, particularly in the treatment of metaphyseal and epiphyseal defects. Unlike methylmethacrylate, SRS and injectable hydroxyapatite do not heat up as they harden; therefore, they do not act as an adjuvant for tumor control (as in giant cell tumor treatment).

Bone Morphogenetic Proteins

BMPs are soluble proteins that are very stable and act as local differentiating proteins. They are members of the transforming growth factor-beta (TGF-β) family and act as powerful osteoinductive factors.[27,28] Two human BMP products are currently available, both of which are recombinant human (rh) BMP factors produced by mammalian cells: rhBMP-2 (InFUSE, Medtronic Sofamor Danek, Memphis, TN) and rhBMP-7 (osteogenic protein-1). rhBMP-2 was studied in a randomized, nonblinded 2-year multicenter study of 279 patients who underwent lumbar fusion with threaded fusion cages with either rhBMP-2 on an absorbable collagen sponge or autogenous bone graft.[29] The group of patients treated with rhBMP-2 had less blood loss, shorter surgical time, and a higher fusion rate at 24 months than those treated with autogenous bone graft (94.5%

versus 88.7%). Based on these findings, the FDA approved rhBMP-2 for single-level interbody fusions of the lumbar spine.

rhBMP-7 was tested in a prospective, randomized clinical trial involving 122 patients with tibial nonunions. Nonunions were treated using intramedullary rods and grafting with either autogenous bone or rhBMP-7. The healing rates of the autogenous bone group and rhBMP-7 group were similar (81% versus 85%). As a result, the FDA issued a humanitarian device exemption for rhBMP-7 as an alternative to autograft for the treatment of recalcitrant long bone nonunions in which use of autograft is not feasible and alternative treatments have failed.[30] Although BMPs at this point seem very promising as a bone graft substitute, results have not yet been reported in the treatment of defects after benign bone tumor excision. Improved delivery systems and exact dosing need to be addressed before their role in bone tumor surgery can be verified.

Summary

Several bone graft substitutes are currently available for skeletal reconstruction after bone tumor surgery. Osteoset and Vitoss are currently approved by the FDA as implants for this use, whereas allografts and demineralized bone matrix are tissue-derived products that can also be considered. Coralline hydroxyapatite has also been shown to have good results in skeletal reconstruction after bone tumor surgery. The future use for newer products such as BMPs will improve as better delivery systems are developed and appropriate dosages are determined. Several reports have demonstrated adequate outcomes for patients treated with these alternative products. Unfortunately, it is difficult to critically compare and contrast the efficacy of these different products with autogenous bone graft because of small sample sizes and other contaminating variables. The functional

timeframes of pain-free status, full weight bearing, and return to full unrestricted activities also need to be better documented with the use of these alternative products. Clearly, all of these products enhance bone healing, but any differences in healing rates are difficult to assess at this time.

References

1. Camper Y: Bone grafts and substitutes. *Orthop Network News* 1995;6:7-9.

2. Younger EM, Chapman MW: Morbidity at bone graft donor sites. *J Orthop Trauma* 1989;3:192-195.

3. Kruez FP, Hyatt GW, Turner TC, Bassett AL: The preservation and clinical use of freeze-dried bone. *J Bone Joint Surg Am* 1951;33:863-872.

4. Spence KF, Sell KW, Brown RH: Solitary bone cyst: Treatment with freeze-dried cancellous bone graft. *J Bone Joint Surg Am* 1969;51:87-96.

5. Glancy GL, Brugioni DJ, Eilert RE, Chang FM: Autograft versus allograft for benign lesions in children. *Clin Orthop* 1991;262:28-33.

6. Urist MR: Bone: formation by autoinduction. *Science* 1965;150:893-899.

7. Prewett AB, Moyer MP, O'Leary RK, Mellonig JT: Decalcification inactivates HIV in spiked and infected bone. *Trans Orthop Res Soc* 1992;17:436.

8. Rougraff BT, Kling TJ: Treatment of active unicameral bone cysts with percutaneous injection of demineralized bone matrix and autogenous bone marrow. *J Bone Joint Surg Am* 2002;84:921-929.

9. Tiedeman JJ, Garvin KL, Kile TA, et al: The role of a composite, demineralized bone matrix and bone marrow in the treatment of osseous defects. *Orthopedics* 1995;18:1153-1158.

10. Tiedeman JJ, Connolly JF, Strates BS, Lippiello L: Treatment of nonunion by percutaneous injection of bone marrow and demineralized bone matrix: An experimental study in dogs. *Clin Orthop* 1991;268:294-302.

11. Hu X, Yao L, Lu C, Wang S, Chen Y: Experimental and clinical investigations of human insoluble bone matrix gelatin: A report of 24 cases. *Clin Orthop* 1993;293:360-365.

12. Whiteman D, Gropper PT, Wirtz P, Monk P: Demineralized bone powder: Clinical applications for bone defects of the hand. *J Hand Surg [Br]* 1993;18:487-490.

13. Erbe EM, Clineff TD, Lavagnino M, Dejardin L, Arnoczky S: Comparison of Vitros and ProOsteon 500R in a canine model at one year. *Trans Orthop Res Soc* 2001;47:975.

14. Bucholz RW, Carlton A, Holmes RE: Hydroxyapatite and tricalcium phosphate bone graft substitutes. *Orthop Clin North Am* 1987;18:323-334.

15. Nicholas RW, Lange TA: Granular tricalcium phosphate grafting of cavitary lesions in human bone. *Clin Orthop* 1994;306:197-203.

16. Chapman M, Bucholz R, Cornell C: Treatment of acute fractures with a collagen calcium phosphate graft material: A randomized clinical trial. *J Bone Joint Surg Am* 1997;79:495-502.

17. Cornell CN, Lane JM, Chapman M, et al: Multicenter trial of Collagraft as bone graft substitute. *J Orthop Trauma* 1991;5:1-8.

18. Gazdag AR, Lane JM, Glaser D, Forster RA: Alternatives to autogenous bone graft: Efficacy and Indications. *J Am Acad Orthop Surg* 1995;3:1-8.

19. Kelly CM, Wilkins RM, Gitelis S, Hartjen C, Watson JT, Kim PT: The use of a surgical grade calcium sulfate as a bone graft substitute: Results of a multicenter trial. *Clin Orthop* 2001;382:42-50.

20. Gitelis S: Use of calcium sulfate-based bone graft substitute for benign bone lesions. *Orthopedics* 2001;24:162-166.

21. Bucholz RW, Carlton A, Holmes R: Interporous hydroxyapatite as a bone graft substitute in tibial plateau fractures. *Clin Orthop* 1989;240:53-62.

22. Holmes RE, Mooney V, Bucholz R, et al: A Coralline hydroxyapatite bone graft substitute. *Clin Orthop* 1984;188:252-262.

23. Kuhne JH, Bartl R, Frisch B, et al: Bone formation in coralline hydroxyapatite. *Acta Orthop Scand* 1994;65:246-252.

24. Uchida A, Araki N, Shinto Y, et al: The use of calcium hydroxyapatite ceramic in bone tumor surgery. *J Bone Joint Surg Br* 1990;72:298-302.

25. Dupoirieux L, Costes V, Jammet P, et al: Experimental study on demineralized bone matrix (DBM) and coral as bone graft substitutes in maxillofacial surgery. *Int J Oral Maxillofac Surg* 1994;23:395-398.

26. Kopylov P, Jonsson K, Thorngren KG, Aspenberg P: Injectable calcium phosphate in the treatment of distal radial fractures. *J Hand Surg [Br]* 1996;21:768-771.

27. Sailer H, Kolb H: Application of purified bone morphogenetic protein (BMP) in craniomaxillo-facial surgery. *J Craniomaxillofac Surg* 1994;22:2-11.

28. Wozney JM: Overview of Bone Morphogenetic Proteins. *Spine* 2002;27:S2-S8.

29. Burkus JK, Gornet MF, Dickman CA, Zdeblick TA: Anterior interbody fusion using rhBMP-2 with tapered interbody cages. *J Spinal Disord Tech* 2002;15:337-349.

30. Friedlaender GE, Perry CR, Cole JD, et al: Osteogenic Protein-1 (BMP-7) in the treatment of tibial nonunions. *J Bone Joint Surg Am* 2001;83(suppl 1):S151-S158.

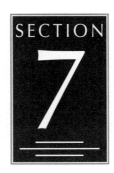

SECTION 7

Miscellaneous Issues in Pediatric Orthopaedics

Miscellaneous Issues in Pediatric Orthopaedics

This group of articles is grouped somewhat pejoratively under the title "Miscellaneous Issues in Pediatric Orthopaedics" because none of them fits neatly into any of the six preceding sections. However, I personally selected these articles because I thought each one ably addresses topics important for all those interested in pediatric orthopaedics.

The most obvious inclusion addresses developments in gene therapy and tissue engineering. Most of us know that gene therapy and tissue engineering eventually will have a startling impact on orthopaedics and all medicine. At one extreme, imagine veritable biologic joints with living articular cartilage grown to fit the recipient on a biocompatible scaffolding. Imagine that these joints are free of all infectious particles and immunogenic proteins with no immunosuppressive medication required and that they bond to and become one with the host, without risk of loosening. The *Journal of Bone and Joint Surgery* recently has described such a prototypical joint. Imagine the transplant possibilities for a mangled or congenitally defective limb.

Turn intracellularly or even intrachromosomally to the truly genetic level and we can see beyond the ability to replenish enzyme and other protein deficiencies to actually replace a defective gene with a proper one that literally cures patients of their ills. Don't give the cell a fish, teach it to fish! Who among us doubts that these capabilities, formerly available only at the science fiction level of imagination, will become viable therapeutic interventions, if not in our lifetime, certainly in that of our children?

The first article by Liu and associates succinctly outlines current research into what promises to be the revolutionary domains of gene therapy and tissue engineering as they relate to orthopaedics. Exciting techniques of enhancing bone, tendon, cartilage healing are outlined. Phase I clinical trials, which are primarily aimed at establishing safety, have been conducted that address the specific gene deficiencies of rheumatoid arthritis and Duchenne muscular dystrophy. Yet, as the authors state in the first few paragraphs, after nearly 40 years of experiments and clinical trials, much remains to be learned, with some sobering obstructions both identified and yet to be identified. Although we can now truly see the mountains in the distance, we are not quite there. This article is beneficial for all orthopaedists in that it helps us to "learn the language," and it is time for us to do so.

The second article by Davids and associates is was another jewel I included in this compendium. The authors neatly summarize the surgical armamentarium and decision-making paradigm in ambulatory cerebral palsy patients in the context of five diagnostic sources of information: the clinical history, physical examination, diagnostic imaging, gait analysis, and examination under anesthesia. The article does not provide an overview of the management of the ambulatory child with cerebral palsy; rather, it presents the rationale for and application of these five sources, particularly as they relate to the indications for common orthopaedic surgical interventions in these children, specifically iliopsoas recession, femoral rotational osteotomy, medial hamstring lengthening, rectus femoris transfer, and gastrocnemius release.

The authors do not address other important modalities in the management of the ambulatory children with cerebral palsy and related disorders, including selective dorsal rhizotomy, baclophen and related tone-reducing medication, botulinum toxin type A (Botox), and other nonsurgical modalities. In the end, without minimizing the positive impact that well-planned, well-executed, and well-indicated orthopaedic surgical procedures can have on these patients, all parties must not lose sight of the fact that these interventions represent relatively primitive muscle-compromising surgical events used to treat a primarily neurologic disorder.

Controversies still exist regarding the precise indications for these surgical techniques and their impact on ambulation and quality of life. The pivotal role of instrumented qualitative gait analysis as used in the decision-making paradigm also remains somewhat controversial. Many surgeons do not have easy access to experienced, expert movement science laboratories. Therefore, they may not have the ability or luxury to follow the authors' recommendation of participating in an interpretation session with clinical and technical members of a motion analysis laboratory team. However, the authors' review of current indications for the five previously mentioned surgical techniques in the context of the diagnostic sources of the decision-making paradigm are of great value.

The least obvious article selected for this volume addresses physician communication skills. Although Tongue and associates obviously wrote this article to hone the communications skills of orthopaedists who treat adult patients, those of us who devote a substantial portion of our practice to the care of children are acutely aware of the special requirements or "art" of examining children of different ages, demeanors, and clinical settings. We also are faced with the unique challenge of balancing those requirements with our interactions with very involved, questioning parents and grandparents. We should assess the quality and effectiveness of our communications with patients, and particularly, parents, in the context of this article. As the authors point out, it takes a degree of humility to acknowledge that we can improve our communications skills.

One survey cited in the article reports that 85% of "customers" but only 56% of orthopaedic surgeons rate a physician's ability to listen to patients as a very important quality. The Academy has reported that the public views orthopaedic surgeons as highly skilled technically but poorly skilled as communicators. As a profession, we should strive to change that perception, particularly when it also has been identified that effective communication results in improved patient and physician satisfaction, better compliance and outcomes, and fewer malpractice suits. Beyond simply reducing the risk of litigation however, a communicative, positive physician can favorably influence a patient's response to intervention.

I recently learned of an investigation that documented a stronger placebo effect in patients when their physicians believed that they were administering a therapeutic agent compared with patients whose physicians knowingly administering the same placebo. In other words, a physician can *communicate* a positive outcome, just in the communication alone. This article provides refreshing insights into how to conduct the new patient medical interview, break bad news regarding unexpected adverse outcomes, and become a more effective, culturally sensitive communicator. The points made here are of direct relevance to our communication with the adults, who almost always are the surrogate providers of consent and evaluators of outcomes for our pediatric patients.

So there you have it, three seemingly unrelated articles, linked by their outstanding quality, clarity, and informative value. They very ably round out the breadth of material provided in this collection of special lectures.

John Birch, MD
Assistant Chief of Staff
Texas Scottish Rite Hospital for
 Children
Dallas, Texas

Gene Therapy and Tissue Engineering in Orthopaedic Surgery

Tzu-Shang Thomas Liu, MD, PhD
Kurt R. Weiss, MD
Freddie H. Fu, MD
Johnny Huard, PhD

Abstract

Despite setbacks in other fields, gene therapy in orthopaedic surgery continues to serve as the basis for novel treatments of various musculoskeletal disorders. Even in the brief time since the last review of scientific progress in this area, another orthopaedic-related disease has joined the ranks of those studied in gene therapy clinical trials. Armed with new techniques and new reagents, and committed to the increased use of tissue engineering, physicians and scientists continue to work together to accelerate tissue repair and reverse the course of chronic debilitating diseases.

The core concept of gene therapy is simple: a gene is introduced to compensate for a defective endogenous gene to induce a desired response. This idea was suggested as early as 1968 by researchers performing a plant cell experiment.[1] With its increasing popularity in the early 1990s, gene therapy was heralded as a means toward the development of potential cures for numerous diseases. However, after nearly 40 years of experiments and clinical trials, much remains to be learned. Indeed, a widely publicized and scrutinized clinical trial resulted in the death of a young patient,[2] and some patients in the clinical trial who were once believed to be "cured" have recently begun to exhibit previously unknown side effects.[3]

The immune system has posed some of the primary obstacles hindering the success of gene therapy; it is ironic that the system designed to protect people from disease or infection can also preclude efficient applications of gene therapy. One major obstacle is the immunogenicity of the vectors, the vehicles used for gene delivery. The transient effects of the transgene, the packaged gene used to achieve therapeutic effects, can be problematic.[4] The immunogenicity of the vectors is usually problematic only during applications involving viral vectors, but such vectors are still the most popular means of transgene delivery because of their high efficiency. Researchers may attenuate or even circumvent difficulties associated with the use of viral vectors by choosing a different vector or mode of transduction, the term for gene delivery. The transient effect of transgenes is a less publicized albeit important issue that is a genuine theoretical and practical concern. However, because a transgene typically is selected on the basis of its therapeutic potential, and because no other proteins may convey the same desired effects, switching to a different transgene may not be ideal.

Despite numerous setbacks in the field of gene therapy, there is still a promising future for the use of gene therapy in orthopaedic surgery because the treatment of many of the clinical diseases encountered by orthopaedic surgeons requires only transient expression of a therapeutic transgene to achieve the desired tissue repair. For example, healing may begin in a nonunion if bone morphogenetic proteins (BMPs) are delivered to initiate the osteoinductive pathway.[5] Muscle injuries may heal faster and more completely if scar

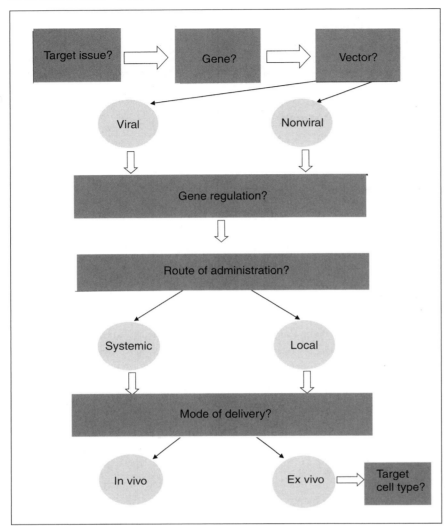

Figure 1 The steps in designing a gene therapy experiment.

formation is minimized.[6] Enhanced ligamentization may extend the life of anterior cruciate ligament (ACL) reconstructions.[7] With additional research and advances, perhaps these successes can be extended to other applications and eventually to those chronic diseases whose treatment requires transgene expression of longer duration.

Pursuit of Gene Therapy

Gene therapy is an extension of the traditional protein therapy in which therapeutic proteins are delivered to attain a desired effect. However, the delivered proteins are usually metabolized shortly after administration. Therefore, the dosage required for effective treatment may be extremely expensive or toxic, or its administration may require multiple surgeries or other invasive efforts. An example is the recent United States Food and Drug Administration approval of the concomitant use of recombinant BMP-2, a collagen sponge, and a titanium cage to treat anterior lumbar interbody fusion. The amount of protein required in humans was sig-

nificantly more than expected when compared with animal studies. Similar findings were noted in a clinical trial focused on posterolateral lumbar spine fusion in humans.[8] Specifically, the amounts of protein required to achieve fusion were 4 to 10 times higher in humans than in rodents, which made the process cost-prohibitive as a treatment of multilevel spine fusions.[9] Gene therapy has the theoretical advantage of incorporating the desired gene directly into the targeted cells and, by so doing, enables more specific targeting, has more enduring results, and achieves more successful treatment of chronic diseases. Several steps are involved in designing a gene therapy experiment (Figure 1).

Experimental Design: Definitions and Strategies
Target

It may be easy to identify the injured or diseased organ, but deciding on a target cell can be surprisingly difficult. Somatic gene therapy and germ line gene therapy are the two broad subsets of gene therapy. Somatic gene therapy targets the nonreproductive cells in the body; any alterations or manipulations are lost when the cells die. Either the injured organ itself can be targeted directly or an immature stem cell population can be isolated, engineered to express a transgene, and then transferred back into the injury site. Such choices may be necessary because some cells are not amenable to certain forms of gene therapy in vivo. For example, skeletal muscle cells are postmitotic, which prevents retroviruses from integration because transduction requires proliferation. Skeletal muscle cells also are surrounded by basal lamina, which precludes all but the adeno-associated virus from penetration

Table 1
Growth Factors in Orthopaedic Surgery

	Skeletal Muscle	Articular Structures	Meniscus	Ligament or Tendon	Bone
Insulin-like growth factor-1[32-34,132-148]	+	+	NA	+	+
Basic fibroblast growth factor[32-34,82,135,140,141,149-156]	+	+	+	+	+
Nerve growth factor[32-34,157,158]	+	NA	NA	NA	NA
Platelet-derived growth factor[82,90,159-162]	+	NA	+	+	±
Endothelial growth factor[82,140,141,144,163-165]	NA	+	+	NA	−
Transforming growth factor-β[33,81,124,141-142,149,166-168]	−	+	+	NA	
BMP-2[5,7,95,142,169-174]	NA	+	NA	+	+
BMP-4[175,176]	NA	NA	NA	NA	+
BMP-7[177,178] (osteogenic protein-1)	NA	NA	NA	NA	+
Vascular endothelial growth factor[36,179,180]	+	NA	NA	NA	±
DEcoRIn[86,166]	+	NA	NA	−	NA
Hepatocyte growth factor[83]	NA	NA	+	NA	NA

Some important growth factors in orthopaedic surgery and their net effects on various tissues of the musculoskeletal system. +, positive effect; −, negative effect; ±, neutral or equivocal; BMP, bone morphogenetic protein; NA = not applicable

and transduction of mature muscle fibers.[10]

Germ line gene therapy targets gamete cells (sperm or egg cells) such that the manipulation will be passed on to the patient's progeny. Because germ line gene therapy raises obvious ethical concerns, and no clinical trial to date has involved germ line gene therapy, the topic is beyond the scope of this chapter.

Gene

After deciding which tissue or organ is the intended target of therapy, choosing the candidate gene is perhaps the most important decision in gene therapy. Over the past 5 years, innumerable recombinant proteins have been shown to have at least some effect on targeted tissues. However, a gene or protein that has a desired or beneficial effect on one target tissue will not necessarily have the same effect on another. For instance, transforming growth factor (TGF)-β is important for cartilage development and regeneration.[11] However, TGF-β also appears to promote fibrosis during regeneration of skeletal muscle, leading to incompletion of the healing process.[12] Thus, it is important to carefully consider which gene to deliver and how this gene might affect the surrounding microenvironment. Table 1 summarizes the effects of many popular transgenes used in orthopaedic gene therapy. Not all transgenes are necessarily designed to be therapeutic; some are simply markers to judge transduction success or follow the fate of the engineered cells.

Vector

There are two broad categories of vectors used to deliver a gene to the targeted cells. Viral vectors dominate most of the experimental and clinical trials focused on gene therapy because their use results in the highest rates of transduction and in persistent transgene expression. Nonviral vectors, which are used infrequently, are less immunogenic but result in less efficient transduction and more transient transgene expression. Table 2 highlights the salient features of each vector used thus far in orthopaedic surgery-related research.

Promoter and Gene Regulation

After choosing the target cells, the gene of interest, and the vector, concern can be turned to the regulation of the desired gene's expression. Transient gene expression is desired in most instances, as oncologic transformation might occur in response to the expression of a particular growth factor at high levels for an indefinite length of time. Gene expression can be regulated by altering sequences upstream of the protein sequence at the promoter region.

The promoters most commonly used in gene therapy are those that activate viral genes, such as the cytome-

Table 2
Viral and Nonviral Vectors Used in Gene Therapy for the Musculoskeletal System

Vector	Description	Capacity	Advantages	Disadvantages
Viral				
Adenovirus	Infects many cell types (dividing and nondividing cells) Inserted gene remains episomal	8 kb (replication defective capacity[181]) 35 kb(helper-dependent capacity)	Large capacity Easy to manufacture	Highly immunogenic. DNA remains episomal and can be lost with time.
AAV	Infects both dividing and nondividing cells Not known to cause any disease in humans Replication competent AAV is inserted into chromosome 19	4 to 5.2 kb	Considered safest of the viral vectors Wildtype virus can integrate into host cell's genome, but most recombinant AAV used in research is replication-defective	Difficult to manufacture Small capacity Most need helper virus to infect noninjured and nondividing cells
Herpes simplex virus	Infects both dividing and nondividing cells Latency in neuronal cells	30 to 40 kb (replication defective capacity) 150 kb (amplicon capacity[181])	Highly infective Large capacity	Cytotoxic Immunogenic
Moloney murine leukemia virus/oncoretrovirus (retrovirus)	Inserted gene is randomly incorporated into host cell's genome Infects dividing cells only	8 kb	Can integrate into host cell's genome Low immunogenicity	Concern of lymphoma and other insertional mutagenesis.
Nonviral				
Lentivirus (retrovirus)	Can integrate with host cell's genome Infects dividing and non-dividing cells	8 kb	Can integrate into host cell's genome Low immunogenicity	Concerns over HIV derivation or relation Concern of insertional mutagenesis
Naked DNA	Naked DNA taken up by host cell Naked DNA can be used with a scaffold (GAM) or coupled with a receptor/ligand		Easy to manufacture Nonimmunogenic	Low gene transfer efficiency
Liposomes	Gene delivered in a phospholipid vesicle that merges with host cell		Easy to manufacture Nonimmunogenic	Low gene transfer efficiency Transient expression
Biolistics (gene gun)	Particle-coated DNA propelled into cell		Low immunogenicity	Low gene transfer efficiency Technically difficult

AAV = Adeno-associated virus

galovirus promoter. However, the regulation of gene expression when using these viral promoters is relatively difficult. Two classes of regulated promoters are commonly used in gene therapy. The first type is activated upon exposure of the transduced cell to a particular drug such as tetracycline; the promoter becomes inactive upon cessation of the drug treatment. Because the most widely used regulatory transcription systems include the tetracycline-dependent constructs developed by Gossen and Bujard,[13] these promoters are often called "tet-on" and "tet-off" promoters. Other promoters within this class are activated by different drugs[14,15] or by irradiation.[16] A single promoter actually can simultaneously drive both the gene of interest and a reporter gene, such as *lacZ*.[17] However, "leakage" sometimes associated with the activity of such promoters can cause gene regulation to be imperfect.[18]

The second class of promoters involves a more complex system based on DNA recombination. The Cre/loxP system uses the machinery in the bacteriophage P1.[19] Cre recombinase is an enzyme that cleaves DNA between highly specific sequences called loxP sites and recombines the DNA strand around them. When the Cre recombinase is active, the sequence between the loxP sites is cleaved and inactivation results. This system can be used to either activate or inactivate a gene. For instance, placing the gene of interest between the loxP sites and subsequently activating Cre can result in "knockout" of the gene, and thereby provides a way to halt gene expression permanently. Alternatively, it is possible to design constructs containing polyadenylation or stop sequences between the loxP sites. If placed between a promoter and the protein-encoding sequences, the construct would be constitutively silent. However, upon activation of Cre recombinase, the spliced product would place the promoter and the protein sequence in proximity and thus enable transcription. A similar system based on the Flp/FRT system from *Saccharomyces cerevisiae* has also been described.[20]

Two additional methods of gene regulation are emerging as powerful new tools for gene therapy: RNA interference and exon skipping. RNA interference uses either short interfering RNAs (siRNA) or short hairpin RNAs (shRNA), short strands of RNA that come from cleavage of double-stranded RNA that is homologous to the targeted gene. The subsequent products mediate the destruction of the endogenous RNA and result in gene suppression.[21] The second technique, exon skipping, has already been shown to be important in the treatment of muscular dystrophy.[22,23] Exon skipping also uses short RNA sequences, but this technique targets endogenous enhancer sequences and thus prevents specific intron and/or exon splicing. Exon skipping has been shown to convert an out-of-frame mutation into an in-frame mutation and can potentially convert a crippling phenotype into a milder one, such as converting Duchenne muscular dystrophy to Becker muscular dystrophy.[24,25]

Table 3
Comparisons of Modes of Delivery

	In Vivo	Ex Vivo
Administration and timing	Easy to administer; one-step injection	Technically more demanding, as process requires at least three steps (harvest, modification, and reimplantation)
Efficacy	No assurance of efficacy before administration	Can test cells for transduction efficacy as well as monitor safety (tumorigenic behavior) before implantation
Cost	Cheaper	More expensive
Target specificity	Only as specific as injection allows	Can target specific tissues
Target choice	Only as specific as injection allows	Can use a variety of cells for transduction
Vector choice	Limits use of certain subsets (eg, oncoretrovirus)	No limitations on vector choice

Route of Administration
The routes of administration for gene therapy also can be categorized into two broad subsets: systemic and localized. Systemic approaches target all systems, can be administered easily through intravenous access, and can be used to treat multiple sites. However, if the goal is to target specific organs or tissues, the efficacy of systemic therapy is questionable. Furthermore, the use of a systemic approach to target tissues with a poor blood supply, such as the central part of the meniscus or the articular cartilage, may not be effective. In addition, dangerous reactions may ensue after the systemic administration of dosages calculated on the basis of theoretical usefulness.[2] Localized administration into a specific organ is preferable for maximum targeted efficacy. However, the invasive procedures required to access certain sites to perform localized administration may be problematic, especially when repeated administrations are necessary. Localized administration also is implausible for systemic disorders such as muscular dystrophies.

Mode of Delivery
The last step of designing an experiment involves choosing how to deliver the engineered constructs. Again, modes of delivery fall into one of two broad categories: in vivo and ex vivo. In vivo approaches involve delivery of the therapeutic construct into the organism itself, whereas ex vivo approaches involve the initial transduction of the therapeutic gene outside of the organism and subsequent transfer of the transduced cells back into the host. Table 3 presents the primary advantages and disadvantages of both approaches. In short, the in vivo approach offers ease of delivery but poor control of the transduction process. The ex vivo approach offers more ensured transduction of the intended tissue and improved safety but also involves significantly greater cost and effort.

Update on Specific Tissues and Diseases
Skeletal Muscle
Gene therapy to muscle is hindered by two major barriers.[10] First, mature muscle fibers are postmitotic

and thus cannot be transduced by retroviruses such as the Mo-MLV, which only infect actively dividing cells.[26] Second, mature muscle fibers are surrounded by the basal lamina, which limits accessibility to vectors smaller than 40 nm.[27] The first barrier is overcome by targeting skeletal muscle while it is in the immature myoblast stage, during which active cell division takes place and allows the integration of retroviruses into the genome. This approach enables the use of ex vivo or in vivo gene therapy in patients with acute injuries or chronic diseases.[26,28-30] The second barrier can be overcome in two ways. Adeno-associated virus vectors can be successful because they are only 20 nm in size and can effectively penetrate the pores of the basal lamina.[31] It is also possible to fenestrate the basal lamina to allow larger viral vectors to bypass that barrier.[29,30]

Several growth factors, including insulin-like growth factor (IGF)-1, basic fibroblast growth factor, and nerve growth factor, have exhibited the ability to improve muscle healing in vivo after contusion, laceration, or strain.[32-34] When compared with control treatment or in vivo gene therapy with adenovirus-IGF1 (Ad-IGF1) alone, ex vivo gene therapy using muscle cells transduced by Ad-IGF1 has improved muscle healing after laceration.[35] Vascular endothelial growth factor, an angiogenic growth factor, has also been shown to enhance muscle regeneration in vivo.[36] Impeding scar formation during muscle recovery is perhaps equally as important as promoting muscle regeneration.[6] Ironically, TGF-β1, the protein most responsible for scar formation in skeletal muscle, is the same growth factor that is integral to cartilage and ligament healing.[37] This fact illustrates a potential pitfall in systemic gene therapy: a single gene with beneficial effects in one tissue may have deleterious effects in another.

Novel techniques in transcriptional modification, such as exon skipping, may be powerful tools with which to target deadly diseases such as Duchenne muscular dystrophy.[24,25] As previously mentioned, exon skipping involves using short RNA sequences to target specific parts of a gene to affect translation and subsequent processing. This action enables the generation of less truncated and more functional dystrophin than formed by the mutated genes that lead to Duchenne muscular dystrophy. Researchers in multiple laboratories have used variations of this technique to "rescue" large sections of muscles in vivo.[22,38]

Perhaps the most important recent findings are the results from the phase I gene therapy trial for Duchenne and Becker muscular dystrophy.[39] Duchenne muscular dystrophy, the most prevalent form of muscular dystrophy, is caused by errors in expression of the dystrophin gene.[40] This very large gene (14 kb) encodes a 3,685 amino acid protein that stabilizes the muscle cell membrane.[41] Patients with Becker muscular dystrophy also have mutations in dystrophin but exhibit a milder phenotype. This gene therapy trial involved injection of a full-length human dystrophin cDNA plasmid into patients diagnosed with Duchenne or Becker muscular dystrophy. Previous studies performed by using similar vector constructs in animals resulted in successful dystrophin expression for 6 months.[42,43] In this trial of nine patients, the extensor carpi radialis longus muscles were injected with various doses of the plasmid. Biopsy specimens obtained 3 weeks later indicated dystrophin expression in two thirds of the patients, and the procedure was well tolerated by all patients. None developed detectable immune responses against the plasmid or the dystrophin during the 180-day study.[39] Because this trial focused on safety, no definitive conclusions regarding efficacy were drawn. Nevertheless, the addition of Duchenne muscular dystrophy to the list of orthopaedic-related diseases that have been studied in gene therapy trials is an important step for the field.

Muscle-derived cells and muscle-derived stem cells are relatively new and powerful additions to the arsenal of gene therapy. These cells' pluripotency, or ability to differentiate into a variety of tissues, is an attribute that uniquely qualifies them as potential target cells for a variety of gene therapy applications. For instance, muscle-derived stem cells can differentiate into hematopoietic lineages while retaining their myogenic potential.[44] Both muscle-derived cells and muscle-derived stem cells have been used for a variety of orthopaedic applications, including the restoration of dystrophin to defective muscles[45,46] and the promotion of bone healing[47,48] and cartilage repair.[49,50]

Rheumatoid Arthritis

Rheumatoid arthritis (RA) is a chronic and systemic inflammatory disease that affects almost 1% of the world's population. Its most prominent clinical features are chronic synovial inflammation of the distal diarthrodial joints that proceeds to articular cartilage and bone destruction and eventual joint ankylosis. RA is thought to be an autoimmune disease, and several animal models involve induction of this disease with type II collagen or lipopolysaccharide autoantigens.[51] Most gene therapy experiments have focused on the immunologic aspects of RA and have demonstrated the important roles of cytokines such as tumor necrosis factor (TNF)-α,[15,52] interleukin-1 (IL-1),[53-55] and IL-4.[56,57] The importance of other critical immunoregulatory molecules such as Fas ligand have also been demonstrated in the treatment of this disease.[58,59]

RA was the first orthopaedic disease to be treated with human gene therapy.[60,61] The original phase I trial used a retroviral vector encoding the IL-1 receptor antagonist, which had previously been shown to be helpful in alleviating the disease in animal models.[62,63] All nine patients enrolled in the trial had joint disease from the second through fifth metacarpophalangeal (MCP) joints and in at least one other joint. Two MCP joints were injected with IL-1 receptor antagonist-transduced synoviocytes, whereas the other two MCP joints were injected with cells from a control model. All four MCP joints, which were scheduled to be replaced 1 week later, were harvested and analyzed for expression of the transgene. The main focus of this trial was safety, and the patients tolerated the procedures well and have had no adverse reactions to date. A phase II protocol is reportedly in place.[64]

Several authors have described the "contralateral effect" in which therapeutic improvements occur in both treated and nontreated limbs of animals modeling inflammatory arthritis.[65-67] Ghivizzani and associates have illustrated this interesting phenomenon by transducing both soluble IL-1 receptor and soluble TNF receptor into rabbit knees.[65] In addition to observing a synergistic effect between the IL-1 receptor antagonist and anti-TNF therapy, they

also observed beneficial effects in the contralateral, nontreated limbs. Further analysis indicates that the dendritic cell, a specialized antigen-presenting cell, may play an important role in this immunomodulation.[68] Other experiments involving transduction of dendritic cells with IL-4,[69] Fas ligand,[70] and TNF-related apoptosis-inducing ligand[71] have generated results supporting the important roles of these special cells.

Articular Cartilage

Both osteoarthritis and RA result in the loss of articular cartilage. The environment in which chondrocytes reside is aneural, avascular, and sequestered in a dense extracellular matrix. The chondrocytes' nondividing status also contributes to the poor healing and resulting continued degeneration of the articular surface.

Numerous growth factors, particularly TGF-β, are beneficial for articular cartilage healing in vivo. Lee and associates[72] demonstrated that fibroblasts transduced with TGF-β1 can promote healing of cartilage defects after transplantation into rabbit knees. A subsequent experiment showed that these cells are still able to promote cartilage healing within femoral defects even after lethal irradiation of the cells,[73] further promoting safety to hosts.

Researchers recently developed a new technique to augment direct gene therapy for cartilage. Light-activated gene transduction uses ultraviolet light as an adjuvant for recombinant adeno-associated virus transduction in human articular chondrocytes.[74] This technique significantly improves the efficiency of transduction of chondrocytes in the superficial layer and enables the use of a significantly lower multiplicity

of infection or doses of virus to achieve a similar level of transduction. Thus, light-activated gene transduction offers the obvious advantages of lower cost of production and a decreased chance of immune reaction to the vector. The amount of ultraviolet light needed to attain this effect does not appear to induce significant morbidity in vivo.

Because of their pluripotency, progenitor cells and stem cells are also used to heal cartilage defects. Genetically engineered myoblasts have been shown to adhere to various structures in rabbit and mouse joints.[75] In that study, the reporter gene was detected for up to 35 days, signifying promising long-term expression by the cellular vehicle. Muscle cells transduced with IGF-1 were also able to partially restore excised tibial growth plates in rabbits and performed better than either muscle cells transduced with BMP-2 or untreated control cells, as determined by histologic and radiologic parameters.[50] Muscle-derived cells have also been shown to be as effective as chondrocytes in restoring cartilage when transplanted into full-thickness osteochondral defects in animals.[49] The transplanted cells were detectable for 4 weeks and, when examined histologically with microscopy, the repaired tissues in the muscle-derived stem cell and chondrocyte groups were similarly better than those of control groups.

Using a combined tissue engineering and gene therapy approach, Mason and associates[76] cultured periosteal-derived cambium-layer cells in a polyglycolic scaffold after transduction with BMP-7. After transplantation, these cells repaired rabbit osteochondral defects, whereas transplantation of control cells resulted in poor cartilage healing, as assessed macroscopically and microscopically. In a follow-up study, the same cells were transduced with either BMP-7 or sonic hedgehog,[77] a protein that plays a key role in limb formation and differentiation.[78] As opposed to the inferior fibrocartilaginous control cells that formed tissue, the cells transduced with BMP-7 or sonic hedgehog protein repaired osteochondral defects by forming more hyaline-like cartilage.

Meniscus

Even as recently as a few decades ago, some researchers and clinicians viewed the meniscus as an unimportant vestigial structure.[79] Its importance in load distribution in the knee is now realized. Meniscal repairs, especially those involving the central avascular white zone, continue to pose difficulties.

Like articular cartilage, the meniscus has proved challenging to treat via gene therapy. However, proof-of-concept experiments have demonstrated that meniscal gene therapy is possible. Goto and associates[80] used both lapine and canine models to transduce the lacZ marker gene into the meniscus. In vitro, transgene expression persisted for more than 20 weeks, and lacZ expression persisted for 3 to 6 weeks after transplantation in the two animal models. Human menisci were also successfully transfected in vitro. A subsequent study using TGF-β1 demonstrated increased collagen synthesis after the transduction of human and canine meniscal cells,[81] further validating the potential use of this novel technology to accelerate meniscal healing.

Kasemkijwattana and associates[82] examined the effect of various growth factors on meniscal fibrochondrocyte proliferation and collagen deposition in vitro. Among

them, endothelial growth factor, TGF-α, basic fibroblast growth factor, and platelet-derived growth factor-AB were identified as candidate molecules for improving meniscal healing. Direct injection of adenovirus encoding β-galactosidase or ex vivo gene therapy using lacZ-expressing myoblasts led to gene expression for up to 6 weeks. These findings demonstrate the feasibility of using this technology to deliver targeted therapeutic genes.

Another study, performed by Hidaka and associates[83] demonstrated that hepatocyte growth factor might also be useful in the treatment of meniscal injuries. Bovine meniscal cells were transduced with lacZ or hepatocyte growth factor while grown on polyglycolic acid felt scaffolds. Expression of both transgenes was detectable for several weeks. The meniscal cells transduced with hepatocyte growth factor had formed significantly more blood vessels at both 2 and 8 weeks than the nontransduced cells. This combined application of tissue engineering and gene therapy suggests that healing of white zone meniscal tears may one day be possible.

Ligaments and Tendons

Although some ligaments and tendons are able to undergo self-repair, there are two major problems with the repaired tissue. First, a significant portion of the healed tissue is replaced by scar tissue, which is biomechanically inferior to noninjured tissue. Healed ligaments have lower load-to-failure strength and more creep than noninjured ligaments. Healed tendons have shown a similar trend but also have exhibited inferior crosslink formation.[84] Second, adhesions can arise from the scar tissue. Inhibited range of motion can be particularly deleterious

in areas such as the flexor tendons of the hand.[85]

Martinek and associates[7] have performed key studies focused on ligament repair. They demonstrated that the administration of an adenoviral construct encoding BMP-2 during ACL reconstruction enhanced the integration of semitendinosus tendon grafts with bone. In control specimens, the insertion site resembled Sharpey fibers. However, specimens treated with the adenoviral BMP-2 construct developed a broad transition zone of bone to mineralized cartilage to nonmineralized fibrocartilage, which resembled the insertion of a normal ACL. These histologic data were corroborated by biomechanical testing that revealed superior stiffness and a higher load-to-failure strength in the BMP-2-treated constructs.

Nakamura and associates[86] demonstrated that antisense dEcoRIn can also be a useful agent for ligament repair. The treatment of injured ligaments with antisense dEcoRIn oligodeoxynucleotides resulted in larger collagen fibrils, increased pullout strength, and decreased creep. However, additional microarray analysis performed by the same group of researchers demonstrated that the injections affected multiple genes, a finding that suggests that this treatment results in complex interactions among more proteins than originally expected.[87]

Recent research has demonstrated that three molecules play important roles in tendon healing. Focal adhesion kinase, a protein implicated in inducing scar formation, has been demonstrated to increase the amount of adhesions in a chicken tendon sheath model.[88] The same research group also demonstrated that BMP-12 cannot only induce soft tissue to form tendon-

and ligament-like structures but also increase the amount of in vitro collagen I production by tenocytes transduced with an adenoviral vector.[89] In vivo data also showed greater strength of repaired tendons treated with adenoviral BMP-12 and compared with controls. Several research groups also have shown that platelet-derived growth factor-B can increase angiogenesis and promote tendon healing in various environments.[90-92]

Bone Healing

Because most facets of orthopaedic surgery involve bone healing, strides made in this area could have tremendous impact in various orthopaedic subspecialties. The study of gene therapy in bone began with Urist's discovery of BMPs in 1965; his description of these novel growth factors launched a completely new area of research.[93]

BMPs delivered by gene therapy are the first proteins to improve the outcome of fracture healing. Early experiments with BMP-2 unequivocally showed bone formation in many instances, but they also revealed complications associated with the immune system's reaction to first-generation adenoviral vectors, reactions that resulted in decreased gene expression and reduced efficacy after subsequent injections.[94-97] Immunosuppression of the animals increased the bone-forming potential of the constructs.[97,98] To avoid the complications associated with immune reactions, researchers began using nonviral vectors that demonstrated early success when used to deliver BMP-4 and parathyroid hormone.[99,100] More recently, researchers have used BMP-7 to induce bone formation in various animal models.[101,102] In one experiment,

skin fibroblasts were transduced with BMP-7 and used to promote bone formation.[103] However, using fibroblasts for such applications may be problematic because fibrous tissue, which is predominant in nonunion sites, can inhibit bone formation.[104]

Stem cells are being used with increasing frequency in the area of bone healing. Stem cells from a plethora of sources, including bone marrow[105] and fat,[106] have been shown to enhance fracture healing. Even without further engineering, these stem cells have demonstrated the ability to heal critical-sized defects in various models.[105,107] When transduced with the genes for osteoinductive factors, stem cells used for such applications yield even better outcomes. BMP-2-engineered mesenchymal stem cells have been used to heal critical defects in the femur,[108] whereas BMP-2-, BMP-4-, and vascular endothelial growth factor-expressing muscle-derived stem cells have been demonstrated to promote the healing of calvarial defects.[5,47,48] Mesenchymal stem cells containing inducible BMP-2 constructs[109] and muscle-derived stem cells containing inducible BMP-4 constructs[110] have also achieved bone formation. Furthermore, periosteal cells transduced with BMP-7 have been shown to repair rabbit calvarial defects,[111] and adipose stem cells transduced with adenoviral BMP-2 have been shown to form bone and cartilage.[112,113]

Spine Fusion

Spine fusion is one of the most common procedures performed in orthopaedic surgery, with an estimated 250,000 procedures performed annually. However, the rate of pseudarthrosis resulting from such fusions ranges from 30% to

40% and may be even higher with multilevel fusions and revisions.[9,114]

The possible therapeutic effects of members of the BMP family have been tested in various animal models of spine fusion. However, the first attempt at gene therapy for spine fusion used a portion of the gene encoding parathyroid hormone.[99] BMP-2 gene therapy was later shown to induce bone formation in the spines of different animal models.[115,116] Although the initial work did not result in solid fusions, it formed the basis for subsequent research that led to the induction of solid fusions.[117] Gene therapy based on adenoviral transduction with BMP-9 was also able to induce solid fusions.[118]

Stem cell-based gene therapy has also been tested in preclinical models of spine fusion. Wang and associates[117] demonstrated successful induction of spine fusion by rat bone marrow cells transduced with adenoviral BMP-2 and placed in rat spine. In two separate experiments, Riew and associates[115,119] demonstrated that BMP-2-transduced mesenchymal stem cells can induce fusion in rabbits and pigs; the researchers successfully used a minimally invasive thorascopic technique in the pigs. BMP-9-transduced mesenchymal stem cells also induced spinal fusion in rats.[120] Similarly, bone marrow and bone marrow-derived cells, both transduced with an adenoviral construct containing LIM mineralization protein-1, a novel transcription factor, induced spine fusion in both rats and rabbits.[121,122]

Intervertebral Disk

Low back pain is one of the most common reasons for medical office visits. A significant portion of people who report this ailment have degenerative disk disease. The intervertebral disk, similar to cartilage, is a relatively avascular structure surrounded by abundant extracellular matrix, including the anulus fibrosus. This structure also contributes to the relatively immunoprivileged status of the disks. Although the exact etiology and pathophysiology of degenerative disk disease remain unclear, loss of proteoglycan content, especially aggrecan, is believed to be a primary contributor to the degradation of the disks' biomechanical properties.[123]

Several experiments have shown that TGF-β can be useful in disk repair. Thompson and associates[124] reported increased proteoglycan production in canine disks treated with TGF-β. Subsequent studies by Nishida and associates[125,126] demonstrated the efficient TGF-β transduction of disk cells in vivo; the transgene expression persisted for up to 12 weeks in rabbits, and proteoglycan synthesis increased by 100%. Combination therapy with TGF-β, BMP-2, and IGF-1 also appears to significantly increase proteoglycan synthesis in a dose-dependent manner while minimizing vector exposure.[123] LIM mineralization protein-1 has recently been shown to increase the production of proteoglycans and the levels of BMP-2 and BMP-7 in rabbit models.[127] A novel study by Wallach and associates[128] have shown that inhibiting matrix degradation by transduction with tissue inhibitor of metalloproteinase significantly increased proteoglycan production in human nucleus pulposus cultures. This finding has important ramifications with regards to targeting both the anabolic and catabolic aspects of degenerative disk disease.

Although the central nervous system was previously viewed as a relatively immunoprivileged site, the ex-act reason for this characteristic remains unclear. Several molecules are thought to mediate this immunoprivileged status, but the system's complexity is magnified because proteins such as Fas ligand can play dual roles in the central nervous system.[129,130] Given the sensitive nature of the spine, preliminary animal studies assessing safety have been performed by researchers using adenoviral vectors with *lacZ*, TGF-β, and BMP-2 transgene constructs.[131] To demonstrate the effects of ectopic gene therapy injections and overdosing in the degenerative spine model, these injections were administered to the epidural space. Within standard doses for disk therapy, injections into the epidural space did not cause significant deleterious sequelae. However, when the doses of gene therapy were increased 100-fold, paralysis and systemic illnesses were observed, particularly in rabbits injected with Ad-TGFβ and Ad-BMP2 constructs. This finding suggests that although standard therapeutic doses may tolerate some degree of misplacement in terms of safety, further increases in vector dose will also significantly decrease the margin for error. The results also indicate that the central nervous system might not be as immunoprivileged as was once believed. The immunologic responses to particular transgenes in the central nervous system warrant further attention.

Summary

There has been significant progress in the study of gene therapy in orthopaedics. It is anticipated that clinical trials of gene therapy for diverse orthopaedic applications will be forthcoming. Although the ultimate goal of gene therapy is to provide cures for lethal pathologies such as orthopaedic malignancies, advances in the study of tissue repair are also important. It is crucial to remember that extreme caution must be exercised in these endeavors because even minor risks are unacceptable for treating nonlethal diseases. With recent advances in tissue engineering and an ever-increasing understanding of stem cell biology, the future of gene therapy in orthopaedic surgery is bright and promising.

References

1. Rogers S, Pfuderer P: Use of viruses as carriers of added genetic information. *Nature* 1968;219:749-751.

2. Raper SE, Chirmule N, Lee FS, et al: Fatal systemic inflammatory response syndrome in a ornithine transcarbamylase deficient patient following adenoviral gene transfer. *Mol Genet Metab* 2003;80:148-158.

3. Hacein-Bey-Abina S, von Kalle C, Schmidt M, et al: A serious adverse event after successful gene therapy for X-linked severe combined immunodeficiency. *N Engl J Med* 2003;348:255-256.

4. Hackett NR, Kaminsky SM, Sondhi D, Crystal RG: Antivector and antitransgene host responses in gene therapy. *Curr Opin Mol Ther* 2000;2:376-382.

5. Lee JY, Musgrave D, Pelinkovic D, et al: Effect of bone morphogenetic protein-2-expressing muscle-derived cells on healing of critical-sized bone defects in mice. *J Bone Joint Surg Am* 2001;83-A:1032-1039.

6. Huard J, Li Y, Fu FH: Muscle injuries and repair: Current trends in research. *J Bone Joint Surg Am* 2002;84-A:822-832.

7. Martinek V, Latterman C, Usas A, et al: Enhancement of tendon-bone integration of anterior cruciate ligament grafts with bone morphogenetic protein-2 gene transfer: A histological and biomechanical study. *J Bone Joint Surg Am* 2002;84-A:1123-1131.

8. Boden SD, Kang J, Sandhu H, Heller JG: Use of recombinant human bone morphogenetic protein-2 to achieve posterolateral lumbar spine fusion in humans: A prospective, randomized clinical pilot trial. *Spine* 2002;27:2662-2673.

9. Yoon ST, Boden SD: Spine fusion by gene therapy. *Gene Ther* 2004;11:360-367.

10. Cao B, Mytinger JR, Huard J: Adenovirus mediated gene transfer to skeletal muscle. *Microsc Res Tech* 2002;58:45-51.

11. O'Keefe RJ, Puzas JE, Brand JS, Rosier RN: Effects of transforming growth factor-beta on matrix synthesis by chick growth plate chondrocytes. *Endocrinology* 1988;122:2953-2961.

12. Li Y, Huard J: Differentiation of muscle-derived cells into myofibroblasts in injured skeletal muscle. *Am J Pathol* 2002;161:895-907.

13. Gossen M, Bujard H: Tight control of gene expression in mammalian cells by tetracycline-responsive promoters. *Proc Natl Acad Sci USA* 1992;89:5547-5551.

14. van der Kraan PM, van de Loo FA, van den Berg WB: Role of gene therapy in tissue engineering procedures in rheumatology: The use of animal models. *Biomaterials* 2004;25:1497-1504.

15. Gould DJ, Bright C, Chernajovsky Y: Inhibition of established collagen-induced arthritis with a tumour necrosis factor-alpha inhibitor expressed from a self-contained doxycycline regulated plasmid. *Arthritis Res Ther* 2004;6:R103-R113.

16. Hallahan DE, Mauceri HJ, Seung LP, et al: Spatial and temporal control of gene therapy using ionizing radiation. *Nat Med* 1995;1:786-791.

17. Lewandoski M: Conditional control of gene expression in the mouse. *Nat Rev Genet* 2001;2:743-755.

18. Blesch A, Conner JM, Tuszynski MH: Modulation of neuronal survival and axonal growth in vivo by tetracycline-regulated neurotrophin expression. *Gene Ther* 2001;8:954-960.

19. Sauer B, Henderson N: Cre-stimulated recombination at loxP-containing DNA sequences placed into the mammalian genome. *Nucleic Acids Res* 1989;17:147-161.

20. O'Gorman S, Fox DT, Wahl GM: Recombinase-mediated gene activation and site-specific integration in mammalian cells. *Science* 1991;251:1351-1355.

21. Elbashir SM, Harborth J, Lendeckel W, Yalcin A, Weber K, Tuschl T: Duplexes of 21-nucleotide RNAs mediate RNA interference in cultured mammalian cells. *Nature* 2001;411:494-498.

22. Goyenvalle A, Vulin A, Fougerousse F, et al: Rescue of dystrophic muscle through U7 snRNA-mediated exon skipping. *Science* 2004;306:1796-1799.

23. Surono A, Van Khanh T, Takeshima Y, et al: Chimeric RNA/ethylene-bridged nucleic acids promote dystrophin expression in myocytes of Duchenne muscular dystrophy by inducing skipping of the nonsense mutation-encoding exon. *Hum Gene Ther* 2004;15:749-757.

24. Aartsma-Rus A, Janson AA, Kaman WE, et al: Therapeutic antisense-induced exon skipping in cultured muscle cells from six different DMD patients. *Hum Mol Genet* 2003;12:907-914.

25. De Angelis FG, Sthandier O, Berarducci B, et al: Chimeric snRNA molecules carrying antisense sequences against the splice junctions of exon 51 of the dystrophin pre-mRNA induce exon skipping and restoration of a dystrophin synthesis in Delta 48-50 DMD cells. *Proc Natl Acad Sci USA* 2002;99:9456-9461.

26. Dunckley MG, Love DR, Davies KE, Walsh FS, Morris GE, Dickson G: Retroviral-mediated transfer of a dystrophin minigene into mdx mouse myoblasts in vitro. *FEBS Lett* 1992;296:128-134.

27. Yurchenco PD: Assembly of basement membranes. *Ann N Y Acad Sci* 1990;580:195-213.

28. Dunckley MG, Wells DJ, Walsh FS, Dickson G: Direct retroviral-mediated transfer of a dystrophin minigene into mdx mouse muscle in vivo. *Hum Mol Genet* 1993;2:717-723.

29. van Deutekom JC, Floyd SS, Booth DK, et al: Implications of maturation for viral gene delivery to skeletal muscle. *Neuromuscul Disord* 1998;8:135-148.

30. van Deutekom JC, Hoffman EP, Huard J: Muscle maturation: Implications for gene therapy. *Mol Med Today* 1998;4:214-220.

31. Pruchnic R, Cao B, Peterson ZQ, et al: The use of adeno-associated virus to circumvent the maturation-dependent viral transduction of muscle fibers. *Hum Gene Ther* 2000;11:521-536.

32. Kasemkijwattana C, Menetrey J, Somogyl G, et al: Development of approaches to improve the healing following muscle contusion. *Cell Transplant* 1998;7:585-598.

33. Kasemkijwattana C, Menetrey J, Bosch P, et al: Use of growth factors to improve muscle healing after strain injury. *Clin Orthop Relat Res* 2000;370:272-285.

34. Menetrey J, Kasemkijwattana C, Day CS, et al: Growth factors improve muscle healing in vivo. *J Bone Joint Surg Br* 2000;82:131-137.

35. Lee CW, Fukushima K, Usas A, et al: Biological intervention based on cell and gene therapy to improve muscle healing after laceration. *J Musculo Res* 2000;4:265-277.

36. Arsic N, Zacchigna S, Zentilin L, et al: Vascular endothelial growth factor stimulates skeletal muscle regeneration in vivo. *Mol Ther* 2004;10:844-854.

37. Li Y, Foster W, Deasy BM, et al: Transforming growth factor-beta1 induces the differentiation of myogenic cells into fibrotic cells in injured skeletal muscle: A key event in muscle fibrogenesis. *Am J Pathol* 2004;164:1007-1019.

38. Lu QL, Rabinowitz A, Chen YC, et al: Systemic delivery of antisense oligoribonucleotide restores dystrophin expression in body-wide skeletal muscles. *Proc Natl Acad Sci USA* 2005;102:198-203.

39. Romero NB, Braun S, Benveniste O, et al: Phase I study of dystrophin plasmid-based gene therapy in Duchenne/Becker muscular dystrophy. *Hum Gene Ther* 2004;15:1065-1076.

40. Hoffman EP, Brown RH Jr, Kunkel LM: Dystrophin: The protein product of the Duchenne muscular dystrophy locus. *Cell* 1987;51:919-928.

41. Selkirk SM: Gene therapy in clinical medicine. *Postgrad Med J* 2004;80:560-570.

42. Zhang G, Ludtke JJ, Thioudellet C, et al: Intraarterial delivery of naked plasmid DNA expressing full-length mouse dystrophin in the mdx mouse model of duchenne muscular dystrophy. *Hum Gene Ther* 2004;15:770-782.

43. Liang KW, Nishikawa M, Liu F, Sun B, Ye Q, Huang L: Restoration of dystrophin expression in mdx mice by intravascular injection of naked DNA containing full-length dystrophin cDNA. *Gene Ther* 2004;11:901-908.

44. Cao B, Zheng B, Jankowski RJ, et al: Muscle stem cells differentiate into haematopoietic lineages but retain myogenic potential. *Nat Cell Biol* 2003;5:640-646.

45. Ikezawa M, Cao B, Qu Z, et al: Dystrophin delivery in dystrophin-deficient DMDmdx skeletal muscle by isogenic muscle-derived stem cell transplantation. *Hum Gene Ther* 2003;14:1535-1546.

46. Gussoni E, Soneoka Y, Strickland CD, et al: Dystrophin expression in the mdx mouse restored by stem cell transplantation. *Nature* 1999;401:390-394.

47. Peng H, Wright V, Usas A, et al: Synergistic enhancement of bone formation and healing by stem cell-expressed VEGF and bone morphogenetic protein-4. *J Clin Invest* 2002;110:751-759.

48. Wright V, Peng H, Usas A, et al: BMP4-expressing muscle-derived stem cells differentiate into osteogenic lineage and improve bone healing in immunocompetent mice. *Mol Ther* 2002;6:169-178.

49. Adachi N, Sato K, Usas A, et al: Muscle derived, cell based ex vivo gene therapy for treatment of full thickness articular cartilage defects. *J Rheumatol* 2002;29:1920-1930.

50. Lee CW, Martinek V, Usas A, et al: Muscle-based gene therapy and tissue engineering for treatment of growth plate injuries. *J Pediatr Orthop* 2002;22:565-572.

51. Firestein GS: The T cell cometh: interplay between adaptive immunity and cytokine networks in rheumatoid arthritis. *J Clin Invest* 2004;114:471-474.

52. Zhang HG, Xie J, Yang P, et al: Adeno-associated virus production of soluble tumor necrosis factor receptor neutralizes tumor necrosis factor alpha and reduces arthritis. *Hum Gene Ther* 2000;11:2431-2442.

53. Fontana A, Hengartner H, Weber E, Fehr K, Grob PJ, Cohen G: Interleukin 1 activity in the synovial fluid of patients with rheumatoid arthritis. *Rheumatol Int* 1982;2:49-53.

54. Horai R, Saijo S, Tanioka H, et al: Development of chronic inflammatory arthropathy resembling rheumatoid arthritis in interleukin 1 receptor antagonist-deficient mice. *J Exp Med* 2000;191:313-320.

55. Evans CH, Ghivizzani SC, Robbins PD: Blocking cytokines with genes. *J Leukoc Biol* 1998;64:55-61.

56. Lubberts E, Joosten LA, Chabaud M, et al: IL-4 gene therapy for collagen arthritis suppresses synovial IL-17 and osteoprotegerin ligand and prevents bone erosion. *J Clin Invest* 2000;105:1697-1710.

57. Boissier MC, Bessis N: Therapeutic gene transfer for rheumatoid arthritis. *Reumatismo* 2004; 56(suppl 1)51-61.

58. Zhang H, Yang Y, Horton JL, et al: Amelioration of collagen-induced arthritis by CD95 (Apo-1/Fas)-ligand gene transfer. *J Clin Invest* 1997;100:1951-1957.

59. Okamoto K, Asahara H, Kobayashi T, et al: Induction of apoptosis in the rheumatoid synovium by Fas ligand gene transfer. *Gene Ther* 1998;5:331-338.

60. Kang R, Ghivizzani SC, Muzzonigro TS, Herndon JH, Robbins PD, Evans CH: Orthopaedic applications of gene therapy: From concept to clinic. *Clin Orthop Relat Res* 2000;375:324-337.

61. Evans CH, Robbins PD, Ghivizzani SC, et al: Clinical trial to assess the safety, feasibility, and efficacy of transferring a potentially anti-arthritic cytokine gene to human joints with rheumatoid arthritis. *Hum Gene Ther* 1996;7:1261-1280.

62. Wooley PH, Whalen JD, Chapman DL, et al: The effect of an interleukin-1 receptor antagonist protein on type II collagen-induced arthritis and antigen-induced arthritis in mice. *Arthritis Rheum* 1993;36:1305-1314.

63. Schwab JH, Anderle SK, Brown RR, Dalldorf FG, Thompson RC: Pro- and anti-inflammatory roles of interleukin-1 in recurrence of bacterial cell wall-induced arthritis in rats. *Infect Immun* 1991;59:4436-4442.

64. Evans CH, Ghivizzani SC, Robbins PD: Orthopaedic gene therapy. *Clin Orthop Relat Res* 2004;429:316-329.

65. Ghivizzani SC, Lechman ER, Kang R, et al: Direct adenovirus-mediated gene transfer of interleukin 1 and tumor necrosis factor alpha soluble receptors to rabbit knees with experimental arthritis has local and distal anti-arthritic effects. *Proc Natl Acad Sci USA* 1998;95:4613-4618.

66. Boyle DL, Nguyen KH, Zhuang S, et al: Intra-articular IL-4 gene therapy in arthritis: Anti-inflammatory effect and enhanced th2activity. *Gene Ther* 1999;6:1911-1918.

67. Chan JM, Villarreal G, Jin WW, Stepan T, Burstein H, Wahl SM: Intraarticular gene transfer of TNFR:Fc suppresses experimental arthritis with reduced systemic distribution of the gene product. *Mol Ther* 2002;6:727-736.

68. Whalen JD, Thomson AW, Lu L, Robbins PD, Evans CH: Viral IL-10 gene transfer inhibits DTH responses to soluble antigens: Evidence for involvement of genetically modified dendritic cells and macrophages. *Mol Ther* 2001;4:543-550.

69. Kim SH, Kim S, Evans CH, Ghivizzani SC, Oligino T, Robbins PD: Effective treatment of established murine collagen-induced arthritis by systemic administration of dendritic cells genetically modified to express IL-4. *J Immunol* 2001;166: 3499-3505.

70. Kim SH, Kim S, Oligino TJ, Robbins PD: Effective treatment of established mouse collagen-induced arthritis by systemic administration of dendritic cells genetically modified to express FasL. *Mol Ther* 2002;6:584-590.

71. Liu Z, Xu X, Hsu HC, et al: CII-DC-AdTRAIL cell gene therapy inhibits infiltration of CII-reactive T cells and CII-induced arthritis. *J Clin Invest* 2003;112:1332-1341.

72. Lee KH, Song SU, Hwang TS, et al: Regeneration of hyaline cartilage by cell-mediated gene therapy using transforming growth factor beta 1-producing fibroblasts. *Hum Gene Ther* 2001;12:1805-1813.

73. Song SU, Hong YJ, Oh IS, et al: Regeneration of hyaline articular cartilage with irradiated transforming growth factor beta1-producing fibroblasts. *Tissue Eng* 2004;10:665-672.

74. Ulrich-Vinther M, Maloney MD, Goater JJ, et al: Light-activated gene transduction enhances adeno-associated virus vector-mediated gene expression in human articular chondrocytes. *Arthritis Rheum* 2002;46:2095-2104.

75. Day CS, Kasemkijwattana C, Menetrey J, et al: Myoblast-mediated gene transfer to the joint. *J Orthop Res* 1997;15:894-903.

76. Mason JM, Grande DA, Barcia M, Grant R, Pergolizzi RG, Breitbart AS: Expression of human bone morphogenic protein 7 in primary rabbit periosteal cells: Potential utility in gene therapy for osteochondral repair. *Gene Ther* 1998;5:1098-1104.

77. Grande DA, Mason J, Light E, Dines D: Stem cells as platforms for delivery of genes to enhance cartilage repair. *J Bone Joint Surg Am* 2003;85-A(suppl 2):111-116.

78. Borycki AG, Brunk B, Tajbakhsh S, Buckingham M, Chiang C, Emerson CP Jr: Sonic hedgehog controls epaxial muscle determination through Myf5 activation. *Development* 1999;126:4053-4063.

79. McCarty EC, Marx RG, DeHaven KE: Meniscus repair: Considerations in treatment and update of clinical results. *Clin Orthop Relat Res* 2002;402:122-134.

80. Goto H, Shuler FD, Lamsam C, et al: Transfer of lacZ marker gene to the meniscus. *J Bone Joint Surg Am* 1999;81:918-925.

81. Goto H, Shuler FD, Niyibizi C, Fu FH, Robbins PD, Evans CH: Gene therapy for meniscal injury: Enhanced synthesis

of proteoglycan and collagen by meniscal cells transduced with a TGFbeta(1)gene. *Osteoarthritis Cartilage* 2000;8:266-271.

82. Kasemkijwattana C, Menetrey J, Goto H, Niyibizi C, Fu FH, Huard J: The use of growth factors, gene therapy and tissue engineering to improve meniscal healing. *Mater Sci Eng C* 2000;13:19-28.

83. Hidaka C, Ibarra C, Hannafin JA, et al: Formation of vascularized meniscal tissue by combining gene therapy with tissue engineering. *Tissue Eng* 2002;8:93-105.

84. Hildebrand KA, Frank CB, Hart DA: Gene intervention in ligament and tendon: Current status, challenges, future directions. *Gene Ther* 2004;11:368-378.

85. Beredjiklian PK: Biologic aspects of flexor tendon laceration and repair. *J Bone Joint Surg Am* 2003;85-A:539-550.

86. Nakamura N, Hart DA, Boorman RS, et al: Decorin antisense gene therapy improves functional healing of early rabbit ligament scar with enhanced collagen fibrillogenesis in vivo. *J Orthop Res* 2000;18:517-523.

87. Hart DA, Nakamura N, Marchuk L, et al: Complexity of determining cause and effect in vivo after antisense gene therapy. *Clin Orthop Relat Res* 2000;(suppl 379):S242-S251.

88. Lou J, Kubota H, Hotokezaka S, Ludwig FJ, Manske PR: In vivo gene transfer and overexpression of focal adhesion kinase (pp125 FAK) mediated by recombinant adenovirus-induced tendon adhesion formation and epitenon cell change. *J Orthop Res* 1997;15:911-918.

89. Lou J, Tu Y, Burns M, Silva MJ, Manske P: BMP-12 gene transfer augmentation of lacerated tendon repair. *J Orthop Res* 2001;19:1199-1202.

90. Hildebrand KA, Woo SL, Smith DW, et al: The effects of platelet-derived growth factor-BB on healing of the rabbit medial collateral ligament: An in vivo study. *Am J Sports Med* 1998;26:549-554.

91. Nakamura N, Shino K, Natsuume T, et al: Early biological effect of in vivo gene transfer of platelet-derived growth factor (PDGF)-B into healing patellar ligament. *Gene Ther* 1998;5:1165-1170.

92. Wang XT, Liu PY, Tang JB: Tendon healing in vitro: Genetic modification of tenocytes with exogenous PDGF gene and promotion of collagen gene expression. *J Hand Surg [Am]* 2004;29:884-890.

93. Urist MR: Bone: Formation by autoinduction. *Science* 1965;150:893-899.

94. Alden TD, Pittman DD, Hankins GR, et al: In vivo endochondral bone formation using a bone morphogenetic protein 2 adenoviral vector. *Hum Gene Ther* 1999;10:2245-2253.

95. Musgrave DS, Bosch P, Ghivizzani S, Robbins PD, Evans CH, Huard J: Adenovirus-mediated direct gene therapy with bone morphogenetic protein-2 produces bone. *Bone* 1999;24:541-547.

96. Baltzer AW, Lattermann C, Whalen JD, et al: Genetic enhancement of fracture repair: Healing of an experimental segmental defect by adenoviral transfer of the BMP-2 gene. *Gene Ther* 2000;7:734-739.

97. Okubo Y, Bessho K, Fujimura K, Iizuka T, Miyatake SI: Osteoinduction by bone morphogenetic protein-2 via adenoviral vector under transient immunosuppression. *Biochem Biophys Res Commun* 2000;267:382-387.

98. Okubo Y, Bessho K, Fujimura K, Iizuka T, Miyatake SI: In vitro and in vivo studies of a bone morphogenetic protein-2 expressing adenoviral vector. *J Bone Joint Surg Am* 2001;83-A(suppl 1):S99-104.

99. Fang J, Zhu YY, Smiley E, et al: Stimulation of new bone formation by direct transfer of osteogenic plasmid genes. *Proc Natl Acad Sci USA* 1996;93:5753-5758.

100. Bonadio J, Smiley E, Patil P, Goldstein S: Localized, direct plasmid gene delivery in vivo: Prolonged therapy results in reproducible tissue regeneration. *Nat Med* 1999;5:753-759.

101. Franceschi RT, Wang D, Krebsbach PH, Rutherford RB: Gene therapy for bone formation: In vitro and in vivo osteogenic activity of an adenovirus expressing BMP7. *J Cell Biochem* 2000;78:476-486.

102. Krebsbach PH, Gu K, Franceschi RT, Rutherford RB: Gene therapy-directed osteogenesis: BMP-7-transduced human fibroblasts form bone in vivo. *Hum Gene Ther* 2000;11:1201-1210.

103. Rutherford RB, Moalli M, Franceschi RT, Wang D, Gu K, Krebsbach PH: Bone morphogenetic protein-transduced human fibroblasts convert to osteoblasts and form bone in vivo. *Tissue Eng* 2002;8:441-452.

104. Baltzer AW, Lieberman JR: Regional gene therapy to enhance bone repair. *Gene Ther* 2004;11:344-350.

105. Bruder SP, Kurth AA, Shea M, Hayes WC, Jaiswal N, Kadiyala S: Bone

regeneration by implantation of purified, culture-expanded human mesenchymal stem cells. *J Orthop Res* 1998;16:155-162.

106. Zuk PA, Zhu M, Mizuno H, et al: Multilineage cells from human adipose tissue: implications for cell-based therapies. *Tissue Eng* 2001;7:211-228.

107. Bruder SP, Kraus KH, Goldberg VM, Kadiyala S: The effect of implants loaded with autologous mesenchymal stem cells on the healing of canine segmental bone defects. *J Bone Joint Surg Am* 1998;80:985-996.

108. Lieberman JR, Daluiski A, Stevenson S, et al: The effect of regional gene therapy with bone morphogenetic protein-2-producing bone-marrow cells on the repair of segmental femoral defects in rats. *J Bone Joint Surg Am* 1999;81:905-917.

109. Moutsatsos IK, Turgeman G, Zhou S, et al: Exogenously regulated stem cell-mediated gene therapy for bone regeneration. *Mol Ther* 2001;3:449-461.

110. Peng H, Usas A, Gearhart B, Young B, Olshanski A, Huard J: Development of a self-inactivating tet-on retroviral vector expressing bone morphogenetic protein 4 to achieve regulated bone formation. *Mol Ther* 2004;9:885-894.

111. Breitbart AS, Grande DA, Mason JM, Barcia M, James T, Grant RT: Gene-enhanced tissue engineering: Applications for bone healing using cultured periosteal cells transduced retrovirally with the BMP-7 gene. *Ann Plast Surg* 1999;42:488-495.

112. Dragoo JL, Choi JY, Lieberman JR, et al: Bone induction by BMP-2 transduced stem cells derived from human fat. *J Orthop Res* 2003;21:622-629.

113. Dragoo JL, Samimi B, Zhu M, et al: Tissue-engineered cartilage and bone using stem cells from human infrapatellar fat pads. *J Bone Joint Surg Br* 2003;85:740-747.

114. Boden SD: Biology of lumbar spine fusion and use of bone graft substitutes: present, future, and next generation. *Tissue Eng* 2000;6:383-399.

115. Riew KD, Wright NM, Cheng S, Avioli LV, Lou J: Induction of bone formation using a recombinant adenoviral vector carrying the human BMP-2 gene in a rabbit spinal fusion model. *Calcif Tissue Int* 1998;63:357-360.

116. Alden TD, Pittman DD, Beres EJ, et al: Percutaneous spinal fusion using bone morphogenetic protein-2 gene therapy. *J Neurosurg* 1999;90(suppl 1):109-114.

117. Wang JC, Kanim LE, Yoo S, Campbell PA, Berk AJ, Lieberman JR: Effect of regional gene therapy with bone morphogenetic protein-2-producing bone marrow cells on spinal fusion in rats. *J Bone Joint Surg Am* 2003;85-A:905-911.

118. Helm GA, Alden TD, Beres EJ, et al: Use of bone morphogenetic protein-9 gene therapy to induce spinal arthrodesis in the rodent. *J Neurosurg* 2000;92(suppl 2):191-196.

119. Riew KD, Lou J, Wright NM, Cheng SL, Bae KT, Avioli LV: Thoracoscopic intradiscal spine fusion using a minimally invasive gene-therapy technique. *J Bone Joint Surg Am* 2003;85-A:866-871.

120. Dumont RJ, Dayoub H, Li JZ, et al: Ex vivo bone morphogenetic protein-9 gene therapy using human mesenchymal stem cells induces spinal fusion in rodents. *Neurosurgery* 2002;51:1239-1244.

121. Boden SD, Titus L, Hair G, et al: Lumbar spine fusion by local gene therapy with a cDNA encoding a novel osteoinductive protein (LMP-1). *Spine* 1998;23:2486-2492.

122. Viggeswarapu M, Boden SD, Liu Y, et al: Adenoviral delivery of LIM mineralization protein-1 induces new-bone formation in vitro and in vivo. *J Bone Joint Surg Am* 2001;83-A:364-376.

123. Sobajima S, Kim JS, Gilbertson LG, Kang JD: Gene therapy for degenerative disc disease. *Gene Ther* 2004;11:390-401.

124. Thompson JP, Oegema TR Jr, Bradford DS: Stimulation of mature canine intervertebral disc by growth factors. *Spine* 1991;16:253-260.

125. Nishida K, Kang JD, Suh JK, Robbins PD, Evans CH, Gilbertson LG: Adenovirus-mediated gene transfer to nucleus pulposus cells: Implications for the treatment of intervertebral disc degeneration. *Spine* 1998;23:2437-2442.

126. Nishida K, Kang JD, Gilbertson LG, et al: Modulation of the biologic activity of the rabbit intervertebral disc by gene therapy: An in vivo study of adenovirus-mediated transfer of the human trans-forming growth factor beta 1 encoding gene. *Spine* 1999;24:2419-2425.

127. Yoon ST, Park JS, Kim KS, et al: ISSLS prize winner: LMP-1 upregulates inter-vertebral disc cell production of pro-teoglycans and BMPs in vitro and in vivo. *Spine* 2004;29:2603-2611.

128. Wallach CJ, Sobajima S, Watanabe Y, et al: Gene transfer of the catabolic inhibitor TIMP-1 increases measured proteoglycans in cells from degenerated human intervertebral discs. *Spine* 2003;28:2331-2337.

129. Shimer AL, Chadderdon RC, Gilbertson LG, Kang JD: Gene therapy approaches for intervertebral disc degeneration. *Spine* 2004;29:2770-2778.

130. Liu TS, Hilliard B, Samoilova EB, Chen Y: Differential roles of Fas ligand in spontaneous and actively induced autoimmune encephalomyelitis. *Clin Immunol* 2000;95:203-211.

131. Kim JS, Sobajima S, Wallach CJ, et al: A profile of safety: The potential hazards of intradiscal gene therapy, in *Transactions of the 51st Annual Meeting of the Orthopaedic Research Society*. Paper No: 0042. Washington, DC, 2005.

132. Barton-Davis ER, Shoturma DI, Musaro A, Rosenthal N, Sweeney HL: Viral mediated expression of insulin-like growth factor I blocks the aging-related loss of skeletal muscle function. *Proc Natl Acad Sci USA* 1998;95:15603-15607.

133. Baudry A, Lamothe B, Bucchini D, et al: IGF-1 receptor as an alternative receptor for metabolic signaling in insulin receptor-deficient muscle cells. *FEBS Lett* 2001;488:174-178.

134. Herndon DN, Ramzy PI: DebRoy MA, Zheng M, Ferrando AA, Chinkes DL, Barret JP, Wolfe RR, Wolf SE. Muscle protein catabolism after severe burn: Effects of IGF-1/IGFBP-3 treatment. *Ann Surg* 1999;229:713-720.

135. Johnson SE, Allen RE: The effects of bFGF, IGF-I, and TGF-beta on RMo skeletal muscle cell proliferation and differentiation. *Exp Cell Res* 1990;187:250-254.

136. Musaro A, McCullagh K, Paul A, et al: Localized Igf-1 transgene expression sustains hypertrophy and regeneration in senescent skeletal muscle. *Nat Genet* 2001;27:195-200.

137. Renganathan M, Messi ML, Delbono O: Overexpression of IGF-1 exclusively in skeletal muscle prevents age-related decline in the number of dihydropyridine receptors. *J Biol Chem* 1998;273:28845-28851.

138. Ashton IK: A recombinant IGF-1 analogue stimulates [3H]thymidine incorporation in human epiphyseal growth cartilage in vitro. *Bone Miner* 1986;1:211-216.

139. Makower AM, Wroblewski J, Pawlowski A: Effects of IGF-I, rGH, FGF, EGF and NCS on DNA-synthesis, cell proliferation and morphology of chondrocytes isolated from rat rib growth cartilage. *Cell Biol Int Rep* 1989;13:259-270.

140. Makower AM, Wroblewski J, Pawlowski A: Effects of IGF-I, EGF, and FGF on proteoglycans synthesized by fractionated chondrocytes of rat rib growth plate. *Exp Cell Res* 1988;179:498-506.

141. Osborn KD, Trippel SB, Mankin HJ: Growth factor stimulation of adult articular cartilage. *J Orthop Res* 1989;7:35-42.

142. Smith P, Shuler FD, Georgescu HI, et al: Genetic enhancement of matrix synthesis by articular chondrocytes: Comparison of different growth factor genes in the presence and absence of interleukin-1. *Arthritis Rheum* 2000;43:1156-1164.

143. Verschure PJ, van Marle J, Joosten LA, van den Berg WB: Chondrocyte IGF-1 receptor expression and responsiveness to IGF-1 stimulation in mouse articular cartilage during various phases of experimentally induced arthritis. *Ann Rheum Dis* 1995;54:645-653.

144. Hunziker EB, Rosenberg LC: Repair of partial-thickness defects in articular cartilage: Cell recruitment from the synovial membrane. *J Bone Joint Surg Am* 1996;78:721-733.

145. Nixon AJ, Fortier LA, Williams J, Mohammed H: Enhanced repair of extensive articular defects by insulin-like growth factor-I-laden fibrin composites. *J Orthop Res* 1999;17:475-487.

146. Lynch SE, Williams RC, Polson AM, et al: A combination of platelet-derived and insulin-like growth factors enhances periodontal regeneration. *J Clin Periodontol* 1989;16:545-548.

147. Lynch SE, de Castilla GR, Williams RC, et al: The effects of short-term application of a combination of platelet-derived and insulin-like growth factors on periodontal wound healing. *J Periodontol* 1991;62:458-467.

148. Isgaard J, Nilsson A, Lindahl A, Jansson JO, Isaksson OG: Effects of local administration of GH and IGF-1 on longitudinal bone growth in rats. *Am J Physiol* 1986;250(4 Pt 1):E367-E372.

149. Barbero A, Benelli R, Minghelli S, et al: Growth factor supplemented matrigel improves ectopic skeletal muscle

formation: A cell therapy approach. *J Cell Physiol* 2001;186:183-192.

150. Cuevas P, Burgos J, Baird A: Basic fibroblast growth factor (FGF) promotes cartilage repair in vivo. *Biochem Biophys Res Commun* 1988;156:611-618.

151. Schofield JN, Wolpert L: Effect of TGF-beta 1, TGF-beta 2, and bFGF on chick cartilage and muscle cell differentiation. *Exp Cell Res* 1990;191:144-148.

152. Sah RL, Chen AC, Grodzinsky AJ, Trippel SB: Differential effects of bFGF and IGF-I on matrix metabolism in calf and adult bovine cartilage explants. *Arch Biochem Biophys* 1994;308:137-147.

153. Fukui N, Katsuragawa Y, Sakai H, Oda H, Nakamura K: Effect of local application of basic fibroblast growth factor on ligament healing in rabbits. *Rev Rhum Engl Ed* 1998;65:406-414.

154. Kobayashi D, Kurosaka M, Yoshiya S, Mizuno K: Effect of basic fibroblast growth factor on the healing of defects in the canine anterior cruciate ligament. *Knee Surg Sports Traumatol Arthrosc* 1997;5:189-194.

155. Nagai H, Tsukuda R, Mayahara H: Effects of basic fibroblast growth factor (bFGF) on bone formation in growing rats. *Bone* 1995;16:367-373.

156. Wiltfang J, Merten HA, Wiltfang J: Ectopic bone formation with the help of growth factor bFGF. *J Craniomaxillofac Surg* 1996;24:300-304.

157. Rende M, Brizi E, Conner J, et al: Nerve growth factor (NGF) influences differentiation and proliferation of myogenic cells in vitro via TrKA. *Int J Dev Neurosci* 2000;18:869-885.

158. Capsoni S, Ruberti F, Di Daniel E, Cattaneo A: Muscular dystrophy in adult and aged anti-NGF transgenic mice resembles an inclusion body myopathy. *J Neurosci Res* 2000;59:553-560.

159. Yablonka-Reuveni Z, Balestreri TM, Bowen-Pope DF: Regulation of proliferation and differentiation of myoblasts derived from adult mouse skeletal muscle by specific isoforms of PDGF. *J Cell Biol* 1990;111:1623-1629.

160. Letson AK, Dahners LE: The effect of combinations of growth factors on ligament healing. *Clin Orthop Relat Res* 1994;308:207-212.

161. Horner A, Bord S, Kemp P, Grainger D, Compston JE: Distribution of platelet-derived growth factor (PDGF) A chain mRNA, protein, and PDGF-alpha receptor in rapidly forming human bone. *Bone* 1996;19:353-362.

162. Zhang Z, Chen J, Jin D: Platelet-derived growth factor (PDGF)-BB stimulates osteoclastic bone resorption directly: The role of receptor beta. *Biochem Biophys Res Commun* 1998;251:190-194.

163. Nonaka K, Shum L, Takahashi I, et al: Convergence of the BMP and EGF signaling pathways on Smad1 in the regulation of chondrogenesis. *Int J Dev Biol* 1999;43:795-807.

164. Bernier SM, Goltzman D: Effect of protein and steroidal osteotropic agents on differentiation and epidermal growth factor-mediated growth of the CFK1 osseous cell line. *J Cell Physiol* 1992;152:317-327.

165. van der Zee E, Jansen I, Hoeben K, Beertsen W, Everts V: EGF and IL-1 alpha modulate the release of collagenase, gelatinase and TIMP-1 as well as the release of calcium by rabbit calvarial bone explants. *J Periodontal Res* 1998;33:65-72.

166. Fukushima K, Badlani N, Usas A, Riano F, Fu F, Huard J: The use of an antifibrosis agent to improve muscle recovery after laceration. *Am J Sports Med* 2001;29:394-402.

167. Shuler FD, Georgescu HI, Niyibizi C, et al: Increased matrix synthesis following adenoviral transfer of a transforming growth factor beta1 gene into articular chondrocytes. *J Orthop Res* 2000;18:585-592.

168. Hunziker EB, Driesang IM, Morris EA: Chondrogenesis in cartilage repair is induced by members of the transforming growth factor-beta superfamily. *Clin Orthop Relat Res* 2001;(suppl 391):S171-S181.

169. Sellers RS, Peluso D, Morris EA: The effect of recombinant human bone morphogenetic protein-2 (rhBMP-2) on the healing of full-thickness defects of articular cartilage. *J Bone Joint Surg Am* 1997;79:1452-1463.

170. Sellers RS, Zhang R, Glasson SS, et al: Repair of articular cartilage defects one year after treatment with recombinant human bone morphogenetic protein-2 (rhBMP-2). *J Bone Joint Surg Am* 2000;82:151-160.

171. Erickson DM, Harris SE, Dean DD, et al: Recombinant bone morphogenetic protein (BMP)-2 regulates costochondral growth plate chondrocytes and induces expression of BMP-2 and BMP-4 in a cell maturation-dependent manner. *J Orthop Res* 1997;15:371-380.

172. Yamaguchi A, Ishizuya T, Kintou N, et al: Effects of BMP-2, BMP-4, and BMP-6 on osteoblastic differentiation of bone marrow-derived stromal cell lines, ST2 and MC3T3-G2/PA6. *Biochem Biophys Res Commun* 1996;220:366-371.

173. Lieberman JR, Le LQ, Wu L, et al: Regional gene therapy with a BMP-2-producing murine stromal cell line induces heterotopic and orthotopic bone formation in rodents. *J Orthop Res* 1998;16:330-339.

174. Boden SD, Zdeblick TA, Sandhu HS, Heim SE: The use of rhBMP-2 in interbody fusion cages. Definitive evidence of osteoinduction in humans: A preliminary report. *Spine* 2000;25:376-381.

175. Li G, Berven S, Simpson H, Triffitt JT: Expression of BMP-4 mRNA during distraction osteogenesis in rabbits. *Acta Orthop Scand* 1998;69:420-425.

176. Watanabe Y, Le Douarin NM: A role for BMP-4 in the development of subcutaneous cartilage. *Mech Dev* 1996;57:69-78.

177. Cook SD, Dalton JE, Tan EH, Whitecloud TS III, Rueger DC: In vivo evaluation of recombinant human osteogenic protein (rhOP-1) implants as a bone graft substitute for spinal fusions. *Spine* 1994;19:1655-1663.

178. Cook SD, Salkeld SL, Brinker MR, Wolfe MW, Rueger DC: Use of an osteoinductive biomaterial (rhOP-1) in healing large segmental bone defects. *J Orthop Trauma* 1998;12:407-412.

179. Gerber HP, Vu TH, Ryan AM, Kowalski J, Werb Z, Ferrara N: VEGF couples hypertrophic cartilage remodeling, ossification and angiogenesis during endochondral bone formation. *Nat Med* 1999;5:623-628.

180. Nakagawa M, Kaneda T, Arakawa T, et al: Vascular endothelial growth factor (VEGF) directly enhances osteoclastic bone resorption and survival of mature osteoclasts. *FEBS Lett* 2000;473:161-164.

181. Thomas CE, Ehrhardt A, Kay MA: Progress and problems with the use of viral vectors for gene therapy. *Nat Rev Genet* 2003;4:346-358.

Optimization of Walking Ability of Children With Cerebral Palsy

Jon R. Davids, MD
Sylvia Õunpuu, MSc
Peter A. DeLuca, MD
Roy B. Davis III, PhD, PE

Abstract

A new paradigm based on an appreciation of the biomechanics of normal and pathologic gait and a better understanding of muscle-tendon unit anatomy and physiology has emerged for orthopaedic clinical decision making to optimize the ambulatory abilities of children with cerebral palsy. This quantitative, biomechanically based approach has been accepted as a research and teaching tool and as an instrument of outcome assessment; however, controversy remains concerning the expense of using this approach and about its accuracy and repeatability.

This paradigm is used within a diagnostic matrix consisting of five data sources. Members of the clinical and technical teams from the motion analysis laboratory intrepret data from the clinical history, physical examination, diagnostic imaging, quantitative gait analysis, and examination under anesthesia. The certainty of intervention selection is proportional to the consistency of the data within the diagnostic matrix. When inconsistencies in the data exist, input from both the clinical and technical teams is needed to resolve discrepancies.

Working within the framework of the diagnostic matrix, it is possible to identify the indications used in the selection and recommendation of musculoskeletal surgical interventions to optimize gait in children with cerebral palsy. It is important to examine indications and controversies for surgical intervention related to iliopsoas recession, femoral rotational osteotomy, medial hamstring lengthening, rectus femoris transfer, and gastrocnemius recession.

In the past 15 years, a new paradigm has emerged for orthopaedic clinical decision making to optimize the walking ability of children with cerebral palsy. This paradigm is based on the biomechanics of normal gait, pathologic gait, and gait disruptions associated with distinct clinical disease processes as well as on a greater understanding of the anatomy and physiology of the muscle-tendon unit and the importance of skeletal alignment.[1]

Normal gait has been studied, and with current technology we are now able to quantitatively measure the normal movements associated with gait (kinematics) and to objectively assess the principal applied moments acting about the joints (kinetics) during the gait cycle.[1,2] This information, coupled with the electrical potentials generated by individual muscles during the gait cycle (dynamic electromyography), has documented the maturation of normal gait in children and led to the development of age-matched normal profiles for walking.[3]

Careful quantitative analysis of pathologic gait and gait disruption associated with a variety of clinical disease processes has led to the development of classification schemes for gait deviations and to the recognition of common pathologic gait patterns.[2-10] It has become clear that the pathomechanics of various gait deviations are often disease-specific, and therefore

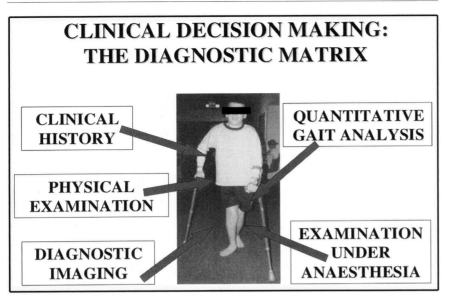

Figure 1 The diagnostic matrix.

the underlying causes and appropriate treatments of similar gait deviations in children with poliomyelitis, cerebral palsy, myelodysplasia, or a spinal cord injury are distinct.[11]

Investigation of the anatomy and physiology of the muscle-tendon unit has revealed numerous variables that can influence the unit's ability to generate a moment about a joint during the gait cycle. These variables include aspects of myoarchitecture such as muscle mass, fiber length, and pennation angle, which are used to determine the physiologic cross-sectional area, a value that is a predictor of the maximum force that can be generated by the muscle-tendon unit.[12-21] Skeletal alignment affects the function of the muscle-tendon unit because the ability of a muscle to generate a moment (moment = force × distance) is related to the distance from the joint center about which the force is applied.[1,12,22-24] Skeletal malalignment generally shortens the available lever arm, placing the muscle-tendon unit at a biomechanical disadvantage and compromising its

ability to generate an optimal moment.

This quantitative, biomechanically based approach has been accepted as a research and teaching tool and as an instrument of outcome assessment. The clinical orthopaedic community has not fully embraced this new paradigm, and its role in clinical decision making remains controversial, with critics expressing concerns about expense and about accuracy and repeatability.[11,25-28] The goals of this review are to: (1) describe this new paradigm and its application to orthopaedic clinical decision making for children with cerebral palsy and (2) present the current indications for the most common orthopaedic operations performed to optimize the walking ability of children with cerebral palsy.

Clinical Decision Making

Orthopaedic clinical decision making to optimize the walking ability of children with cerebral palsy should be based on five sources of information (Figure 1).

Clinical History

The clinical history is obtained by reviewing the patient's medical record and interviewing the child and his or her care providers. The medical history identifies associated medical problems and all previous treatments. The social history assesses the family dynamics and support resources required to undertake the arduous rehabilitation that is required after musculoskeletal surgery. A functional assessment of both the cognitive and the motor neurodevelopment is performed. Finally, the child's and care providers' perceived functional problems and goals for interventions to improve gait should be identified.

Physical Examination

The physical examination begins with observing the patient's gait. This should be done in a systematic fashion in two planes. The ranges of motion of all major joints from the pelvis to the foot are measured. The accuracy and repeatability of these measurements are improved by using standardized techniques of limb-segment manipulation and using a goniometer and an angle guide.[29-33] Skeletal alignment in the transverse, coronal, and sagittal planes is assessed in a similar systematic fashion. A neurologic examination is performed to identify any deficits of selective control of muscle activation, muscle strength, and balance.

Diagnostic Imaging

Diagnostic imaging is used to better assess skeletal alignment. It is most valuable for evaluation of the foot and ankle and for assessment of the alignment of the lower extremity in the coronal and sagittal planes. It is best to make these radiographs while the patient is standing. Common patterns of malalignment of the foot and ankle include ankle valgus, pes equinus, pes planovalgus, and pes equinovarus.[1,7] Rotational malalignments, which are common in the femur and tibia, cannot be evaluated well on plain radiographs. The value of CT in the assessment of rotational malalignment of the femur and tibia is more controversial.[34] Concerns about the accuracy of this measurement technique are related to the difficulty in defining and determining the axis of the proximal part of the femur, the femoral neck, and the femoral head.

Quantitative Gait Analysis

Quantitative gait analysis uses high-speed motion-picture cameras, retro-reflective markers on the surface of the skin aligned with palpable skeletal landmarks, and force platforms to measure various aspects of gait.

Kinematic data, presented as a waveform, describe the motion occurring simultaneously in three planes. Kinetic data (moments and powers), also presented as a waveform, define the motion occurring about the joints during the gait cycle. Analysis of kinetic data provides a biomechanical basis for the understanding of pathologic gait and helps to provide a rationale for the selection of various orthopaedic, neurosurgical, and orthotic interventions.

Dynamic electromyography documents the timing of individual muscle activation during the gait cycle. Other modalities that may be used include pedobarography (dynamic assessment of foot pressure distribution and progression) and energetics (dynamic assessment of oxygen consumption, reflecting the physiologic costs associated with walking).

Interpretation of these data are improved by understanding the technologies and techniques used to measure movement. Kinematic calculations assume a constant relationship between the skin surface marker and the underlying skeletal landmark.[2,7,35] However, this relationship varies depending on the patient's soft-tissue and bone anatomy. Kinetic data require determination of the relationship between the ground reaction force vector and the joint center. The location of the joint center is estimated from the skin surface markers. The model that is most widely used to make these estimates for the pediatric population is based on the measurement of 25 hip and pelvic radiographs of children of unstated age with presumably normal hip joints.[35] The effects of hip joint pathoanatomy and skin surface-marker motion artifact on kinetic calculations have not been systematically established.[36]

Dynamic electromyography measures the electrical potential generated by a muscle when it is activated. The magnitude of the electrical signal is related to the force being generated by the muscle. This relationship can be determined when the magnitude of that potential can be normalized to that associated with a maximum manual muscle contraction. However, children with cerebral palsy may have impaired selective control of muscle activation, compromising the ability to assess a maximum manual muscle contraction. In such a situation, the dynamic electromyography data can be normalized to the maximum value occurring during the gait cycle, or more commonly presented as a raw signal.[2,37] In this circumstance, the dynamic electromyography data can provide valuable information concerning the timing of muscle activation but cannot indicate relative muscle strength or weakness. An appreciation of these limitations greatly enhances the critical and correct application of the quantitative data to the clinical decision-making process.

Quantitative analysis of normal gait has identified four important components or prerequisites: (1) stability of the limb in stance phase, (2) clearance of the limb in swing phase, (3) effective shifts of the limb from stance to swing and from swing to stance phases, and (4) occurrence of these components in a fashion that promotes maximum efficiency of energy expenditure.

In pathologic gait, these four components are disrupted to varying degrees and in varying combinations. Gait deficits or deviations, as identified by quantitative gait analysis, associated with the pathologic gait of children with cerebral palsy may be classified as primary, secondary, or tertiary.[2,4,7,38] Primary deficits are directly related to the underlying disorder of the central nervous system and include spasticity, impaired balance, and impaired motor control. In general, orthopaedic interventions do not directly address these primary deficits. Secondary deficits or deviations occur as a consequence of growth and development of the musculoskeletal system and are generally sequential and progressive over time. Such deficits result in greater disability as children grow into young adults. Examples include the progression of deformity of muscle-tendon units from completely dynamic deformity (overactivity with no fixed shortening) in early childhood to myostatic deformity (fixed or structural shortening or contracture) seen in later childhood and preadolescence. The same sequential progression is true for skeletal deformities, in which flexible and passively correctable segmental malalignment at the foot and ankle is followed in time by rigid skeletal deformity. Finally, the interpretation of quantitative gait data are facilitated by the recognition of common patterns of pathologic gait of children with cerebral palsy. The most common patterns—jump gait, crouch gait, stiff gait, recurvatum gait, and intoeing or outtoeing gait—have distinct kinematic and kinetic profiles.[2,5,7,9,10,39,40-44]

Examination Under Anesthesia

The clinical assessment of whether a muscle-tendon unit deformity is dynamic or myostatic is best performed when the child is examined under general anesthesia. When the child is awake, the presence of spasticity can limit the distinction between dynamic overactivity and fixed shortening of the muscle-tendon unit. Because spasticity is not present under general anesthesia, any limitation of range of motion is caused by a myostatic deformity (contracture) of the muscle-tendon unit or intra-articular pathology such as adhesions or bone deformity.

The Diagnostic Matrix

Clinical decision making with use of the diagnostic matrix is best performed at an interpretation session attended by clinical and technical members of the motion analysis laboratory team. The certainty of selecting the best intervention is proportional to the consistency of the data within the diagnostic matrix. The selection and results of a specific treatment are optimized when the problems being considered are common and the data from all sources are consistent. It is not possible to be as confident about the selection of intervention or its results when the problems are unusual and the data within the matrix are not consistent. This inconsistency may be a consequence of attempts to classify the continuous

spectrum of a clinical disease process into a categorical framework and/or deficiencies in the technology and techniques of quantitative gait analysis. Sorting out these inconsistencies frequently involves the input of members of both the clinical and the technical team. For example, discrepancies concerning motion about the hip and pelvis between observational gait analysis and quantitative gait analysis are generally resolved by giving greater weight to the quantitative data. This is done because visual assessment of the movement about the hip and pelvis during the gait cycle is difficult and frequently misleading, whereas the accuracy of the kinematic assessment is much greater in all three planes.[24,35,42,45,46] On the other hand, discrepancies among the clinical examination, diagnostic imaging, and quantitative gait analysis data about the foot and ankle should be resolved in favor of the data derived from the clinical examination and diagnostic imaging. The reason for this is that the foot and ankle model used in quantitative gait analysis is simplistic.[35,47-49] For example, ankle dorsiflexion is defined by the relative alignment of the shank and foot axes in the sagittal plane, and the foot axis is defined by a single marker over the forefoot that combines the movements occurring through multiple foot segments into a single measure. With a major skeletal segmental malalignment, such as pes planovalgus, the model overestimates the amount of ankle dorsiflexion occurring during midstance, giving inaccurate kinematic data.

Current Indications for Common Musculoskeletal Surgical Interventions

With use of the diagnostic matrix, it is possible to identify the indications for the selection of specific muscu-

loskeletal surgical interventions to optimize the gait of children with cerebral palsy.

Iliopsoas Recession

Clinical History The most common symptom indicating the need for this procedure is the inability to stand straight and walk with the upper body erect.

Physical Examination A hip flexion contracture (> 30°) is an indication for iliopsoas resection. The patient should be examined in the supine position (Thomas test) and the prone position (Staheli test).[29] The magnitude of a hip flexion contracture is frequently overestimated by these techniques because of the difficulty in stabilizing the pelvis, and the measurements are inconsistent because of variability in pelvic positioning. The current recommendation is to position the pelvis so that the line connecting the anterior-superior and posterior-superior iliac spines is vertical.[50] This technique facilitates more consistent positioning of the pelvis and ensures that the angle measured during the clinical examination is the same as that used in the kinematic model in gait analysis for the calculation of hip motion in the sagittal plane. Observing the child while he or she walks in a high kneel pattern (ie, walks on the knees) removes the influence of tight hamstrings on pelvic alignment (Figure 2). This will unmask any tightness of the hip flexors.

Diagnostic Imaging No imaging studies are required.

Quantitative Gait Analysis With this analysis, which identifies kinematic and kinetic indicators (Figure 3), pelvic motion in the sagittal plane shows an anterior tilt with a "double bump" waveform pattern during stance phase. Hip motion in the sagittal plane shows diminished extension in terminal stance, with a decreased dynamic range throughout the gait cycle. Kinetic analysis of the hip moment in the sagittal plane shows an increased internal extension moment in midstance, with delayed crossover to an internal flexion moment in midstance or terminal stance.

Examination Under Anesthesia This is frequently required to resolve the roles of dynamic and myostatic deformities of the hip flexor muscles.

Management There is considerable controversy concerning the appropriate indications for iliopsoas recession to improve gait in children with cerebral palsy.[40,50-56] A better understanding of the biomechanics of hip, pelvic, and trunk motion is needed to clarify the indications for this procedure in these children. When hip flexion contractures are present, they are seldom an important problem for a child with cerebral palsy who is able to walk. In addition, these contractures are frequently overestimated on clinical examination. The kinematic and kinetic variables identified as indications for this procedure are frequently the consequence of other primary gait deficits, such as weakness of the abdominal and hip extensor muscles and impaired balance and position senses. Similar quantitative profiles may be seen as tertiary or compensatory deviations, such as in a severe crouch gait because of insufficiency of the ankle plantar flexors and overactivity of the knee flexors. These disorders increase hip flexion and possibly anterior pelvic tilt, shifting the body's center of gravity forward relative to the hip center, increasing the external hip flexor moment and delaying the flexor-to-extensor moment crossover in stance phase. Such compensatory gait patterns resolve spontaneously

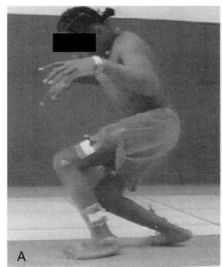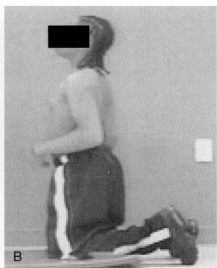

Figure 2 A, Sagittal plane view of a subject walking with a crouch gait pattern. Note the greatly increased hip flexion, anterior pelvic tilt, and anterior trunk tilt. **B,** Sagittal plane view of the same subject performing high kneel walking. Note the greatly improved alignment of the hips, pelvis, and trunk. This improvement suggests that these deviations are compensatory in nature.

following correction of the underlying primary or secondary deficits.

Femoral Rotation Osteotomy
Clinical History Candidates for this procedure or their parents report in-toeing, knee knocking, and tripping.

Physical Examination The patient has increased femoral anteversion, which is best appreciated when he or she is examined in the prone position with the hip in full extension. Hip rotation is abnormal, with increased internal rotation and limited external rotation, indicating increased femoral anteversion.[24,29] The value of another physical examination maneuver, the trochanteric prominence angle test, has recently been shown to be limited by obesity, scarring associated with previous surgery, and variable alignment of the greater trochanter with respect to the axis of the femoral neck.[57,58] Observational gait analysis may reveal internal rotation of the patella relative to the line of progression when the child walks.

This visual assessment is often confounded by increased, asymmetric pelvic rotation during the gait cycle.[24,42]

Diagnostic Imaging CT scans may be used to assess femoral anteversion when the findings of the clinical examination are compromised or confusing. The most widely accepted techniques are done in either two-dimensional or three-dimensional (volumetric reconstruction) formats.[34]

Quantitative Gait Analysis Kinematic data reveal increased internal hip rotation throughout the gait cycle (Figure 4).

Examination Under Anesthesia Anesthesia may be necessary to evaluate a patient with suspected femoral anteversion. Relative internal-external rotation of the hip is tested as described above, and when necessary, the examination can be augmented by the use of fluoroscopy to visualize the alignment of the femoral head and neck.[59]

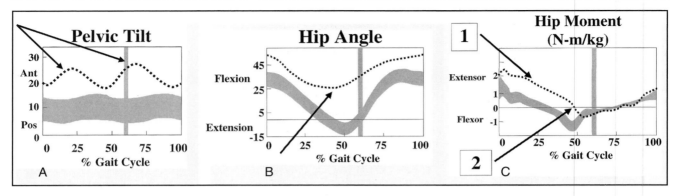

Figure 3 Findings on quantitative gait analysis that serve as indicators for iliopsoas recession at the pelvic brim. The normal ranges of the kinematic and kinetic data for the pelvis and hip are indicated by the gray band on each plot. **A,** Kinematic analysis of pelvic tilt in the sagittal plane. Note the anterior tilt with a "double bump" waveform pattern during stance phase (*arrows*). **B,** Kinematic analysis of hip flexion-extension in the sagittal plane shows diminished extension in terminal stance (*arrow*), with a decreased dynamic range throughout the gait cycle. **C,** Kinetic analysis of hip moment in the sagittal plane shows an increased internal extension moment in midstance (*arrow 1*), with delayed crossover to an internal flexion moment in midstance or terminal stance (*arrow 2*).

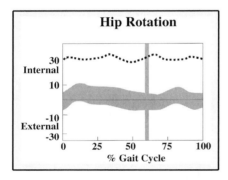

Figure 4 Findings on quantitative gait analysis that serve as indicators for femoral rotation osteotomy. Kinematic analysis of hip rotation in the transverse plane shows increased internal hip rotation throughout the gait cycle. Normal hip motion is indicated by the gray band.

Management There is a relationship between increased femoral anteversion (a static, structural skeletal deformity) and increased internal hip rotation (a dynamic gait deviation). The latter occurs as a compensation to restore the lever arm available for the hip abductor muscles, which is diminished by the former. When both are present, surgical correction of the increased femoral anteversion will result in resolution of the gait deviation and normalization

of hip rotation during walking.[24] Not all children with cerebral palsy and increased femoral anteversion exhibit increased internal hip rotation when walking, and not all children with cerebral palsy and increased internal hip rotation during the gait cycle have increased femoral anteversion.

Medial Hamstring Lengthening
Clinical History The patient or parents may report that the child cannot stand up straight, walks with the knees bent, and has anterior knee pain with fatigue when walking a distance.

Physical Examination Straight-leg raising is limited (< 60°), the popliteal angle is diminished (< 130° when measured within or behind the popliteal space), and there is a spastic response to a fast stretch of the hamstrings.[29]

Diagnostic Imaging Patella alta with elongation and fragmentation of the inferior pole of the patella is frequently seen on lateral radiographs of the knee. These changes are presumably a consequence of

chronic overload of the extensor mechanism as a result of an increased and prolonged external knee flexion moment occurring throughout stance phase.[60]

Quantitative Gait Analysis Kinematic, kinetic, and dynamic electromyography data are useful (Figure 5). Knee motion in the sagittal plane shows increased knee flexion during the loading response, variable knee alignment in midstance and terminal stance, and decreased knee extension in terminal swing. The knee moment in the sagittal plane shows an increased internal extension moment throughout stance phase. Dynamic electromyography shows prolonged activity of the medial hamstrings into midstance.

Examination Under Anesthesia The relative contribution of dynamic and myostatic components of hamstring deformity is determined with this examination. It is best done by measuring the popliteal angle, with direct palpation of both the medial and the lateral hamstrings.

Management The hamstring muscles cross both the hip and the knee joint, and appropriate medial hamstring lengthening will improve knee extension at initial contact and in terminal swing.[6,40,52,54,56,60-63] Increased anterior pelvic tilt is not seen following unilateral or bilateral medial hamstring lengthening.[50,64] Lateral hamstring lengthening is necessary only in teenagers with a severe crouch gait (> 40° of knee flexion in stance) and should otherwise be avoided to minimize the risk of excessive weakness following surgery. Severe hamstring tightness may cause posterior pelvic tilt.[50] In this situation, the increased anterior pelvic tilt that may occur following bilateral medial and lateral hamstring lengthening is not harmful. Knee flexion contractures that exist following hamstring lengthening are best corrected by the use of serial casts in the postoperative period.

Rectus Femoris Transfer

Clinical History The patient or parents report that the child has stiff knees, toe dragging, and tripping.

Physical Examination The patient has a positive prone rectus test (Duncan-Ely test).[1,7,29-31] The child is placed in the prone position with the hips and knees fully extended. The test is considered positive when the pelvis elevates (as a result of hip flexion) as the knee is slowly passively flexed and/or there is a "catch" on rapid passive knee flexion.

Diagnostic Imaging No imaging studies are required.

Quantitative Gait Analysis Kinematic and dynamic electromyographic data are useful (Figure 6). Knee motion in the sagittal plane shows a diminished dynamic range of motion (< 80% of normal), delayed and diminished peak flexion in swing phase, and a blunting of the flexion wave in swing phase. Dynamic electromyography shows an

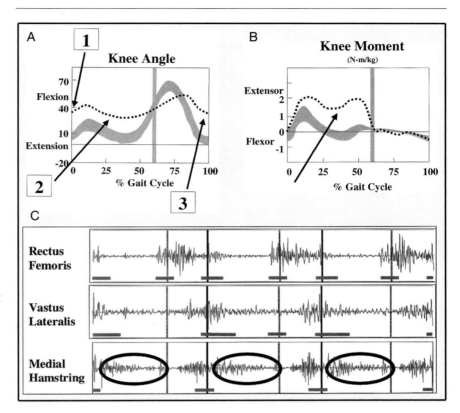

Figure 5 Findings on quantitative gait analysis that serve as indicators for medial hamstring lengthening. The normal ranges of the kinematic and kinetic knee data are indicated by the gray band on each plot. **A,** Kinematic analysis of knee flexion-extension in the sagittal plane shows increased knee flexion on initial contact (*arrow 1*), variable knee alignment in midstance and terminal stance (*arrow 2*), and decreased knee extension in terminal swing (*arrow 3*). **B,** Kinetic analysis of knee moment in the sagittal plane shows an increased internal extension moment throughout stance phase (*arrow*). **C,** Dynamic electromyography of the muscles about the knee over three gait cycles shows prolonged activity of the medial hamstrings into midstance (*circles*).

inappropriate midswing phase of the rectus femoris.[65] Coactivation of the vastus lateralis in midswing may or may not be present and does not seem to affect the outcome of a rectus femoris transfer.[66]

Examination Under Anesthesia No additional information is gained from an examination under anesthesia.

Management Diminished and delayed peak knee flexion in swing phase may be the consequence of decreased velocity and diminished stride length. In addition, a combination of factors occurring during stance phase,

at the stance-to-swing interval, as well as abnormal activity of the rectus femoris in midswing can all contribute to the disruption of knee flexion in swing phase. Currently, the rectus femoris transfer is indicated to maintain or improve the magnitude and timing of peak knee flexion in swing phase when hamstring lengthening is being performed.[6,62,63,66-74] The rectus femoris transfer is best performed at the time of hamstring lengthening, but it may also be done following inappropriate isolated hamstring lengthening that has resulted in a stiff knee gait pattern. Although it is con-

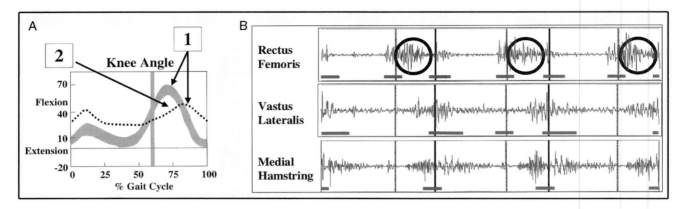

Figure 6 Findings on quantitative gait analysis that serve as indicators for rectus femoris transfer. Normal knee motion is indicated by the gray band on each plot. **A,** Kinematic analysis of knee flexion-extension in the sagittal plane shows a diminished dynamic range of motion (< 80% of normal), delayed and diminished peak flexion in swing phase (*arrow 1*), and a blunting of the flexion wave in swing phase (*arrow 2*). **B,** Dynamic electromyography of the muscles about the knee over three gait cycles shows inappropriate activity of the rectus femoris in the midswing phase (*circles*).

sidered a component of the quadriceps femoris muscle group, the rectus femoris is actually a two-joint muscle (the other three components are single-joint muscles) whose activation timing and functional importance during the gait cycle are distinct from those of the remainder of the quadriceps. For this reason, transfer of the rectus femoris does not compromise knee extensor function in stance phase.[71,72]

Gastrocnemius Lengthening

Clinical History Patients and their families report toe walking, toe dragging, tripping, and intoeing.

Physical Examination The patient has a diminished passive range of ankle dorsiflexion, a sustained spastic response to an applied fast stretch of the gastrocnemius muscle (clonus), and an increased deep tendon reflex at the ankle.[29] It is helpful to consider the foot and ankle as consisting of three segments (hindfoot, midfoot, and forefoot) and two columns (medial and lateral). The alignment of each segment is described relative to the adjacent proximal segment. The three most common patterns of seg-

mental malalignment of the foot and ankle in children with cerebral palsy are equinus (seen most commonly in younger children), planovalgus (seen most commonly in children with spastic diplegia), and equinovarus (seen most commonly in children with spastic hemiplegia).[1,4,7,8,49,75,76] Equinus malalignment consists of plantar flexion deformity of the hindfoot, with the other segments in normal alignment and the columns having an appropriate length. Planovalgus malalignment consists of hindfoot plantar flexion and eversion, midfoot pronation, and forefoot supination. The lateral column is functionally shorter than the medial column. Equinovarus malalignment consists of hindfoot equinus and inversion, midfoot supination, and forefoot pronation. The lateral column is functionally longer than the medial column.

Diagnostic Imaging Weight-bearing plain radiographs of the foot and ankle are routinely used. When malalignment is found on physical examination, it is evaluated further on the radiographs, for structural abnormalities.

Quantitative Gait Analysis Kinematic, kinetic, and dynamic electromyographic data are routinely obtained (Figure 7). Ankle motion in the sagittal plane shows excessive plantar flexion in stance and swing phases. All three ankle rockers in stance phase are disrupted, with an absence of the first (or heel) rocker, flattening or inversion of the second (or ankle) rocker, and a premature, diminished third (or forefoot) rocker. The ankle moment in the sagittal plane shows an absence of the internal dorsiflexion moment in the loading response, an increased internal plantar flexion moment in midstance (the "double bump" pattern), and a decreased internal plantar flexion moment in terminal stance. The ankle power in the sagittal plane shows premature power generation in midstance and diminished power generation in terminal stance. Dynamic electromyography of the gastrocnemius is notable for premature activation of the stance-phase burst, beginning at initial contact or in terminal swing.

Examination Under Anesthesia The relative contributions of the gas-

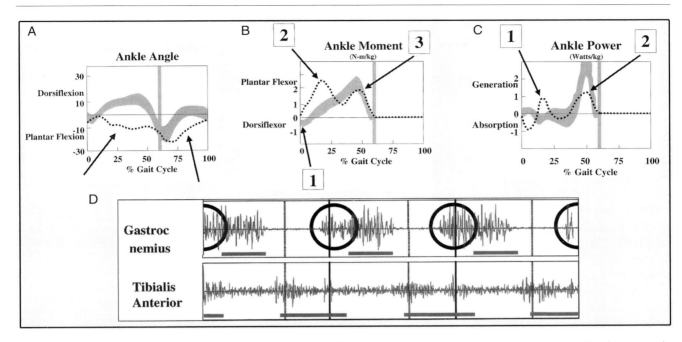

Figure 7 Findings on quantitative gait analysis that serve as indicators for gastrocnemius recession. Normal ankle data are indicated by the gray band on each plot. **A,** Kinematic analysis of ankle plantar flexion-dorsiflexion in the sagittal plane shows excessive plantar flexion in stance and swing phases (*arrows*). **B,** Kinetic analysis of ankle moment in the sagittal plane shows an absence of the internal dorsiflexion moment in the loading response (*arrow 1*), an increased internal plantar flexion moment in midstance (the "double bump" pattern, *arrow 2*), and a decreased internal plantar flexion moment in terminal stance (*arrow 3*). **C,** Analysis of ankle power in the sagittal plane shows premature power generation in midstance (*arrow 1*) and diminished power generation in terminal stance (*arrow 2*). **D,** Dynamic electromyography of the muscles about the ankle over three gait cycles shows premature activation of the gastrocnemius in terminal swing, with premature activity in the loading response (*circles*).

trocnemius and soleus muscles to tightness of the ankle plantar flexors are best determined with an examination under anesthesia. These contributions are assessed by measuring ankle dorsiflexion with the knee flexed (which relaxes the gastrocnemius and allows evaluation of the soleus) and extended (greater reduction in ankle dorsiflexion motion with the knee extended, compared with the motion when the knee is flexed, is attributed to myostatic deformity of the gastrocnemius).[29]

Management Discrepancies between the passive range of motion of the ankle noted on physical examination and the dynamic ankle motion measured during gait may be the consequence of (1) an increased spastic response following the dis-

rupted first rocker, which further limits the dynamic range of motion at the ankle in the second rocker; (2) the fact that the external forces applied about the ankle during gait (particularly in adolescence and the teenage years, primarily as a result of increased body weight) are greater than those that can be applied by the examiner during the clinical assessment; or (3) the fact that foot and ankle segmental alignment during the clinical examination may not be consistent with dynamic foot and ankle segmental alignment during gait (because of variable lever arm alignment). Discrepancies between the findings of observational gait analysis and those of quantitative gait analysis at the foot and ankle may be the result of the assumption that a toe

strike at initial contact, easily appreciated visually, implies increased or excessive ankle plantar flexion. However, increased knee flexion, with neutral ankle alignment, also results in a toe-strike pattern at initial contact.[4,7,49,56,77,78] Quantitative gait analysis (kinematic data) effectively documents the absence or presence of excessive ankle plantar flexion in this situation.

Summary

The acceptance and integration of quantitative gait analysis into clinical decision making for children with cerebral palsy will occur as pediatric orthopaedic surgeons move away from opinion-based practices toward evidence-based medicine.[79] Good clinical practice involves the interpretation of evidence from a variety of sources, with application of the results of population-based studies to the individual patient.[80-82] With technological improvements and greater clinical experience with their applications, issues related to the accuracy and reliability of quantitative gait analysis will be resolved, greatly facilitating the collaboration required for multicenter studies.[27,45] Comprehensive assessment of outcome in multiple domains (technical, functional, patient satisfaction, and cost) will determine the true costs of performing the correct (or incorrect) surgery to improve walking for children with cerebral palsy.[11,25,26,28,83] Utilization of a diagnostic matrix that includes quantitative gait analysis will play a central role in the incorporation of an evidence-based−medicine paradigm for clinical decision making to optimize the walking ability of children with cerebral palsy.

References

1. Chambers HG, Sutherland DH: A practical guide to gait analysis. *J Am Acad Orthop Surg* 2002;10:222-231.

2. Perry J (ed): *Gait Analysis: Normal and Pathological Function.* Thorofare, NJ, Slack Inc, 1992.

3. Sutherland DH, Olshen R, Biden E, Wyatt M (eds): *The Development of Mature Walking.* New York, NY, Cambridge University Press, 1998.

4. Davids JR, Foti T, Dabelstein J, Bagley A: Voluntary (normal) versus obligatory (cerebral palsy) toe-walking in children: A kinematic, kinetic, and electromyographic analysis. *J Pediatr Orthop* 1999;19:461-469.

5. Fabry G, Liu XC, Molenaers G: Gait pattern in patients with spastic diplegic cerebral palsy who underwent staged operations. *J Pediatr Orthop Br* 1999;8:33-38.

6. Gage JR: Surgical treatment of knee dysfunction in cerebral palsy. *Clin Orthop* 1990;253:45-54.

7. Gage JR (ed): *Gait Analysis in Cerebral Palsy.* London, England, Mac Keith Press, 1991.

8. Hullin MG, Robb JE, Loudon IR: Gait patterns in children with hemiplegic spastic cerebral palsy. *J Pediatr Orthop Br* 1996;5:247-251.

9. O'Byrne JM, Jenkinson A, O'Brien TM: Quantitative analysis and classification of gait patterns in cerebral palsy using a three-dimensional motion analyzer. *J Child Neurol* 1998;13:101-108.

10. Õunpuu S, DeLuca PA, Davis RB: Gait analysis, in Neville B, Goodman R (eds): *Congenital Hemiplegia.* London, England, Mac Keith Press, 2000, pp 81-97.

11. Mulder T, Nienhuis B, Pauwels J: Clinical gait analysis in a rehabilitation context: Some controversial issues. *Clin Rehabil* 1998;12:99-106.

12. Delp SL, Zajac FE: Force- and moment-generating capacity of lower-extremity muscles before and after tendon lengthening. *Clin Orthop* 1992;284:247-259.

13. Delp SL, Statler K, Carroll NC: Preserving plantar flexion strength after surgical treatment for contracture of the triceps surae: A computer simulation study. *J Orthop Res* 1995;13:96-104.

14. Lieber RL: Skeletal muscle adaptability: I. Review of basic properties. *Dev Med Child Neurol* 1986;28:390-397.

15. Lieber RL: *Skeletal Muscle Structure, Function and Plasticity: The Physiological Basis of Rehabilitation,* ed 2. Philadelphia, PA, Lippincott Williams & Wilkins, 2002.

16. Moseley CF: Physiologic effects of soft-tissue surgery, in Sussman MD (ed): *The Diplegic Child: Evaluation and Management.* Park Ridge, IL, American Academy of Orthopaedic Surgeons, 1992, pp 259-269.

17. O'Dwyer NJ, Neilson PD, Nash J: Mechanisms of muscle growth related to muscle contracture in cerebral palsy. *Dev Med Child Neurol* 1989;31:543-547.

18. Perry J: Determinants of muscle function in the spastic lower extremity. *Clin Orthop* 1993;288:10-26.

19. Reimers J: Functional changes in the antagonists after lengthening the agonists in cerebral palsy: I. Triceps surae lengthening. *Clin Orthop* 1990;253:30-34.

20. Tardieu C: Huet de la Tour E, Bret MD, Tardieu G: Muscle hypoextensibility in children with cerebral palsy: I. Clinical and experimental observations. *Arch Phys Med Rehabil* 1982;63:97-102.

21. Ziv I, Blackburn N, Rang M, Koreska J: Muscle growth in normal and spastic mice. *Dev Med Child Neurol* 1984;26:94-99.

22. Abel MF, Damiano DL, Pannunzio PI, Bush J: Muscle-tendon surgery in diplegic cerebral palsy: Functional and mechanical changes. *J Pediatr Orthop* 1999;19:366-375.

23. Arnold AS, Delp SL: Rotational moment arms of the medial hamstrings and adductors vary with femoral geometry and limb position: Implications for the treatment of internally rotated gait. *J Biomech* 2001;34:437-447.

24. Ounpuu S, DeLuca P, Davis R, Romness M: Long-term effects of femoral derotation osteotomies: An evaluation using three-dimensional gait analysis. *J Pediatr Orthop* 2002;22:139-145.

25. DeLuca PA, Davis RB III, Õunpuu S, Rose S, Sirkin R: Alterations in surgical decision making in patients with cerebral palsy based on three-dimensional gait analysis. *J Pediatr Orthop* 1997;17:608-614.

26. Morton R: New surgical interventions for cerebral palsy and the place of gait analysis. *Dev Med Child Neurol* 1999;41:424-428.

27. Skaggs DL, Rethlefsen SA, Kay RM, Dennis SW, Reynolds RA, Tolo VT: Variability in gait analysis interpretation. *J Pediatr Orthop* 2000;20:759-764.

28. Watts HG: Editorial: Gait laboratory analysis for preoperative decision making in spastic cerebral palsy: Is it all it's cracked up to be? *J Pediatr Orthop* 1994;14:703-704.

29. Greene WB, Heckman JD (eds): *The Clinical Measurement of Joint Motion* ed 1. Rosemont, IL, American Academy of Orthopaedic Surgeons,1994.

30. Hislop HJ, Montgomery J, Connolly BH, Daniels L (eds): *Daniels and Worthingham's Muscle Testing: Techniques of Manual Examination,* ed 6. Philadelphia, PA, WB Saunders, 1995.

31. Kendall FP, McCreary EK, Provance PG (eds): *Muscles, Testing and Function: With Posture and Pain,* ed 4. Baltimore, MD, Williams & Wilkins, 1993.

32. McDowell BC, Hewitt V, Nurse A, Weston T, Baker R: The variability of goniometric measurements in ambulatory children with spastic cerebral palsy. *Gait Posture* 2000;12:114-121.

33. McMulkin ML, Gulliford JJ, Williamson RV, Ferguson RL: Correlation of static to dynamic measures of lower extremity range of motion in cerebral palsy and control populations. *J Pediatr Orthop*

2000;20:366-369.

34. Davids JR, Marshall AD, Blocker ER, Frick SL, Blackhurst DW, Skewes E: Femoral anteversion in children with cerebral palsy: Assessment with two and three-dimensional computed tomography scans. *J Bone Joint Surg Am* 2003;85:481-488.

35. Davis RB III, Õunpuu S, Tyburski D, Gage JR: A gait analysis data collection and reduction technique. *Hum Mov Sci* 1991;10:575-587.

36. Stagni R, Leardini A, Cappozzo A, Grazia Benedetti M, Cappello A: Effects of hip joint centre mislocation on gait analysis results. *J Biomech* 2000;33:1479-1487.

37. Perry J, Hoffer MM: Preoperative and postoperative dynamic electromyography as an aid in planning tendon transfers in children with cerebral palsy. *J Bone Joint Surg Am* 1977;59:531-537.

38. Gage JR, Õunpuu S: Surgical intervention for the correction of primary and secondary gait abnormalities, in Patla AE (ed): *Adaptability of Human Gait: Implications for the Control of Locomotion.* Amsterdam, Netherlands, North-Holland, 1991, pp 359-385.

39. Davids JR, Foti T, Dabelstein J, Blackhurst DW, Bagley A: Objective assessment of dyskinesia in children with cerebral palsy. *J Pediatr Orthop* 1999;19:211-214.

40. Hoffinger SA, Rab GT, Abou-Ghaida H: Hamstrings in cerebral palsy crouch gait. *J Pediatr Orthop* 1993;13:722-726.

41. Lin CJ, Guo LY, Su FC, Chou YL, Cherng RJ: Common abnormal kinetic patterns of the knee in gait in spastic diplegia of cerebral palsy. *Gait Posture* 2000;11:224-232.

42. Õunpuu S, Thomson JD, Davis RB, DeLuca PA: An examination of the knee function during gait in children with myelomeningocele. *J Pediatr Orthop* 2000;20:629-635.

43. Segal LS, Thomas SE, Mazur JM, Mauterer M: Calcaneal gait in spastic diplegia after heel cord lengthening: A study with gait analysis. *J Pediatr Orthop* 1989;9:697-701.

44. Sutherland DH, Davids JR: Common gait abnormalities of the knee in cerebral palsy. *Clin Orthop* 1993;288:139-147.

45. Gorton GE, Hebert D, Goode B: Assessment of the kinematic variability between 12 Shriners motion analysis laboratories. *Gait Posture* 2001;13:247.

46. Hillman SJ, Hazlewood ME, Loudon IR, Robb JE: Can transverse plane rotations be estimated from video tape gait analysis? *Gait Posture* 1998;8:87-90.

47. Etnyre B, Chambers CS, Scarborough NH, Cain TE: Preoperative and postoperative assessment of surgical intervention for equinus gait in children with cerebral palsy. *J Pediatr Orthop* 1993;13:24-31.

48. Leardini A, Benedetti MG, Catani F, Simoncini L, Giannini S: An anatomically based protocol for the description of foot segment kinematics during gait. *Clin Biomech (Bristol, Avon)* 1999;14:528-536.

49. Steinwender G, Saraph V, Zwick EB, Uitz C, Linhart W: Fixed and dynamic equinus in cerebral palsy: Evaluation of ankle function after multilevel surgery. *J Pediatr Orthop* 2001;21:102-107.

50. DeLuca PA, Õunpuu S, Davis RB, Walsh JH: Effect of hamstring and psoas lengthening on pelvic tilt in patients with spastic diplegic cerebral palsy. *J Pediatr Orthop* 1998;18:712-718.

51. Delp SL, Arnold AS, Speers RA, Moore CA: Hamstrings and psoas lengths during normal and crouch gait: Implications for muscle-tendon surgery. *J Orthop Res* 1996;14:144-151.

52. Nene AV, Evans GA, Patrick JH: Simultaneous multiple operations for spastic diplegia: Outcome and functional assessment of walking in 18 patients. *J Bone Joint Surg Br* 1993;75:488-494.

53. Novacheck TF, Trost JP, Schwartz MH: Intramuscular psoas lengthening improves dynamic hip function in children with cerebral palsy. *J Pediatr Orthop* 2002;22:158-164.

54. Saraph VZ, Zwick EB, Zwick G, Steinwender C, Steinwender G, Linhart W: Multilevel surgery in spastic diplegia: Evaluation by physical examination and gait analysis in 25 children. *J Pediatr Orthop* 2002;22:150-157.

55. Schutte LM, Hayden SW, Gage JR: Lengths of hamstrings and psoas muscles during crouch gait: Effects of femoral anteversion. *J Orthop Res* 1997;15:615-621.

56. Zwick EB, Saraph V, Linhart WE, Steinwender G: Propulsive function during gait in diplegic children: Evaluation after surgery for gait improvement. *J Pediatr Orthop Br* 2001;10:226-233.

57. Davids JR, Benfanti P, Blackhurst DW, Allen BL: Assessment of femoral anteversion in children with cerebral palsy: Accuracy of the trochanteric prominence angle test. *J Pediatr Orthop* 2002;22:173-178.

58. Ruwe PA, Gage JR, Ozonoff MB, DeLuca PA: Clinical determination of femoral anteversion: A comparison with established techniques. *J Bone Joint Surg Am* 1992;74:820-830.

59. Bobroff ED, Chambers HG, Sartoris DJ, Wyatt MP, Sutherland DH: Femoral anteversion and neck-shaft angle in children with cerebral palsy. *Clin Orthop* 1999;364:194-204.

60. Thometz J, Simon S, Rosenthal R: The effect on gait of lengthening of the medial hamstrings in cerebral palsy. *J Bone Joint Surg Am* 1989;71:345-353.

61. Granata KP, Abel MF, Damiano DL: Joint angular velocity in spastic gait and the influence of muscle-tendon lengthening. *J Bone Joint Surg Am* 2000;82:174-186.

62. Hadley N, Chambers C, Scarborough N, Cain T, Rossi D: Knee motion following multiple soft-tissue releases in ambulatory patients with cerebral palsy. *J Pediatr Orthop* 1992;12:324-328.

63. Rethlefsen S, Tolo VT, Reynolds RA, Kay R: Outcome of hamstring lengthening and distal rectus femoris transfer surgery. *J Pediatr Orthop B* 1999;8:75-79.

64. Kay RM, Rethlefsen SA, Skaggs D, Leet A: Outcome of medial versus combined medial and lateral hamstring lengthening surgery in cerebral palsy. *J Pediatr Orthop* 2002;22:169-172.

65. Õunpuu S, DeLuca PA, Bell KJ, Davis RB: Using surface electrodes for the evaluation of the rectus femoris, vastus medialis and vastus lateralis muscles in children with cerebral palsy. *Gait Posture* 1997;5:211-216.

66. Chambers H, Lauer A, Kaufman K, Cardelia JM, Sutherland D: Prediction of outcome after rectus femoris surgery in cerebral palsy: The role of cocontraction of the rectus femoris and vastus lateralis. *J Pediatr Orthop* 1998;18:703-711.

67. Damron TA, Breed AL, Cook T: Diminished knee flexion after hamstring surgery in cerebral palsy patients: Prevalence and severity. *J Pediatr Orthop* 1993;13:188-191.

68. Gage JR, Perry J, Hicks RR, Koop S, Werntz JR: Rectus femoris transfer to improve knee function of children with cerebral palsy. *Dev Med Child Neurol* 1987;29:159-166.

69. Miller F, Cardoso Dias R, Lipton GE, Albarracin JP, Dabney KW, Castagno P: The effect of rectus EMG patterns on the

outcome of rectus femoris transfers. *J Pediatr Orthop* 1997;17:603-607.

70. Nene A, Mayagoitia R, Veltink P: Assessment of rectus femoris function during initial swing phase. *Gait Posture* 1999;9:1-9.

71. Õunpuu S, Muik E, Davis RB III, Gage JR, DeLuca PA: Rectus femoris surgery in children with cerebral palsy: Part I. The effect of rectus femoris transfer location on knee motion. *J Pediatr Orthop* 1993;13:325-330.

72. Õunpuu S, Muik E, Davis RB III, Gage JR, DeLuca PA: Rectus femoris surgery in children with cerebral palsy: Part II. A comparison between the effect of transfer and release of the distal rectus femoris on knee motion. *J Pediatr Orthop* 1993;13:331-335.

73. Perry J: Distal rectus femoris transfer. *Dev Med Child Neurol* 1987;29:153-158.

74. Sutherland DH, Santi M, Abel MF: Treatment of stiff-knee gait in cerebral palsy: A comparison by gait analysis of distal rectus femoris transfer versus proximal rectus release. *J Pediatr Orthop* 1990;10:433-441.

75. Graham HK, Fixsen JA: Lengthening of the calcaneal tendon in spastic hemiplegia by the White slide technique: A long-term review. *J Bone Joint Surg Br* 1988;70:472-475.

76. Olney BW, Williams PF, Menelaus MB: Treatment of spastic equinus by aponeurosis lengthening. *J Pediatr Orthop* 1988;8:422-425.

77. Rose SA, DeLuca PA, Davis RB III, Õunpuu S, Gage JR: Kinematic and kinetic evaluation of the ankle after lengthening of the gastrocnemius fascia in children with cerebral palsy. *J Pediatr Orthop* 1993;13:727-732.

78. Simon SR, Ryan AW: Biomechanical/neurophysiologic factors related to surgical correction of equinus deformity, in Sussman MD (ed): *The Diplegic Child: Evaluation and Management.* Park Ridge, IL, American Academy of Orthopaedic Surgeons, 1992, pp 365-382.

79. Narayanan UG, Wright JG: Editorial: Evidence-based medicine: A prescription to change the culture of pediatric orthopaedics. *J Pediatr Orthop* 2002;22:277-278.

80. Carey TS: Randomized controlled trials in surgery: An essential component of scientific progress. *Spine* 1999;24:2553-2555.

81. Laupacis A, Rorabeck CH, Bourne RB, Feeny D, Tugwell P, Sim DA: Randomized trials in orthopaedics: Why, how, and when? *J Bone Joint Surg Am* 1989;71:535-543.

82. Winter RB: The fallacy of short-term outcomes analysis in pediatric orthopaedics. *J Bone Joint Surg Am* 1999;81:1499-1500.

83. Kay RM, Dennis S, Rethlefsen S, Skaggs DL, Tolo VT: Impact of postoperative gait analysis on orthopaedic care. *Clin Orthop* 2000;374:259-264.

Communication Skills

John R. Tongue, MD
Howard R. Epps, MD
Laura L. Forese, MD, MPH

Abstract

Surveys of American Academy of Orthopaedic Surgeons members and patients indicate that orthopaedic surgeons are "high tech, low touch." According to patients and colleagues surveyed, orthopaedic surgeons are given high ratings by patients and colleagues for their skills in the operating room, but their listening and communication skills can be improved upon; they could listen better and show more empathy for their patients. Communication affects patient satisfaction, adherence to treatment, and physician satisfaction. Communication problems have also been cited as the most common factor in the initiation of malpractice suits. All orthopaedic surgeons can benefit from improving their communication skills.

Orthopaedic surgeons perform one procedure over 100,000 times throughout their careers: the medical interview. Improving skills during these patient interactions and with office staff, surgical teams, and colleagues directly improves patient outcomes, reduces medical errors, and makes the specialty of orthopaedic surgery more enjoyable.[1,2]

Addressing the need to study and improve communications, the American Academy of Orthopaedic Surgeons (AAOS) developed a partnership with the Bayer Institute for Health Care Communication (BIHCC), a nonprofit foundation with 15 years of experience teaching the art behind the science of medicine. The BIHCC has trained more than 90,000 physician participants to engage, empathize, educate, and enlist the patient, a clinical model known as the four Es. The BIHCC has also estab-

lished partnerships with over 100 medical organizations. Whereas the biomedical tasks of finding the problem (diagnosis) and fixing the problem (treatment)—the two Fs—are critical, the BIHCC educational model defines the four Es as equally important communication tasks (Figure 1).

AAOS Communication Skills Mentor Program

The AAOS has combined the BIHCC educational model with jointly developed orthopaedic-specific video vignettes and has trained a select group of 23 orthopaedic surgeons as mentors to serve as facilitators of interactive workshops that teach communication skills. This project is called the AAOS Communication Skills Mentor Program (CSMP). To develop and evaluate the most meaningful curriculum possible, the AAOS

Board of Directors approved a 3-year pilot program that includes training for more than 1,600 orthopaedic surgeons. Mentors have already completed nearly 100 highly rated 4-hour workshops across the country. The initial phase of the program was completed in July 2004. The success of this collaborative effort was recognized by the 2003 Partner Award, which was presented by the BIHCC.

AAOS CSMP workshops are limited to 30 participants to allow interaction for adult learning through a comparison of differences. Discussions of each segment produce relevant and lively conversation because each participant brings considerable experience and knowledge. Each workshop is therefore unique. After completing these workshops, participants have learned specific techniques they can apply immediately in everyday conversations as well as difficult patient situations. Workshops receive overwhelmingly positive evaluation rankings, averaging 3.7 out of 4.0 points.

For orthopaedic surgeons with full waiting rooms and busy surgical schedules, it takes a degree of humility to acknowledge that everyone can improve their communication skills. Because effective communication skills play an important role in achieving successful medical outcomes, an outline for new

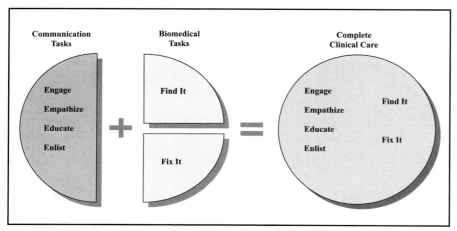

Figure 1 The BIHCC educational model.

orthopaedic patient medical interviews has been developed as have guidelines for communicating unanticipated adverse outcomes and dealing with ethnic and culturally related disparities in health care. (Additional information can be obtained at http://www.aaos.org by scrolling down the Continuing Medical Education (CME) tab and clicking on the Communication Skills Mentoring Program. The AAOS CSMP Website includes valuable outlines and tips sheets, the names and locations of all CSMP mentors, and a current schedule of dates and locations of workshops across the country.)

New Orthopaedic Patient Medical Interviews
The Greeting
Physicians should wear professional attire for new orthopaedic patient medical interviews. Before entering the examination room, it is important that physicians clear their thoughts and smile before knocking and opening the door. Care should be taken to enter the examination room at a deliberate pace so as not to give the impression of being rushed.

Welcoming Statement
The welcoming statement should begin with a greeting (for example, "good morning") as appropriate. Physicians should smile, make eye contact, use a consistent vocal tone, focus attention, and be calm, pleasant, appropriate, and not rushed. The patient should be addressed as Mr. or Ms., and the pronunciation of the patient's name should be checked, if necessary. Physicians should introduce themselves as "Doctor." Even in an emergency department, introductions are important. With the initial introduction, physicians should say "Welcome" or "Good to see you" and combine these statements with a handshake and eye contact.

Physicians should then sit down approximately 2 to 4 feet across from the patient and maintain eye contact at the same level. If the patient continues to look the physician over in an attempt to estimate the physician's pace and the warmth of the initial greeting, the physician should try a simple, normalizing comment such as "How were the roads this afternoon?" or "How do you like this hot/cold/wet weather?" Physicians are cautioned against asking patients "How are you today?" Although this is more of a greeting than a question in the United States, it can put ill or injured patients in the awkward position of responding that they are "fine" just before relating their story and/or medical problem(s). Phy-

sicians should not stand while the patient is seated during the medical interview.

The Patient's Story
Physicians should lean forward, maintain eye contact, smile, and inquire "How can I help you today?"—six simple, powerful, empowering words. Open-ended questions allow the patient the opportunity to define the conversation. Although it is hard to do, physicians should continue to lean forward and wait until the patient finishes speaking. Information should be taken in without trying to organize it. It takes most patients 2 minutes to tell their stories and/or explain why they are seeking medical attention; however, the average physician interrupts the patient within 18 to 23 seconds. At this point in the evolution of managed care, many patients expect to be interrupted or have little time to tell their stories. They may simply respond to open-ended questions with a single sentence answer and stop (for example, "I'm here because my right shoulder hurts"). If this occurs, physicians should respond by saying "Fine. Tell me about it," in which instance patients will typically tell their stories. Most patients who see orthopaedic surgeons have two or more musculoskeletal problems they wish to discuss; knowing all of the patient's problems early helps physicians prioritize the time and negotiate the agenda for the current visit. Physicians should listen to the patient's exact words and key phrases, which can often be repeated later to the patient to demonstrate understanding, listening ability, and caring. Physicians have the opportunity to facilitate the telling of the story with nodding, facial expression, voice inflections, or repetition of a key phrase.

Physicians should avoid asking "What seems to be the problem today?" Patients sometimes react defensively to this question, and they may be thinking "That's what you're supposed to tell me." Physicians should also avoid saying "Tell me about your shoulder pain." Although this statement is open ended, it may convey the impression that the physician is interested in a body part and not the patient. This statement also implies that only one complaint can be discussed.

Once a patient has finished telling his or her story, the next step is to ask questions about it rather than provide an immediate interpretation of the orthopaedic condition. Physicians should be as curious about the person as they are about the presenting medical problem. Care should be taken to resist the urge to jump into an orthopaedic fix-it mode by interrupting with how, what, when, and where questions at this time. Rather than write and listen at the same time, physicians should look at the patient while listening and then write. Additional questions that may be used to probe the patient's story include "I'm curious about...", "Tell me more about...", or "That must have been very painful/frightening/frustrating." It is also helpful to name the patient's expressed or nonverbal emotion and acknowledge stressful situations. Acknowledgment of patient emotions and values by the physician helps patients understand that the physician is someone who values them as individuals, rather than, for example, the sore shoulder in room three. Unfortunately, orthopaedic surgeons rarely use empathic statements for fear of getting into a long discussion or when uncomfortable relating the patient's emotions. Patients will appreciate a physician's empathy and, as a result, typically not tell their life stories. When physicians are uncomfortable relating to the emotions of patients, it is helpful to recall that a little human kindness may make a patient the physician's best advocate.

Negotiating an Agenda
Physicians should reflect on their understanding of the patient's story by summarizing what they have heard. Some of the patient's own words should be repeated, feelings should be normalized, and it may

help the patient's well being to share a story from the physician's own life that relates to the patient's condition.

Physicians should then explain any necessary additional information and/or discuss any diagnostic tests that will be done, taking care to orient patients to these processes and limit the scope of the day's evaluation, if necessary. Orienting statements and offering to reschedule time for complete consideration of secondary complaints shows consideration and respect for the patient. For example, after completing the medical history and initial physical examination, physicians should briefly explain what is next by saying: "With your permission, we can now take x-rays of your shoulder for more information." If the patient agrees, physicians should then say: "Wait here for a few minutes. The technician will take the pictures here in this office. Then I'll show you the films and discuss them with you shortly. Thank you."

Educate
After completing the medical history and physical examination, physicians should ask patients what they know. Physicians should explain their thoughts with clear, direct words that suit the patient's style and values. Analogies and simple drawings should be used to give patients perspective and reduce the chance that they do not understand what physicians are explaining. Because patients normally will forget 50% of what physicians tell them the moment they leave the office, patient information brochures can be effective supplements. Humor is also important, but it can cause misunderstandings and possibly result in patients judging physician behavior as being patronizing or arrogant. Physicians should interact with patients during any discussion to ensure that patients understand what is being explained. This can be done by encouraging questions and discussion by asking: "What questions do you have?" "Is there anything else you

have been wondering about?" Physicians should avoid asking: "Do you have any questions?" with a hurried glance, a low "I sure hope not" tone of voice, or a nod of the head indicating "no."

Physicians should enlist patients as partners. Patients typically have a self-diagnosis; therefore, after presenting a professional opinion, physicians should always ask: "How does this fit with what you've been thinking?" This question can help avoid a great deal of misunderstanding and may reveal that patients have a different agenda or a deep concern that they have been hesitant to share. The treatment regimen should be discussed in simple terms, emphasizing benefits, explaining potential obstacles, and offering a specific time frame. Goals linked to future results should be offered that put patients in control. To improve treatment compliance, physicians should write treatment instructions down and schedule a follow-up appointment to monitor progress. Physicians should then say: "When you return, I'll ask you whether you are better. If so, I'll ask you how much: 10%, 50%, or 90%? So be thinking about this until I see you next time." This positively framed request encourages patients to participate in evaluating their own course of treatment and helps motivate them to be accountable to the treatment program.

Closing
Physicians should conclude by reviewing the diagnosis, treatment, and prognosis. With a sincere, uplifting tone of voice, physicians should say good-bye and, while shaking hands and maintaining eye contact, express an expectation for a positive outcome.[3]

Breaking Bad News: Unanticipated Adverse Outcomes
An adverse outcome is a serious injury or death resulting from medical management rather than from the underlying condition of the patient. Patients and

their families, who experience feelings of fear, isolation, and mistrust from adverse outcomes, often feel that communication of the incident is insensitive and inadequate. Although breaking bad news is always difficult and stressful, a systematic approach can improve the communication process and reduce the overall negative impacts. Honest, timely disclosure of errors strengthens the physician-patient relationship and can reduce the risk of litigation.

Plan to Disclose

Although physicians have been trained to be perfectionists, most have experienced sudden emotional shock—even nausea—after a medical mistake. Immediate feelings of anxiety and defensiveness are normal. Discussing the incident with members of the patient's health care team and other supportive staff members can ease the burden, help prepare an appropriate response, and help determine who should break the news. Immediate family members should be included, and both parents should be present when the patient is a minor. Care should be taken to avoid interruptions by pagers and phone calls. The exact content of the disclosure and the order in which statements will be given should be carefully considered. All pertinent data and test results should be readily available. Physicians should avoid distancing themselves from those who are affected by a bad mistake. Although it is common and instinctive to do so, such reactions lead patients and families to perceive those involved to be arrogant and disinterested.

Dialogue With Patients

Physicians should deliver bad news in person. Sometimes errors can be forgiven when the key issue of caring for the patient is fully addressed. Direct, clear statements are important as well as how those statements are made, particularly the tone of voice used.

Communication in such instances

should be open, compassionate, and timely. Accurate, clear-cut statements should be made, and care should be taken to avoid any defensive explanation of what has happened. Short statements are best, and physicians should frequently pause to ask the patient and/or family members whether they understand what is being said. Overly technical descriptions and vocabulary should be avoided, and emotional responses should be expected and acknowledged. Complex and even severe reactions of fear, anger, mistrust, and hopelessness are common in such instances, to which it is advisable to reply by saying: "You sound very upset with this news." Physicians should apologize when appropriate by saying: "We are sorry this has happened to you." This is an apology, but it is not an admission of liability. Physicians should avoid saying: "We are sorry that we did this to you." The disease, not the doctor, should be the focus. Physicians should keep in mind that because communication is primarily nonverbal the participants in such a meeting should sit together in a quiet, private room. Barriers such as desks and tables should be avoided, and physicians should face the people with whom they are speaking, maintain eye contact, speak with an even tone of voice, and appear calm rather than hurried or irritated. The content of the initial discussion may be less important than how it is said. Physicians should provide ample time for such meetings; and as would typically occur for a difficult emergency surgical procedure, other commitments should be rescheduled to properly organize and address the communication needs of this unexpected event. Physicians should take care to avoid offering opinions regarding possible causes of the adverse event. Criticism by members of the health care team should also be avoided because it may create misunderstandings and detract from the essential goal of caring for the patient.

Emotional Support for Patients

The most common deficiency in daily patient interviews is a failure to demonstrate an empathic response to patients. Although it is difficult to predict the severe emotional reactions of patients and families to adverse outcomes, physicians should prepare for an emotional outpouring of fear, anger, disappointment, and mistrust. Because strong emotions are gradually sorted out before they are expressed, special care should be taken by physicians to tolerate silence as a patient reaction. Physicians should take the time to reflect on and acknowledge those emotions that are expressed, listen carefully for concerns that can be clarified and values that can be confirmed, and offer to listen to other members of the family who were not present during the initial disclosure. Physicians should avoid making defensive comments when confronted by fearful or angry patients. Instead, it is advisable to say: " I understand that you feel very sad and angry in this situation." Concise explanations should be repeated, and the physician's commitment to helping the patient deal with the illness or injury should be emphasized.

Provide Direction

To provide direction for additional treatment, physicians should summarize an explicit, proactive plan for the care and support for the patient, solicit the patient's and/or family's understanding and acceptance of this plan, make a list of tasks and instructions (drawings can also be helpful), avoid delays in the completion of subsequent tests and consultations, review progress of the care plan directly with the patient and/or family, recognize and respect shifting complex emotions as care continues, express hope in each encounter with the patient and/or family, and document discussions and care plans. Physicians should keep in mind that failure to execute the care plan or failure to effectively communicate will cause the patient and/or family to lose trust. Promises must be kept in a timely manner to ensure the primary goal of providing appropriate care for the patient.[4]

Communications—Bridging the Disparities Gap

Nearly 20 years ago, Katz[5] first articulated the premise that effective communication between physicians and patients builds essential mutual trust and facilitates medical decision making. Orthopaedic surgeons currently encounter three communication barriers in the effort to better understand and accommodate diversity among patients. First, everyday communication skills must be acquired to effectively interact with all patients. Second, there is a growing language divide between physicians and patients who do not share a common language. Third, cultural competency issues often lead to distrust that can adversely affect patient outcomes, particularly for patients with musculoskeletal conditions.

Communication Skills

The need for everyday communication skills was made evident by a comprehensive public survey completed by the AAOS in 1998, which suggested that orthopaedic surgeons overall are "high tech, low touch"[6] (Table 1). A "significant gulf" was identified between physicians' self-perception and public perception of physicians' effectiveness in listening, care, and compassion.[7] As discussed previously, the AAOS partnered with the BIHCC to form the CSMP to address this challenge and teach effective communications skills to physicians by using an educational model of interactive adult learning based on the comparison of differences.[8] Because strong evidence shows that effective communication skills improve health outcomes for patients and reduce the risk of malpractice suits for physicians,[9] the medical interview should be considered an orthopaedic surgeon's

Table 1
Attribute Ratings of "Very Important" and Performance Ratings of "Excellent"

Attribute	Consumer Ratings of Orthopaedists (%)	Important to Customers (%)	Important to Orthopaedists (%)
Listens to patients	NA	**84.7**	56.2
Level of medical training	35.2	**85.6**	70.9
Prestige of specialty	28.3	33.0	NA
Research orientation	22.4	38.5	NA
Successful medical results	18.4	**83.7**	**88.4**
Caring and compassionate	17.7	**76.7**	63.8
Spending enough time to listen	13.3	73.5	47.8
Ease of scheduling an appointment	12.8	64.6	24.0
Value for cost of service	12.7	70.4	50.2
Physician of choice for musculoskeletal surgery	NA	NA	75.0

Source: Consumer survey question 10: "How important is it that your health care professional...?" (N = 807) and fellows' survey questions 59-67: "Please rate how important it is to have patients associate each of the following characteristics with orthopaedists...." (N = 700). Both based on a 5-point scale on which 5 = very important and 1 = not at all important.

Bold type indicates communications messages for public relations program.

Reproduced from the American Academy of Orthopaedic Surgeons: *1999 Public Image Investigation, Second Report.* Rosemont, IL, American Academy of Orthopaedic Surgeons, May 1999.

NA = not applicable.

most important procedure. Because orthopaedic surgeons typically conduct over 100,000 patient interviews during their careers, they should continue to review, evaluate, and improve the communication skills needed for these patient interactions.[10]

The Language Divide

In the United States, the disparity between the languages understood by physicians and those spoken by their patients continues to grow. The number of immigrants has nearly tripled since 1970, increasing from 9.6 to 26 million.[11] More than 20 million people living in the United States have limited English language proficiency. In Portland, Oregon, 210 languages are spoken. The University of California–Davis Medical Center Hospital in Sacramento employs translators for 57 different languages. Few orthopaedic surgeons, however, have access to such broad translation services.

The scope of the language divide is qualitative as well as quantitative. Lin-

guistic minorities report worse care than ethnic or racial minorities.[12] Patients using interpreters require more physician time than those who are proficient in English,[9] and they also require more visits.[13] Decision making may be more cautious and expensive when non–English-speaking patients are treated in the absence of a bilingual physician or professional interpreter.[14]

The Office of Civil Rights of the US Department of Health and Human Services has issued final policy guidance (regulation) that requires physicians who receive reimbursement from Medicaid or state-run Children's Health Insurance Programs to provide competent translation services when requested by all patients who claim to have limited English proficiency.[15] According to this regulation, any reimbursement for medical services provided to Medicaid patients (and, if applicable, Medicare Part A) constitutes "federal financial assistance" to the physician under provisions of Title VI of the Civil Rights Act of 1964.

Table 2	
Costs for Medical Interpreter Services	
Setting	**Cost**
Emergency department	$8.6 million
Community health centers	$11.5 million
Hospital outpatient	$12.4 million
Hospital inpatient	$78.2 million
Physician office	$156.9 million
Total	$276.6 million

(Reproduced with permission from Hawryluk M: HHS eases interpreter mandate but doctors must pay bills: New guidance on serving patients with limited English skills grants physicians more flexibility. *American Medical News*, October 13, 2003. Available at: http://www.ama-assn.org/amednews/2003/10/13/gvl11013.htm. Accessed July 9, 2004.)

Table 3
The Six Realities of Cultural Programming
Culture is not obvious.
Each individual believes that his or her own culture is the best.
Individuals misinterpret the actions of others when their interpretations of their own observations are not understood.
Individuals may not know when they are offending others.
Awareness of differences and possible barriers improves the chances for successful interactions.
Understanding one's own "software" or value system is a crucial step in providing culturally competent care.

(Adapted with permission from Gardenswartz L, Rowe A: *Managing Diversity in Health Care*. San Francisco, CA, Josey-Bass Inc, 1998.)

Physicians can comply by retaining employees who are fluent in English and a second language to perform the translation services, by using commercially available telephonic services, or by hiring professional translators. In some communities, volunteer translators for certain languages are available as an alternative.

The Office of Civil Rights strongly suggests that it is inappropriate for family members to act as translator for the patient and physician and other medical office staff for reasons of confidentiality. If the patient offers or agrees to use a family member or friend to translate, the practice is acceptable; however, it is not acceptable when the patient requests an independent translator. The rule also specifically bars physicians from discriminating against patients with limited English proficiency by refusing to see them or discharging them from their practices.

Because these regulations make no provision to pay for translators, several specialty medical associations and nearly 40 states have signed letters in opposition. These physician groups argue that these regulations are unreasonable. Also, they express concern that the effect of such regulations will be to drive physi-cians away from accepting patients who participate in insurance programs that already reimburse physicians at a low rate. On September 23, 2003, the Practicing Physicians Advisory Council recommended that physicians be exempted from these Office of Civil Rights regulations and that translators be allowed to bill third-party carriers or patients directly for their services (Table 2).

Cultural Competence

Cultural competence as it relates specifically to the medical interview refers to effective communication of the patient's diagnosis and treatment plans in a manner that is acceptable to patients from different cultural backgrounds.[16] The American Medical Association's Cultural Competence Compendium defines a culture as any group of people who share experiences, language, and values that permit them to communicate knowledge not shared by those outside the culture.[17] Because individual physicians reflect individual cultural values as well as the culture of medicine, they must be aware of their own culture, belief systems, and values and acknowledge that their own biases can affect interactions with patients. If disparities in medical care access and outcomes are to be reduced, cross-cultural communication must be learned by physicians and other health care workers.

Misunderstandings in cross-cultural communication commonly arise regarding the following six topics: authority, physical contact, communication styles, gender, sexuality, and family.[18] To avoid misunderstandings, Gardenswartz and Rowe[19] suggest that physicians consider the six realities of cultural programming as listed in Table 3. Additionally, Bulger[20] argues that a science-based clinician healer must be both scientifically and ethnically competent. This requires physicians to be calm, understanding, knowledgeable about the placebo effect, able to deal with death and dying, and especially be able to listen.

Ethnicity-specific information for several different disease states is available in a series of booklets entitled *A Provider's Handbook on Culturally Competent Care*.[21] Sections of these handbooks are devoted to major diseases and areas of special clinical focus; however, there are no specific references to musculoskeletal conditions. Recently, Jimenez[22] reported on specific communication issues for Hispanic/Latino orthopaedic patients and concluded that patients with musculoskeletal conditions must actively participate in their treatment programs to achieve favorable outcomes. Whaley[23] has suggested that patients must understand and accept their diagnoses as well as believe that the recommended treatment programs offer them hope for satisfactory recovery.

Although every physician can improve communications with patients of different cultural backgrounds by being exposed to specific cultural norms, care must be taken to guard against stereotyping. The learning process should broaden the cultural horizons of physicians and improve their ability to meet the needs of their patients. Nonetheless, physicians must also acknowledge that education, occupation, economics, spiritual values, lifestyle, and family background may be as important in determining culture as ethnicity.

Summary

Communication skills have recently been identified as being increasingly important for achieving successful patient outcomes, particularly those needed for the most common procedure in orthopaedics—the medical interview. The award-wining CSMP workshops of the AAOS represent a new and successful response to this challenge.

References

1. Tongue JR: Communicating: The most important procedure you'll ever perform, in *AAOS Orthopaedic Legal Advisor*. Rosemont, IL, American Academy of Orthopaedic Surgeons, 2004.

2. Herndon JH, Pollick KJ: Continuing concerns, new challenges, and next steps in physician-patients communication. *J Bone Joint Surg Am* 2002;84:309-315.

3. Tongue JR: Approaching new orthopaedic patients: Enhanced communications lead to better outcomes. *AAOS Bulletin*. Rosemont, IL, American Academy of Orthopaedic Surgeons, 2003. Available at: http://www.aaos.org/wordhtml/bulletin/aug03/comm.htm. Accessed January 10, 2005.

4. Epps HR, Tongue JR: Communicating adverse outcomes. *AAOS Bulletin*. Rosemont, IL, American Academy of Orthopaedic Surgeons, 2003.

5. Katz J: *The Silent World of Doctor and Patient*, ed 2. Baltimore, MD, The John Hopkins University Press, 2002.

6. American Academy of Orthopaedic Surgeons: *1999 Public Image Investigation, Second Report*. Rosemont, IL, American Academy of Orthopaedic Surgeons, May 1999.

7. Frymoyer JW, Frymoyer NP: Physician-patient communication: A lost art? *J Am Acad Orthop Surg* 2002;10:95-105.

8. Keller VF, Carroll JG: A new model for physician-patient communication. *Patient Educ Couns* 1994;23:131-140.

9. Levinson W, Roter DL, Mullooly JP, Dull VT, Frankel RM: Physician-patient communication: The relationship with malpractice claims among primary care physicians and surgeons. *JAMA* 1997;277:553-559.

10. Kundhal KK, Kundhal PS: Cultural diversity: An evolving challenge to physician-patient communication. *JAMA* 2003;289:94.

11. Weech-Maldonado R, Morales LS, Elliott M, Spritzer K, Marshall G, Hays RD: Race/ethnicity, language, and patient's assessment of care in Medicaid managed care. *Health Serv Res* 2003;38:789-808.

12. Kravitz RL, Helms LJ, Azari R, Antonius D, Melnikow J: Comparing the use of physician time and health care resources among patients speaking English, Spanish, and Russian. *Med Care* 2000;38:728-738.

13. Derose KP, Baker DW: Limited English proficiency and Latinos' use of physician services. *Med Care Res Rev* 2000;57:76-91.

14. Hampers LC, McNulty JE: Professional interpreters and bilingual physicians in a pediatric emergency department: effect on resource utilization. *Arch Pediatr Adolesc Med* 2002;156:1108-1113.

15. HHS Office for Civil Rights: Guidance to Federal Financial Assistance Recipients Regarding Title VI Prohibition Against National Origin Discrimination Affecting Limited English Proficient Persons. Available at: http://www.hhs.gov/ocr/lep/revisedlep.html. Accessed July 9, 2004.

16. Misra-Hebert AD: Physician cultural competence: Cross-cultural communication improves care. *Cleve Clin J Med* 2003;70:289-303.

17. *Cultural Competence Compendium*. American Medical Association Web site. Available at: http://www.ama-assn.org/ama/pub/category/4848.html. Accessed October 4, 2003.

18. Carrillo JE, Green AR, Betancourt JR: Cross-cultural primary care: A patient-based approach. *Ann Intern Med* 1999;130:829-834.

19. Gardenswartz L, Rowe A: *Managing Diversity in Health Care*. San Francisco, CA, Josey-Bass Inc, 1998.

20. Bulger RJ: The quest for the therapeutic organization. *JAMA* 2000;283:2431-2433.

21. *A Provider's Handbook on Culturally Competent Care*. Oakland, CA, Kaiser Permanente National Diversity Council, 1999.

22. Jimenez R: Culturally competent patient encounter tips: Enhance communications with your Hispanic and Latino patients. *AAOS Bulletin*. Rosemont, IL, American Academy of Orthopaedic Surgeons, 2002. Available at: http://www.aaos.org/wordhtml/bulletin/oct02/comm.htm. Accessed January 10, 2005.

23. Whaley BB: *Explaining Illness: Research, Theory, and Strategies*. Mahwah, NJ, Lawrence Erlbaum Associates Publishers, 2000.

Index

Page numbers with *f* indicate figures
Page numbers with *t* indicate tables

A